COMPARATIVE IMMUNOLOGY

COMPARATIVE IMMUNOLOGY

EDITED BY JOHN J. MARCHALONIS

The Walter and Eliza Hall Institute of Medical Research
P.O. Royal Melbourne Hospital, Victoria 3050, Australia

A HALSTED PRESS BOOK

JOHN WILEY & SONS

NEW YORK TORONTO

Published in the U.S.A. and
Canada by Halsted Press, a
Division of John Wiley & Sons, Inc.,
New York.

First published 1976

Library of Congress Cataloging in Publication Data
Main entry under title:

Comparative immunology.
Includes bibliographical references and index.
1. Immunology, Comparative. I. Marchalonis, John J., 1940– [DNLM: 1. Immunity. QW504 C737]
QR181.C72 591.2'9 76-18782
ISBN 0-470-15160-9

Printed in Great Britain.

Contents

Preface *by J. J. Marchalonis* ix

1 Phylogenetic origins of the vertebrates *by Sue Rosser* 1

2 The Nature of Immune Phenomena in Mammals: (a) Cellular Immunity; (b) Antibody Formation *by G. J. V. Nossal* 20

3 Cellular Recognition of Allografts and Xenografts in Invertebrates *by Edwin L. Cooper* 36

4 Factors Involved in the Recognition of Foreign Material by Phagocytic Cells from Invertebrates *by C. R. Jenkin* 80

5 Phylogeny of Cellular Immunity Among Vertebrates *by M. R. Tam, A. L. Reddy, R. D. Karp & W. H. Hildemann* 98

6 Phylogeny of Cell–Cell Cooperation in Immunity *by Laurens N. Ruben* 120

7 Phylogeny of Neoplasia and Immune Reactions to Tumours *by Michael Balls & Laurens N. Ruben* 167

8 Immunologic Diversity Within the Class Amphibia *by Nicholas Cohen* 209

9 Regulatory Effects of Temperature upon Immunity in Ectothermic Vertebrates *by R. R. Avtalion, E. Weiss & T. Moalem* 227

10 Physical Properties of Immunoglobulins of Lower Species: A comparison with immunoglobulins of mammals *by Gary W. Litman* 239

11 Immunoglobulin Class of Lower Vertebrates distinct from IgM Immunoglobulin *by John L. Atwell & John J. Marchalonis* 276

12 Immunoglobulins and Antibody Production in Reptiles *by H. Ambrosius* 298

13 Immunoglobulins and Antibody Production in Avian Species *by Albert A. Benedict & Karen Yamaga* 335

14 Immunity in Prototherian and Metatherian Mammals *by David T. Rowlands Jr* 376

15 Amphibian Models for Study of the Ontogeny of Immunity *by Louis Du Pasquier* 390

16 Ontogenetic Development of Lymphoid Tissues in Avian Species *by A. Szenberg* 419

17 Ontogeny of Immunity in Mammals *by David T. Rowlands Jr* 432

Index 447

Contributors

H. AMBROSIUS, Sektion Biowissenschaften, Karl-Marx-Universitat, 701 Leipzig, Talstrasse 33, D.D.R.

JOHN L. ATWELL, The Walter and Eliza Hall Institute of Medical Research, P.O. Royal Melbourne Hospital, Victoria 3050, Australia.

R. R. AVTALION, Rapaport Laboratory for Microbiology, Department of Life Sciences, Bar-Ilan University, Ramat-Gan, Israel.

MICHAEL BALLS, Department of Human Morphology, The University of Nottingham University Hospital and Medical School, Clifton Boulevard, Nottingham N67 2UH, U.K.

ALBERT A. BENEDICT, Department of Microbiology, University of Hawaii, Honolulu, Hawaii 96822, U.S.A.

NICHOLAS COHEN, Department of Microbiology, University of Rochester, School of Medicine and Dentistry, Rochester, New York 14642, U.S.A.

EDWIN L. COOPER, Department of Anatomy, School of Medicine, University of California, Los Angeles, California 90024, U.S.A.

W. H. HILDEMANN, Department of Biology, Hilo College, University of Hawaii, Hilo, Hawaii 96720, U.S.A.

C. R. JENKIN, Department of Microbiology, University of Adelaide, South Australia 5000, Australia.

R. D. KARP, Department of Microbiology and Immunology, School of Medicine, University of California, Los Angeles 90024, U.S.A.

GARY W. LITMAN, Memorial Sloan-Kettering Cancer Center, New York, New York 10021, U.S.A.

JOHN J. MARCHALONIS, The Walter and Eliza Hall Institute of Medical Research, P.O. Royal Melbourne Hospital, Victoria 3050, Australia.

T. MOALEM, Rapaport Laboratory for Microbiology, Department of Life Sciences, Bar-Ilan University, Ramat-Gan, Israel.

G. J. V. NOSSAL, The Walter and Eliza Hall Institute of Medical Research, P.O. Royal Melbourne Hospital, Victoria 3050, Australia.

LOUIS DU PASQUIER, Basel Institute for Immunology, 487, Grenzacherstrasse, CH4058 Basel, Switzerland.

A. L. REDDY, Department of Microbiology and Immunology, School of Medicine, University of California, Los Angeles 90024, U.S.A.

SUE ROSSER, Department of Genetics, University of Wisconsin, Madison, Wisconsin, U.S.A.

DAVID T. ROWLANDS JR, Department of Pathology, School of Medicine, University of Pennsylvania, Philadelphia, Pennsylvania 19174, U.S.A.

LAURENS N. RUBEN, Department of Zoology, Reed College, Portland, Oregon, U.S.A.

A. SZENBERG, The Walter and Eliza Hall Institute of Medical Research, P.O. Royal Melbourne Hospital, Victoria 3050, Australia.

M. R. TAM, Department of Microbiology and Immunology, School of Medicine, University of California, Los Angeles, 90024, U.S.A.

E. WEISS, Rapaport Laboratory for Microbiology, Department of Life Sciences, Bar-Ilan University, Ramat-Gan, Israel.

KAREN YAMAGA, Department of Microbiology, University of Hawaii, Honolulu, Hawaii 96822, U.S.A.

Preface

John J. Marchalonis

Phylogenetic studies and the mechanisms of immune functions

The subject matter of concern to comparative immunologists is far-ranging in scope, encompassing analyses of the recognition of non-self by circulating cells of vertebrates and invertebrates and the defence reactions of these organisms to foreign challenge. The overall objects of the phylogenetic studies are (1) to synthesize the diverse observations into an evolutionary pattern which provides meaningful insight into the mechanisms underlying functional differentiation of immunologically competent cells and (2) to obtain simplified experimental models which facilitate investigations which are extremely difficult, if not impossible, using the usual mammalian systems. The importance of the phylogenetic approach to the elucidation of complex immunological mechanisms was recognized more than 70 years ago by Metchnikoff (1893) and Noguchi (1903). Yet workers today (see Du Pasquier, Chapter 15) complain of a 'phylogenetic prejudice' towards results of lower species. The unsoundness of this prejudice has clearly been shown by studies in molecular biology and neurophysiology where major contributions resulted from experiments using the gut bacterium *Escherichia coli* and the humble horseshoe crab *Limulus polyphemus*. Studies of lower species as primitive as the earthworm (Chapter 3) and sea stars (Chapter 4) will likewise result in important contributions to our knowledge of the origins of immunological recognition and differentiation.

Chapters 1 and 2 of this volume provide an introduction first to principles of phylogeny and then to an exposition of present thinking regarding the immune system of mammals. Chapters 3–9 generally reflect cell-mediated immune reactions which are considered to be functions of thymus-derived lymphocytes (T cells) acting in some association with phagocytic cells. Chapters 10–13 are concerned with the structure of immunoglobulins synthesized by vertebrate species and chapters 14–17 illustrate the advantages of various lower vertebrates to the study of the ontogeny of immune function. Du Pasquier (Chapter 15) reports on the use of larval amphibians which possess few lymphocytes and develop in the absence of maternofetal interactions as models to study the generation of antibody diversity and the differentiation of functional thymus lymphocytes. Szenberg (Chapter 16) describes the development of lymphoid cells of the chicken and the clear demarcation between thymus-derived cells and B cells of the bursa of Fabricius. Rowlands (Chapters 14 & 17) discusses immune responses of the primitive mammalian suborders, prototheria and metatheria and their relevance to investigations of the ontogeny of mammalian immune reactivity. 'Pouch Young' of metatherians such as the opossum offer a very convenient model because these creatures are 'born' at a stage of hematopoietic development comparable to that of a 10-day mouse embryo (Block 1967).

Just as the genetic code is universal, it is now clear that virtually all living organisms can differentiate self from non-self to some degree (Chapters 3–5). However, it is obvious that not all such reactions are homologous to specific immunological recognition and response. Persuasive evidence is accumulating that invertebrates related to the stream of chordate emergence, e.g. echinoderms and tunicates, reject allografts and might be considered to express a primitive form of cellular or T-cell immunity. Further study is required to elucidate the mechanisms of recognition and effector functions in invertebrates, particularly inasmuch as the recognition molecules of protolymphocytes and their interactions with macrophages might prove extremely relevant to a variety of similar cellular reactions of mammals where classical antibody is not involved. Analysis of recognition in echinoderms and protochordates bears directly upon allogeneic responses of certain subsets of T lymphocytes which mount graft-versus-host reactions and mixed-leucocyte reactions (Chapters 2, 3 & 5).

The organization of this volume reflects the major revolution in immunological thought which has been established in the last decade; namely, the recognition of two major functional classes of lymphocytes, T cells and B cells, and their separate and also collaborative roles in immune processes (Miller 1972). Two chapters (6 & 9) maintain that cells with specific functional properties of mammalian B and T cells occur within fishes and amphibians and collaborate in the elaboration of immune responses to antigens considered thymus-dependent in mammals. Even the effect of temperature on immune function (Chapter 9), a characteristic property of ectothermic vertebrates, is probably related to the cooperation of B- and T-type cells. The presently available data indicate that T-type cells can be primed or made tolerant at low temperatures but the collaborative interaction which activates B-type cells into antibody-secreting cells requires higher temperatures.

I use the terms T-type and B-type here because exact identifications of lymphocytes of a fish, for example, as comparable to murine T cells are difficult to make. Thymus function in lower species parallels that in well-characterized mammals as demonstrated by repeated observations that thymectomy of larval or neonatal animals usually reduces the capacity to reject allografts and to form antibodies. Positive identification of T and B cells of lower species requires the development of markers characteristic for certain cell types, e.g. the Thy 1 (θ) alloantigen of murine thymus cells, and the application of separation techniques to obtain pure populations of the different lymphocyte types.

Certain apparent differences between lymphocytes of lower species and those of mammals have already been established. One generally used means of distinguishing T and B cells of man or mouse is the detection of surface immunoglobulin by immunofluorescence. Conditions can be readily established where B cells bear immunoglobulin by this technique but T cells apparently lack this surface marker. Studies of thymus lymphocytes of larval amphibians (*Xenopus*, Chapter 15) and adult carp (Emmrich *et al.* 1975) however, establish that the majority of lymphocytes possess membrane immunoglobulin. These results might suggest that T cells of lower species are functionally distinct or more primitive than those of mammals and birds. However, these observations serve as a further illustration of the utility of lower vertebrate models for the resolution of complex immunological problems; in this case, the nature of the T-cell receptor for antigen. It has been extremely difficult to detect and isolate surface immunoglobulin of mammalian T cells and some workers vehemently maintain that it does not exist (see Marchalonis 1975, Warner 1974 for reviews). By contrast, a number of workers have now isolated a low molecular weight (180,000) immunoglobulin from T cells which shows receptor and collaborative function. The immunoglobulin-bearing thymus lymphocytes of lower vertebrates clearly are relevant to the question of the relationship of T-cell antigen receptors to immunoglobulins. Since antigen specific cooperation occurs in forms as low as fishes (Chapters 6 & 9), functional T- and B-type cells must have diverged early in vertebrate evolution. Moreover, the gene encoding T-type immunoglobulin must have diverged from the surface receptor immunoglobulin (7S IgM sub-unit) of B cells. This event probably involved the tandem duplication of the gene encoding the primordial μ chain gene. It stands to reason that surface receptors would most closely resemble IgM because the first immunoglobulins to appear in evolution are extremely similar to mammalian IgM molecules. Furthermore, 7S IgM molecules occur in large amounts in the serum of species such as sharks (Chapter 10).

The general pattern of the evolutionary emergence of immunoglobulins is now fairly well established even though extensive primary amino acid sequence data are lacking. All true vertebrates can form circulating antibodies to diverse antigens. Consistent with this observation, limited N-terminal sequence data coupled with analyses of binding affinities for haptens indicate substantial homologies on the V regions of antibodies of species ranging from fish to mammals (Chapters 10, 12 & 13). All vertebrates possess an antibody comparable to mammalian IgM in a variety of physiochemical properties (Chapters 10 & 11). In placoderm-derived species, the light and heavy chains are joined by inter-chain disulphide bonds. The immunoglobulin of cyclostomes (ostracoderm-derived) contain light chains and μ-like heavy chains, but are not covalently linked. Classes of immunoglobulin distinct from IgM as characterized by the presence of a heavy chain distinct from μ chain emerged in lungfish and occur in amphibians, reptiles, birds and mammals. Although it was once thought that the low molecular weight (7S) immunoglobulins of amphibians, reptiles and birds were homologous to mammalian IgG, evidence presented in Chapters 11–13 establishes that this is not the case. In fact, it now appears that IgG probably emerged during the evolution of the therapsid reptiles which were ancestral to mammals. All three mammalian groups possess IgG immunoglobulin as the major class (Chapter 11). The emergence of immunoglobulins distinct from IgM raises a number of important questions because the appearance of these molecules, e.g. IgG and IgE, in the immune response of mammals is considered to require the functional interaction of T and B cells. In contrast, IgM antibodies to certain antigens can be synthesized by B cells in the absence of T-cell influence. The genetic mechanism by which non-μ heavy chains arose probably consisted of tandem duplication of the gene encoding the μ chain. The non-μ chains, like the μ chains, are composed of domains of approximately 110 amino acids which form a compact spatial unit and are specialized for some biological function.

Immunoglobulins of two classes of vertebrates, namely reptiles and birds, have received little attention in the past. Chapters 12 and 13 rectify this situation providing detailed descriptions of the biology of antibody production and the physicochemical properties of the antibodies. Ambrosius (Chapter 12) demonstrates that reptiles possess multiple classes of immunoglobulin and can mount clear-cut secondary responses involving shifts in antibody class and an increase in binding affinity. Therefore, the secondary response in these species meets rigorous criteria for immunological memory.

Taken as a whole, this volume maintains that the basic aspects of cellular and humoral immunity are present in all vertebrate species. In addition, there is an increasing sophistication of certain elements of the lymphoid system (e.g. the emergence of lymph nodes in mammals), antibody forming cells (e.g. the appearance of plasma cells in advanced sharks and teleosts) and in types of antibodies (e.g. the appearance of multiple classes of antibodies representing constant region divergence and the increase in binding affinity representing V region divergence). Much work remains in order to develop a complete evolutionary pattern of immune recognition and effector function. It is clear that the continued effort is worthwhile, both as a challenging set of biological problems and as a useful approach to elucidating the mechanisms which underlie those aspects of immunity relevant to disease.

References

BLOCK M. (1967) The 'fetal' opossum, as an experimental tool in ontogeny of immunologic competence, p. 150. In *Ontogeny of Immunity*, eds Smith R.T., Good R.A. & Miescher P.A. University of Florida Press, Gainesville.

EMMRICH F., RICHTER R.F. & AMBROSIUS H. (1975) Immunoglobulin determinants on the surface of lymphoid cells of carp. *Eur. J. Immunol.* **5,** 76.

MARCHALONIS J.J. (1975) Lymphocyte surface immunoglobulins. *Science* **190,** 20.

METCHNIKOFF E. (1893) *Lectures on the comparative pathology of inflammation.* Dover Publications, New York, 1968, re-publication of 1893 edition, 224 pp.

MILLER J.F.A.P. (1972) Lymphocyte interactions in antibody responses. *Int. Rev. Cytol.* **33,** 77.

NOGUCHI H. (1903) A study of immunization—haemolyins, agglutinins, precipitins and coagulins in cold-blooded animals. *Centralbl. f. Bakt. Abt. Orig.* **33,** 353.

WARNER N.L. (1974) Membrane immunoglobulins and antigen receptors on B and T lymphocytes. *Adv. Immunol.* **19,** 67.

Chapter 1. Phylogenetic Origins of the Vertebrates

Sue Rosser

Introduction

A phylogeny of the animal kingdom
The invertebrates
The protochordates

A phylogeny of the animal kingdom *continued*
The vertebrates

Some principles of evolution

Introduction

'Let it be borne in mind how infinitely complex and close-fitting are the mutual relations of all organic beings to each other and to their physical conditions of life.' (Darwin 1859, p. 80.)

In order to interpret data concerning the phylogeny of immunity, a clear understanding of the phylogeny of the animal kingdom is necessary. The purpose of this introductory chapter is to discuss some evolutionary principles and relationships among members of the animal kingdom. It is hoped that the immunological data given in subsequent chapters concerning particular classes and species can subsequently be considered and correlated in light of the phylogenetic framework provided here.

This discussion of the evolution of the animal kingdom may be separated into two parts. A phylogeny of the animal kingdom comprises the first; some principles of evolution comprise the second.

The discussion here will be very brief, giving the general information necessary to understand the reasons for the choice of the particular ancestor–descendant relationship presented. Besides being brief, the phylogeny given here will be biased towards the vertebrates, with the vertebrates and invertebrates being discussed on two different taxonomic levels. More is known about the immunology of the vertebrates, particularly mammals, than of invertebrates, and most of the techniques for detecting an immune response were developed for the higher vertebrates. The rest of this volume deals primarily with vertebrate immunity. Furthermore, the invertebrates are composed of many diverse groups, most of which are not on the main line to vertebrate evolution. Thus, the invertebrates will be dealt with primarily at the taxonomic level of the phylum, with particular emphasis being given to those phyla that have been considered to be ancestral to vertebrates. In contrast, the vertebrates will be discussed primarily at the level of the class, with the main emphasis given to those orders and genera considered to be transitional between one class and another.

The principles of evolution which are the basis for the phylogeny of the animal kingdom comprise the second part of this chapter. The principles of evolution will also be presented in a brief, undetailed form. Particular emphasis will be placed on principles which might prove helpful in interpreting some of the data dealing with the phylogeny of immunity.

A phylogeny of the animal kingdom

The invertebrates

The invertebrates consist of a large and diverse number of phyla which have been grouped together primarily because they do not have backbones. Because the phyla are so diverse, it is especially difficult to assess the relationships among them and to draw a phylogenetic tree that accurately represents these relationships. Although Nursall (1962) has suggested that the phyla evolved in parallel and should not be depicted by a 'tree' at all, a tree image will be used here because it more clearly demonstrates the origins of vertebrate ancestry. (See Fig. 1.1.)

Almost all of the invertebrate phyla have been proposed as the ancestors for the vertebrates at one time or another. Embryological, anatomical, and biochemical evidence now indicate that one phylum is more likely to have been the one that was ancestral to the vertebrates than the others.

The basic ancestral stock of the invertebrates lies in the phylum Protozoa, the one-celled organisms. Although the Protozoa represent a very primitive level of organization, contained within their one cell is all the machinery that is necessary for life.

The Protozoa were ancestral to the sponges. Consisting of many cells which function essentially independently while grouped together in a colony, the sponges represent a more advanced form than the one-celled Protozoa, but perhaps at a parazoan rather than metazoan level of organization. The sponges are an evolutionary dead end.

The evolutionarily important phylum arising from the Protozoa was the Coelenterata. The corals, jellyfish, and sea anemones of this group have a tissue level of organization with cooperation occurring between the two layers of cells. With their muscle and nerve tissue, radial symmetry, digestive cavity with mouth, and larval form, the coelenterates represent an ancestral group from which the two main lines of invertebrates arose.

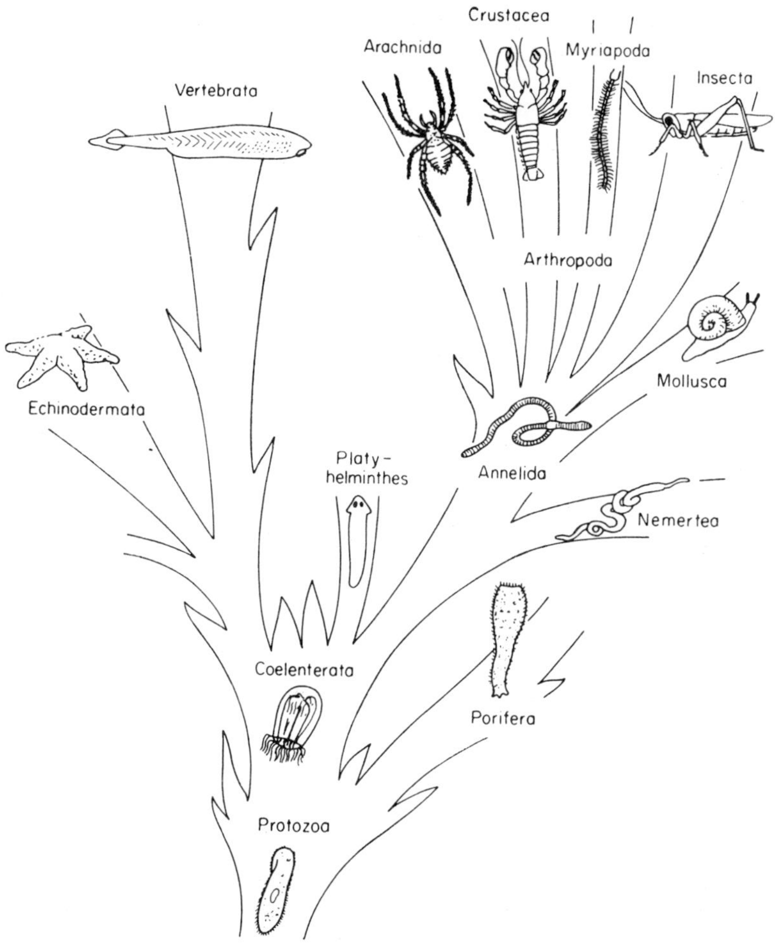

Fig. 1.1. Invertebrate evolution (modified after Buchsbaum 1948, p. 334).

The distinctions between the two main lines of invertebrate evolution are made on the basis of the different ways in which the mesoderm layer and the coelom are formed in the two groups. In thc arthropod line, the mesoderm develops from two special cells, which are equal in size and set aside during the early gastrula stage of development. The coelom is formed in the arthropod line from splits in the bands of mesoderm budded off from the primitive mesoderm cells. In the chordate line, in contrast, the mesoderm is formed from outpocketings of the primitive endoderm, and the coelom is developed from hollow mesodermal pouches.

The arthropod line consists of a large number of phyla in which many evolutionary advances have occurred. The Platyhelminthes (or flatworms) use mesoderm in their organ systems. The Nemerteans (or marine worms) have the beginnings of a circulatory system and a digestive tract with two openings. The molluscs, including the oysters, clams, and snails, have a free swimming trochophore larva.

The Annelida (or earthworms) with their bilateral symmetry, segmented body, nerve cord, and excellent circulatory system actually seem to have many chordate-like characteristics. Because of these characteristics, they have often been proposed as the ancestors of the vertebrates. Certain of the vertebrate-like adaptive immune responses of the annelids may be dependent upon the annelid circulatory system, which in some respects resembles the closed system found in vertebrates. The annelid humoral immunity is extensively used, as it is in the vertebrates, for protection against penetration of foreign antibodies and bacteria (Chateaureynaud-Duprat 1973).

However, the annelid nerve cord is ventral, rather than dorsal, as in the chordates. The blood in the annelid circulatory system flows in the opposite direction from the blood in the chordate system. Finally, the annelids show no notochord or gill slits, both of which are considered to be important chordate characteristics. Thus, the annelids are rejected by most students as ancestors of the chordates.

The phylum Arthropoda, which is thought to be descended from the annelids, includes a large, diverse number of species. The crustaceans (lobsters and crabs), insects, centipedes, and arachnids are included in the Arthropoda. The arthropods encompass forms which have attained a high degree of organization. In terms of absolute numbers and number of species, the Arthropoda constitutes by far the most successful phylum today. It is thus not unreasonable to assume that the vertebrate ancestry might be found in this group. The arachnid stock is the group of arthropods which has been proposed as vertebrate ancestors (Patten 1912). The arachnids include spiders, mites, scorpions, the horseshoe crab *Limulus*, and the extinct eurypterids or water scorpions. The external skeleton or 'armour' of the eurypterids resembled the 'armour' of some of the early vertebrate fish. On this basis, it has been suggested that a eurypterid-type invertebrate might have been the vertebrate ancestor. However, the eurypterids had no internal skeleton and did have jointed limbs. Furthermore, the nerve cord was ventral in eurypterids while the top of the arachnid was comparable to the top of the vertebrate. Thus, in turning the arachnid over to obtain the dorsal chordate nerve cord, the resemblance to the vertebrates is largely destroyed. Neither the arachnids nor any other creature in the arthropod line has the characteristics of a good vertebrate ancestor.

As the name indicates, it is from the chordate line of invertebrates that the vertebrate ancestors came. The chordate line of invertebrates includes the phylum Echinodermata and the protochordate members of the phylum Chordata. Although Barrington (1965) gives the hemichordates phylum status while keeping the other protochordates as subphyla within the phylum Chordata, here all protochordates will be considered as subphyla within the Chordata after Halstead (1968). Romer (1959) suggests that a 'stalked sessile animal, making its living from tiny food particles gathered by ciliary currents along its outspread arms' was probably the ancestral type for both the echinoderms and the protochordates. (See Fig. 1.2.)

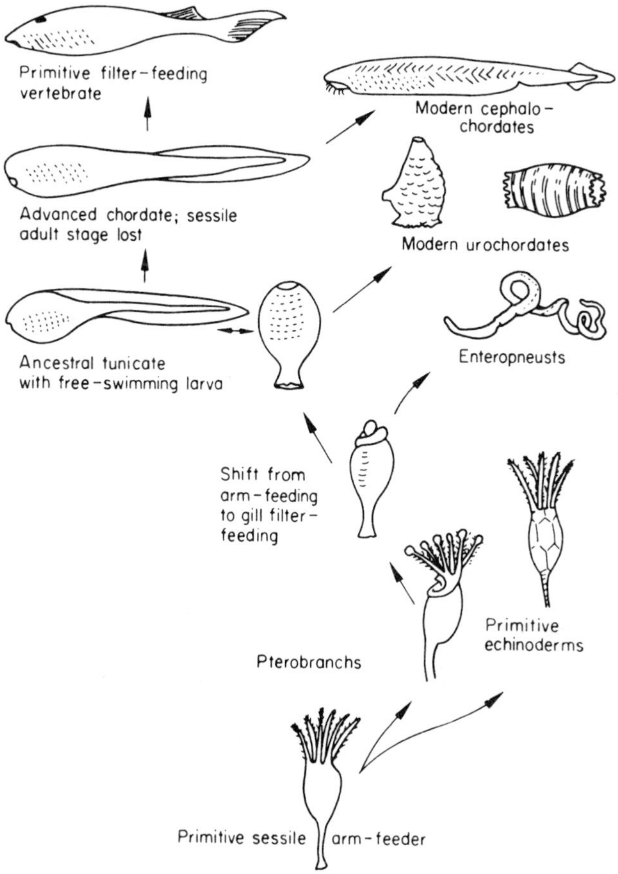

Fig. 1.2. Protochordate evolution (modified after Romer 1959, p. 30).

Upon first appearance, it seems unlikely that the echinoderms would be the invertebrate phylum most closely related to the chordates. The echinoderms have radial symmetry, instead of the bilateral symmetry found in the vertebrates. The echinoderms also show no trace of the three defining chordate characteristics—notochord, dorsal tubular nerve chord, or pharyngeal gill slits. They have no internal skeleton. In these respects, the echinoderms seem less suited to be vertebrate ancestors than do the annelids or arthropods.

However, the embryology of the echinoderms suggests that they are related to the protochordates. The early embryo of the echinoderms is known as the tornaria larva. This is a bilateral, free-swimming form with longitudinal, looped ciliated bands that are used for locomotion. 'There is evidence that some of the earliest fossil echinoderms probably made use of external ciliated grooves for feeding' (Barrington 1965, p. 9). The tornaria very much resembles the larval stage of some of the protochordates. Furthermore, the order and mode in which the main structural elements of the body are laid down embryologically in echinoderms is similar to that of the vertebrates, but different from that of other invertebrates.

Biochemical and immunological evidence also indicate that the echinoderms are closely related to the vertebrates. The haemoglobin of the blood and the chemistry of muscle action in the echinoderms and vertebrates is more similar than that of other invertebrate phyla and the vertebrates. The recent demonstration of immunity in echinoderms with host cell reactions and questionable memory responses is more similar to vertebrate immunity than that found in most other invertebrates (Bailey *et al.* 1971). Thus, it seems likely that a stalked sessile form was indeed ancestral to both the echinoderms and protochordates.

The protochordates

Although many groups such as the Calcichordata (Jefferies 1967) and Pogonophora (Halstead 1965) are often considered as protochordates, only the Hemichordata, Urochordata, and Cephalochordata will be discussed here. The subphylum Hemichordata consists of the pterobranchs and enteropneusts or acorn worms. The hemichordates resemble the echinoderms so closely that when the first enteropneust was discovered in 1821 it was originally thought to be an echinoderm holothurian (Barrington 1965). The larval form of the hemichordates also was thought to be an echinoderm larva at first. Although the close relationship of the enteropneusts to echinoderms was recognized immediately, it was not until 1886 that Bateson explained the affinities between the enteropneusts and the chordates. He recognized the pharyngeal openings as gill slits, the tubular nervous system of the collar as being dorsal, and the stomochord as a possible homologue of the vertebrate notochord.

The pterobranchs, in contrast, have no trace of a hollow nerve cord, nor any notochord. One of the two groups of pterobranchs has no gill openings at all; the other group retains only one small pair of gill openings. For a long time, it was believed that the pterobranchs were a modern, degenerate form of hemichordate, which had lost all chordate characteristics. Recently, however, the pterobranchs have been recognized as being affiliated with the fossil graptolites which were present long before the first vertebrates. Thus, pterobranchs are now considered to be a truly primitive group of chordates from which the more typical chordates were derived by progressive development of a gill-filtering system.

From the pterobranchs evolved the Urochordata or tunicates, the next step towards the vertebrates. The adult tunicate or sea squirt is a sessile form which has few chordate characteristics, with the exception of the gill system it uses for breathing and feeding. The larval form of the tunicates, however, does have chordate characteristics. The larva is motile, having a dorsal nerve cord and a well developed notochord in the tail. Garstang (1928), Berrill (1955), and Romer (1955) have emphasized the importance of this larval stage for vertebrate evolution. They suggest that the chordate ancestor of the vertebrates was a sessile feeder on tiny food particles somewhat like the adult tunicate. The ancestor presumably had a motile larva with a swimming tail complete with muscle, notochord, and nerve cord. The ability to swim allowed the species to be dispersed. The evolution of the cephalochordates and vertebrates could have occurred by paedogenesis or neoteny of the larval form. According to this view, the subsequent evolution of the vertebrates rested on the ability of the larval form to obtain reproductive maturity. Since neoteny does occur in modern tunicates, the hypothesis is more plausible than it might seem at first glance.

If one accepts the hypothesis of neoteny of the tunicate larva, then the transition can be made from a sessile form to a motile, advanced chordate. The cephalochordate *Amphioxus* is probably only slightly more specialized than the motile advanced chordate from which the first true vertebrates arose. *Amphioxus* has all the chordate characteristics—a highly developed notochord, a dorsal hollow nerve cord running the length of the body, and gills. The several dozen gills in *Amphioxus* are used for feeding and breathing. Van Wijhe (1923) attempted to homologize the excretory ducts in the gill region of *Amphioxus* with the vertebrate thymus. *Amphioxus* has even developed the closed circulatory system. In fact, the main characteristic preventing *Amphioxus* from being designated as a vertebrate is its lack of a backbone.

The vertebrates

The first true vertebrates that appear in the known fossil record belong to the fish class Agnatha. Although the Agnatha have no true jaws or paired limbs and are primitive in this respect, they are quite advanced compared to the protochordates.

Essentially nothing is known about the transitional forms between the protochordates and the Agnatha. The Ostracoderms, extinct fossilized fish of the class Agnatha, were heavily armoured fish which showed little resemblance to the protochordates. Except for the absence of jaws and paired appendages, the Ostracoderms also showed little resemblance to the modern Agnatha, the cyclostomes.

The cyclostomes, the lamprey and hagfish, have completely cartilaginous skeletons. Stensio (1968) suggests that the cyclostomes are diphyletic in origin and that the hagfish and lamprey are not very closely related. Stensio's theory might explain some of the immunological evidence such as the presence of the thymus in the lamprey but not in the hagfish. Because the cyclostomes are parasites, many of their 'primitive' features are often considered to be

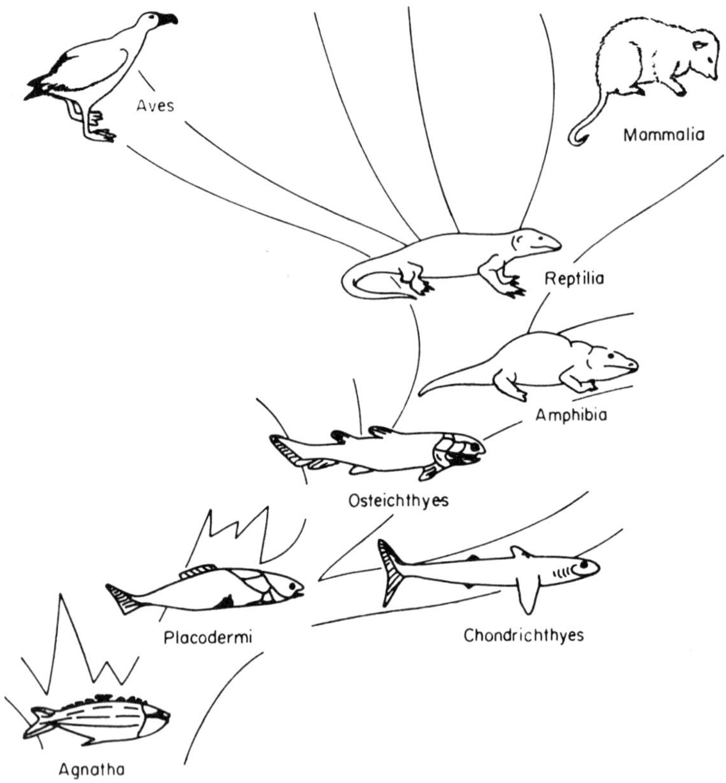

Fig. 1.3. Vertebrate evolution (adapted from Romer 1959, p. 37).

degenerate specializations. Jarvik (1968) suggests that they are not the most primitive group of fish from which the other fish classes evolved. In contrast, Romer (1966) and many other authors consider the Agnatha to be a primitive basal stock from which the placoderms evolved. (See Fig. 1.3.) Thoenes (1972) suggests that the hagfish stands at the juncture to the immunology of the vertebrates since it shows concurrent cellular and humoral immunity for the first time.

The placoderms constitute the only class of vertebrates of which all members are extinct. The placoderms are generally considered to be an evolutionary headache. They include a group of grotesque, armoured fish with true jaws and strange, paired fins. No one has been able to determine from which group of the Agnatha they evolved; nor is there much proof that the placoderms were ancestral to any groups of higher fishes. Romer (1966) states that they might have been antecedent to the sharks and chimaeras of the class Chondrichthyes. Relationships among the various orders are vague.

The class Chondrichthyes includes the cartilaginous jawed fishes. The Chondrichthyes are divided into two subclasses: the Elasmobranchii, including the sharks, skates, and rays, and the Holocephali, including the chimaeras or ratfishes. Romer (1966) believes that the two subclasses may have evolved independently from placoderm-like ancestors and, thus, may not constitute a natural evolutionary class. However, all Chondrichthyes are marine, have no lungs, and have paired claspers on the pelvic fins of the male. Much argument has centred around the question of whether the cartilaginous skeleton is a primitive characteristic or a degenerate characteristic from an ossified ancestral type (Moy-Thomas 1939). If one considers that sharks came from a placoderm-like ancestor (Romer 1966) in which bone was present, and their late appearance in the geologic record, then it seems likely that the cartilaginous skeleton is a degenerate feature paralleling the bone reduction seen in the evolution of other fish groups.

The other class of fish, the Osteichthyes or bony fish, includes the most successful group of fish living today. Unlike the Chondrichthyes, the early Osteichthyes had an ossified skeleton, scales, and lungs or air sacs. Although the actual ancestor of the bony fish is unknown, they are assumed to have evolved from a gnathostomous type, much like the early placoderms.

There are two groups of Osteichthyes: the Actinopterygii and the Sarcopterygii. The Actinopterygii are ray-finned fishes with ganoid scales and a single dorsal fin. The ray-finned fishes may be further divided into three groups: The Chondrostei, the Holostei, and the Teleostei. The Chondrostei, as the name indicates, have experienced a reduction in the degree of ossification of the skeleton. The Chondrostei have primitive characteristics such as ganoid scales, the way the plates are arranged in the head skeleton, and a heterocercal tail. Although most of the members of the Chondrostei are extinct, surviving degenerate species include the sturgeons, paddlefish, and *Polypterus*. The early members of the Chondrostei were ancestral to the other two groups of Actinopterygii.

The Holostei represent another group of nearly extinct ray-finned fishes. Today the Holostei are represented by only the bowfin (*Amia*) and the garpike. The early forms had structural features which were intermediate between those of the Chondrostei and the Teleostei.

The teleosts are the most successful of all fishes today. They are the dominant fish of fresh and marine waters. The teleostean features show the culmination of phylogenetic trends seen in the earlier chondrosteans and holosteans. The ganoine layer of the scale is lost, and the number of bones in the head skeleton is reduced. The tail has become homocercal. The teleosts show tremendous variation with respect to body shape and the habitats into which they have evolved. They represent a group which shows great evolutionary diversity today but which has not been ancestral to any other vertebrate group.

It is in the subclass Sarcopterygii that we find the stem group for the other vertebrates. The Sarcopterygii are distinguished from the Actinopterygii because they have fleshy fins, cosmoid scales, two dorsal fins, and a diphycercal tail. Although Jarvik (1968) implies that the Sarcopterygii may be the most primitive vertebrates of all, most students believe that they had a placoderm-like ancestor. The subclass may be divided into two additional groups, the Dipnoi and the Crossopterygii.

The Dipnoi constitute a group of primitive freshwater lungfish. They are extinct today with the exception of three tropical forms, *Neoceratodus*, *Protopterus*, and *Lepidosiren*. Although they are fairly closely related and similar in structure to the crossopterygians, they are not ancestral to any other vertebrate groups.

The crossopterygians include the ancestors of the first vertebrates that made the transition from water to land. In addition to their sharp, pointed teeth and cosmine scales, the crossopterygians had two important characteristics which made them uniquely suited for the transition from water to land. They had a short, basal fleshy lobe, with a bony skeleton, in their fins which allowed them to use these fins as limbs. A second characteristic, equally as important as the lobed fins, was lungs which allowed the crossopterygians to breathe air. Thus, during the Devonian when continental uplift was common, when the ponds in which the fish were living dried up, while other fish died, the crossopterygians could survive by breathing air and 'walking' overland to another pond.

The crossopterygians are divided into two groups, the Rhipidistia and the Coelacanthini. The coelacanths were a group long thought to be extinct until the modern form *Latimeria* was discovered in 1938 off the coast of southern Africa. The coelacanths are distinguished from the rhipidistians by the absence of internal nostrils.

The rhipidistian crossopterygians with their lobed fins and lungs were ancestral to the amphibians. In many respects the rhipidistian skull and tooth structure was very similar to that of the amphibians. The extinction of the rhipidistians is usually attributed to the fact that they were replaced as freshwater predators by their descendants, the amphibians (Romer 1966).

The amphibians were the first land vertebrates. Evolving as they did from the crossopterygians, perhaps diphyletically (Jarvik 1942), these tetrapods had lungs and limbs that gave them the potential to breathe the air and walk on the land. However, amphibians are still dependent upon an aquatic environment. Most amphibians must return to the water to reproduce; some are fully aquatic; and many amphibians go through an aquatic larval stage.

These groups of amphibians are distinguished on the basis of their skull and vertebral constructions. The most primitive amphibians were the Labyrinthodontia. Although labyrinthodonts are extinct, they were an important group which exhibited a structural transition from the crossopterygians to tetrapods. Also, they were ancestral to the other amphibians and the reptiles. The Lepospondyli are a second extinct group which arose from the labyrinthodonts and were ancestral to the modern amphibians. The Lissamphibia are the only group of amphibians with any living representatives. The Lissamphibia have been further separated into three divisions: the Salientia or Anura, including the frogs and toads; the Urodela or Caudata, including the salamanders and newts; and the Apoda or Caecilia, including some rare, limbless, wormlike types. Colbert (1961) suggests that the three groups of Lissamphibia may not be closely related to each other. This theory may help to explain the differences in immune response found in anurans and urodeles (Cohen 1970). Although the Lissamphibia are the only amphibians surviving today, they are a relatively unimportant group evolutionarily.

Thus, the amphibians were the first vertebrate group to leave the water and make the transition to the tetrapod mode of life on the land. The labyrinthodont group served as the stem group from which the other tetrapods evolved. The transition from the amphibian mode of life with its dependency on the water for reproduction, to the reptilian mode of life, with the amniotic egg removing the necessity to return to the water to reproduce, was a gradual one. The fossil form *Seymouria* attests to the fact that the change was gradual and that the main distinction between the amphibians and reptiles is, indeed, mode of reproduction. *Seymouria* has some skeletal characteristics of reptiles and some of amphibians. *Seymouria* stands so exactly on the dividing line between the amphibian and reptilian classes that it would be impossible to classify it were it not for the fact that fossilized larvae with preserved gill structures of a species closely related to *Seymouria* have been found. Thus, *Seymouria* is believed to have been an amphibian, although it had many reptilian characteristics.

The reptiles, with their characteristic amniotic egg, were at last totally free from the water and fully able to exploit the different habitats available on the land. Not only did they diversify and occupy the land and the air, but some reptiles also reverted to an aquatic existence. A very successful group for millions of years in the past, the reptiles were also the ancestors of the successful land vertebrates of today, the birds and mammals. The relationships among the immune systems of the diverse reptilian species are complex. The cloacal tissue of the snapping turtle has been shown to be lymphoid and has been suggested to be similar to the bursa of Fabricius in avian species

(Sidky & Auerbach 1968). Although the cloacal tissue of the lizard is also lymphoid, Muthukarrupan (1972) has shown that splenectomy in *Callotes versicolor* removes the lizard's ability to respond to sheep red blood cells. Further study of the reptilian immune systems is necessary to understand their complexities and relationships to the avian and mammalian immune systems.

Although the reptiles are a very diverse class which encompasses 15 or 20 taxonomic orders, they are often clustered into five basic groups on the basis of the number and position of temporal openings in the skull:

1. The Anapsida are those reptiles with a solidly built skull with no temporal openings. The anapsids include the order Cotylosauria, the stem group from which most other reptiles developed. Today the anapsids are represented by the turtles.

2. The Lepidosauria are the scaly reptiles. This group includes the lizards, snakes, and *Sphenodon*, a rhyncocephalian. The lepidosaurs are one of the most successful groups of reptiles today.

3. The Euryapsida are an extinct group of aquatic reptiles. They are relatively uninteresting evolutionarily, since they were ancestral to no other vertebrate forms.

4. The Archosauria were the so-called ruling reptiles. The dinosaurs, crocodiles, and flying reptiles of this group are the exciting animals that school children recall when they hear the word 'reptile'. The Archosauria, too, are an evolutionarily exciting group because they are the group from which the birds evolved. The transition between the reptiles and birds was gradual and only partially documented by the fossil record. Birds remain so closely related to reptiles that some students even believe that they should simply be classified as another reptilian order, rather than having the taxonomic status of class. *Archaeopteryx* is the fossilized transitional form between the reptiles and birds. It retains the reptilian features of a long bony tail, teeth, and claws, while adding the avian feature of feathers and an expanded braincase. No one is ever likely to know whether *Archaeopteryx* had achieved the changes in the circulatory and respiratory systems necessary for the warm-blooded condition, nor the nesting habit and care of the young found in modern birds. Behavioural features and soft anatomy are rarely fossilized. However, *Archaeopteryx* does provide the transitional link between reptiles and birds.

5. The Synapsida represent another group of reptiles evolving from the anapsid cotylosaurs. Although all synapsids are extinct today, they are the group from which the mammals evolved. The synapsids are divided into two groups, the Pelycosauria and the Therapsida. The pelycosaurs include the primitive forms such as *Dimetrodon* in which the vertebral spines were extended vertically to form great 'sails' on their backs. Although these sails have been interpreted in many different ways, Romer (1948) suggests that

they were an attempt to regulate the thermal temperature of the body. The sails might represent an evolutionary attempt at achieving the warm-blooded condition found in mammals.

The pelycosaurs became the stock from which the Therapsida or mammal-like reptiles evolved. The therapsids were an advanced, varied group of reptiles which spanned the entire evolutionary gap between reptiles and mammals. In one group or another of the more advanced therapsids almost every diagnostic feature of the mammalian skeleton in terms of loss of skull elements, palate, teeth, and limb structure was realized. Marchalonis and Atwell (1972) have shown that the G immunoglobulins of mammals emerged within the therapsid line of reptiles before the divergence of the three modern mammalian subclasses. (Unfortunately there is no perfect transitional form such as *Archeopteryx* or *Seymouria* to serve as the link between reptiles and mammals. Although in a number of cases forms are known having both the reptilian and the mammalian form of jaw articulation operative at the same time.) A polyphyletic origin of the mammals from the reptiles has been suggested (Simpson 1959). However, most of the diagnostic features of mammals lie in their soft anatomy and reproductive processes, which are never fossilized. Thus, one must be content knowing that although the details of the phylogenetic history are still uncertain, the therapsid ancestry of mammals is established.

By many criteria the mammals are the most successful of all vertebrates living today. In terms of exploiting different ecological habitats, the mammals are certainly successful. Not only have they competed more successfully than most of the reptiles and amphibia on the land but, in forms such as the whale and the bat, they have attempted to invade the sea and air. Many characteristics of the mammals which seem more advanced than those of the other vertebrates make them particularly well-adapted to cope with their environment. With the exception of the primitive forms, the mammals nourish their young via the placenta and retain the young inside the mother before birth. After the live birth, the mother suckles the infants. During this time, the infant usually receives some guidance from the parents which presumably helps it to survive in the physical environment. The mammals are warm-blooded with a four-chambered heart that completely separates the oxygenated from the deoxygenated blood; the presence of hair aids in the preservation of body heat. The warm-blooded condition coupled with an increase in relative size and convolution of the brain have allowed the mammals to become a very active and intelligent group. These behavioural and internal anatomical characteristics along with the characteristics of the teeth, ear ossicles, and jaw articulation are used to separate the mammals from the reptiles.

Very little is known about the early mammals. Because of their small size and the scarcity of geological deposits, early mammals are known principally from their dental anatomy. Teeth from several different evolutionary lineages such as the triconodonts, multituberculates, symmetrodonts, and pantotheres have been discovered. Of these, the pantotheres show the greatest similarity to later mammals.

The living mammals may be separated into three groups on the basis of their mode of bearing young:

1. The Prototheria or monotremes lay eggs. The duckbill and spiny anteater of Australia are monotremes living today. They represent a primitive or highly specialized offshoot of the mammals, which originated separately from, and was not ancestral to, the higher mammals. The evolutionary history of the monotremes is essentially unknown.

2. The Metatheria or marsupials bear their young alive at an immature stage. These include the opossums, South American forms, and many Australian forms. Although marsupials are considered to share a common ancestor with the placentals, the marsupials themselves were probably not ancestral to placentals, except possibly in an ecological sense (Romer 1966).

3. The Eutheria or placentals retain the young in the mother's body for a longer time than marsupials, nourishing the fetus via the placenta. The placentals include most of the common animals with which one is familiar. A primitive insectivore stock is usually considered to be the stem group from which the rodents, edentates, rabbits, primates, bats, whales, carnivores, and several other, now extinct, orders arose. Arising also from the same basal insectivore stock were the condylarths, another basal stock. From the condylarths evolved the ungulate groups: artiodactyls, including pigs and cows; perissodactyls, including horses; elephants; Sirenia; and several other now extinct ungulate groups. Volumes have been written on the different placental orders and their relationships to each other. No attempt will be made to discuss the various orders here, other than to say that they are many, and that each is well adapted to its particular environment.

Some principles of evolution

After considering the phylogeny of the animal kingdom, one is impressed by the many complex and diverse species present on the earth. The question which comes to mind next concerns the mechanism by which all these different species evolved. Several theories such as inheritance of effects of use and disuse, orthogenesis, vitalism, catastrophism, and telefinalism have been suggested and accepted in certain circles at various times. Today the evolutionary theory which is accepted by most scientists is Darwin's theory of natural selection. Only a brief outline will be given here of Darwin's theory with particular emphasis placed upon points that are especially relevant to immunology.

Perhaps the easiest way to understand Darwin's theory is to consider one species (a population of individuals that can interbreed and produce fertile offspring) in one particular environment. If limited resources (especially food) along with ever increasing numbers of individuals of the species exist in the environment, then competition for the available limited resources and a struggle for survival will ensue among the members of the species. All of the individuals of one species will be similar to each other and distinguishable from members of other species. However, individuals of the same species will differ from each other with respect to minor characteristics. The intraspecific variability makes some individuals better adapted to live in a particular environment and other individuals less adapted to live in that same environment. The source of the variability within the species population is in the genotypes of the individuals. (Darwin, of course, was not aware of genetics. Thus, although he recognized the variability, he was not aware of its exact source, though he did develop a theory of inheritance of his own.)

An individual of the species that is better adapted to the environment is more likely to survive and reproduce, thus passing its genes on to its offspring, than is an individual that is less adapted to the environment. A continuation of this process over time results in the survival of the fittest members of the species, with individuals of the species being well adapted for their particular environment.

New variations may be introduced into the population via recombinations and mutations of the genes. If the mutation is beneficial in helping the individual adapt to the environment, the chances of that individual surviving to reproduce and pass the favourable gene on to its offspring will be increased. In this manner, beneficial mutations may be preserved in the population and harmful ones eliminated. It has been suggested and experimentally demonstrated that even genes controlling very minor characteristics are acted upon by the force of natural selection.

Recently, evidence has been garnered (Kimura 1968) for a non-Darwinian evolution that operates by random drift of mutants whose effects are very minute. This non-Darwinian theory suggests that most DNA changes and amino acid substitutions in evolution have been so nearly neutral that their fate was determined mainly by random processes. Thus, observed molecular evolution is caused by random fixation of neutral mutations. This view does not compete with the Darwinian view of natural selection for most observed characters, since the effect of the non-Darwinian evolution on fitness is probably negligible (Kimura 1971).

Normally the non-Darwinian theory might not be mentioned in a brief discussion of evolution such as this. However, immunology may provide examples of non-Darwinian evolution. The transplantation or histocompatibility antigens (H-2 in mice, HLA in humans, Rh-LA in rhesus monkeys, etc.) are highly polymorphic antigens at two closely linked loci. No particular survival benefit seems to be conferred on any individual by its possession of one particular antigen or another, as long as it has histocompatibility antigens (Burnet 1973). Nevertheless, selection seems to favour a high mutation rate for the histocompatibility loci. Thus, the presence of histocompatibility antigens is probably controlled by Darwinian natural selection, since the ability to distinguish self from other members of the same species must be important for survival (Burnet 1973). However, the particular antigens that any one individual possesses are probably controlled by non-Darwinian evolution.

So far, our discussion of evolution has considered one species in one particular environment. But how did the diversity of species present in our modern world arise? If new, different environments or 'ecological niches' were to open up to the species, some individuals in the species might move in to the niche, taking over the opportunity presented by this new environment. The forces of natural selection would operate on the variations in the genotype of the population so that individuals moving into the new environment would become more and more adapted to the new environment. Eventually, structural and functional changes might occur in the individuals in the new environment such that they could no longer breed with the individuals still present in the old environment. Thus, a new species would evolve. Sometimes a variety of major environmental opportunities might open up for members of a group, with the result that a whole series of diversified descendants might rapidly evolve to occupy, with appropriate adaptations, a series of varied ecological niches. This phenomenon is termed adaptive radiation or divergent evolution.

In a very broad sense, the phylogeny of the animal kingdom is the result of many adaptive radiations. The final result is a series of widely separated forms in different environments which appear to have little or no relationship to each other.

The adaptive radiation of a number of groups may result in two unrelated species occupying similar ecological niches. When this happens, the two species may develop similar structural features which are necessary for survival in similar modes of life. An example of an analogous structure resulting from convergent evolution would be the wing of a bird and the wing of a bat. Perhaps certain aspects of the immune response of annelids (Bailey *et al.* 1971) and amphibians might represent convergent evolution in unrelated groups adapting to a moist environment.

A tangential point which may be raised here, while discussing unrelated species, is Haeckel's law: Ontogeny recapitulates phylogeny. The law, often used as an aid in determining relationships among groups, is incorrect in many respects. During development, an individual does not retrace its phylogenetic history exactly. Certain parts of the history are skipped; other parts are done in reverse order. Some stages of embryological development have no counterpart in phylogeny. Embryos of some species may even go through developmental stages similar to phylogenetic stages of their descendants rather than their ancestors. However, despite its problems, Haeckel's law still is used to aid in determining relationships because the ontogeny of an individual does have a superficial resemblance to the phylogenetic history of that species. Recently Hildemann and Reddy (1973) have suggested that, in immunology, ontogeny appears to recapitulate phylogeny in the sense that mixed leukocyte culture-type reactivity precedes other correlates of cellular immunity both phylogenetically and developmentally.

An obvious conclusion that can be drawn after studying vertebrate evolution is that the phylogeny of the animal kingdom is the result of a complex interaction between the animal and its environment. The forces of natural selection operate on the population to make it well adapted to its particular environment. Characters will be selected which allow the individual to survive and produce viable offspring in the environment.

In the light of natural selection, one must reconsider the meaning of such questions as whether the invertebrates and lower vertebrates have an immune system. In the broadest sense of the term 'immune system', the invertebrates and lower vertebrates are able to survive and defend themselves against invasion from 'foreign' matter. Many times the question that the immunologist is really asking is do the invertebrates and lower vertebrates have a mammalian- or avian-type immune system? The criteria and tests for immune responses were developed in mammals and birds. Thus, it is natural that these tests and criteria should be the ones first used when attempting to detect immune responses in other classes and phyla. However, it is important to remember that natural selection is concerned with having the population function efficiently in its environment. Different ways of maintaining this function may have been developed by different species at different times. The immune system should not be thought of as evolving orthogenetically towards the mammalian type, just because the mammalian structured immune system is the one which immunologic tests were developed to detect. Ernst Mayr expressed this idea very beautifully in the following discussion: 'It is not strictly correct to ask whether selection acts on structure or on function. Selection responds to the total phenotype, and any genetic component that improves the viability of the phenotype will be selected. Usually this is something functional, although in most cases it is quite impossible to make a clean separation of function and structure. In different organisms evolution often finds independent (and different) answers to the same challenges of the environment. It is not necessary for the elasmobranch, the bony fish, and the birds to evolve the same defense mechanisms as the mammals. There is even the uncomfortable possibility that a defense mechanism present in the ancestral form is replaced by different mechanisms in some of the descendant lines.' (Mayr 1966, p. 129).

Thus it is important to remember when interpreting data on phylogeny of immunity that natural selection will operate to defend and adapt the population in the best way possible for that particular species in that particular environment.

Acknowledgments

This work was done in the laboratory of Dr Robert Auerbach at the University of Wisconsin and was supported partially by grant number CA 14520–01 from the National Cancer Institute and partially by grant number GB 3667 from the National Science Foundation. I would like to thank Dr Robert Auerbach, Dr David Clark, and Dr J. T. Robinson for their suggestions and criticisms of the manuscript. I would like to thank Miss Cheryl Hughes and Mr Francis McCormick for assistance in assembling the manuscript.

References

Bailey S., Miller B.J. & Cooper E.L. (1971) Transplantation immunity in annelids. II. Adoptive transfer of xenograft reaction. *Immunology* **21,** 81–6.

Barrington E.J.W. (1965) *The Biology of Hemichordata and Protochordata.* Oliver & Boyd, Edinburgh and London.

Bateson W. (1886) The ancestry of the chordata. *Quart. Journ. Micr. Sci.* **26,** 535–71.

Berrill N.J. (1955) *The Origin of Vertebrates.* Clarendon Press, Oxford.

Buchsbaum R. (1948) *Animals Without Backbones.* University of Chicago Press, Chicago.

Burnet F.M. (1973) Multiple polymorphism in relation to histocompatibility antigens. *Nature,* **245,** 359–61.

Chateaureynaud-Duprat P. (1973) Mise en evidence et etude de l'immunite chez les vers. *L'etude phylogenique et ontogenique de la response immunitaire et son apport a la theorie immunologique.* Editions Inserm, Paris.

Cohen N. (1970) Tissue transplantation immunity and immunologic memory in Urodela and Apoda. *Transpl. Proc.* **2**(2), 275–81.

Colbert E.H. (1961) *Evolution of the Vertebrates.* John Wiley & Sons, Inc. New York.

Darwin C. (1859) *On the Origin of Species.* Atheneum, New York.

Garstang W. (1928). The morphology of the Tunicata, and its bearings on the phylogeny of the Chordata. *Quart. Journ. Micr. Sci.* **72,** 51–187.

Good R.A., Finstad J., Pollara B., & Gabrielsen A. (1966) Morphologic studies on the evolution of the lymphoid tissues among the lower vertebrates. *Phylogeny of Immunity,* eds Smith R.T., Miescher P.A. & Good R.A. Univ. of Florida Press, Gainesville.

Halstead L.B. (1968) *The Pattern of Vertebrate Evolution.* W. J. Freeman & Co., San Francisco.

Hildemann W.H. & Reddy A.L. (1973) Phylogeny of immune responsiveness in marine invertebrates. *Fed. Proc.* **32,** 2188–94.

Jarvik E. (1942) On the structure of the snout of crossopterygians and lower gnathostomes in general. *Zool. Bidrag Uppsala* **21,** 235–675.

JARVIK E. (1968) Aspects of vertebrate phylogeny. In *Current Problems of Lower Vertebrate Phylogeny*, ed. Tor Orvig. Nobel Symposium 4. Interscience Publishers, Almquist & Wiksell, Stockholm.

JEFFERIES R.P.S. (1968) The subphylum Calcichordata (Jefferies 1967) primitive fossil chordates with echinoderm affinities. *Brit. Mus. Nat. Hist. Geol.* **16,** 6.

KIMURA M. (1968) Genetic variability maintained in a finite population due to mutational production of neutral and nearly neutral isoalleles. *Genet. Res.* **11,** 247–69.

MARCHALONIS J.J. & ATWELL J.L. (1972) Phylogenetic emergence of distinct immunoglobulin classes. *L'etude phylogenique et ontogenique de la reponse immunitaire et son apport a la theorie immunologique.* Editions Inserm, Paris.

MAYR E. (1966) Interpretation of phylogenetic data. *Phylogeny of Immunity*, eds Smith R.T., Miescher P.A. & Good R.A. Univ. of Florida Press, Gainesville.

MOY-THOMAS J.A. (1939) The early evolution and relationships of the elasmobranchs. *Biol. Rev.* **14,** 1–26.

MUTHUKARRUPAN V.R. (1972) Effect of splenectomy on the immune response in the lizard, *Calotes versicolor. Experentia* **28,** 1225.

NURSALL J.R. (1962) On the origins of the major groups of animals. *Evolution* **16,** 118–23.

PATTEN W. (1912) *The Evolution of the Vertebrates and their Kin.* Blakiston, Philadelphia.

ROMER A.S. (1948) Relative growth in pelycosaurian reptiles. *Roy. Soc. South Africa, Spec. Publ. Robt. Broom Comm. Vol.*, 45–55.

ROMER A.S. (1955) The primitive vertebrate as a dual animal—somatic and visceral. *Proc. Zool. Soc. London* **125,** 81.

ROMER A.S. (1959) *The Vertebrate Story.* University of Chicago Press, Chicago.

ROMER A.S. (1966) *Vertebrate Paleontology*, 3rd edition. University of Chicago Press, Chicago.

SIDKY Y.A. & AUERBACH R. (1968) Tissue culture analysis of immunological capacity of snapping turtles. *J. exp. Zool.* **167,** 187–96.

STENSIO E. (1968) The cyclostomes with special reference to the diphyletic origin of the Petromyzontida and Myxinoidea. *Current Problems of Lower Vertebrate Phylogeny*, ed. Tor Orvig. Nobel Symposium 4. Interscience Publishers, Almquist & Wiksell, Stockholm.

THOENES G.H. (1972) The hagfish at the phylogenetical juncture towards immunological response. *L'etude phylogenique et ontogenique de la response immunitaire et son apport a la theorie immunologique.* Editions Inserm, Paris.

VAN WIJHE J.W. (1923) Thymus, spiracular sense organ and fenestra vestibuli (ovalis) in a 63 mm long embryo of *Heptanchus cinereus. Proc. Sci. Akad. Wetensch. Amsterdam* **26,** 727.

Chapter 2. The Nature of Immune Phenomena in Mammals: (a) Cellular Immunity; (b) Antibody Formation

G. J. V. Nossal

Introduction

T and B lymphocyte families in mammals

The role of macrophages in immunity

Interaction between antigens and lymphocyte receptors

T and B lymphocyte receptors and collaboration

Genetic factors in immune responsiveness

Immunological memory

Immunological tolerance

Summary

Introduction

The wide-ranging panoply of phenomena which constitutes the mammalian adaptive immune response falls conveniently into two distinct but closely interrelated sets of reactions that are termed cellular immunity (or cell-mediated immunity) and humoral immunity (or antibody formation). The student of these phenomena finds himself humbled by their complexity, and looks longingly towards his colleagues in phylogenetic research to provide simpler model systems. The purpose of the present chapter is to provide a brief outline of cellular and humoral immunity in mammals, as a preface to the chapters which will deal with lower species. This should help to show both the similarities and the differences in defence functions between mammals, lower vertebrates and invertebrates.

We must first seek to find common ground between cellular and humoral immunity before defining the distinction between them. In either case, the central fact is that the introduction of some foreign ('non-self') molecule into the body is followed by a series of cellular events, designed to aid the elimination of the foreign molecule, which render the animal capable of reacting in a specifically heightened way to a second encounter with the foreign molecule. It is this characteristic of specificity, and the acquired nature of immunity, that distinguish adaptive immune responses from more primitive innate defence functions. The specific recognition of foreign molecules, or portions of molecules termed antigenic determinants, depends on sets of complementary recognition molecules within the mammal, either free in the serum or attached as receptors to the surface of lymphocyte cells. The essence of the mammalian immune response is selection (Burnet 1959). Cells bearing receptors appropriate to the antigen entering the body are stimulated to

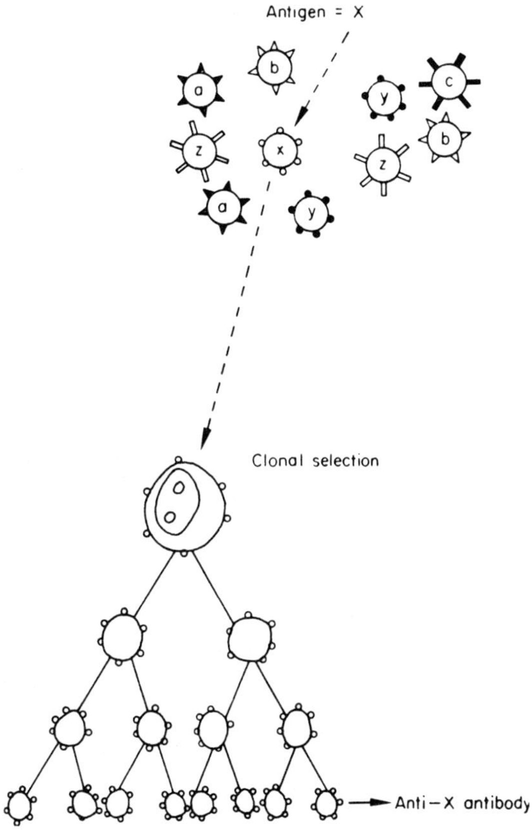

Fig. 2.1. The clonal selection theory of antibody formation. Antigen is seen as entering the body and stimulating selectively lymphocytes bearing pre-existing receptors with capacity to unite specifically with that antigen. Stimulation causes the cell to embark on clonal proliferation and simultaneous differentiation into cells specialized for high-rate antibody secretion.

divide and differentiate, greatly amplifying the proportionate representation of particular elements amongst the recognition molecules (Fig. 2.1). Thus, the immune response increases greatly the concentration of certain antibodies, the capacity to synthesize which was nevertheless already present in the animal prior to the introduction of the antigen. In order for such a selective system to work at all, the pre-existent set of recognition units ('natural' antibodies and cell receptors) must be sufficiently large to allow at least a reasonable degree of heterogeneity. Perhaps the most important single challenge facing the immunophylogenist is to understand the evolution of these recognition sets, that is, the ancestors of the variable portions of antibody chains. A deep clue may be contained in the fact that portions of the molecules determining histocompatibility, e.g. the HLA complex in man, may be evolutionarily related to portions of immunoglobulin heavy chains. The outright speculation that the immune system and the intraspecies polymorphisms due to histocompatibility genes both arose as an elaboration of some system needed for intercellular recognition and collaboration within a given animal is raised.

Historically, the chief difference between cellular and humoral immunity lies in the capacity to transfer the latter immune state from animal to animal by immune serum, whereas the former state can be transferred only by actual transplantation of living lymphoid cells from the immune to the non-immune animal. Both types of immunity are due to the activity of lymphoid cells. For humoral immunity, the activated cell (termed a plasma cell in its most specialized state of differentiation) secretes antibody. For cellular immunity, the immune state depends not on serum antibody but on a family of specifically activated lymphocytes with the capacity to recognize the antigen concerned and to react to contact with antigen by releasing a variety of pharmacological mediators of cell damage and inflammation. This cellular immunity aids elimination of foreign entities, either through their direct cytotoxic destruction (as in the case of grafted cells or parasitic metazoans) or through indirect means via chronic inflammation.

A major step forward in the understanding of cellular versus humoral immunity came, curiously enough, not from mammals but from birds (Warner & Szenberg 1964). The chicken has been extensively used in immunological research, and it possesses two kinds of primary lymphoid organs, that is organs where lymphocytes are formed through antigen-independent cell proliferation but where antigens do not normally penetrate or cause immunocyte activation. These are the thymus, which is bilaterally distributed and segmented; and the bursa of Fabricius, attached to the cloaca. It was found that ablation of the bursa in embryonic life prevented the later development of the capacity to form circulating antibody. In contrast, ablation of the thymus, if achieved early enough, had its dominant effect on cell-mediated immunity. This suggested the presence of two separate families of lymphoid cells, one, under the control of the bursa, mediating humoral immunity; the other, under the control of the thymus, responsible for cellular immunity.

T and B lymphocyte families in mammals

A decade's further work (see Nossal & Ada 1971, Miller 1972 for reviews) has shown that this dichotomy applies also to mammals. In fact, two broad classes of lymphocytes exist, which have come to be termed T and B lymphocytes. T lymphocytes (often called T cells) are formed in the thymus, through the immigration into that organ of multipotential haemopoietic stem cells. These cells receive some inductive stimulus through the thymic microenvironment, perhaps through the production of a humoral inducer by thymic epithelial cells, which commits them to a pathway of lymphoid differentiation (Metcalf & Moore 1971). A proportion of them leave the thymus and colonize the peripheral or secondary lymphoid organs such as lymph nodes, spleen, Peyer's patches and other lymphoid collections. There, they constitute the pool of immunocompetent T cells. There is no strict mammalian analogue to the avian bursa of Fabricius, but bone marrow contains cells capable of differentiating into 'bursal equivalent' or B lymphocytes (Metcalf & Moore 1971). B lymphocytes act as the cells which, on appropriate activation by antigen, turn into antibody-forming cells (Fig. 2.2).

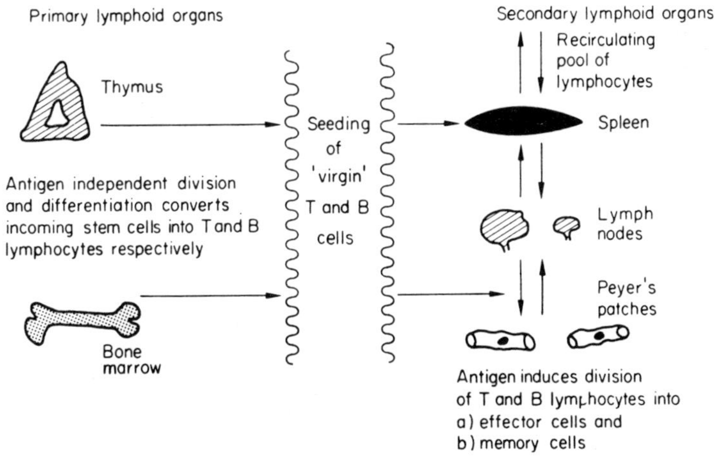

Fig. 2.2. An overview of the various compartments of the lymphoid system.

T and B lymphocytes can be distinguished from each other through various sets of characteristics, some of which are listed on Table 2.1. It is now clear, however, that each of the two major types can be further broken down into subtypes (e.g. high-θ versus low-θ T cells; spleen-seeking versus lymph node-seeking T cells, etc.). Unfortunately, definitions of subtypes retain a strong operational component, and it will be some time before a clear picture relating origins, structure and function emerges. A detailed documentation of the many phenomena listed in Table 2.1 has been presented elsewhere (Nossal & Ada 1971, Miller 1972). For the present purposes, suffice it to say that sufficient markers exist not only to distinguish T and B cells from each

Table 2.1. Some characteristics differentiating mouse T and B lymphocytes

Broad function Origins	T cells Cell-mediated immunity Thymus	B cells Humoral immunity Fetal liver; adult bone marrow
Examples of function	(i) Delayed hypersensitivity. (ii) Antibody and complement-independent. cytotoxicity against grafts or tumours. (iii) Graft versus host reactions. (iv) Helper functions, aiding B cells to respond to antigens. (v) Suppressor functions, inhibiting B cell responses.	Secretion of antibody of different classes.
Function mediated by	(i) Direct cell-to-cell contact. (ii) Secretion of lymphokines which activate other cells. (iii) Possibly shedding of specific IgM-like receptors.	Antibody acting directly on antigen, or via the macrophage ('opsonization') or the complement system.
Surface characteristics and antigenic markers	(i) Surface relatively smooth and featureless on scanning electron-microscopy. (ii) θ antigen present. (iii) MBL antigen absent. (iv) Anti-immunoglobulin (Ig) bound very weakly by living cells. (v) Receptor for Fc piece of Ig and for C3 component of complement absent. (vi) High mobility in electrophoretic field.	(i) Surface covered by numerous filamentous projections. (ii) θ antigen absent. (iii) MBL antigen present. (iv) Anti-immunoglobulin bound strongly by most B cells. (v) Fc and C3 receptors present on some B cells. (vi) Most cells possess low electrophoretic mobility.

	(vii) In general, non-adherent to glass or plastic. Exceptions occur. (viii) Ir gene associated cell surface antigen present in small amounts.	(vii) In general, greater tendency to adhere than T cells. Exceptions occur. (viii) Ir gene associated cell surface antigen present in large amounts.
Activation markers	(i) Phytohaemagglutinin (PHA) and pokeweed mitogen (PWM) stimulate division in some T cells. (ii) Anti-Ig does not stimulate division.	(i) PWM stimulates division; PHA does not unless bound to a solid phase. (ii) Anti-Ig can stimulate division.
In vivo habitat	(i) Constitute about 85 per cent of the recirculating pool of lymphocytes, 75 per cent of lymph node lymphocytes, 50 per cent of spleen lymphocytes and <5 per cent of bone marrow lymphocytes. (ii) Live in and traffic through certain 'T-dependent' areas of lymphoid tissue, such as lymph node paracortical nodules and spleen white pulp periarteriolar region.	(i) Constitute about 15 per cent of recirculating pool, 25 per cent of lymph node lymphocytes, 50 per cent of spleen lymphocytes and a majority of bone marrow lymphocytes. All organs contain a small proportion of lymphocytes which are neither typical B nor T; some of these are probably 'pre-B' cells. (ii) Live in and around primary lymphoid follicles and germinal centres; also prominent in lymph node medullary cords and splenic red pulp. Demarcation into T and B areas in lymphatic tissue is not absolute.

other, but also to allow their partial, and at times complete, biophysical separation from each other.

Use of biophysically purified T or B cell sub-populations is not yet widespread, but certain models in the mouse have served extensively to aid our understanding of differences between T and B cells. For example, a certain gene mutation has occurred which, in the homozygous form (*ν/ν*) causes early arrest of thymus development and produces mice which lack T cells completely or almost completely. As such mice also lack body hair, they are frequently referred to as 'nude' mice. Another good source of B-cell enrichment is the so-called 'ATXBM' mouse. Here, adult mice are thymectomized, given a lethal dose of whole body X-irradiation, and a restorative inoculum of bone marrow or fetal liver stem cells. The T-cell contamination of bone marrow and the persistence of small numbers of radio-resistant T cells can be a problem in such animals. A relatively pure T-cell source is provided by animals that are given lethal X-irradiation followed by a thymus cell infusion and an antigen (Miller 1972). The spleen and/or the lymph of such animals provides a source of relatively pure T cells activated against the antigen concerned (ATC).

In man, nature has provided models of 'thymusless' or 'bursaless' individuals. Thus, certain forms of agammaglobulinaemia represent children lacking B cells but with normal T-cell function, whereas di George syndrome represents failure of T cells with residual B-cell function. Thymus grafts have been rewarding in a proportion of such patients.

Some of the literature on T and B cells may confuse the student or worker entering this field in not clarifying sufficiently the difference between central or peripheral T or B cells. The central or primary lymphoid organs, namely thymus and bone marrow, contain relatively few cells that are ready and competent to respond, and a larger proportion of cells that are not able to respond to antigen but represent less differentiated precursors. Furthermore, the thymus contains certain cells that appear not to be destined for export at all, but which die locally. In contrast, secondary lymphoid organs contain various later differentiation stages of T and B lymphocytes. These include 'virgin' cells that have not yet met antigen; 'memory' cells that have been through one or more cycles of antigen-induced proliferation and are capable of further response to antigen; and executive or effector cells actively mediating cellular immunity or secreting antibody. Each sub-category of cells will display its special characteristics. Therefore, the classification of T and B cells into sub-types is likely to require extensive continued modification over the years ahead.

The role of macrophages in immunity

Phagocytic cells are phylogenetically much older than lymphocytes and play a major but still controversial role in immunity (Warner & Szenberg 1964, Feldman & Nossal 1972). Certainly, when immunogenic antigen is injected into an animal, most of what is stably trapped is retained in and on the cells of the reticulo-endothelial system. There appear to be two largely separate types of cells involved, namely macrophages, which sequester antigen into inclusions (phagolysosomes) and dendritic cells which retain antigen on their surface, though the distinction between the two is not absolute. Macrophages help the induction of the immune response in at least three ways. First, they may digest particulate antigens such as bacteria or foreign erythrocytes into smaller antigenic fragments, more capable of interacting with lymphocytes. Secondly, surface-retained material may represent a concentrated focus of antigen, with the presentation of an array of antigenic determinants to lymphocyte receptors, the resulting antigen-receptor union being more effective in triggering than that between a single receptor and a univalent antigen. Thirdly, macrophages, particularly after activation, may secrete substances or factors which facilitate lymphocyte triggering (Schrader 1973). Finally, a long and somewhat controversial series of experiments suggests that RNA derived from macrophages that have ingested antigen can aid antibody formation (Fishman 1969). The most likely explanation of this is that certain antigen-RNA complexes are particularly efficacious in lymphocyte triggering. None of these explanations are mutually exclusive and all may play a part in the complex *in vivo* events preceding T- and B-lymphocyte activation.

While most immune responses require the participation of macrophages, there are some in which the requirement may be by-passed. For example, B lymphocytes from the thoracic duct lymph can be stimulated to form antibody by presenting to them the multivalent antigens polymerized flagellin or sonicated extracts of sheep erythrocytes. Here the important feature appears to be the multi-point binding of lymphocyte receptors to a single particle of antigen. This can induce a surface rearrangement of receptors into, first, aggregated patches and, later, into cap-like aggregates over one pole of the cell (Raff *et al.* 1973). This may be an important early event in triggering. However, experiments purporting to show macrophage independence involve tissue cultures of *relatively* pure B-cell populations, and the absence of a small residuum of macrophages or macrophage precursors is difficult to prove. Physiologically, most immune induction probably involves macrophage-lymphocyte contact.

Interaction between antigens and lymphocyte receptors

Consideration of the role of the macrophage serves to introduce the general question of interaction between antigens and lymphocyte receptors. We have already seen that the immune response is selective (Fig. 2.1) and that the main job of antigen is to trigger into proliferative activity and further differentiation that sub-set of lymphocytes carrying receptors capable of reacting with that antigen. Two further concepts need to be introduced at this point, namely affinity and immunogenicity.

The secret of the immune system is that the sets of recognition units, namely the lymphocyte receptors, do not know in advance what it is that they must recognize. The library of receptors possessed by the whole animal must be large enough to encompass all imaginable antigens. Evolution has coped with this requirement by constructing a recognition system which is degenerate and redundant. Each antibody can recognize more than one antigen; each antigen can be recognized by more than one antibody. When an antigenic determinant enters the body, it can interact with receptors of many different specificities. In each case, the union will involve a reaction of a given affinity. The association constants of reactions which clearly belong into the category of immune recognition vary over a range of at least one million fold. Furthermore, to the concept of affinity we must add the closely allied one of avidity. Affinity refers to the strength of union of a single antigenic determinant with a single receptor site, whereas avidity is the term used to embrace both the binding constant and the gain in strength of union resulting from multivalency. As we now know that cell receptors are mobile in the plane of the membrane, it is clear that the physical chemistry of lymphocyte-antigen interactions is very complex. The central point is that whether a particular immunoglobulin molecule is an antibody for a particular antigen will depend frequently on the methodology used for assay.

This leads on to the idea that immunogenicity and antigenicity are not necessarily identical. Immunogenicity is that operationally defined property of an antigen molecule which allows it to induce an active immune response on injection. The avidity of union between lymphocyte and antigen will be an important, but by no means the sole, determining factor. Others may include the possession of more than one antigenic determinant, encouraging T–B lymphocyte cooperation (*vide infra*); prior exposure of the animal concerned to related antigens; physical state of the antigen (particulate entities being, in general, more immunogenic than soluble molecules) and a variety of other circumstances. Not infrequently, the end result of the union of a soluble, monomeric antigen with a lymphocyte receptor is the very reverse of triggering. In that case, the cell is rendered refractory to the inductive influence of subsequently administered antigen. This is known as immunological tolerance, and will be discussed in a separate section.

T and B lymphocyte receptors and collaboration

It is clear that the receptor for antigen present on B lymphocytes is immunoglobulin (Ig) (Marchalonis & Cone 1973). The operative portions in antigen recognition are combining sites, the specificity of which depends on the amino acid sequences of the variable (V) portions of Ig light and heavy chains. While a given B cell may carry more than one class of heavy chain on its surface, the evidence is strong (Nossal 1974a) that each B cell only expresses one unique type of combining specificity, i.e. a single pair of Ig V regions, one from either κ or λ light chains, and one coded for by the heavy chain V gene, common to all heavy chains. Activation of a B cell results in the secretion at high rate by its clonal progeny of antibody molecules bearing the combining specificity of the original receptor. There is some evidence that the primordial receptor in most species is IgM and that certain lymphocytes undergo an IgM to IgG transition after activation. Whether that is so or not, it is clear that the production of IgG antibody is intimately dependent on T-cell activation under most experimental circumstances.

T cells do not secrete large quantities of antibody. Their defence function against antigenic microorganisms or cells depends on close contact between antigen and lymphocyte. It is generally believed that such close contact is mediated by an interaction between T lymphocyte receptors and antigenic determinants. Various pharmacologically active substances, collectively termed lymphokines, are released on such contact, and these are profoundly important in cellular immunity. They promote chemotaxis, cause macrophage activation, and potentiate B-cell responses to antigen. The molecular mechanisms by which T lymphocytes kill antigenic cells and collaborate with B cells are not fully elucidated.

The chemical nature of T-cell receptors for antigen, both those responsible for the initial activation of the cell and those (perhaps identical) receptors permitting close contact between activated T lymphocytes and their target antigens, is the subject of much current debate. One line of experimentation suggests that the receptor is an IgM-like molecule, perhaps consisting of standard κ or λ light chains, and a μ-chain like heavy chain which might be coded for by a fourth set of V genes linked to separate c genes, i.e. a fourth 'translocon'. The second line of experimentation argues for a family of recognition molecules that are not Ig at all. The suggestion is that the T-cell receptor is coded for by a set of immune response (Ir) genes that are closely linked to the major histocompatibility genes of the species. A compromise suggestion recently proposed was that there are two kinds of T cells, one working through IgM-like receptors and the other through Ir gene products, which collaborate in many T cell responses. In the light of this uncertainty, it is not possible to be dogmatic about the question of whether a given T cell displays only a single receptor specificity, but fair arguments in favour of this view can be mustered. Many immunologists assume that T lymphocytes undergo a somatic diversification process comparable with that of B lymphocytes, with the production of mature T cells, each with a single receptor specificity.

For T cells to act as 'helper' cells in antibody formation, i.e. as cells which allow B cells to respond to an antigen, they must recognize some determinant on the antigen *different* from that to which a particular B cell is responding. This is frequently referred to as a 'carrier' determinant, and artificial reconstruction experiments are best performed with hapten-protein conjugates as antigens, antibody-formation being measured against the hapten, and the protein being the carrier antigen recognized by T cells. In many models, B cells will form anti-hapten antibody only in the presence of T cells actively responding to the carrier. Furthermore, the carrier and the hapten must be on the same molecule. The details of how T cells exert their helper effects are not yet clear. According to one theory (Feldman & Basten 1972, Marchalonis & Cone 1973), the T cell recognizes antigen by its IgM-like receptor (IgT) and sheds complexes of antigen-IgT which rapidly become adsorbed to the surface of macrophages. The resulting depot of antigen, tethered to the macrophage via the carrier determinants linked to IgT, is seen as favourable for B cell triggering. Other theories (e.g. Katz & Benacerraf 1972) see the T cell as releasing mitogenic factors helpful in B-cell triggering, which under physiological circumstances act only over a short range. The antigen is then seen as a bridge, holding B and T cells close together, either attached to each other or both close to the surface of a macrophage. This is a very active field of current research, and the true mechanism should emerge over the next few years.

Genetic factors in immune responsiveness

Genetic factors influence immune responses at least as profoundly as prior antigenic load (McDevitt & Landy 1973). Three main streams of investigation document this. First, outbred individuals can be selectively mated to produce lines of animals that are either good or poor producers of antibody to a wide variety of antigens. This can be shown to depend on a multiplicity of genes, which influence *inter alia*, macrophage performance and B cell mitotic rate. Secondly, there exists a series of genes linked to the major histocompatibility locus which determine how well the T cells of an individual can respond to a given antigen. These are termed Ir or immune regulatory genes, which, as discussed above may function in T-cell recognition of antigen. Thirdly, the immunoglobulin structural genes present in the germ line of an animal may determine the efficiency of antibody production to particular antigens. These genetic influences may not be evident in many cases where animals are given powerful antigens like bacterial or viral vaccines, where a multiplicity of different antigenic determinants contributes to the overall response as usually titrated. They may be most important in responses to tumour antigens, where the critical period of immune defence involves low concentrations of poorly immunogenic molecules.

This area of immune response genes is also moving rapidly, not only because of its great intrinsic interest, but also because it now appears certain that quite a variety of human diseases occur only or much more frequently in individuals of a given Ir genotype. The nature of the products of the Ir genes is under vigorous investigation.

Immunological memory

In most immune responses of mammals, the second injection of an antigen evokes a larger immune response than the first. This is referred to as immunological memory. The memory state can be at the level of the T cell, the B cell, or both. It has quantitative as well as qualitative implications. Quantitatively, the first encounter with antigen results in an increase in the number of lymphocytes with capacity to recognize that particular antigen. The exact relationship of these memory cells to the effector cells which actually form antibody or mediate cellular immunity is not known. They may be by-products of the antigen-induced clonal expansion, or it is even possible that effector cells complete their executive function and revert to being memory cells. Whether the factorial increase in antigen-binding cells is greater for T cells or for B cells depends on details of antigen dosage and timing. Qualitatively, it appears that memory cells differ from virgin cells, having, in all probability, a longer median life-span, a greater tendency to recirculate, a lower degree of adhesiveness to glass or plastic, and a higher buoyant density. Furthermore, studies with B cells indicate that the median avidity of memory cells for antigen is higher than that of virgin cells. This parallels the known increase in the affinity of serum antibody with increasing time of immunization. This is readily understood when one realizes that, in the pre-immunized animal, the further injection of antigen leads to a competition between free serum antibody and lymphocyte surface receptor for the available antigen. Only the lymphocytes with receptors of highest affinity will be able to capture antigen, so only they will be triggered into proliferation. This sequential preferential stimulation leads to further and further selection of the best-fitting cells.

Immunological tolerance

Immunological tolerance can be considered as the exact opposite of immunological memory. It is a specific diminution in the expected immune response to an antigen, brought about through prior exposure of the animal to that antigen. Again, tolerance can affect the T-cell compartment, the B-cell population, or both. Tolerance is a necessary alternative, because of the need to avoid immune responses against autologous components. It is now clear that self-tolerance is acquired during embryonic life and maintained in later life through the continued presence of 'self' antigens, rather than being an innate, genetic property of the lymphoid system.

Neither self-tolerance nor experimentally-induced tolerance is due to a single, unique causal mechanism. Rather, tolerance should be seen as a quantitative concept which is just one facet of the wide problem of immunoregulation. Model systems provide us with a plausible series of mechanisms, the relative importance of each of which in self-tolerance is unknown (Nossal 1974b). Of these, four warrant a brief description here. These can be listed as (i) the 'Signal 1 only' theory; (ii) excessive receptor cross-linkage; (iii) suppressor T cells and (iv) clonal abortion. More detailed description and correct citation of the relevant references have been given elsewhere (Nossal 1974b, Nossal & Pike 1974).

The 'signal 1 only' theory of tolerance (Cohn 1971) is an elaboration in more precise terms of previous views which stated that soluble antigen, meeting a lymphocyte, would tend to cause tolerance, whereas macrophage-associated antigen would cause immunity. The theory holds that triggering requires two signals, signal 1 being union of antigen and receptor, and signal 2 being a T-cell derived stimulus, dependent on the recognition by T cells of some carrier determinant on the antigen molecule. Some versions of the theory place emphasis on the macrophage, perhaps after appropriate activation by T cells, as the source of the signal 2 substance. The theory predicts that signal 1 alone, unaided by signal 2, will lead to tolerance. Certainly, experimental models abound to show that particulate-free antigens which permeate widely through the extracellular fluids and are not extensively taken up by the reticulo-endothelial system make good tolerogens for T or B cells, and that such tolerance induction can be prevented by adjuvant-like agents which might be thought of as mimicking or producing signal 2.

The excessive receptor cross-linkage theory notes that highly polymeric antigens can be good B-cell tolerogens, as can antigen–antibody complexes. It envisions an excessive cycle of receptor patch-formation, capping and subsequent pinocytosis eventually wearing out the antigen-specific lymphocyte, leading to its depression or even destruction. New light has been shed on this theory by the recent finding that such multivalent antigens can even cause fully differentiated effector cells to reduce their functioning, e.g. to slow down their rate of antibody secretion (Schrader & Nossal 1974). This effector cell blockade could masquerade as tolerance under some circumstances, or could affect B-cell precursors of antibody-forming cells as well.

Some forms of tolerance appear to require an active process. An example is tolerance in B-cell populations due to suppressor T cells. Such T cells could simply be 'helper' T cells producing an excess of those factors responsible (in lower concentration) for triggering. It is not unusual for pharmacological agents to be stimulatory at one concentration but suppressive at another.

Alternatively, suppressor T cells could represent a different sub-population. Undoubtedly, suppressor T cells are causative in some models of tolerance, but cannot be the chief mechanism responsible for self-tolerance, as congenitally athymic mice manifest both self-tolerance and experimentally-induced tolerance to the same extent as do normal mice.

One of the oldest theories of tolerance, which we have termed clonal abortion, has recently received some experimental support (Nossal & Pike 1974). It states that lymphocytes mature from a state of ready tolerizability, where virtually any contact with antigen leads to tolerance, to a more differentiated state, when they can be readily immunized. Lymphocytes with potential self-reactivity are 'nipped in the bud' through reaction with self-antigen while in this early differentiation phase. Thus, mature cells competent for auto-reactivity never emerge. This theory sees the other mechanisms of tolerance essentially as 'fail-safe' mechanisms, which come into operation to cope with cells that, for any reason, escape clonal abortion, and which operate as useful negative feedback mechanisms in some situations.

There is good evidence to suggest that T cells are tolerized rather more readily than B cells, and that B cells of low avidity against self-components about in healthy animals and humans. There has even been some speculation that anti-self antibodies of low avidity may serve useful physiological functions. This concern demonstrates again the absence of 'absolutes' in the immune system. Recognition of foreignness and the whole antibody problem can be understood only if the relative nature of antibody–antigen interactions is borne constantly in mind.

Summary

This chapter has taken a broad look at the anatomical and functional elements of the mammalian immune system. Typical immune responses involve the activation of two separate types of response, namely cell-mediated immunity which is due to thymus-derived (T) lymphocytes, and antibody formation, which is the province of bone marrow-derived (B) lymphocytes. Both systems work on a selective basis, with antigen acting essentially as a derepressive trigger allowing the preferential proliferation and differentiation of certain sub-sets of T and B cells, possessing receptors capable of recognizing the particular antigen. The T- and B-lymphocyte systems work in concert rather than separately, each being related to the other by collaborative and feedback links.

T and B cells differ from each other by a large number of markers and characteristics. Each family is separable into sub-types representing progressive differentiation stages. The third category of cell important to an understanding of the immune system is the macrophage, which is crucially involved in antigen capture and in the triggering of lymphocytes. Lymphocytes recognize antigen via receptors, which are immunoglobulin (largely IgM) in nature in the case of B cells and probably Ig in the case of T cells also, though this point is still controversial.

Genetic factors are important in determining the level of immune responses of mammals to particular antigens. Some of these work largely through the T-cell system. The most interesting regulatory genes are those linked to the major histocompatibility genes of species. Pre-exposure of an animal to an antigen will alter its capacity to react to that antigen when re-introduced. This first contact may heighten the responsiveness, and this is referred to as immunological memory. In some cases, particularly when the antigen is not taken up by the reticulo-endothelial system, the pre-exposure specifically lowers or abolishes responsiveness. This is referred to as immunological tolerance. Memory and tolerance can affect T cells, B cells or both. The detailed mechanisms of each phenomenon are poorly understood, though it is known that they involve quantitative and qualitative changes in the sub-sets of lymphocytes capable of recognizing the particular antigen concerned.

Acknowledgments

Original work referred to in this Chapter was supported by the National Health and Medical Research Council, Canberra, Australia; by the Volkswagen Foundation (Grant No. 11 2147); and by the United States Public Health Service (Grant AI-0-3958) and Contract No. NO1-CB-23889 with the National Cancer Institute, National Institutes of Health, Department of Health, Education and Welfare, U.S.A.

References

Burnet F.M. (1959) *The Clonal Selection Theory of Acquired Immunity.* Cambridge University Press, Cambridge.

Cohn M. (1971) The take-home lesson. *Ann. N. Y. Acad. Sci.* **190,** 529.

Feldmann M. & Basten A. (1972) Cell interactions in the immune response *in vitro.* IV. Comparison of the effects of antigen-specific and allogeneic thymus-derived cell factors. *J. exp. Med.* **136,** 722.

Feldmann M. & Nossal G.J.V. (1972) Cellular basis of antibody production. *Quart. Rev. Biol.* **47,** 269.

Fishman M. (1969) Induction of antibodies *in vitro. Ann. Rev. Microbiol.* **23,** 199.

Goding J.W., Nossal G.J.V., Shreffler D.C. & Marchalonis J.J. (1974) Cellular localization of an I-Associated antigen. *J. Immunogenetics* (in press).

Katz D.H. & Benacerraf B. (1972) The regulatory influence of activated T cells on B cell responses to antigen. *Advances in Immunol.* **15,** 1.

McDevitt H.O. & Landy M. (eds) (1973) Brook Lodge Conference on Genetic Control of Immune Responsiveness. Academic Press, New York.

MARCHALONIS J.J. & CONE R.E. (1973) Biochemical and biological characteristics of lymphocyte surface immunoglobulin. *Transplant. Rev.* **14,** 3.

METCALF D. & MOORE M.A.S. (1971) *Haemopoietic Cells.* North-Holland, Amsterdam. *Frontiers of Biology*, **24,**

MILLER J.F.A.P. (1972) Lymphocyte interactions in antibody responses. *Intern. Rev. Cytol.* **33,** 77.

NOSSAL G.J.V. (1974a) Various forms of specialization in cells which synthesize immunoglobulins. A contribution to the Pasteur Institute Symposium on the occasion of the 150th Anniversary of Louis Pasteur 'The Genetics of Immunoglobulins and of the Immune Response', ed. Oudin J., Paris, May 1973. *Ann. Immunol.* (*Inst. Pasteur*) **125C,** 239.

NOSSAL G.J.V. (1974b) Principles of immunological tolerance and immunocyte receptor blockade. In: *Advances in Cancer Research* **20,** 93.

NOSSAL G.J.V. & ADA G.L. (1971) *Antigens, Lymphoid Cells and the Immune Response.* Academic Press, New York and London.

NOSSAL G.J.V. & PIKE B.P. (1974) Unifying concepts in tolerance induction for various T and B cell sub-populations. Brook Lodge Conference on Immunological Tolerance, eds Katz D. and Benacerraf B. Academic Press, New York (in press).

OSMOND D.G. & NOSSAL G.J.V. (1974) Differentiation of lymphocytes in mouse bone marrow. II. Kinetics of maturation and renewal of antiglobulin-binding cells studied by double labeling. *Cell. Immunol.* (in press).

POLLIAK A., LAMPEN N., CLARKSON B.D. DE HARVEN E., BENTWICK Z., SIEGEL F.P. & KUNKEL H. (1973) Identification of human T and B lymphocytes by scanning electron microscopy. *J. exp. Med.* **138,** 607.

RAFF M.C., FELDMANN M. & DE PETRIS (1973) Monospecificity of bone marrow-derived lymphocytes. *J. exp. Med.* **137,** 1024.

SCHRADER J.W. (1973) Mechanism of activation of the bone marrow-derived lymphocyte. III. A distinction between a macrophage-produced triggering signal and the amplifying effect on triggered B lymphocytes of allogeneic interactions. *J. exp. Med.* **138,** 1466.

SCHRADER J.W. & NOSSAL G.J.V. (1974) Effector cell blockade—a new mechanism of immune hyporeactivity induced by multivalent antigens. *J. exp. Med.* (in press).

WARNER N.L. & SZENBERG A. (1964) The immunological functions of the Bursa of Fabricius in chickens. *Ann. Rev. Microbiol.* **18,** 253.

Chapter 3. Cellular Recognition of Allografts and Xenografts in Invertebrates

Edwin L. Cooper

Quasi-immunorecognition
Introduction
Organelle transplantations in protozoans
Aggregation in Porifera
Instances of incompatibility in Cnidaria
Platyhelminthes: union of developmental and primitive immunologic events
Sipunculida: eggs as foreign grafts
Unexplained incompatibilities in Mollusca
Arthropoda: pests as clues to beginning events in transplantation immunology
Urochordata: genetic control
Summary of quasi-immunorecognition

Primordial cell-mediated immunity
Short-term immunologic memory in echinoderms
Short- and long-term memory in annelid worms
First-set allograft rejection

Primordial cell-mediated immunity *continued*
Rejection of xenografts exchanged between *Lumbricus* and *Eisenia*
Histopathology of graft rejection
Evidence for coelomocyte-mediated memory after xenografting revealed by adoptive transfer
Regulation of long-term xenograft memory by temperature revealed in differential coelomocyte activity and typical anamnestic responses
Summary of primordial cell-mediated immunity best exemplified by earthworms

Summary of quasi-immunorecognition, primordial cell-mediated immunity and relation to immunologic theory

Quasi-immunorecognition

Introduction

The invertebrates are a vast and relatively unexplored subject with much to contribute to our knowledge of the immune response (Bang 1967, Hildemann & Cooper 1970, Cooper 1974a, in press). Characteristics of immunity are usually defined in terms of a vertebrate's response to antigen, or not-self. According to this definition, if reference is made to cell or tissue antigens, animals accept autografts (self), but reject allo- or xenografts (not-self). Allografts are exchanged between members of the same genus and species; xenografts involve related members of different genera and species. The vertebrate response, very simply stated, is characterized by specificity and anamnesis. *Specificity* is evident when animals respond precisely to individual antigens. For example, animals made immune to foreign graft A can only give heightened responses to a second challenge of A, not B. *Anamnesis* or memory occurs when animal responses to a second antigen are accelerated; second grafts from the same donors are rejected more rapidly than first grafts. Another indisputable characteristic is the fact that vertebrates produce specific antibodies against antigens.

Unlike the vertebrate's response, for most invertebrates, *recognition*, only, of not-self, seems to constitute the sole event in ancestral immune responsiveness. Presently, there are no reports that any invertebrate synthesizes specific antibodies, though as this chapter will reveal, a specific cellular immune response is evident. The origin of specific cellular immunity can be traced to primordial recognition phenomena. Lagging far behind, neither the invertebrate receptor cell nor its recognition unit have been identified as has been determined for vertebrates although invertebrate coelomocytes and hemocytes are prime candidates (Burnet 1968, 1974).

Hildemann and Reddy (1973), in a recent review, postulate three phylogenetic levels of immuno-evolution involving some few representative members of the animal kingdom and their characteristic responses. These three levels are *Quasi-immunorecognition* in coelenterates (cnidarians), tunicates and mammals; *primordial cell mediated immunity*, echinoderms and annelids; *integrated cell and humoral antibody immunity* in all vertebrates. In this chapter I propose that, in addition, examples of quasi-immunorecognition are demonstrable in protozoans, sponges and numerous other invertebrates. These observations emanate from studies restricted to first experimental encounters designed to demonstrate self-, not-self recognition. Secondly, the echinoderms will be treated separately since the works are extended, designed to reveal short-term memory. Finally, the annelid worms are described last because of diverse approaches devoted to demonstrating the characteristics of cell recognition and immunity.

Organelle transplantations in protozoans

INTRODUCTION

This section describes the reactions of protozoan and certain metazoan species (Acoelomates) to organelle transplantation, tackling the problem in species where technical failures abound and where explanations related to immunologic concepts are more often conflicting than clear. Although there is evidence of organelle transplantation among the Protozoa and tissue incompatibilities among several metazoan invertebrate groups, these are at best only initial efforts. A mere demonstration of first-set transplant destruction or cell incompatibilities is insufficient proof of immune capacity (Hildemann

1972). In advanced metazoan groups manifestations of non-specific phenomena, such as inflammation and wound healing, should not be confused with specific graft rejection resulting from immune responses. To determine whether an invertebrate exhibits an immune reaction to transplants the precise series of events leading to its rejection of cell or tissue grafts must be thoroughly examined in the light of immunologic concepts.

SARCODINA

This group, especially the amoebae, has greatly facilitated organelle transplantation studies, nuclear transfers, in particular. It is technically easy to remove the 'heart' of a cell, its nucleus, and transfer it to the enucleated cytoplasm of another cell (Goldstein 1970). The results reflect an amoeba's capacity for specificity. When transfers are incompatible, recipients die, thus clones are not produced. As an example, when the nuclei of *Amoeba discoides* are transferred into the enucleated cytoplasm of *A. proteus*, the cytoplasm may divide several times but a viable clone rarely develops. Such unsuccessful xeno- or heterotransfers support the idea of protozoan recognition. Allo- or homotransfers, transplants of nuclei to cytoplasm of the same strain are, on the other hand, at least 90 per cent successful in yielding viable mass cultures. Autogeneic transfers, where the nucleus is replaced in the same cytoplasm, always produce viable cells. These reactions, even at the unicellular level, clearly provide evidence of a universal example of self-, not-self recognition.

When carried to technical perfection, cell reassembly is possible and even adequate enough so that combinations of nucleus, cytoplasm and cell membranes can be reutilized to fashion new and different cells (Jeon *et al.* 1970). Presumably the efficacy of clone reproduction is directly dependent upon the degree of relatedness of transferred parts between clones. For example, when nucleus, cytoplasm, and membranes are derived from three different amoebae of the same strain, 85 per cent viability can be achieved. This contrasts markedly with the lack of any viable clones when these three cellular components originate from amoebae of three different strains, still another example of specific recognition even at the cell organelle level.

CILIATA

In his work with ciliates Tartar (1964, 1970) recognized the evolutionary implications of protozoan incompatibilities. He believed that as primordial immune phenomena, they may provide 'evidence at the unicellular level of an anticipation of those specificities which so sharply limit the interindividual grafting of tissues in man.'

Inter-racial, or allografts between *Stentor*, reveal many affinities between animals from different localities; many combinations are compatible. Although interspecific, hetero- or xenografts produce some permanent chimeras, there are also incompatibilities, easily measureable by abnormal physiologic reactions. For example, cytoplasm from *S. coeruleus* causes ejection of the symbiotic *Chlorella*, characteristic of *Stentor polymorphus*. In a reciprocal combination *S. polymorphus* cytoplasm leads to depigmentation or loss of the blue-green stentorin in *S. coeruleus* cytoplasm followed by death of the chimera.

Aggregation in Porifera

SPECIFICITY OF REAGGREGATION IN SPONGES

As one diploblastic animal group and taxonomically first among metazoans, sponges are important to understanding phylogeny of specific cell recognition, immune responses, and differentiation. In his classic studies on regeneration from dissociated sponge cells Wilson (1907) observed that when mixed, cells of a given species aggregate with like kind. Galtsoff (1925) later demonstrated that cell sorting occurs between different cell types of *Microciona prolifera* during reformation of dissociated sponges.

The precise causes of cell aggregation are still unknown. Humphreys (1967) believes that a large glycoprotein molecule is probably a component of the cell's surface coat; this glycocalix may be responsible for aggregation of dissociated sponge cells. If cell-surface material does indeed promote reaggregation, then cell surface specificity is the basis for species-specific sorting and binding together of sponge cell types. These cell-surface materials may have, in addition, other cell-surface properties enabling cells to carry antigenic determinants such as those on red cells or to be sources of transplantation antigens in other cells.

Spiegel (1954) compared invertebrate recognition reactions to aspects of vertebrate immunity in his analysis of sponge aggregation. According to his hypothesis, cells are held together by specific macromolecules with precise stereochemical properties. These are arranged on the cell surface to make combinations possible. When injected experimentally into a vertebrate these macromolecules are, therefore, able to act as antigens that lead to antibody production. Resulting antisera are likely, then, to affect cell aggregations. Antisera were prepared in rabbits against *Microciona prolifera* (a large encrusting red sponge), *Cliona celata* (a yellow sulphur sponge), and a mixture of these cells from both species. Reaggregation of dissociated cells is reversibly inhibited in the first two antiserums. Aggregates formed in normal serum containing cells of both species are of either one cell species or the other, never of both species. Aggregates in antiserum against both species are composed of cells of both species but distributed randomly throughout. In addition, Spiegel found, surprisingly, that calcium-free and high calcium media has no effect on reaggregation. These results, although equivocal, confirm the hypothesis that contiguous cell surfaces are normally held together by forces similar to those between antigens and antibodies as proposed by Tyler 1947 and Weiss 1947.

LACK OF SPECIFIC AGGREGATION

Contrary to earlier observations (Humphreys 1963), aggregation of sponges is not always species-specific. In other words, bispecific sponge cell aggregates may be obtained easily by mixing cell suspensions of two species simultaneously, even if they belong to different classes (*Calcispongiae* and *Demonspongiae*). To test this, Sara *et al.* (1966a) used dissociated, vitally stained (neutral red) cells of several sponge species from the above classes. In numerous combinations, bispecific aggregations were always observed. This represents but one example of other similar approaches often leading to conflicting interpretations of sponge cell reaggregation (Gasic & Galanti 1966, MacLennan & Dodd 1967, MacLennan 1969, 1970, John *et al.* 1971). This exception of non-specific aggregation should not be viewed with alarm but with caution as with diverging views resulting from any investigation. The merits of these sponge studies rest with their wide applicability not only to specific cell recognition as *Quasi-immunorecognition* but to specific cell sorting and its extreme importance in differentiation and morphogenesis. Whether the promoting or inhibiting substances affecting aggregation are at all related to prototypic immunoglobulin receptors is in the realm of total speculation. Regardless of the outcome of experiments and justified musing, specific recognition is fundamental and represents another built-in natural device for preserving a balanced internal milieu.

Instances of incompatibility in Cnidaria

INTRODUCTION

Loeb's (1945) accounts of tissue incompatibilities among the Cnidaria (formerly the Coelenterates) is an important contribution to the study of self-, not-self specificity, and how it evolved, though his terminology may be confusing. His 'organismal differentials', can be interpreted as antigens or gene products, that determine self-, or not-self specificity. This applies with equal force to primitive animals. He states, for example, that 'in adult birds and mammals there is a very strong reaction against . . . strange organismal differentials in general; the normal equilibrium is strictly autogenous (self); it depends upon the presence of the same individuality differential in all the important tissues and organs . . . Notable reactions (result) if small parts of tissues possessing a strange individuality differential are introduced into the animal body.' Prior to the time of information on immune responses it is noteworthy that his interpretations seem timely even if couched in romantic terms.

HYDROZOA

The observations of Campbell and Bibb (1970) are more recent, still substantiating the predicted terminologies of Loeb. *Hydra*, too, accepts autografts but rejects other types of transplants. Some unsuccessful transplantations result when natural or characteristic developmental patterns are severely disturbed by grafting, such as changing positions (orthotopic or heterotopic). Yet others arise because of genetic incompatibilities between host and donor tissues. Such evidence suggests that reasonably simple allelic differences between animals are sufficient to produce graft incompatibility. However, this may be even more complex as revealed in the extensive genetic analyses of incompatibilities in *Hydractinia echinata*, a marine colonial encrusting hydroid, performed by Hauenschild (1954, 1956) and recently resurrected in a review by Du Pasquier (1974, in press). There may exist at least one locus with 6 alleles, conclusions derived from precise matings over several generations.

In his studies of tissue compatibility in *H. echinata*, Toth (1967) ruled out the action of complementary divalent cations or intercellular matrices. In regenerating explants, fusion fails to occur if the opposing explants are of different sex, from different individuals of the same sex, or if peripheral explant contact occurs after free stolons have begun to form. He based compatibility on a temporal factor. It is interesting that Ivker (1972), contrary to Toth, found a hierarchy of histoincompatibility in *Hydractinia*; thus her views are apparently more contiguous with our current thesis of progressive phylogenetic immuno-differentiation and also to those of Hauenschild. According to her interpretation, in *Hydractinia*, tissue incompatibility develops after mutual contact resulting in hyperplastic stolon (overgrowth) production. She suggests that this overgrowth may involve surface bound molecules produced by the ectoderm, but ultimately referable to genes that control histoincompatibility and hyperplastic growth. This is based on her observations of consistent morphology and intermediate forms of incompatibility between related strains (i.e. parent-offspring, half-sibs).

By means of light and electron microscopy Bibb and Campbell (1973) found several interesting observations. Using seven species of the genera *Hydra*, *Chlorohydra*, and *Pelmatohydra* in various allograft and xenograft combinations, they found, after allografting, that the so-called edge cells show pseudopodial activity, attach and heal quickly. By contrast, even xenografts do show some normal healing but they eventually dissolve. In xenograft combinations with satisfactory healing, cell attachments develop which resemble septate desmosomes, adequate to preserve healing for several days. Incompatibility is signalled by the formation of a constriction at the graft site that progresses until the incompatible tissues are divorced. Unlike the thesis of this chapter, Bibb and Campbell advance an alternative interpretation accounting for rejection. It is not due to immunological rejection but it results from replacement of xenotypic cell junctions by allospecific attachments leading to gradual tissue separations.

ANTHOZOA

Theodor (1966, 1969, 1970) studied invertebrate tissue recognition in the arborescent coelenterates, the Gorgonacea. His works contradict the notion that allogeneic ectoderm histoincompatibility developed late in evolution. More specifically, he found that branches taken from two individuals belonging to the same species fail to fuse with the host. Thus genetic control of compatibility may not be due to few genetic loci nor to level of phylogeny. As would be expected, autografts do succeed, surviving indefinitely. In xenogeneic cultures of gorgonian tissue, mutual damage or histotoxicity occurs within 1–4 days after contact, but allogeneic combinations are considerably slower for tissue disintegration to occur. Theodor's interpretations are provocative if the gorgonian immune response is not a conventional one. He believes that instead it represents a kind of '*pre immunology*'. Gorgonian histotoxicity is 'induced suicide' that might explain cell destructions mediated by cytotoxic or 'non-immune' reactions in vertebrate cell cultures (Möller & Möller 1966). Preliminary evidence using earthworm coelomocytes in xenogeneic combinations, likewise, reveals a cytotoxic reaction (Cooper 1973). Thus, at all phylogenetic levels, at least one manifestation of incompatibility seems to result in cytotoxicity. Whether this involves the liberation of mediating substances is unknown (Lemmi *et al.* 1973a,b, Cooper 1974b, Cooper *et al.* 1974).

Despite the technical difficulties involving anaesthesia, surgery, reactions to injury, Hildemann, Dix and Collins (1974) were successful in exchanging grafts in staghorn corals *Acropora* originating from the bays around Magnetic Island, Australia. A staghorn branch can be broken off as a graft and brought into intimate contact with recipient soft tissues (i.e. coenenchyme). If graft and recipient are derived from the same colony as branches of the same original clone then the resulting fusions (autogeneic, isogeneic) are entirely compatible for as long as 300 days. At 25°C, fusion of soft tissue and skeletal tissue occurs in 6–8 days. Such fusion happens in nature, normally, after accidental breakage; it serves to protect the structural integrity of an entire colony against occasional destructive waves. Confidence in the assumption of healing of unseen naturally-occurring grafts, can be tested by several experimental approaches. First, at the graft–host contact zone, intact polyps and pigmented zooanthellae persist. Moreover, because of the nerve net, gentle probing of polyp tentacles leads to withdrawal responses perceived and immediately transferred across the graft–recipient contact zone. Hildemann *et al.* considered this a sensitive and unequivocal test for functional graft survival. After studying preliminary intercolonial allografts, they found only moderate incompatibilities. That morphologic and functional fusion occurs is real but healing is always followed, after several to many weeks, by destruction of soft tissue and frequent death at the graft–host contact zone. Heterografts involving several species of *Acropora* heal rapidly but after one week, a region of cell death quickly develops, preceding obvious regression of soft tissues.

MIXED CELL AGGREGATION BETWEEN SPONGES AND AN ANTHOZOAN CNIDARIAN

Sponge cells were the first dissociated metazoan cells used for studying specific reaggregation at this second phylogenetic step. By contrast, species specificity may not always occur. Indeed, it is possible to demonstrate mixed aggregates formed from the dissociated cells of both sponges and cnidarians. Sara *et al.* (1966b) used the sponges *Clathrina coriacea* (Montagu) (*Calcispongiae*), *Tethya aurantium* (Pallas) Gray, *Haliclona elegans* (Bow) and the anthozoan, *Anemonia sulcata* (Pennant). Cells previously pressed through bolting cloth were stained vitally with neutral red to identify living sponge cells after aggregation. Examinations up to 72 hours after cell mixing revealed the presence of well-formed mosaics composed of sponge and sea anemone cells. Viable cell aggregates can therefore form after cell mixtures from species of the phyla Porifera and Cnidaria. As revealed earlier, at certain points it is not possible to declare, with absolute surety, that self does not always separate with self. Obviously this is due to lack of specificity, but how it occurs, and how long it lasts is still a mystery.

Platyhelminthes: union of developmental and primitive immunologic events

Lindh's (1959) transplantation experiments using flatworms were, from the viewpoint of developmental biology, supporting his concern for events associated with induction and regeneration. His results, nevertheless, are important to an understanding of the phylogeny of transplantation reactions if interpreted differently; for his observation period auto- and allotransplants succeed. Although some heterotransplants behave as allotransplants, most grafts involving the same genus but different species result only in temporary regeneration. For example, heterotransplants between *Planaria dorotocephala* and *P. maculata* are not permanent. Animals with tissues derived from three germ layers and possessing a pseudocoel show specific recognition.

Sipunculida: eggs as foreign grafts

Exhaustive studies on this small group of largely marine, worm-like creatures reveal certain superficial resemblances to annelids. For example, in both *Dendrostomum zostericolum* and the annelids, the sexes are separate but each retains its gametes in the coelom for long periods of time. Thus, technically, transplantations can be made by injecting the eggs, sperm, or even minced tentacles, for example, of one individual into the coelom of another (Cushing *et al.* 1965). Following such transplantations, both auto- and allograft tentacles are encapsulated by host coelomocytes at similar rates. Quite to the contrary, eggs seem to be 'immune' and neither sex recognizes normal eggs as foreign. However, eggs stained with eosin are encapsulated. Furthermore, other treatments such as washing, heating, and sonication destroy the capacity for self-recognition, resulting also in encapsulation and death of the eggs. Nothing akin to antibody is demonstrable after cellular or protein antigens are injected into the coelom, nor does acceleration of the encapsulation rate or phagocytosis occur in response to repeat transplants. This approach for demonstrating incompatibility seems unclear and such animals should be examined once again.

Unexplained incompatibilities in mollusca

PELECYPODA

Drew and de Morgan (1910) were among the first to report on the fate of transplanted tissues in molluscs. According to their results, autogeneic gills implanted in the adductor muscle of *Pecten maximus* are eventually isolated by encapsulation. This information on *Pecten* is equivocal since auto- and allotransplants behave similarly. Such encapsulation of autotransplants is probably not an example of the animal recognizing not-self; it probably results, instead, from faulty grafting techniques that damage the grafts; the cells undoubtedly react to the product of autolysis. This drastic kind of heterotopic surgery involving gills into muscles is objectionable and grafts should be placed in as natural an environment as possible. Half of the transplantations of mantle strips and female gonads in grafts from *P. irradians* heal after 49 hours. However, none do if male gonads are used or transplantations are performed under the mantle. Well healed autografts retain eyes, tentacles, and contractility for over a month. These findings point out clearly that our knowledge of molluscan transplantation reactions is still hampered by lack of appropriate techniques. Cushing (1957) found, also, minimal cell responses when allografts were performed.

Des Voigne and Sparks (1969) allografted small portions of the mantle to slits in the connective tissue near the palps in the oyster, *Crassostrea gigas.*

Some allografts are rejected by the host, but others remain viable and appear normal throughout the observation period. Even those implants that initially seem to inhibit wound healing ultimately follow the pattern typical of the species: leucocytes delineate the wound and form a union with the implants; the implant finally fuses and becomes contiguous with the host. Their experiment points out that the molluscs are valuable to invertebrate transplantation studies. The rejections they observed are, however, not examples of an immune response, for the observation time was short. Moreover, they made no comparison with autograft controls.

Canzonier (1963) reports 50 per cent rejection of normal and diseased implants of allogeneic tissues in *C. virginica.* Once the implants were healed, there seemed to be no later indication of host rejection. The blood spaces joined with those of the host, but Canzonier observed no establishment of any cross circulation.

In comparison studies to those performed on coelenterates, Hildemann, Dix and Collins (1974) began transplantation studies in the pearl oyster, *Pinctada margaritifera.* They chose mantle tissue because its accessibility and texture are amenable to surgery. Furthermore, the orange versus black colour dimorphism of the marginal mantle of individual oysters provides a sure indication of viability. Apparently, technical difficulties were formidable, making it almost impossible to be unequivocal when viewing the fate of transplants. The orthotopic technique, as they initiated it, is a promising approach to assessing the true condition of grafts after healing. In locations other than natural micro-environments (heterotopic positions) destruction is not attributed to qualities of the immune system but to other unknown factors related solely to technique.

GASTROPODA

Tripp (1961) transplanted pedal tissue of *Australorbis glabratus.* Allografts placed in the cephalopedal sinus (the space between the anterior cerebral region and the foot) are successful if layers of the two tissues are joined. Implantation of fresh allogeneic tissue elicits only a transient coelomocytic infiltration but formalin-fixed allogeneic tissue is encapsulated. Xenogeneic tissues from the planorbid species, *Planorbarius corneus,* elicits a marked cellular response followed by graft destruction. Formalin-fixed xenogeneic tissue is encapsulated within 24 hours by fibroblasts originating from the nearby connective tissue.

Cheng and Galloway (1970) transplanted digestive gland tissues from the gastropods *Helisoma duryi* normale (strain HI-3), *H. trivolvis*, *Tarebia granifera*, and *Melania newcombi* into the cephalopedal sinuses of *Helisoma duryi normale* (strain HI-2). Implants were later studied histologically and revealed that host reactions to xenografts are more rapid and generally more severe than reactions to allografts. Although this suggests that recipients are capable of differentiating between allografts and xenografts, no distinction is made between autografts, allografts, and other necessary controls.

CEPHALOPODA

In his work with the octopus Cushing (1962) made auto- and allo-skin transplants. During the observation period he found no differences in the behaviour of autografts or allografts. Except for a few technical failures both survive as long as the hosts.

Arthropoda: pests as clues to beginning events in transplantation immunology

Experiments with arthropods have often yielded conflicting reports on the outcome of transplants. This is especially true where grafts involved embryonic primordia such as imaginal discs (Spinner 1969, Bhaskaran & Sivasubramanian 1969). Some transplantation studies of certain inbred arthropod species demonstrate that many investigators are careless observers but still two aims have been uppermost: highly inbred species have, in the past, been of greater interest to those trying to determine the genes which control recognition phenomena and immune reactions in the invertebrates.

DIPTERA

Kambysellis (1968, 1970) analysed differences between populations of *Drosophila* by performing interspecific (xeno-) transplants of larval ovaries. His concern was to expose genetic differences revealed by the fate of transplantations; thus he gave no consideration to the possibility of immune phenomena regulating host response to donor tissue. According to his conclusions 'the degree of gonadal development . . . is highly dependent on the genetic relationship of host environment and hybrid embryos or hybrid larvae can be produced between distantly isolated species'.

Hadorn's (1937) early studies of ovarian transplants in *Drosophila* also reveal the viewpoint of the geneticist and embryologist rather than the immunologist. Using the transplantation methods of Ephrussi and Beadle (1936) which allows full development of normal ovaries and testes so that immune interference cannot curtail development, Hadorn transplanted ovaries and testes into genetically normal larvae of the same age. Many transplants grow and elongate, the egg strings differentiate, and their apical ends contract as they do in normal larvae. But development is incomplete, and the transplants never reach sizes of full grown normal ovaries. Although eggs are formed, they degenerate before reaching their full size. According to Hadorn's interpretation, the distinct but limited development of transplanted ovaries confirms that ovaries have inherent developmental potencies unlike those of other organs, such as the imaginal discs. It is the lethal genetic constitution that prevents further development in different organs at different periods of time. My alternative interpretation, limited not to development, assumes that the presence of gene-determined foreign antigens are eventually recognized by the host's immune response which then acts to arrest development by rejection of the foreign graft.

ORTHOPTERA

In another approach to cell recognition, Scott (1971) made recent attempts to determine what constitutes foreignness to an invertebrate by implanting foreign tissues into the hemocoel of the American cockroach, *Periplaneta americana*. The nylon monofilaments that he implanted were completely encapsulated by haemocytes of the host's body fluid, a kind of response studied in detail by Salt (1970). Scott found a multilayered capsule that forms and isolates particles from the blood circulation. Furthermore, interspecific or xenogeneic implants from *Nauphoeta cineria* are also recognized as foreign and encapsulated. Somewhat related xeno-implants from the blowfly, *Calliphora* of the family Calliphoridae or even implants from distantly related mice are also encapsulated 24 hours after implantation.

In contrast to these findings, allogeneic transplants, as implanted nerve cords, are not encapsulated. However, allogeneic nerve cords can be treated with various enzymes to render them susceptible to encapsulation. Following treatment with collagenase and lecithinase C, encapsulation occurred. Evidently recognition sites on the membrane surface in the form of intact neural lamella are required to prevent the haemocyte reaction. This work strongly suggests that specificity of recognition is, at least partially, determined by properties of the antigenic surface.

From a different point of view, cockroaches have been important to studies of insect hormones. Bell (1972) transplanted ovaries in 18 species of cockroaches. Intraspecific allografts resulted in the initiation of yolk formation and oocyte growth rates comparable to controls. Heterotransplants of roach ovaries led to sequestered host vitellogenins but the grafts grew to terminal stages only when donor and host were closely related. When ovaries were transplanted between species of different superfamilies or families, yolk formation did not occur. Thus, the fate of endocrine glands can be tested after transplantation and the resulting fate reflects the degree of histocompatibility between donor and host.

Urochordata: genetic control

Freeman (1970) recently reviewed the results of Japanese workers on the genetic control of transplantation specificity in *Botryllus*, a colonial ascidian. Working with *B. primigenus*, Oka and Watanabe (1960) showed that if two parental non-fusable colonies are mated, four classes of progeny result in the F_1. Each progeny class then fuses with members of its class, those of two other classes, and with both parents. Assuming that the parents are both heterozygous at a locus for colony specificity with genotypes expressed by the notation AB and CD (with each letter representing one allele), the F_1 generation possesses four classes of progeny: AC, AD, BC and BD. Thus, colonies which have at least one allele in common at the colony specificity locus will fuse with each other; matings of the F_1 progeny producing F_2 and colony fusion tests established that this scheme is correct. According to the genetic analysis of Hildemann and Reddy (1973), these results are surprising; these do not agree with the immunogenetic rules of transplantation established for vertebrates. AD can fuse with BD but not BC colonies.

In a further analysis of recognition events in *Botryllus* Tanaka (1973) and Tanaka and Watanabe (1973) arrived at the following conclusions. They see their non-fusion reaction or NFR as a measure of allogeneic inhibition when two incompatible ascidian colonies were placed in mutual contact: ampullae to ampullae, ampullae to margin without ampullae, and cut surface of one colony to cut surface of another. Incompatible colonies showed the non-fusion reaction. NFR is first manifested by destruction of the test (outer covering) cells around the contact area. This leads to an appearance of filaments around disintegrated test cells, followed by contraction of the ampullae. Constriction and necrosis resulted in severance of distal ampullae. Finally the NFR was complete when the contact areas of both colonies were severed completely. The response is irreversible and progresses to completion even if one participating member is removed. There is one possible interpretation from their works. Colony specific NFR resides in the test matrix and blood, causing death of granular amoebocytes. It is noteworthy that the so-called non-immunologic allogeneic inhibition discovered by the Möllers (1966) was interpreted as an evolutionary precursor of immune type responses probably related to the immunologic surveillance system (to be described in last section).

According to Scott and Schuh (1963) the tunicate *Amaroecium constellatum* has remarkable powers of regeneration, for if parts are separated from the body, detached fragments regenerate all missing members much like sponge cells do after dissociation. Such cells recognize histogenetic affinity or genetic kinship and behave according to the antigenic composition of their cell surfaces. This indicates the tunicate's capacity for specific recognition.

Summary of quasi-immunorecognition

This section has pointed out that the ability to recognize the difference between self-, and not-self is an attribute not restricted to metazoans. Indeed, transplantations of cell organelles in protozoans produces incompatibility reactions that are, by analogy, to immunity, what irritability is to nervous coordination. According to Hildemann and Reddy (1973), '*Quasi immunorecognition* or capacity for non-self recognition of allogeneic tissue followed by incompatibility reactions appears characteristic of coelenterates as shown in colonial hydroids, gorgonians, and hard corals'. The term is appropriate, one which they use 'because of the apparent specificity of the antagonistic reactions and the compatible lag period preceding manifestations of incompatibility. Absence of a memory component enters this kind of surveillance system unlike the vertebrate response'. This does not rule out the possibility that memory could be demonstrable, but one must devise careful techniques for confronting hosts with second transplants of organelles, cells and tissue grafts. I wish to extend their concept, bearing in mind degrees of complexity, to unicellular protozoans. Thus from these simple animals to the most complex, *quasi-immunorecognition* is a universal characteristic.

Primordial cell-mediated immunity

Short term immunologic memory in echinoderms

The echinoderms are important for assessing the evolution of cell recognition mechanisms. According to some taxonomists, echinoderms are close to the vertebrates ancestrally, thus they are excellent for studying immune reactivities intermediate between invertebrates and vertebrates. The phylum Echinodermata includes the sea cucumbers (class Holothuroidea), sea stars (Asteroidea), brittle stars (Ophiuroidea), sea urchins and sand dollars (Echinoidea), sea lilies (Crinoidea) and several extinct classes. The results from two independent earlier studies dealing with allograft recognition in echinoderms are equivocal, mainly due to faulty technique. Transplantations were performed to heterotopic sites and the animals maintained in excessively cold sea water, two parameters that create difficulty in distinguishing between graft acceptance and rejection (Ghiradella 1965, Buslé 1967).

TRANSPLANTATION OF CELLS AND TISSUES IN ASTEROIDEA

Despite the difficulty of the echinoderm transplantation process, Ghiradella (1965) found that the two starfishes, *Patiria miniata* and *Asterias forbesi* discriminate between reciprocal allo- and xenocoelomic implants and heterogeneic pyloric caecum from two other species, *A. vulgaris* and *Henricia sanguinolenta*. Normal allografts, although healthy after five weeks, are surrounded by connective tissue and amoebocyte masses. Although amoebocytes are usually associated with damaged allograft areas, amoebocytic attack, phagocytosis, and encapsulation are, apparently, not associated with the elimination of xenotransplants. Xenografts are eliminated by the hosts one week after transplantation. *Henricia* caecum is extruded through the dermal branchiae by both hosts; *Patiria* disposes of *Asterias* caecum by transferring it from the host ray to the cardiac stomach where it is digested or extruded through the mouth.

CELL RESPONSES AS INDICATORS OF SELF-RECOGNITION IN ASTEROIDEA ECHINOIDEA

Recently, Reinisch and Bang (1971) performed an experiment crucial to understanding cell recognition, but not anamnesis. They injected *Arbacia* (sea urchin) cells, about half of which are deeply pigmented, into *Asterias* (sea star) *in vivo*. The number of circulating amoebocytes in the hosts dropped abruptly. The *Arbacia* cells adhered to and were phagocytosed by host cells which clumped consistently within the papulae—outpushings of the body wall. Injection of *Asterias* cells into *Asterias* does not elicit cell clumping, nor is it followed by a drop in circulating amoebocytes. These results suggest that *Asterias*'s recognition of intact foreign cells evokes a defence mechanism distinct from simple responses to an injected foreign body such as carborundum particles. In fact, this echinoderm response closely resembles the type of self-, not-self cell recognition demonstrable within the vertebrate phylum.

It must be remembered that because of the echinoderm body structure (rigid exoskeleton) enormous technical difficulties must be surmounted before adequate grafting procedures can be undertaken. Despite this, Hildemann and Dix (1972) made substantial progress toward revealing specific recognition as well as a memory component in echinoderms. To define the events in allograft destruction they chose the sea cucumber (*Cucumaria tricolor*) and the horned sea star (*Protoreaster nodosus*) from the Great Barrier Reef. Because of variable colorations, pigment cell destruction is the easiest external criterion of graft rejection.

As in all animals, autografts in both genera heal and are never rejected. In *Cucumaria* three distinct cell layers are evident, the epidermis, an outer muscle layer, and a deep muscle layer. Similarly, *Protoreaster* integumentary autografts show normal morphology characterized by an outer epithelium with secretory cells and muscle fibre bundles. Three layers are distinguishable into epidermis, thick dermis with loose connective tissue, and an underlying muscle layer into which crypts extend. Macrophages and small lymphocytes make up the remainder of the cellular components, undoubtedly those that would eventually evoke allograft rejection in *Cucumaria*.

Allograft destruction does occur in both species and the response is apparently no different from chronic slow allograft destruction in other invertebrates. Rejection, grossly, is heralded by progressive pigment cell destruction. Those microscopic events studied more intensively in the sea cucumber than in the sea star show the following characteristics. Initially the epidermis becomes oedematous with vacuolation and loss of cytoplasm in some areas. Macrophages are abundant at 173 days, although they may have appeared earlier. The most important feature at later rejection stages was the presence of varying leucocyte types, especially macrophages and lymphocytes in association with *Cucumaria* grafts. At terminal stages of rejection *Protoreaster* grafts show less macrophages and more eosinophils infiltrated into the dermis and loose connective tissue. First-set allograft destruction occurs 4–6 months at 21°C.

To test for memory, only a low percentage of second-set grafts were performed, but all showed pronounced accelerated rejection (positive memory). The second-set response was characterized by early inflammatory discoloration and hyperplasia leading to invasive resorption of grafts. This type of response readily occurred and was interpreted as an example of short-term memory since these repeat test grafts were performed when first-set transplants were still in the process of rejection at approximately 50–75 per cent. Even after the destruction of second-sets the first-set response continued unaffected. There is no other evidence for long-term memory in echinoderms, demonstrable by positive memory, i.e. accelerated rejection of second transplants performed after first-set transplant destruction. With echinoderms we now have a second phylum in addition to the annelids (see last sections) that offer evidence for specificity and memory.

Short- and long-term memory in annelid worms

INTRODUCTION

Transplantation has been, historically, a primary tool for studying *in vivo* cellular immunity, although now, there are numerous *in vitro* assays. Nineteenth-century investigators were not so concerned with the immune causes of graft rejections, an unknown fact at that time (Joest 1897, Korschelt 1896–8, 1927a,b, 1929, Leypoldt 1911, Rabes 1902). By observing an animal's response to xenografts, allografts or autografts, investigators now can partially characterize immune responses. Usually, rejection of a repeat graft will be more rapid than that of the first, however some animals, such as earthworms, fishes, newts, legless amphibians or caecilians, iguanas, and hamsters, exhibit negative memory. In other words, the response to the second-set graft is the converse of positive memory, i.e. prolonged and not accelerated (Hildemann & Cohen 1967, Cohen & Borysenko 1970).

As will be explained later, raising the temperature of earthworms from 15°C to 20°C prevents the appearance of both positive and negative responders and results in accelerated rejections of all second-set transplants. This suggests that temperature, true to a physiologist's prediction, is crucial in regulating immune responsiveness like other physiologic responses. Since all positive responders are considered to be like the vertebrates and therefore truly immune, earthworms, capable of both positive and negative reactions at 15°C invited scepticism by mammalian immunologists; prolonged second reactions were not considered as an anamnestic response. Immunologists, unlike biologists, seem to be unaccustomed to thinking of organ systems functioning throughout the animal kingdom and that their efficacy, *vis-à-vis* man, is directly proportional to the level of structural and functional complexity. Although there are numerous examples of vertebrate responses which are essentially similar they escape, somewhat, the alarming outcries of classical immunologists since, unlike the invertebrates, vertebrates synthesize antibody. There is still a general consensus that until antibody is discovered in an animal without a backbone, invertebrates will always be relegated to worthless positions due to their 'poorly' developed immune systems. According to Acton (1972) 'the exact relationship of all aspects of invertebrate immunity to that of the vertebrates will, of course, require much additional study. However it is now clear that these primitive animals not only have cellular capabilities to ward off intrusion by infectious agents, but also have been shown to possess a whole system of components which interact to provide a type of immune response analogous to the vertebrates. While all the criteria established to determine vertebrate immunity cannot be met by the invertebrate species, only the [special] purist would argue that these animals do not possess immune capabilities.'

THE EARTHWORMS

Invertebrate cellular immune responses may, indeed, be the evolutionary precursor of vertebrate responses as revealed by cellular immunity in earthworms. Several laboratories (Cooper, Duprat, Valembois) have demonstrated the earthworm's capacity to show cellular immune responses characterized by specificity and anamnesis. These cellular responses were confirmed since we demonstrated them independently using several criteria. For these reasons the earthworms are discussed in greater detail than the other invertebrates. Other invertebrates of similar structural complexity probably possess the same degree of immune capability as the earthworm, but as of now studies have not been pursued rigorously.

The following technique is from our own laboratory (Cooper *et al.* 1970). Before grafting earthworms, they are anaesthesized in 5 per cent ethanol (*Lumbricus*) and 25 per cent chloroform (*Eisenia*). After becoming sufficiently immobile, worms are placed on the stage of a binocular dissecting microscope and the grafts, usually three segments of body wall, exchanged between host and donor. Sutures or adhesives are unnecessary since the grafts adhere while the worms are anaesthesized. Autografts survive permanently. Autografts are grossly healed after 24 hours and microscopically healed after 48 hours. Allografts, after healing, exhibit varying degrees of incompatibility and are eventually rejected; the same is true for xenografts.

First-set allograft rejection

INTRODUCTION

When the earthworm studies were first done independently during the last 10 years it was evident that earthworms indeed possessed the capacity to recognize and destroy tissue antigens (Cooper 1965, 1966a,b, 1968a,b, Cooper & Baculi 1968a, Winger & Cooper 1968, Cooper & Rubilotta 1969, Cooper 1969a,b, Hostetter & Cooper 1972a,b, 1973a, 1974b, Lemmi *et al.* 1973c, Cooper 1970, 1971, Bailey *et al.* 1971, Du Pasquier & Duprat 1968, Izoard 1964, Duprat 1964, 1967, Duprat & Lasalle 1967, Duprat-Chateaureynaud 1970, 1971, Duprat-Chateaureynaud & Izoard 1972, Valembois 1963, 1968, 1970). Like allografts, xenograft rejection is recognizable by the gradual death of pigment cells, the sole external criterion of rejection.

THE SITUATION IN *LUMBRICUS*

To determine responses to allografts, more than 300 adult *Lumbricus terrestris* from varying locales were used to exchange allografts (Cooper 1969b). Autograft controls always show permanent survival. Allografts, like autografts, heal normally but much later show varying signs of incompatibility measured by pigment cell destruction. Up to 153 days post-grafting, use of different populations of worms proved advantageous since allografts exchanged within populations showed little or no incompatibility. This was presumably due to a lack of recognizable alloantigenic differences. Whether this is a direct result of the earthworm's hermaphroditism, but sexual mode of reproduction, is unknown. Lack of recognizable alloantigenic differences was recognizable by no signs of intrapopulation allograft rejection when earthworms were derived from Oregon. Similarly, only 1 per cent of intrapopulation eastern Canadian allografts were destroyed. Operating on the assumption that within populations there may be, in effect, the manifestation of inbreeding, we exchanged interpopulation allografts, thus increasing the numbers of total rejects to 5 per cent on Oregon recipients and 15 per cent on Canadian recipients.

THE SITUATION IN *EISENIA*

To test whether this apparently sluggish form of graft recognition and rejection was characteristic of all oligochaete annelids we tested for allograft destruction in another earthworm, *Eisenia foetida*, a member like *Lumbricus*, of the family Lumbricidae (Cooper & Rubilotta 1969). Although *Eisenia* shows greater variability in external physical appearance, displaying phenotypic 'red' and 'stripe' worms, according to Dr G. E. Gates, Bangor, Maine, an authoritative earthworm systematist, they are the same species. When allografts are exchanged between *Eisenia* they always heal but eventually a larger percentage show complete destruction than in *Lumbricus*. After 255 days post-transplantation, 23 per cent showed total destruction. Since the period is longer than that for our observations using *Lumbricus*, it might be argued that *Lumbricus*, too, would have shown more rejections had our observation period been extended. After reading the work of Duprat (1964, 1967), we surmised that essentially no rejection of first-set allografts, but destruction of second-sets, occurred. There was no indication of observation period, nor temperature, therefore we do not know if first-set rejections were not augmented by a second transplant. At about three weeks, we had only observed one completely destroyed from a total of 23 grafts and a second at 130 days post-grafting. On the basis of xenograft information to be reported later perhaps her observation periods should have been longer. According to Duprat's latest review (1970), first-set allografts exchanged between *Eisenia foetida* from the same geographical location, like autografts, heal promptly and remain grossly intact. Presumably, a genetic homogeneity results from the inbreeding of worms from the same locale. Normally, both first- and second-set transplants between worms from different regions that are genetically heterogeneous are always rejected.

Rejection of xenografts exchanged between *Lumbricus* and *Eisenia*

INTRODUCTION

Because of the seemingly discouraging allograft information, we decided to try a new approach to the earthworm's capacity for recognition and sequestration of transplantation antigens. This alternative approach took into account the fact that 100 per cent rejection was never observed when allografts were exchanged suggesting:

(1) lack of recognition of strong alloantigenic differences;
(2) lack of the existence of strong alloantigenic differences;
(3) either one and two combined.

Assuming that the immune system was capable of adequate recognition, then absence of complete rejections was probably due to the second alternative. For if there was nothing to recognize then the most efficient of immune systems would also be incapable of responding. Ruling out the existence of strong alloantigenic differences, and to support our contention of a vigorous immune system, we exchanged xenografts between *Eisenia* and *Lumbricus*, and in so doing, confronted each genus with diverse xeno-antigenic differences (Cooper 1968a). Such grafts can be exchanged easily despite the difference in size; this is counteracted by transplanting two-segment *Lumbricus* grafts and three-segment *Eisenia* grafts.

GENERAL CHARACTERISTICS OF HEALING AND AUTOGRAFTS

As Fig. 3.1 reveals, autografts exchanged on earthworms, in this case *Lum-*

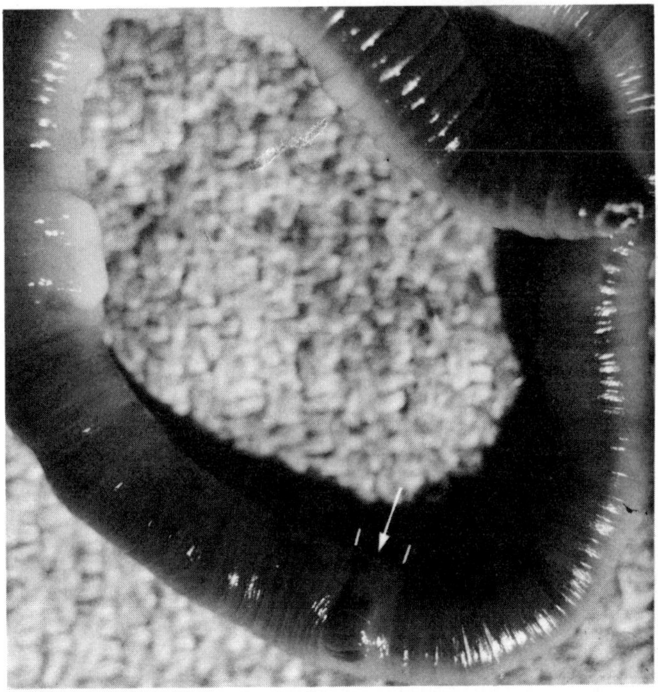

Fig. 3.1. This is a *Lumbricus* bearing a perfectly healed autograft indicated by the arrow. Graft polarity has been rotated so that the graft is healed perpendicular to the antero–posterior axis. This is at 75 days post-grafting, ×2·5 (after Cooper 1968a).

bricus, heal rapidly and are always accepted permanently. This occurs even if the normal graft polarity is rotated. Grafts rotated so that the antero–posterior axis is now perpendicular to the worm's long axis still heal normally. Grossly-healed grafts can be touched with sharp instruments and in response often show immediate contraction, even if healed in the opposite direction. In addition to tactile testing, strong pressure with other instruments never provokes dislodging of firmly healed autografts nor xenografts. At 20 days, one can compare in Fig. 3.2 the situation of an autograft, now indistinguishable from surrounding host tissue and a completely destroyed xenograft. The host is *Lumbricus* and the rejected graft is from *Eisenia*. There are no surviving pigment cells leaving a transplant totally devoid of colour. Heat-killed or alcohol-treated autografts never heal. Strongly distantly unrelated frog skin remains totally unrecognized, the host graft bed remains empty and merely heals together leaving isolated frog skin unaffected.

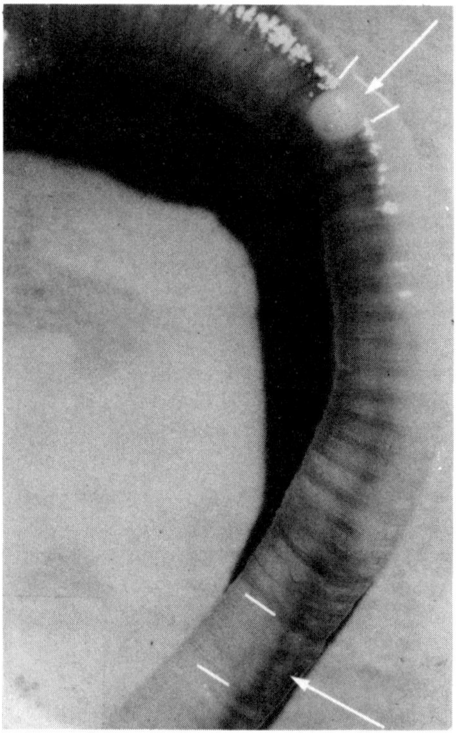

Fig. 3.2. A *Lumbricus* well-healed autograft (bottom arrow) and a rejected xenograft (top arrow). The xenograft shows blanching, swelling, and oedema at 20 days post-grafting, ×2·5 (after Cooper 1968a).

REJECTION OF FIRST-SET INTRAFAMILIAL (LUMBRICIDAE) XENOGRAFTS

Specificity of self-recognition

In order to ascertain whether earthworm coelomocytes do distinguish sharply between autografts and xenografts, an autograft from *Eisenia* and a xenograft from *Lumbricus* can be placed in the same graft bed of an *Eisenia* host. Both heal together and to the surrounding host tissue. However, the xenograft is always destroyed at 33 days; the autograft remaining permanently surviving. It makes no difference whether the position in the bed is autograft, anterior or xenograft, posterior. One can easily imagine coelomocytes 'choosing' between self-, and non-self and ultimately destroying the xenograft. To demonstrate that this confrontation has no effect on the outcome of the rejection time, a single *Lumbricus* graft to *Eisenia* yields a survival time of 34 days (Cooper 1969a).

Diverse intrafamilial specificities

In the opposite direction, *Lumbricus* hosts respond differently to *Eisenia* xenografts, yielding a mean survival time of 26 days. However, an *Allolobophora* graft on a *Lumbricus* host leads to a survival time of approximately 40 days. When *Eisenia* is employed as host and *Allolobophora* as donor, the rejection time is 35 days (Cooper 1969a).

REJECTION OF INTRAFAMILIAL (EUDRILIDAE LUMBRICIDAE) GRAFTS

First-set xenografts

Longer survival times of intrafamilial transplants suggests a greater sharing of cellular and tissue antigens than might be expected, should grafts from more distantly related individuals be exchanged. To test this assumption, grafts from *Eudrilus* to *Lumbricus* yield a survival time of 13 days. Similarly, a graft of *Eudrilus* on to *Eisenia* produces a short survival time of 17 days. Both survive for a significantly shorter time than those involving intrafamilial combinations (Cooper 1969a).

REJECTION OF FIRST-SET *EISENIA* XENOGRAFTS ON *LUMBRICUS* HOSTS

In contrast to allografts which show, maximally, only 20 per cent destruction over prolonged periods, the situation with xenografts is different (Cooper 1968a). All xenografts heal initially but eventually show signs of incompatibility at varying times. At 15°C four groups can be distinguished, based on rejection times. An acute response occurs in 11 days or less and rapid-chronic from 12 to 19 days. Intermediate chronic responses can appear from 20 to 49 days and those in the prolonged chronic class from 50 to more than 100 days. The highest number of rejections fall into the period from 12 to 50 days. All xenografts are always destroyed, confirming our earlier contention that absence of rejections in the allogeneic combinations was not a reflection of defective immune recognition mechanisms; it probably represented absence of recognizable antigens. With these experiments we were closer to defining the existence of an immune system capable of specific recognition and reaction.

POSITIVE AND NEGATIVE MEMORY REVEALED BY ACCELERATED REJECTION AND PROLONGED SURVIVAL OF SECOND-SET *EISENIA* XENOGRAFTS TO *LUMBRICUS* HOSTS

Albeit terribly exciting that an invertebrate simply rejects a graft confirming an important function of an immune system, it was still absolutely necessary to define the events that transpire before, during and after rejection. Thus, are the two main parameters of *specificity* and *anamnesis* demonstrable characteristics of earthworm transplant rejection? If so how are these working? For now we can dismiss with specificity momentarily, and deal with memory, since specificity is already inherent in differential specific recognition and reaction to auto-, allo-, and xenografts. Classically, memory is tested by

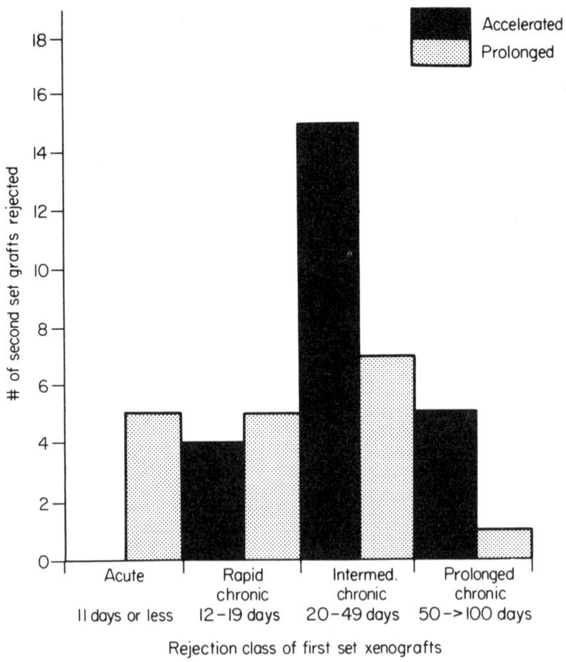

Fig. 3.3. The relationship between rate of rejection of first-set xenografts and rejection of second-set grafts. When first-set grafts are rejected in an acute or rapid-chronic fashion, second-set grafts show prolonged survival (negative responders). First-set grafts, rejected in an intermediate, chronic, prolonged fashion, are always followed by second-set grafts rejected at an accelerated rate (positive responders) (after Cooper 1968a).

a repeat transplantation from the same donor that provided the first transplant. Such second-set transplantations are performed usually after gross signs of first-graft rejection.

When grafted immediately after first-set rejection, second-sets are destroyed at 15°C in a biphasic manner, i.e. most transplant destructions occur faster than the first; however, a significant number are destroyed at times longer than the survival times of the first grafts (Cooper 1968a). We interpret such a response as positive (accelerated) and negative (prolonged) memory. It was obvious (see Fig. 3.3) that there existed a relationship between the first-set xenograft rejection class and the appearance of positive and negative memory. All worms showing acute rejection of first-set grafts always yielded prolonged survival of repeat second-sets. Although all three remaining groups show negative responders, the greatest number of positive responders resulted from those second-sets transplanted to worms that had first-sets destroyed during the intermediate chronic period of 20 to 49 days.

From Fig. 3.4, it is possible to correlate the interval between first-set rejection with the type of memory response to a second graft. Short intervals

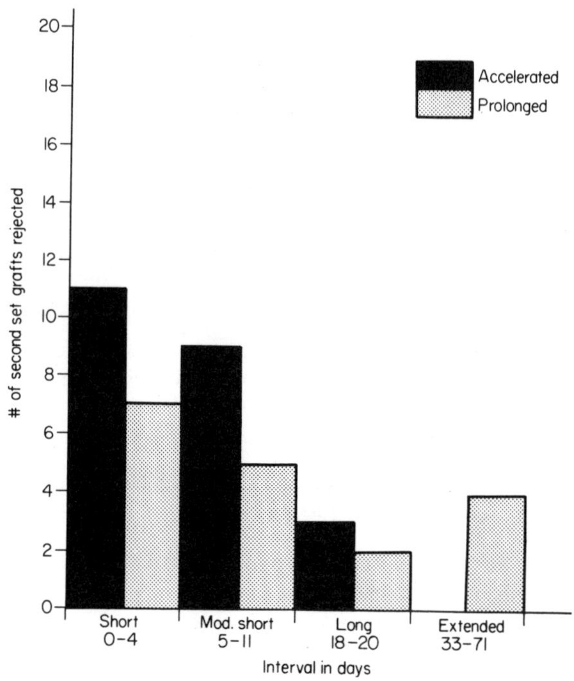

Fig. 3.4. Relationship of first-set graft rejection class to number, interval, and type of second-set rejection. Shorter intervals produced both positive and negative responders in similar proportions; extended intervals yielded only negative and no positive responders (after Cooper 1968a).

tend to produce more positive responders than longer intervals. Secondly, the onset of first-graft rejection seems to affect the time of second-set rejection. For example, moderately short onsets of rejection (e.g. 6 to 12 days) result in slightly more accelerated rejections (positive responders) than prolonged survivors (negative responders). Short intervals of 5 days or less gave significantly more accelerated reactions (positive responders) (Fig. 3.5).

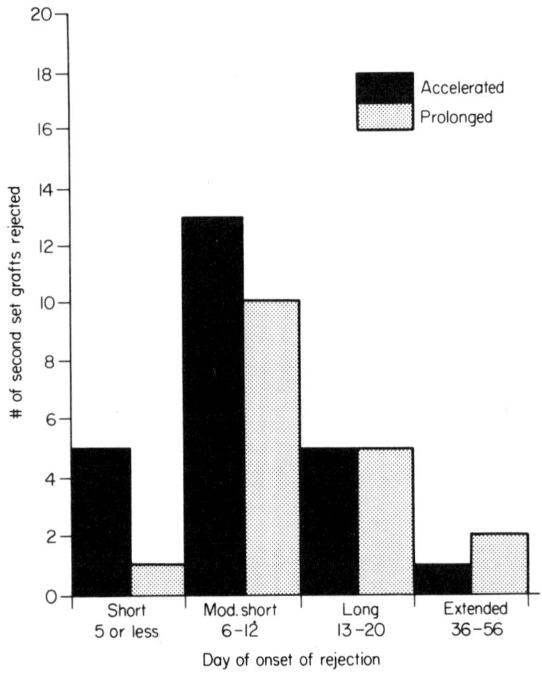

Fig. 3.5. Relationship between onset of second-set graft rejection and rejection type. Shorter onset times generally produced positive responders but extended onsets were followed by negative responders (after Cooper 1968a).

SHORT-TERM POSITIVE MEMORY AND SPECIFICITY DEMONSTRABLE BY EARLY SECOND-SET CHALLENGE

That second-set xenografts are destroyed rapidly, provided evidence that graft rejection mechanisms in earthworms are characterized by a memory component reminiscent of vertebrate anamnesis. Similarly, prolonged survival, interpreted as negative memory, also recalls certain vertebrate-like responses. To manipulate the immune system such that responses were either all positive or all negative was the aim of one very fruitful experiment (Cooper 1969a).

We had determined previously that short intervals between first-set rejection and second-set grafting tended to produce more positive responders.

In addition there occurred a maximal coelomocyte response immediately after first-set grafting and prior to 5 days post-transplantation. This suggested that the memory component was short-lived leading to the following experiment. Control *Lumbricus* hosts were transplanted with two *Eisenia* grafts at 15°C and the transplants then allowed to undergo rejection. Such grafts were destroyed at approximately 33 days. In the second experiment, one group of *Lumbricus* was given a single *Eisenia* graft followed 5 days later by a second-set graft from the same donor as the first. Instead of an accelerated rejection of the second transplant only, the first-set was also destroyed rapidly, a striking, unexpected result. This heightened reactivity to both grafts at 18 and 15 days, respectively, leads to this possible interpretation. The immune response to the first graft was already in progress and the second served as a booster for an already ongoing reaction. Finally, in the third experiment, the plan was the same as the second, with one exception. A group of *Lumbricus* was grafted with a single *Eisenia* transplant. Five days later, a second *Eisenia* transplant was made simultaneously along with a third graft from a completely independent donor, *Allolobophora* (family Lumbricidae). *Eisenia* grafts produced the same survival times as those obtained in Experiment 2, but the rejection time of *Allolobophora* was independent of the two *Eisenia* transplants, at a time equivalent to that of a single *Allolobophora* on a *Lumbricus* host. In Experiment 2 we suggest evidence for memory and in Experiment 3 we confirm anamnesis and show again specificity. If the coelomocytes of *Lumbricus* could not distinguish specifically between *Eisenia*, then the host would have showed confused rejection times when confronted at the same time with a donor graft from *Allolobophora*. This was not the case. Thus, the numbers of positive and negative responders to second-set grafts can be regulated by antigen challenge time. As will be seen later, temperature is also an important regulator of earthworm cellular immunity.

Histopathology of graft rejection

EVENTS DURING THE FIRST TWO WEEKS

It is clear now that the earthworm immune system is sufficiently differentiated to handle the destruction of foreign tissue antigens. We have at hand gross quantifiable criteria for assessing graft destruction. In addition there is strong evidence for active coelomocyte participation in graft destruction. After 24 hours, autografts and xenografts are well healed by histologically identical scar tissue. This is characterized by growing tissue from the severed ends of muscle and the connective tissue between the muscle; it grows to connect with similar graft tissue. In Figs. 3.6 and 3.7 epithelial cells redifferentiate and are obvious as young mucus secreting cells. At 24 hours, coelomocytes

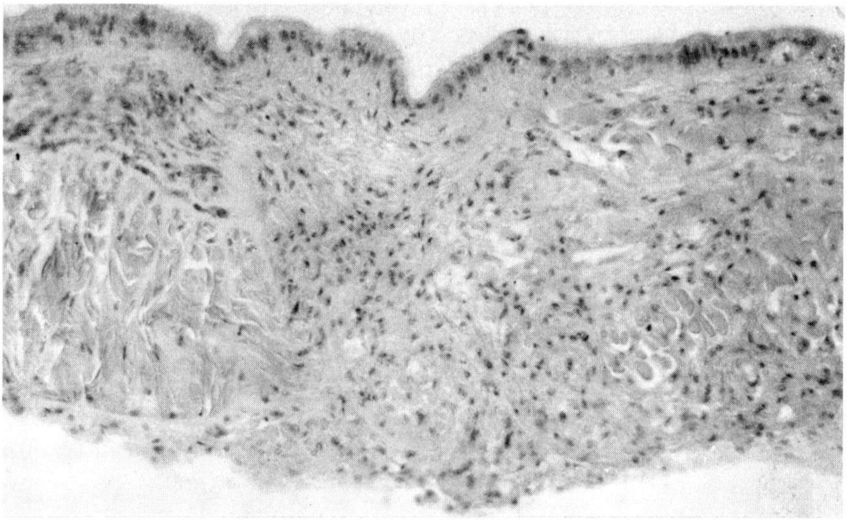

Fig. 3.6. A *Lumbricus* autograft at 11 days' post-grafting, showing host tissue (at left) and graft (at right). The epithelium covering the scar tissue shows differentiation into cell types similar to those seen on host and graft sides, × 320 (after Cooper 1968a).

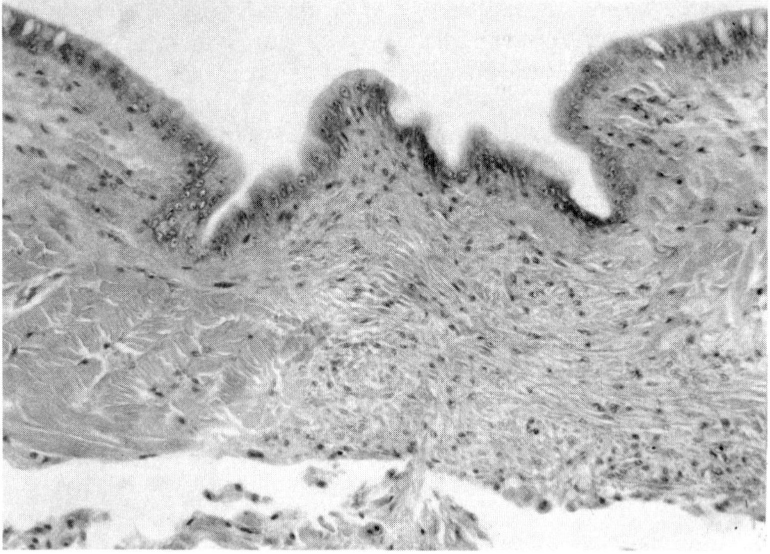

Fig. 3.7. An *Eisenia* xenograft 12 days' post-grafting. Note the scar tissue between the host (at left) and the graft (at right). Many circular and longitudinal muscle bundles and epithelium show essentially no difference on either side. At biopsy this xenograft was well healed with no signs of rejection, × 320 (after Cooper 1968a).

congregate at both autograft and xenograft sites suggesting general non-specific responses to injury and healing. Coelomocyte specificity is inferred by the ultimate rejection of xenografts, and not autografts. The initial response seems to occur primarily at the graft host contact zone represented in association with scar tissue, still, the central portion of grafts were not without profuse coelomocyte activity.

Although there are several suggested origins of coelomocytes, we favour coelomocytes coming from a loose aggregation of acidophilic staining tissue invested in the dorsal gut called 'lymph gland'. Often coelomocytes can be viewed in direct contact with xenografts and emigrating there from the so-called lymph gland. The coelomic cavity is bathed by the fluid and guarded by numerous coelomocytes (Fig. 3.8). New information suggests that coelomocytes divide as revealed by uptake of ^{3}H thymidine by coelomocytes in response to xenografts (Lemmi & Cooper, in preparation).

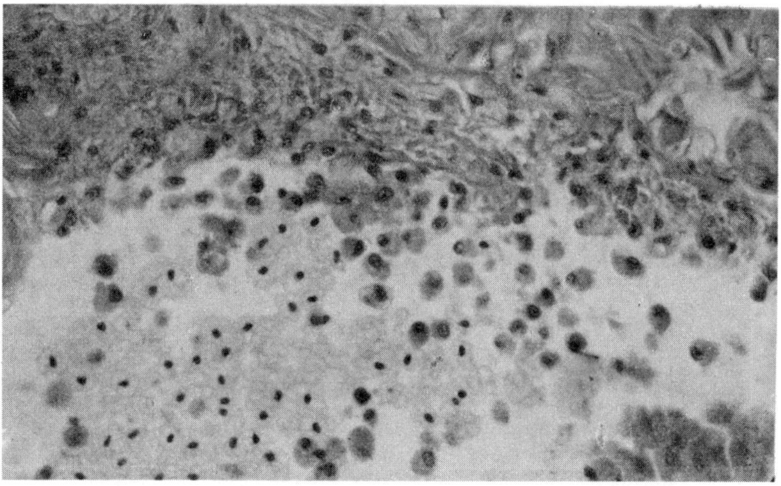

Fig. 3.8. An *Eisenia* xenograft on a *Lumbricus* host 8 days' post-grafting. Note the intense coelomocyte reaction at the base of the graft, ×500 (after Cooper 1968a).

RE-ESTABLISHMENT OF VASCULARIZATION TO TRANSPLANTS

We are not clear on when blood flow ensues to grafts, however vessels are easily observed in transplants as early as day 1. Blood vessels usually occur as extensions from thin sheets of host peritoneal tissue and are found in the surrounding scar tissue (Figs. 3.9, 3.10). There are two possibilities, i.e. growth of host vascular twigs directly into transplants, and secondly, inosculation of host vessels with those in the graft. Tactile sensitivity of transplants suggests at least partial re-establishment of branches of integumentary nerves during the first few days after transplant healing.

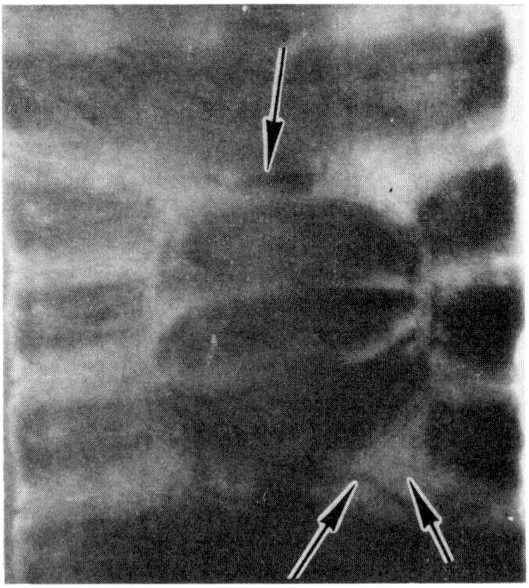

Fig. 3.9. The circulatory pattern is clearly revealed in this *Lumbricus* xenograft on an *Eisenia* host. The arrows indicate vascular twigs grown over from the host side to connect to this well-healed transplant (Cooper, unpublished).

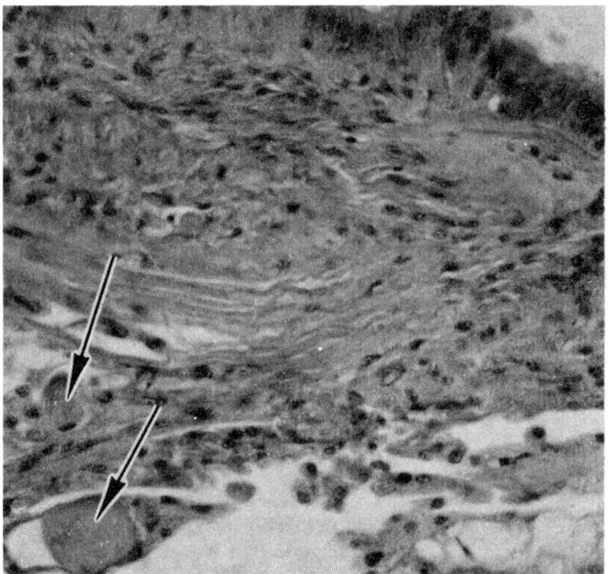

Fig. 3.10. A well-healed *Eisenia* xenograft on a *Lumbricus* host 8 days' post-grafting. Graft tissue is at the left. Arrows indicate a cross-section through two blood vessels at the base of the graft, × 500 (after Cooper 1968a).

Evidence for coelomocyte-mediated memory after xenografting revealed by adoptive transfer

Since coelomocytes aggregate at xenograft sites, it was intriguing to design experiments to test the coelomocyte's capacity, alone, to mediate immunity. Two alternatives were clear, namely that coelomocytes are involved in recognition or that coelomocytes actually effect rejection. To test this assumption, *Lumbricus* hosts were challenged with xenografts and the coelomocyte's capacity to transfer memory was analysed (Bailey *et al.* 1971, Cooper 1973). Host *Lumbricus* (A) were xenografted with *Eisenia*. To confirm short term memory, coelomocytes were harvested at 5 days post-transplantation, and injected into ungrafted *Lumbricus* (A). This second host was then xenografted with the same *Eisenia* donor used to induce immunity in A. Since we had determined previously that *Lumbricus* shows only negligible allograft responses late after transplantation, we suspected no early coelomocyte allo-incompatibility prior to the action of primed coelomocytes against the *Eisenia* graft on *Lumbricus* A. Such was the case, and at 15°C, the second host showed accelerated rejection of its first transplant due to adoptive transfer of graft rejection capacity by primed coelomocytes. The response is cell-mediated since transfer of coelomic fluid alone, free of coelomocytes, is ineffective. Other controls revealed that the coelomocytes from unprimed *Lumbricus* are unable to transfer the response. Similarly, coelomocytes from *Lumbricus* primed with saline are unable to transfer the response which resides, therefore, primarily in the coelomocytes. How specific this adoptive transfer response is remains to be determined. For example, if we graft a *Lumbricus* host with *Eisenia*, then transfer the coelomocytes and graft the new host with *Alloloborphora*, what is the response? Furthermore, how long does this response last and what is the role of temperature in regulating the response? Is memory longer lived at lower temperatures?

Regulation of long-term xenograft memory by temperature revealed in differential coelomocyte activity and typical anamnestic responses

We had previously established two important criteria when studying memory to xenografts. Memory is short-lived at 15°C. Secondly, to achieve all positive responders, it was necessary to challenge with repeat grafts soon after the healing of initial priming grafts. Both positive and negative responders develop when hosts are challenged after first-set grafts are destroyed. To study the role of challenge time (induction) and temperature on regulation of immune responsiveness the ambient temperature was raised to 20°C for all succeeding experiments and second-set transplants were performed after first-set grafts were destroyed. In addition, we developed a technique for harvesting and quantitating coelomocytes from just beneath the surface of grafts (Hostetter & Cooper 1972a,b, 1974a,b). In such enumerations we are able to deduce the specificity of coelomocyte responsiveness. Secondly, gross survival of grafts can be correlated with coelomocyte activity.

The mean survival time of first-set xenografts at 20°C was 17 days, clearly different from previous results at 15°C (Figs. 3.11, 3.12). After receiving second-set xenografts, coelomocytes increase from normal levels of 5,000 cells/mm^3 to 10,000 cells/mm^3 in 24 hours. At 48 hours post-grafting, coelomocytes reach a significantly higher number of 12,000 cells/mm^3. The mean survival time for second-set xenografts is 6 days; a classic type

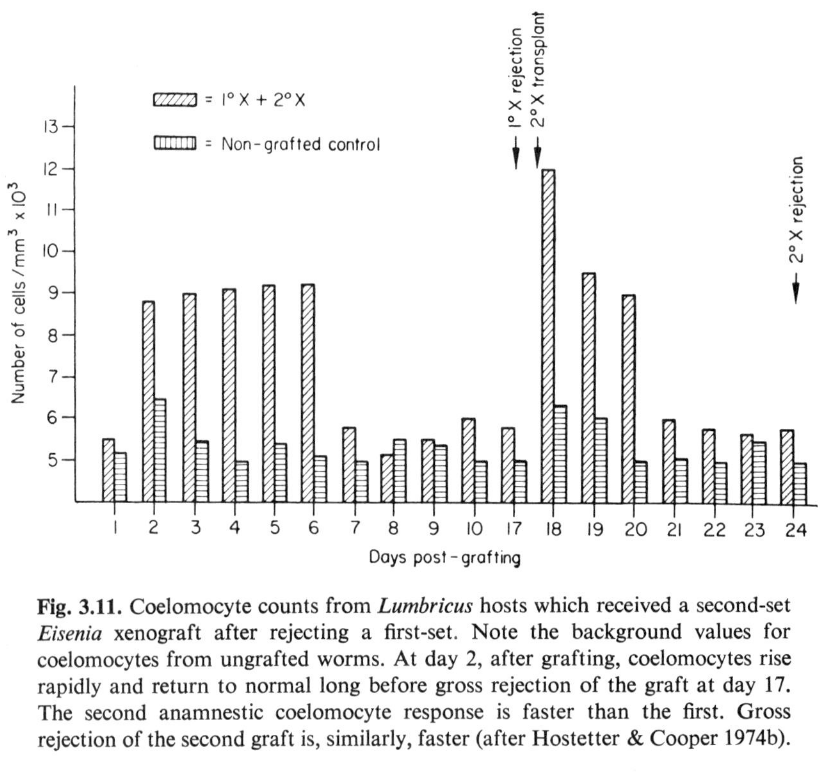

Fig. 3.11. Coelomocyte counts from *Lumbricus* hosts which received a second-set *Eisenia* xenograft after rejecting a first-set. Note the background values for coelomocytes from ungrafted worms. At day 2, after grafting, coelomocytes rise rapidly and return to normal long before gross rejection of the graft at day 17. The second anamnestic coelomocyte response is faster than the first. Gross rejection of the second graft is, similarly, faster (after Hostetter & Cooper 1974b).

anamnestic response occurs at the cellular level and can be correlated with accelerated rejection of a second-set xenograft.

Coelomocytes from *Lumbricus* with first-set xenografts followed by first-set autografts or non-specific injury increase at 24 hours and 48 hours but normal cell counts were attained at the end of 72 hours post-grafting or injury (Fig. 3.12). A non-specific injury causes abrupt increases in coelomocytes during the first 24 hours to 9,000 cells/mm^3 but this response declines rapidly to normal at 72 hours post-injury. If a second injury is inflicted, coelomocytes increase at 24 hours to similar values (10,500 cells/mm^3), maintain until 48 hours, and then return to normal.

At 20°C, the usual widespread survival times of first-set grafts observed previously are narrowed significantly so that second-sets are rejected faster than both accelerated (positive) and prolonged (negative) anamnestic reactions at 15°C. Secondly, second-set tests for *typical memory* were performed *after* rejection of first-sets, not 5 days after first-set transplantation to test for short-term memory. Finally, of obvious significance, coelomocytes respond differently to autografts, non-specific wounds and both first- and second-set xenografts, revealing both non-specific and immunologic reactions. A comparison of coelomocyte numbers from *Lumbricus* with no grafts or only first

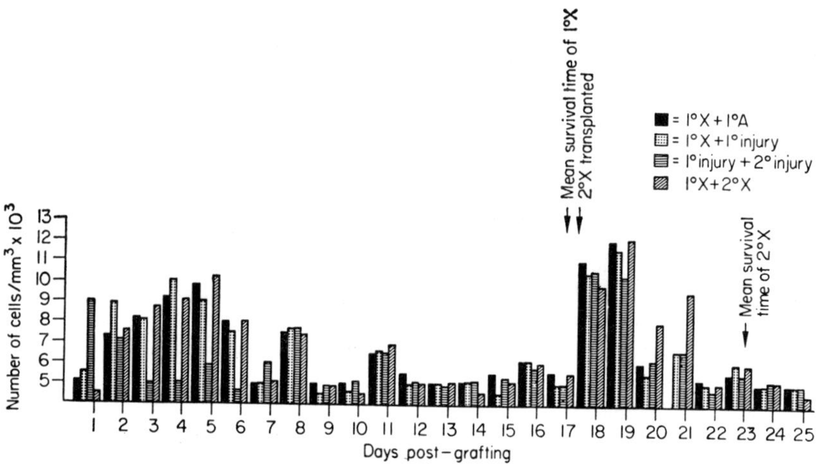

Fig. 3.12. Coelomocyte counts from another group similar to Fig. 3.11. Note the additional number of controls incorporated into the experiment to add further support to specific anamnesis and to rule out non-specific responses (after Hostetter & Cooper 1974).

autografts, with coelomocytes responding to second-set xenografts, reveals a specific heightened cellular response to repeat grafts. In addition, there is a marked difference in the rates of first- and second-set coelomocyte increases. The first coelomocyte increase in response to second-set xenografts is interpreted as general and non-specific since autografts or simple injury provoke similar reactions. Thus a primary phase ensues after any injury during transplantation surgery. The information suggests links between the degree of coelomocyte responses during second reactions and the type of first induction. For example, autografts performed later on hosts bearing first-set xenografts produce counts similar to those from hosts with first-set xenografts and then injured.

Apparently an interdependency exists between first induction and the resulting primary and secondary phases, finalizing the specific end of the anamnestic response. Cellular responses to first xenografts rise and then decline gradually during first-set coelomocyte reactions. Primary xenografts may stimulate the production of specific memory cells, leading to an abrupt increase (secondary phase) in coelomocytes after secondary challenge. This differs considerably from the slow non-specific coelomocyte build-up (primary phase) after first-set xenografts or autografts.

Quantification of coelomocyte responses provides further confirmation for the existence of true immunologic memory in earthworms. Initial cellular reactions are effete by 6 days post-grafting, yet the same first-set xenografts are rejected at 17 days. As an indicator of memory, second-set cellular reactions are spent by 3–4 days and grossly the grafts destroyed at 6 days. This alone is a typical second-set response revealed grossly by accelerated second-set rejection and at the cellular level, by heightened numbers of sensitive coelomocytes.

Summary of primordial cell-mediated immunity best exemplified by earthworms

INTRODUCTION

The earthworm coelomic cavity may be considered a hypothetical precursor of vertebrate immune organs such as bone marrow, thymus, spleen or nodes. In the coelomic cavity, as in these organs, there are several varieties of immunocompetent cells. The coelom is partitioned by septa that form an efficient filtering organ which together with the epithelial lining and phagocytic cells is analogous to the vertebrate reticulo-endothelial system. Earthworm

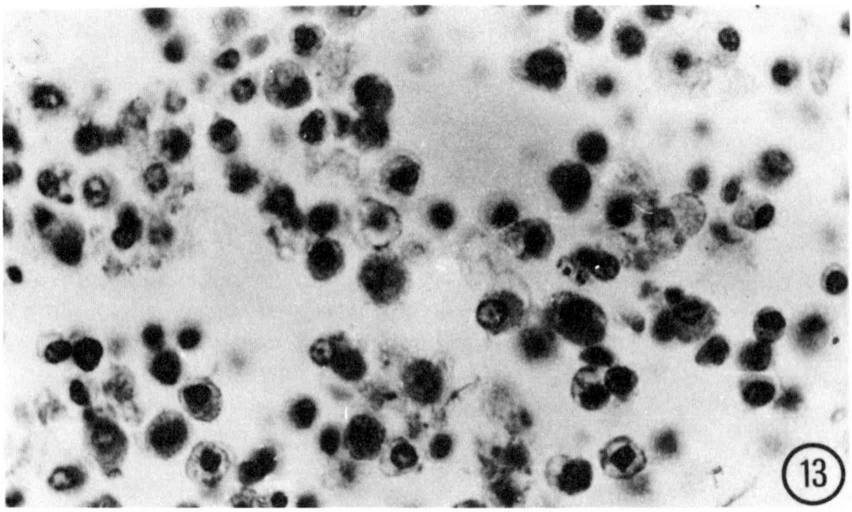

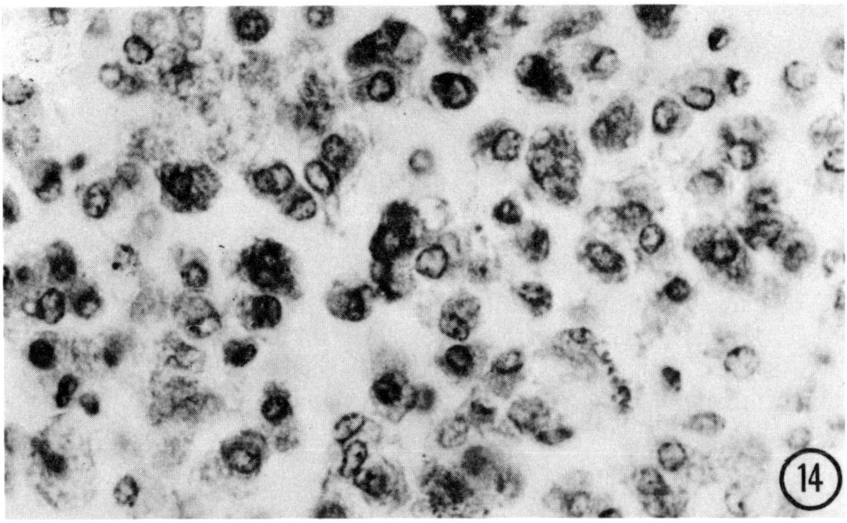

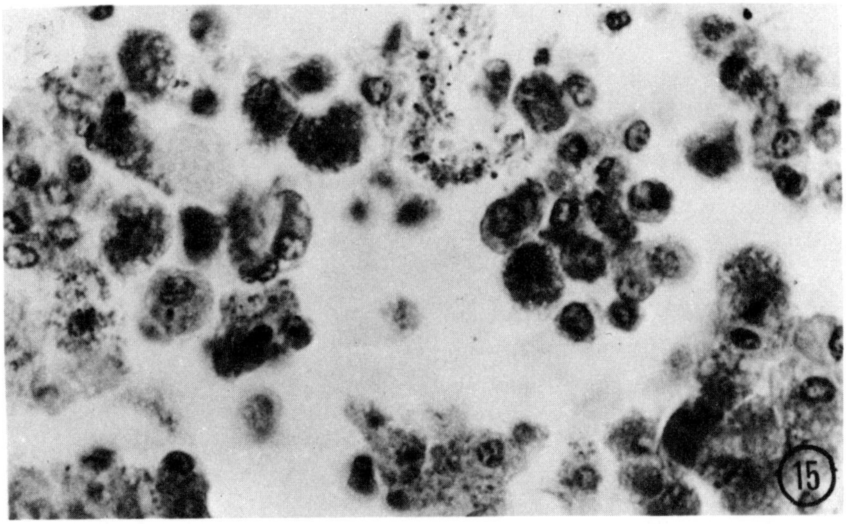

Figs. 3.13, 3.14, 3.15. Coelomocytes, upper, middle and lower layers after differential centrifugation, stained with Harris's haematoxylin and eoxin. Paraffin section, cut at 6 μ, $\times 500$ (Hostetter & Cooper, unpublished).

coelomocytes respond similarly to vertebrate immunocytes by sequestering pathogenic organisms or effecting tissue graft rejection. Coelomocytes are the primary forces in graft destruction, one aspect of immunity for which we have sufficient information. If coelomocytes are harvested from worms and centrifuged differentially, at least three (Figs. 3.13, 3.14, 3.15) distinct morphologic types are distinguishable presumably representing three functional cell types.

HYPOTHETICAL INTERRELATIONSHIPS OF COELOMOCYTES

Considering the above information, we present an hypothetical outline of coelomic cell interrelationships (Hostetter & Cooper 1974b). A small basophilic cell grows and becomes a large phagocytic amoebocyte. Acidophilic granular cells represent a cell line developing from small acidophilic granular cells. Transitions between small acidophilic cells and large acidophilic cells could become modified basophilic cells. Several structures have been suggested as sites from which other coelomic cells might be derived. The epithelial lining of the coelomic cavity, 'lymph glands', other coelomic cells, the nephridia and the alimentary canal may all be involved.

FUNCTIONS OF EARTHWORM COELOMOCYTES

Coelomocytes may utilize the same or similar mechanisms for dealing with allografts and xenografts as those observed during cellular reactions against bacteria and parasites. Phagocytosis and encapsulation result in the clearing of dead and injured tissue from graft or injury sites (Figs. 3.16, 3.17). Upon

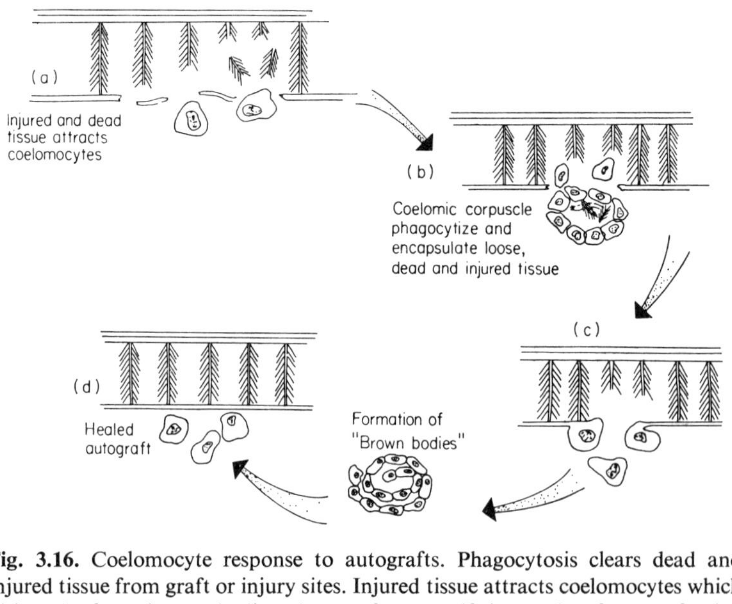

Fig. 3.16. Coelomocyte response to autografts. Phagocytosis clears dead and injured tissue from graft or injury sites. Injured tissue attracts coelomocytes which ultimately form brown bodies. Autografts are self-tissue, therefore no foreign response is evoked and the graft heals without coelomocyte damage (after Hostetter & Cooper 1974a).

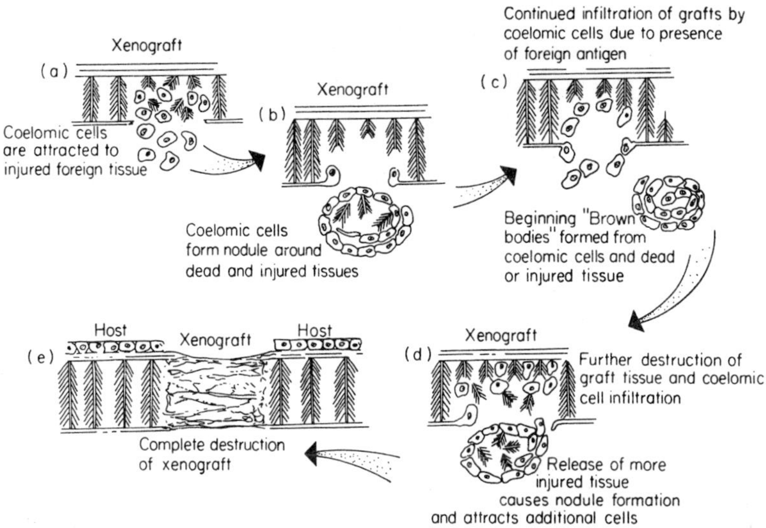

Fig. 3.17. Coelomocyte response to xenografts. Essentially the same first general non-specific reactions occur when coelomocytes recognize a foreign, *not-self* xenograft. However, the response is much more intense. Brown bodies are formed, but at least some of the coelomocytes continue to effect xenograft destruction leaving no transplant and only collagenous scar tissue. Coelomocytes then migrate elsewhere, carrying memory to effect a second-response after second-set transplantation (after Hostetter & Cooper 1974b).

contact with a foreign antigen coelomocytes become immobilized and then they may release various humoral factors such as opsonins, lysins, agglutinins, and substances similar to mammalian migration inhibitory factor (MIF) (Lemmi *et al.* 1974). The presence of antigen or the release of humoral agents causes additional coelomocyte formation by stimulation of coelomocytopoiesis sites. These substances may also lead to accumulations around foreign antigens; thus phagocytosis ensues followed by encapsulation and release of hydrolytic enzymes resulting in antigen destruction. Once foreign antigens are degraded, the stimulus for coelomocytes is removed. Excess coelomocytes produced because of antigen stimulation become attached to surrounding organs and the total coelomocyte population returns to normal.

Upon second challenge with a foreign antigen, the following events take place:

1. coelomocytes in the free circulating pool come in contact with antigen, are immobilized, and release humoral factors;
2. these factors stimulate and cause local accumulations and coelomocyte movements where they attach to various organs.

This results in rapid coelomocyte accumulations at antigen sites and because of greater numbers of coelomocytes, a more rapid destruction of foreign antigens ensues. These proposals certainly take into account the conflicting morphological evidence for the origins of coelomocytes (Stephenson 1930, Stang-Voss 1971, Kindred 1929, Liebman 1942). Perhaps we can be led into a knowledge of the development of coelomocytes by observing them after labelling with tracers in response to foreign grafts. We (Lemmi & Cooper, in preparation) already have information that coelomocytes do incorporate significant amounts of ^{3}H thymidine after transplantation with xenografts.

EARTHWORM COELOMOCYTES

It seems clear now that earthworms are excellent invertebrates for establishing thorough searches of phylogenetic origins of cell-mediated immunity. Their activities are easily measurable in response to foreign tissue antigens such as xenografts. Although the humoral aspects of earthworm immunity reveal a negative response to bacterial antigens (Cooper *et al.* 1969) the coelomocyte may yet yield vital information on its surface properties (Fig. 3.18). This would make it possible for us to know how it recognizes not only foreign antigens introduced experimentally but how coelomocytes may be the earthworm's sole policing system against other natural threats such as tumours and neoplastic changes (Cooper 1968c, 1969c, Cooper & Baculi 1968b).

Summary of quasi-immunorecognition, primordial cell-mediated immunity and relation to immunologic theory

We may assume that recognition, primordial cell mediated immunity and the 'zenith' of vertebrate immune responsiveness are in one form or another characteristic of all animals; these evolved as protective mechanisms against predation by micro-organisms. Unicellular protozoans combine both food-getting, recognition, and ultimate sequestration of harmful micro-organisms (Burnet 1968). This action occurs by combined chemotaxis and phagocytosis. At this phylogenetic level, self-, not-self discrimination presumably occurs by means of 'proto-immunoglobulins' or other substances. These may act like opsonins, if at all existent, and are still unknown chemically (Boyden 1960a,b, 1963, 1966). Primitive metazoans exhibiting, as of now, only quasi-immunorecognition, may be members of the phylogenetic groups that we should examine for the presence of such cellular recognition units. Nossal (1971) believes that the earthworm work should be greatly extended and that the coelomocyte may be one model that holds the key to the 'molecular ancestor of vertebrate immunoglobulins provided certain blocking and binding studies are exploited to the fullest'.

Jerne (1971) proposes that 'cell recognition, which must be fundamental in even the most primitive metazoa [as just described under quasi-immunorecognition] may require the presence of histocompatibility antigens and of

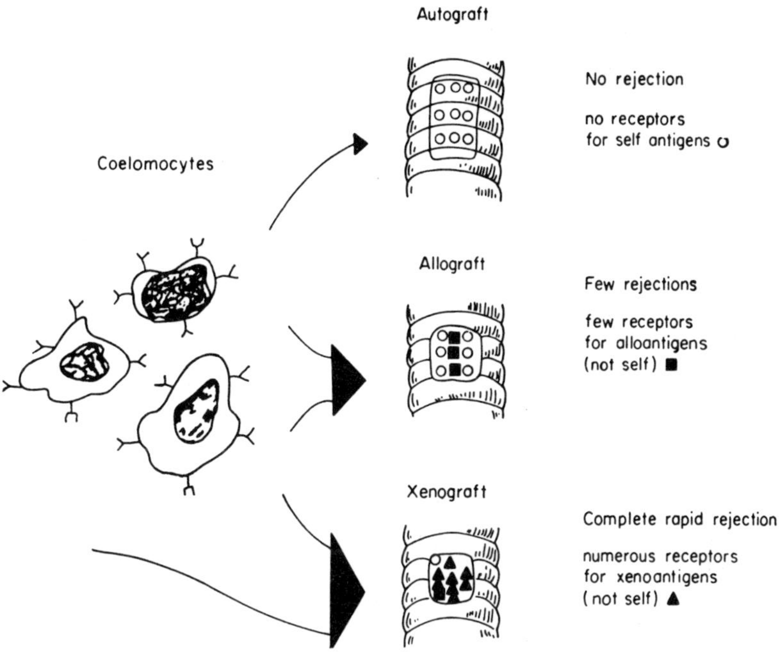

Fig. 3.18. Hypothetical model of coelomocyte recognition of self- versus not-self exemplified by responses to transplants (primordial T-Cell Response). Three representative coelomocyte types bearing receptors for allograft and xenograft antigens are at the left side. Coelomocytes have no receptors for *self* antigens, thus they are unable to recognize autografts. With regard to allografts, only few alloantigens are present and correspondingly few specific coelomocyte receptors. Rejection is slow. Xenografts elicit strong recognition responses and ultimately rejection of all grafts due to many xenogeneic antigens. Such specificity, accompanied by memory, represents a primordial T-cell response. Certain coelomocytes probably divide leaving daughter cells carrying memory information.

complementary "antibody" molecules at cell surfaces'. He further suggests that 'at some stage of metazoan evolution, an immune system of specialized lymphocytes developed, based on this older recognition system, and that a mechanism evolved for suppressing those lymphocytic stem cells that express v-genes of subset S (self), i.e. that produce antibodies against the histocompatibility antigens of the individual'. The complementary subset A (allo) of v-genes determine antibodies directed against all other relevant histocompatibility antigens of a given species absent in a particular animal.

Should we invoke another cause for the development in evolution of cell recognition we can take note of Thomas's (1959) idea, later elaborated by Burnet in his concept of immunologic surveillance (1963, 1970a,b, 1971). According to this view, the fetus as allograft and particularly neoplasia, were strong forces in the evolutionary development of the immune system. Thus, we progress phylogenetically from combined food-getting and defence manifested by simple recognition, to specific primitive cellular immunity with a memory component effected by cells with definable unknown receptors to specific anamnestic immune responses mediated by cells with known receptors (immunoglobulins). The dictum of Haeckel (1891) that 'ontogeny recapitulates phylogeny' may be referable to immune responsiveness if we still are to view such dicta as instructive. Indeed, simplest manifestations of immunity are found throughout the phylogenetic sequence and each level of metazoan complexity yields species adapted to certain environmental niches. Each therefore possesses remnants of the successive steps in the development of immunity in both the ontogenetic and phylogenetic development of animal species in stepwise, ordered fashion.

As an example, non-specific phagocytosis is clearly a universal attribute of all living animals early recognized by Metchnikoff (1892) but primarily through his studies of invertebrates. If we are to develop an encompassing theory of immunity, the gaps from *Amoeba* to *Amaroecium* to *Anadonta* to Apteryx must be filled by the results of intensive investigations which bear in mind, on the one hand, the great strides made by the more mammalian-oriented immunologists (Jerne 1967, 1969) but, on the other, remain coupled with the more biological expertise of the invertebrate and comparative immunologist.

Acknowledgments

Supported by USPHS grant 1RO1 HDO9333–01. The author expresses appreciation to Mrs Lois T. Gehringer and Mrs Pamela Konrad for help in preparing the MS.

References

Acton R.T., Evans E.E., Weinheimer P.F., Cooper E.L., Campbell R.D., Prowse R.H., Bizot M., Stewart J.E. & Fuller G.M. *et al.* (1972) *Invertebrate immune defense mechanisms.* MSS Information Corporation, New York.

Bailey S., Miller B.J. & Cooper E.L. (1971) Transplantation immunity in annelids. II. Adoptive transfer of the xenograft reaction. *Immunology*, **21,** 81.

Bang F.B. (1967) Defense reactions in invertebrates. *Fed. Proc.* **26,** 1964.

Bell W.J. (1972) Yolk formation by transplanted cockroach oocytes. *J. Exptl Zool.* **181,** 41.

Bhaskaran G. & Sivasubramanian P. (1969) Metamorphosis of imaginal disks of the housefly: evagination of transplanted disks. *J. Exptl Zool.* **171,** 385.

Bibb C. & Campbell R.D. (1973) Cell affinity determining heterospecific graft intolerance in Hydra. *Tissue and Cell* **5,** 199.

Boyden S.V. (1960a) Antibody production. *Nature* **185,** 724.

Boyden S.V. (1960b) Cellular discrimination between indigenous and foreign matter. *J. Theor. Biol.* **3,** 123.

Boyden S.V. (1963) Cellular recognition of foreign matter. *Int. Rev. Exptl Pathol.* **2,** 311.

Boyden S.V. (1966) Natural antibodies and the immune response. *Adv. Immunol.* **5,** 1.

Truslé J. (1967) Homogreffes et heterogreffes du tegument et des gonades chez *Asterina gibbosa* et *Asterina pancerii* (Echinodermes, Asterides). *Cahiers de Biologie Marine* **8,** 417.

BURNET F.M. (1963) The evolution of bodily defense. *Med. J. Austr.* **2,** 817.

BURNET F.M. (1968) Evolution of the immune process in vertebrates. *Nature* **218,** 426.

BURNET F.M. (1970a) The concept of immunological surveillance. *Progr. Exptl Tumor Res.* **13,** 1.

BURNET F.M. (1970b) *Immunological Surveillance*. Pergamon, New York.

BURNET F.M. (1971) 'Self-recognition' in colonial marine forms and flowering plants in relation to the evolution of immunity. *Nature* **232,** 230.

BURNET F.M. (1974) Invertebrate precursors to immune responses. In *Contemporary Topics in Immunology*, 4, ed. Cooper E.L. Plenum Press, New York (299 pp.).

CAMPBELL R.D. & BIBB C. (1970) Transplantation in coelenterates. *Transpl. Proc.* **2,** 202.

CANZONIER W.J. (1963) Histological observations on the response of oysters to tissue implants. *Proc. Nat. Shellf. Assoc.* **54,** 1.

CHENG T.C. & GALLOWAY P.C. (1970) Transplantation immunity in mollusks: the histoincompatibility of *Helisoma duryi normale* with allografts and xenografts. *J. Invert. Pathol.* **15,** 177.

COHEN N. & BORYSENKO M. (1970) Acute and chronic graft rejection: possible phylogeny of transplantation antigens. *Transpl. Proc.* **2,** 333.

COOPER E.L. (1965) A method of tissue grafting in the earthworm, *Lumbricus terrestris. Am. Zool.* **5,** 233.

COOPER E.L. (1966a) Algunos aspectos de inmunidad en invertebrados, peces, y anfibios. *Acta Medica* **2,** 1.

COOPER E.L. (1966b) Rechazo de tejidos en la lombriz de tierra una respuesta immunologica? *Arch. Mex. Anat.* **7,** 21.

COOPER E.L. (1968a) Transplantation immunity in annelids. I. Rejection of xenografts exchanged between *Lumbricus terrestris* and *Eisenia foetida. Transplantation* **6,** 322.

COOPER E.L. (1968b) Transplantation immunity in earthworms. *Am. Zool.* **8,** 379b.

COOPER E.L. (1968c) Multinucleate giant cells, granulomata and 'myoblastomas' in annelid worms. *J. Invert. Pathol.* **11,** 123.

COOPER E.L. (1969a) Specific tissue graft rejection in earthworms. *Science* **166,** 1414.

COOPER E.L. (1969b) Chronic allograft rejection in *L. terrestris. J. Exptl Zool.* **171,** 69.

COOPER E.L. (1969c) Neoplasia and transplantation immunity in annelids. *J. Nat. Can. Inst.* **31,** 655.

COOPER E.L. (1970) Transplantation immunity in helminths and annelids. *Transpl. Proc.* **2,** 216.

COOPER E.L. (1971) Phylogeny of transplantation immunity. Graft rejection in earthworms. *Transpl. Proc.* **3,** 214.

COOPER E.L. (1973) Evolution of cellular immunity, pp. 11–23. In *Symposium on Non-Specific Factors Influencing Host Resistance*, eds Braun W. & Ungar J.S. Karger, Basel.

COOPER E.L. (1973) Earthworm coelomocytes: Role in understanding the evolution of cellular immunity. I. Formation of monolayers and cytotoxicity, pp. 381–404. *Proc. III International Colloquium on Invertebrate Tissue Culture*, eds Rehacek J., Blaskovic D. & Hink W.F. Publishing House of the Slovak Academy of Sciences, Bratislava.

COOPER E.L. (1974a) Contemporary Topics in Immunobiology, **4,** Plenum Press (299 pp.).

COOPER E.L. (1974b) Phylogeny of leucocytes: earthworm coelomocytes *in vitro* and *in vivo*. In *Proc. 8th Leukocyte Culture Conference*, University of Uppsala, Academic Press, pp. 155-162.

COOPER E.L. & BACULI B.S. (1968a) Cell responses during xenograft rejection in annelids. *Anat. Rec.* **160,** 335.

COOPER E.L. & BACULI B.S. (1968b) Degenerative changes in the annelid, *Lumbricus terrestris. J. Geront.* **23,** 375.

COOPER E.L. & RUBILOTTA L.M. (1969) Allograft rejection in *Eisenia foetida. Transplantation* **8,** 220.

Cooper E.L., Acton R.T., Weinheimer P. & Evans E.E. (1969) Lack of a bacterial response in the earthworm *Lumbricus terrestris* after immunization with bacterial antigens. *J. Invert. Pathol.* **14,** 402.

Cooper E.L., Beller J. & Hayes S.A. (1970) A successful medium for maintaining earthworms. *Laboratory Animals* **4,** 25.

Cooper E.L., Lemmi C.A.E. & Moore T.C. (1974) Agglutinins and cellular immunity in earthworms. *Ann. New York Acad. Sci.* **234,** 34.

Cushing J.E. (1957) Tissue transplantation in *Pecten irradians. Biol. Bull.* **113,** 327.

Cushing J.E. (1962) Blood groups in marine animals and immune mechanisms of lower vertebrates and invertebrates (comparative immunology). *Proc. Conf. on Immuno-Reproduction,* La Jolla, Calif. The Population Council, New York, N.Y.

Cushing J.E., Boraker D. & Keough E. (1965) Reactions of sipunculid worms to intracoelomic injections of homologous eggs. *Fed. Proc.* **24,** 504.

Des Voigne D.M. & Sparks A.K. (1969) The process of wound healing in the Pacific oysters, *Crassostrea gigas* (Thunberg). *J. Invert. Pathol.* **12,** 53.

Drew G.H. & De Morgan W. (1910) The origin and formation of fibrous tissue produced as a reaction to injury in *Pectin maximus,* as a type of lamellibranchiata. *Quart. J. Micros. Sci.* **55,** 595.

Du Pasquier L. (1974) The genetic control of histo-compatibility reactions: phylogenetic aspects. *Arch. de. Biol.* p. 41.

Du Pasquier L. & Duprat P. (1968) Aspects humoreaux et cellulaires d'une immunité naturelle non spécifique chez l'oligachète *Eisenia foetida* sur (Lumbricidae). *C. R. Acad. Sci. Paris* **266,** 538.

Duprat P. (1964) Mise en evidence de reaction immunitaire dans les homogreffes de paroi du corps chez le Lombricien *Eisenia foetida. C. R. Acad. Sci. Paris* **259,** 4177.

Duprat P. (1967) Etude de la prise et du maintien d'un greffon de paroi du corps chez le lombricien *Eisenia foetida* typica. *Ann. Inst. Past.* **113,** 867.

Duprat P. & Lasalle A.M. (1967) Etude du liquide coelomique du Lombricien *Eisenia foetida* Sav. dans quelques cas experimentaux. *C. R. Acad. Sci. Paris* **264,** 386.

Duprat-Chateaureynaud P. (1970) Specificity of the allograft rejection in *Eisenia foetida.* In Symposium on *Phylogeny of Transplantation Reactions,* eds Hildemann W.H. & Cooper E.L. *Trans. Proc.* **2,** 222.

Duprat-Chateaureynaud P. (1971) Etude des reactions de défense de nature humorale chez le Lombricien *Eisenia foetida. C. R. Acad. Sci. Paris* **273,** 1647.

Duprat-Chateaureynaud P. & Izoard F. (1972) Etude *in vitro* de l'histocompatibilité chez les Lombriciens. *C. R. Acad. Sci. Paris* **275,** 2795.

Ephrussi B. & Beadle G.W. (1936) A technique for transplantation for *Drosophila. Am. Nat.* **70,** 218.

Freeman G. (1970) Transplantation specificity in echinoderms and lower chordates. *Transpl. Proc.* **2,** 236.

Galtsoff P.S. (1925) Regeneration after dissociation (an experimental study on sponges). I. Behavior of dissociated cells of *Microciona prolifera* under normal and altered conditions. *J. Exptl Zool.* **42,** 183.

Gasic G.K. & Galanti N.L. (1966) Proteins and disulfide groups in the aggregation of dissociated cells of sea sponges. *Sci.* **151,** 203.

Ghiradella H.T. (1965) The reactions of two starfishes, *Patiria miniata* and *Asterias forbesi,* to foreign tissue in the coelom. *Biol. Bull.* **128,** 77.

Goldstein L. (1970) Nucleo-cytoplasmic incompatibilities in free-living amoeba. *Trans. Proc.* **2,** 191.

Hadorn E. (1937) Transplantation of gonads from lethal to normal larvae in *Drosophila melanogaster. Proc. Soc. Exptl Biol. Med.* **36,** 632.

HAECKEL E. (1891) Anthropogenic oder Entwicke lungsgeschichte des Menschen. *Keimes- und Stammes-Geschichte*. 4th rev. & enl. ed. Wilhelm Engelmann, Leipzig.

HAUENSCHILD C. (1954) Genetische und entwicklungs-physiologische untersuchungen über intersexualität und gewebeverträglichkeit bei *Hydractinia echinata* Flemm (Hydroz. Baugainvill.) *Roux Arch. Entwick lungsmechanik* **147,** 1.

HAUENSCHILD C. (1956) Ueber die Vererbung einer gewebertiäg lichkeits-Eigenschaft bei dem Hydroidpolypen *Hydractinia echinata. Z. Naturforsch* **2,** 132.

HILDEMANN W.H. (1972) Phylogeny of transplantation reactivity. In *Transplantation Antigens, Markers of Biological Individuality*. Academic Press, Inc., New York and London, pp. 3–73.

HILDEMANN W.H. & COHEN N. (1967) Weak histoincompatibilities: emerging immunogenetic rules and generalizations. In *Histocompatibility Testing*. Munksgaard, Copenhagen 13.

HILDEMANN W.H. & COOPER E.L. (1970) Phylogeny of transplantation reactions. *Trans. Proc.* **2,** 179.

HILDEMANN W.H. & DIX T.G. (1972) Transplantation reactions of tropical Australian echinoderms. *Transplantation* **15,** 624.

HILDEMANN W.H. & REDDY A.L. (1973) Phylogeny of immune responsiveness: marine invertebrates. *Fed. Proc.* **32,** 2188.

HILDEMANN W.H., DIX T.G. & COLLINS J.D. (1974) Tissue transplantation in diverse marine invertebrates. In *Contemporary Topics In Immunobiology*, **4,** ed. Cooper E.L. (299 pp.).

HOSTETTER R.K. & COOPER E.L. (1972a) Coelomocytes as effector cells in earthworm immunity. *Immunol. Comm.* **1,** 155.

HOSTETTER R.K. & COOPER E.L. (1972b) Coelomocytes as effector cells in earthworm immunity. *Fed. Proc.* **31,** 4086.

HOSTETTER R.K. & COOPER E.L. (1974a) Earthworm cellular immunity. In *Contemporary Topics in Immunobiology*, **4,** ed. Cooper E.L. Plenum Press (299 pp.).

HOSTETTER R.K. & COOPER E.L. (1974b) Cellular anamnesis in earthworms. *Cell. Immunol.* **9:** 384.

HUMPHREYS T. (1963) Chemical dissolution and *in vitro* reconstitution of sponge cell adhesions. I. Isolation and functional demonstration of the components involved. *Develop. Biol.* **8,** 27.

HUMPHREYS T. (1967) The cell surfaces and specific cell aggregation, pp. 199–210. In *The Specificity of Cell Surfaces*, eds Davis B.D. & Warren L. Prentice Hall Inc., Englewood Cliffs, N.J.

IVKER F. (1972) A hierarchy of histo-incompatibility in *Hydractinia echinata. Biol. Bull.* **143,** 162.

IZOARD D. (1964) Évolution de greffes hétéroplastiques de paroi du corps realisees, chez les Lombriciens, entre animaux de meme genre mais d'espèces differentes. Recherches sur le genre *Lumbricus. C. R. Acad. Sci. Paris* **258,** 5972.

JEON K.W., LORCH I.J. & DANIELLI J.F. (1970) Reassembly of living cells from dissociated components. *Science* **167,** 1626.

JERNE N.K. (1967) Summary: Waiting for the end. Cold Spring Harbor Symp. *Quant. Biol.* **32,** 591.

JERNE N.K. (1969) The complete solution of immunology. *Aust. Ann. Med.* **4,** 345.

JERNE N.K. (1971) The somatic generation of immune recognition. *Eu. J. Immunol.* **1,** 1.

JOEST E. (1897) Transplantationsversuche an Lumbriciden. Morphologie und physiologie der transplantationen. *Archiv für Entwicklungsmechanik der Organismen* **5,** 419.

JOHN H.A., CAMPO M.S., MACKENZIE A.M. & KEMP R.B. (1971) Role of different sponge cell types in species specific cell aggregation. *Nature* **230,** 126.

KAMBYSELLIS M.P. (1968) Interspecific transplantation as a tool for indicating phylogenetic relationships. *Proc. Nat. Acad. Sci.* **59,** 1166.

KAMBYSELLIS M.P. (1970) Compatibility in insect tissue transplantations. I. Ovarian transplantations and hybrid formation between *Drosophila* species endemic to Hawaii. *J. Exptl Zool.* **175,** 169.

KINDRED J.E. (1929) The leucocytes and leucocytopoietic organs of an oligochaete, *Pheretima indica* (Horst). *J. Morph. Physiol.* **47,** 435.

KORSCHELT E. (1896–8) Über regenerations und transplantations veguche an Lumbriciden. *Verh. Deutsch. Zoolog. Gesellsch* 6–8, 79.

KORSCHELT E. (1927a) Kapital 7 Transplantations versuche an anneliden, pp. 304–79. *Regeneration und Transplantation.* Verlag von Gebrüder Borntraeger, Berlin.

KORSCHELT E. (1927b) *Regeneration und Transplantation,* pp. 332–3. Verlag von Gebrüder Borntraeger, Berlin.

KORSCHELT E. (1929) Zur frage der morphogenetischen induktion nach transplantation. *W. Rous Archiv. f. Entwicklungsmechanik* **117,** 1.

LEMMI C.A., COOPER E.L. & MOORE T.C. (1973a) Histamine and kinin metabolism in earthworms: techniques for their study. *Internat. Res. Comm. Sys.* 29-1-1.

LEMMI C.A., COOPER E.L. & MOORE T.C. (1973b) Immune challenge: effect of histamine and kinin metabolism in earthworms. *Internat. Res. Comm. Sys.* 29-1-2.

LEMMI C.A., COOPER E.L. & MOORE T.C. (1974c) Activity of ^{51}Cr labelled earthworm coelomocytes. In *Contemporary Topics In Immunobiology,* **4,** ed Cooper E.L. Plenum Press (299 pp.).

LEYPOLDT H. (1911) Transplantationsversuche an Lumbriciden. Zur Beeinflussung der Regeneration eines kleinen Pfropfstückes durch einen grösseren Komponenten. *Roux's Archiv. für Entwickelungsmechanik* **31,** 1.

LIEBMANN E. (1942) The coelomocytes of lumbricidae. *J. Morphol.* **71,** 221.

LINDH N.O. (1959) Heteroplastic transplantation of transversal body sections in flatworms. *Arkiv für Zool.* **12,** 183.

LOEB L. (1945) *The Biological Basis of Individuality.* C. C. Thomas, Springfield, Ill.

MACLENNAN A.P. (1969) An immunochemical study of the surfaces of sponge cells. *J. Exptl Zool.* **172,** 253.

MACLENNAN A.P. (1970) Polysaccharides from sponges and their possible significance in cellular aggregation. *Symp. Zool. Soc. Lond.* **25,** 299.

MACLENNAN A.P. & DODD R.Y. (1967) Promoting activity of extra-cellular materials on sponge cell reaggregation. *J. Embryol. Exp. Morph.* **17,** 473.

METCHNIKOFF E. (1892) *Lecons sur la Pathologie Comparee de l'Inflammation,* pp. xi + 239. Paris, Masson.

MÖLLER G. & MÖLLER E. (1966) Interaction between allogeneic cells in tissue transplantation. *Ann. N.Y. Acad. Sci.* **129,** 735.

NOSSAL G.J.V. (1971) Summary of the Third International Congress of The Transplantation Society: A Personal Approach. *Transpl. Proc.* **3,** 967.

OKA H. & WATANABE H. (1960) Problems of colony specificity in compound ascidians. *Bull. Biol.* **10,** 153.

RABES O. (1902) Transplantationsversuche an Lumbriciden. *Archiv. für Entwicklungsmechanik der Organismen.* Verlag von Wilhelm Engelmann **13,** 239.

REINISCH C.L. & BANG F.B. (1971) Cell recognition: Reactions of the sea star (*Asterias vulgaris*) to the injection of amebocytes of sea urchin (*Arbacia puntulata*). *Cell. Immunol.* **2,** 496.

SALT G. (1970) *The Cellular Defence Reactions of Insects.* Cambridge University Press, Cambridge.

SARA M., LIACI L. & MELONE N. (1966a) Bispecific cell aggregation in sponges. *Nature* **210,** 1167.

SARA M., LIACI L. & MELONE N. (1966b) Mixed cell aggregation between sponges and the anthozoan *Anemonia sulcata. Nature* **210,** 1168.

SCOTT F.M. & SCHUH J.E. (1963) Intraspecific reaggregation in *Amaroecium constellatum* labelled with tritiated thymidine. *Acta Emb. Morph. Exp.* **6,** 39.

SCOTT M.T. (1971) Recognition of foreignness in invertebrates. Transplantation studies using the American cockroach, *Periplaneta americana. Transplantation* **11,** 78.

SPIEGEL M. (1954) The role of specific surface antigens in cell adhesion. I. The reaggregation of sponge cells. *Biol. Bull.* **106,** 130.

SPINNER W. (1969) Transplantationsversuche zur blastemgliederung, regenerations und differen zierungsleistung der beinanlagen von *Culex pipiens* (L.). *Wilhelm Roux Archiv.* **163,** 259.

STANG-VOSS C. (1971) Zur ultrastruktur der blutzellen wirbelloser tiere. IV. Die Hämocyten von *Eisenia foetida* L. (Sav) (Annelidae) *Z. Zellforsch* **117,** 451.

STEPHENSON J. (1930) *The Oligochaeta.* Clarendon Press, Oxford.

TANAKA K. (1973) Allogeneic inhibition in a compound ascidian, *Botryllus primigenus* Oka. II. Cellular and humoral responses in 'nonfusion' reaction. *Cell. Immunol.* **7,** 427.

TANAKA K. & WATANABE H. (1973) Allogeneic inhibition in a compound ascidian, *Botryllus primigenus* Oka. I. Processes and features of 'nonfusion' reaction. *Cell. Immunol.* **7,** 410.

TARTAR V. (1964) *Experimental techniques with ciliates in Methods in Cell Physiology.* Vol. 1, pp. 109–125, ed. Prescott D.M. Academic Press, New York.

TARTAR V. (1970) Transplantation in Protozoa. In Symposium on *Phytogeny of Transplantation Reactions,* New York, eds Hildemann W.H. & Cooper E.L. *Trans Proc.* **2,** 183.

THEODOR J. (1966) Contribution à l'étude des gorgones (V) Les greffes chez les gorgones: etude d'un système de reconnaissana de tissu. *Bull. Inst. Oceanogr. Monaco* **66,** 3.

THEODOR J. (1969) Histotoxicité *in vivo* et *in vitro* entre tissue xénogénique et entre tissus allogéniques chez un Invertébré. *C. R. Acad. Sci. Paris* **268,** 2534.

THEODOR J. (1970) Distinction between 'self' and 'not-self' in lower invertebrates. *Nature* **227,** 690.

THOMAS L. (1959) Untitled contribution to the discussion in *Cellular and humoral aspects of the hypersensitive states,* p. 529, ed. Lawrence H.S. Hoeber Harper, New York.

TOTH S.E. (1967) Tissue compatibility in regenerating explants from the colonial marine hydroid *Hydractinia echinata J. Cell. Physiol.* **69,** 125.

TRIPP M.R. (1961) The fate of foreign materials experimentally introduced into the snail *Australorbis glabratus. J. Parasitol.* **47,** 745.

TYLER A. (1947) An auto-antibody concept of cell structure, growth and differentiation. *Symp. Soc. Study Develop. Growth* **6,** 7.

VALEMBOIS P. (1963) Étude anatomique de l'évolution de greffons hétéroplastiques de paroi du corps chez quelques Lombriciens. *C. R. Acad. Sci. Paris* **257,** 3227.

VALEMBOIS P. (1968) Libération de phosphatase acide dans les cellules musculaires d'un greffon de paroi du corps dhez un Lombricien. *J. Microscopic.* **7,** 61a.

VALEMBOIS P. (1970) Etude d'une heterogreffe de paroi du corps chez les Lombriciens. Aspects cytologiques, physiologiques et immunologiques de l'evolution du greffon (*Allolobophora caliginosa* Duges) et de la reaction du porte-greffe *Eisenia foetida* Sav. *Study of heterografts of body wall in earthworms.* Thesis for Doctor of Natural Science, No. 281. Bordeaux.

WEISS P. (1947) The problem of specificity in growth and development. *Yale J. Biol. Med.* **19,** 235.

WILSON H.V. (1907) On some phenomena of coalescence and regeneration in sponges. *J. Exptl Zool.* **5,** 245.

WINGER L.A. & COOPER E.L. (1969) Effect of temperature on the first-set xenograft rejection in the earthworm *Eisenia foetida. Am. Zool.* **9,** 352.

Chapter 4. Factors Involved in the Recognition of Foreign Material by Phagocytic Cells from Invertebrates

C. R. Jenkin

Introduction

The function of phagocytic cells of invertebrates

Factors involved in the recognition of foreign material by phagocytic cells from vertebrates

Removal of foreign particles from the circulation of invertebrates

***In vitro* studies on phagocytosis in invertebrates**

The physico-chemical properties of haemagglutinins in serum from invertebrates

Conclusion

Introduction

One of the striking phenomena in biology and one which must have played an important role in the evolution of multicellular animals was the ability of certain specialized cells, phagocytes, to recognize and remove unwanted material.

These cells are not only capable of discriminating between 'self' components and foreign exogenous materials such as food particles and micro-organisms but also between 'self' components that are functional and those components that are effete or damaged. Indeed, as suggested by Boyden (1963), it is unlikely that the development of animals would have evolved beyond the unicellular stage had it not been for the existence of a discriminatory mechanism capable of distinguishing between functional and damaged indigenous components as well as foreign materials of the environment.

However, despite the importance of this recognition phenomenon in the life and development of invertebrates and vertebrates, we are surprisingly ignorant of the mechanisms involved particularly at the comparative level.

It might be pertinent therefore, to review in a general fashion and from a historical point of view, the function and ability of phagocytic cells of invertebrates to distinguish between self and non-self.

The function of the phagocytic cells of invertebrates

In the invertebrates, phagocytic cells which have been given various names such as coelomocytes, amoebocytes and haemocytes play an important role in the nutrition, differentiation, and defence of the host against potential parasites, as well as repair of tissue damage. Since in each of these roles within any individual the phagocytic cells are merely recognizing a difference between the host's functional tissues and something that is foreign or 'unwanted' it is difficult to envisage a separate recognition mechanism for each. However, until considerably more work is done on these fundamental problems one can only quote examples of the diverse functions of these cells.

In order to develop this theme one might consider first the selective feeding of the Protozoa, for like the phagocytic cells of the Metazoa they are able to discriminate between different kinds of particles. It has been noted for example, that *Amoeba proteus* will ingest either the flagellate Chilomonas or the ciliate Colpidium in preference to the flagellate Monas. The size and form of Chilomonas and Monas is similar yet amoeba given equal amounts of each of these species engulfed almost 100 times as many Chilomonas individuals as they did Monas (Mast & Hahnert 1935). Whilst at present we know little regarding the molecular basis of this phenomenon some lines of evidence would suggest that this recognition may be dependent on the interaction of complementary molecules. Thus Roy (1951) found that *Hartmonella* were capable of capturing large numbers of motile bacteria by a process of agglutination. More recently Jeon and Bell (1965) have suggested that the chemotactic movements of *Amoeba proteus* towards hydra tissues may be dependent on the release of macromolecules from the damaged hydra which combine with the surface of the *Amoeba*. In their initial studies they found that pieces of Hydra elicited a powerful chemotactic response for free-living *A. proteus*. Crude extracts of the hydra tissue were also chemotactic, the substance(s) being non dialysable. The preliminary analysis of the extract indicated that it was rich in basic amino acids. They suggested that the chemotactic principle may be a macromolecule having basic properties which combines with the polysaccharide of the mucous coat of the amoeba. This combination alters the physico-chemical properties of the surface causing the formation of pseudopods on the side of the cell nearest the source of the chemotactic principle.

In many of the other invertebrate phyla the nutrition of the individual depends on the phagocytosis of nutrients by specialized cells (Yonge 1937). In many instances, such as in the coelenterates, intracellular digestion may take place in fixed phagocytic cells of the endoderm lining the coelomic cavity. In other instances wandering amoebocytes digest and transport the products. For example in the sponges (*Porifera*) the choanocytes, cells lining the cavity of the animal, are responsible for capturing the micro-organisms present in the water drawn in through the ostia. However, little or no digestion takes place in these cells, the food being passed to and digested by amoebocytes. In many of the molluscs and echinoderms amoebocytes may pass into the lumen of the gut where they actively ingest food particles which they carry back to the tissues and digest. These are but a few examples, but they serve to illustrate the importance of the wandering phagocytic cells in host nutrition. It would be interesting to know to what extent a similar though perhaps more limited function is performed by the phagocytic cells of vertebrates.

It was Metchnikoff who first focused attention on the role these wandering phagocytes play in host resistance to various infections. He also stressed the importance of these cells as scavengers in areas of tissue damage, and showed by a number of simple experiments the capacity of these cells to surround and ingest non-living particles introduced into the host tissues (Metchnikoff 1907).

In a similar series of experiments with the echinoderm (*Asterias rubins*), Durham (1888) noted that particles of indian ink or aniline blue injected into the coelom were rapidly ingested by coelomocytes which then passed to the exterior of the animal. This method of getting rid of indigestable foreign material appears to be a widespread phenomenon and has been reported for example in the earthworm (*Lumbricus terrestris*), the oyster (*Crassostrea virginica*) and more recently in the clam (*Tridacna maxima*) (Cameron 1932, Tripp 1966, Reade & Reade 1972).

In certain other species of invertebrates, specialized cells known as urn cells seem also to play an important role in host defence. Cantacuzène (1922a) noticed that red cells or bacteria introduced into the cavity of a sipunculid worm (*Sipunculus nudus*) were rapidly agglutinated to the posterior part of the urn cell. This is reminiscent of the reaction observed with certain species of amoebae (Roy 1951). Amoebocytes were then attracted to the agglutinated mass and proceeded to ingest the agglutinate. Cantacuzène observed also that a fine distinction was made between self components injected into the cavity, and the foreign material. No agglutination of the former being noted. In a further extension of these studies he observed that in worms of this species that had been previously vaccinated with living bacteria, there was a marked increase in the number of urn cells. When rechallenged with the vaccinating strain of bacteria the secretion of the urns increased and following the agglutination of bacteria to their surface a much more rapid phagocytosis of the agglutinated mass by the amoebocytes was noted (Cantacuzène 1922b). If the bacteria were mixed with urn cells either from vaccinated worms or from normal worms *in vitro*, then whilst precipitation of urn cells and bacteria took place in both systems, the degree of precipitation was much more marked in the 'immune' system.

Unfortunately, in a great many of these early studies there is a lack of quantitative data, thus in Cantacuzène's investigations no figures are given of the increase in number of urns or how the increased secretion was determined.

An increase in the number of cells participating in the host's response to injected foreign matter has been observed in other species of invertebrates. Cameron (1932) noted a rapid increase in the number of 'lymphocytes' in earthworms that had been injected with particles such as carbon and bacteria. Similar reactions were seen in caterpillars of various species of lepidoptera (Cameron 1934). The increase in the numbers of phagocytic cells following injection of foreign material has its counterpart in the vertebrates.

Echinoderms belonging to the order Apoda of the Class Holothuroidea have specialized arrangements of the citiated urn cells. Thus in some of the Apoda a number of urns may be arranged on mesenterial folds forming what have been called trees of urns. Following injection of carmine there is an accumulation of this material in the cavity of the urns (Schultz 1895, Clark 1899, Cuenot 1902).

The organization of the phagocytic cells is interesting and whilst initially it might have been of equal importance in nutrition as well as defence, once a complete extracellular mode of digestion had developed the retention of such organized structures in situations where they could monitor the body fluids would be clearly of great advantage in host defence. Thus in the crayfish (*Parachaeraps bicarinatus*) specialized phagocytic cells line the sinuses of the hepato-pancreas and remove injected particles such as bacteria and carbon (Reade 1968, McKay & Jenkin 1970a). This situation is very reminiscent of that in vertebrates where fixed phagocytic cells line the liver sinuses.

As well as being of importance in nutrition and defence the phagocytes of invertebrates play an important role in the development and differentiation of the animal.

In freshwater sponges the embryo escapes from the maternal tissues as a completely flagellated larva. After swimming for a few hours to several days, the larva fixes by the anterior pole and the canal system develops. The flagellated cells of the surface are no longer required and are phagocytosed (Hyman 1940). In *Eucumaria laevigeta* and *Mesothuria intestinalis*, both holothuroids, the developing tubules of the gonadial base are sexually indifferent at first but some become female and release eggs as they lengthen. Finally, these female elements are destroyed by coelomocytes and the basal tubules then lengthen and produce sperm. Eventually these tubules are also phagocytosed and replaced by newly transformed female tubules (Ackermann 1902, Theèl 1901). Phagocytosis also plays an important role in the metamorphosis of insects in removing cells that are dead and in the process of autolysis. In the blood of the pupa of the blowfly *Caliphora*, haemocytes may be observed packed with fragments of disintegrated tissue (Wigglesworth 1950). Prior to metamorphosis, in some insects, the numbers of circulating haemocytes may be small, though they may be found adhering to various tissues. At the time of metamorphosis large numbers of cells are released from the haemocytopoietic tissue and there may be occasions when the haemocytes themselves actually divide (Arvy 1953, Harvey Williams 1961, Lea & Gilbert 1961).

From this broad introduction it is clear that the phagocytes of invertebrates are as capable of discriminating between self and unwanted material as are the phagocytes of vertebrates. However, these *in vivo* studies offer little explanation as to the underlying mechanism.

Before considering more recent literature in the field, much of which has been done *in vitro* with cell cultures, it would be valuable to consider what is known about this mechanism in vertebrates so that if possible comparisons may be made.

Factors involved in the recognition of foreign material by phagocytic cells from vertebrates

Based on his studies in the invertebrates Metchnikoff suggested that phagocytic cells were of prime importance in the defence of the organism against disease (Metchnikoff 1907), a hypothesis which Metchnikoff first gave to a meeting at Odessa in 1883. Apparently the important implications of this hypothesis in general passed unnoticed. In a continuation of these studies Metchnikoff in 1884 published two papers concerned with the importance of amoebocytes in protecting Daphnia from a fungal disease and phagocytes in protecting vertebrates from the anthrax bacillus. These investigations were criticized by a number of investigators, perhaps the most vociferous being Baumgarten, and the general hypothesis was at times bitterly attacked. von Behring (1888) showed that the blood of rats destroyed the anthrax bacillus with great rapidity in the absence of phagocytic cells. These observations, which were expanded by a number of investigations, were the basis for the humoral theory of immunity, a theory that received far more acclaim than the phagocytic one. The discovery of antibody by von Behring and Kitasato (1890) in their studies with bacterial toxins further strengthened the humoral hypothesis. However, by the late 1890s much more consideration was given to the thesis of Metchnikoff such that Lord Lister in his Presidential Address to the British Association of the Advancement of Science in 1896, stated that if there was a romantic chapter in pathology it had surely been that of the story of phagocytosis (Lister 1896). This was indeed a far cry from Baumgarten's paper in 1888 in which he said that the arguments that Metchnikoff gives to justify his theory are contrary to logic and the truth (Baumgarten 1888).

These opposite points of view were resolved largely through the work of

Wright and Douglas (1903). They incubated white blood cells in thin capillary tubes with *Staphylococcus aureus* in the presence of serum or plasma. A cell smear was made after fifteen minutes and the number of bacteria ingested by a certain number of phagocytes counted. Significant phagocytosis of *S. aureus* by polymorphonuclear cells occurred only in the presence of serum or plasma.

Wright spoke of this action of serum as an 'opsonic' effect (*opsono*—I cater for; I prepare victuals for), and employed the term 'opsonins' to designate those elements in serum or plasma which promoted phagocytosis. Sera from patients immunized with vaccines prepared from various bacteria were found to have a greater opsonic titre against those strains than sera from normal patients. These *in vitro* tests were carried out with polymorphonuclear cells from normal donors.

More recent research has established that these opsonins are specific antibodies (Benacerraf *et al.* 1959, Cohn & Morse 1959, Mackaness 1960, Jenkin & Benacerraf 1960, Jenkin & Rowley 1961, Biozzi & Stiffel 1961).

While many workers have established that non-living particles such as carbon, carmine, and quartz are readily ingested by phagocytic cells, it is only in the last decade that the mechanism involved in the recognition of these non-living particles has received much consideration. Fenn (1921) found that polymorphonuclear cells ingested carbon and quartz particles only in the presence of serum. Using particles with similar dimensions he showed that carbon was ingested more readily than quartz and suggested that this was related to the greater adsorbtive properties of carbon for serum proteins.

Whilst this particular area is still a matter of controversy a number of investigations indicate that immunoglobulin molecules adsorbed to the surface of the particle are an essential pre-requisite for recognition to take place (Nelson & Lebrun 1956, Jenkin & Rowley 1961, Potter & Stollerman 1961, Murray 1963, Normann & Benditt 1965).

Likewise investigations, beyond the scope of this review, concerned with the cellular events involved in the production of antibody show that the recognition of antigen may be mediated by specific immunoglobulins either on the surface of cells or free in the serum.

Whilst these experiments demonstrate that a specific group of proteins, the immunoglobulins play an important role in recognition, they offer no explanation as to the mechanism which enables phagocytic cells to recognize the antigen/antibody complex. However, studies by Berken and Benacerraf (1966) would suggest that when the immunoglobulin reacts with foreign material there is some distortion of the molecule in the Fc region which opens up a site complementary to a receptor site on the membrane of the phagocyte. These observations are substantiated by the finding that (Fab)2 fragments are not opsonic (Spiegel *et al.* 1963). Thus the final phase of recognition involves a binding between these two sites.

A further interesting aspect regarding this reaction is that the number of antibody molecules required to initiate recognition is small and varies according to the immunoglobulin class. Rowley and Turner (1966) calculated that one bacterium need have only nine molecules of 19S IgM antibody or 2,200 molecules of 7S IgG on its surface. A similar order of magnitude for IgG antibody was found by Jackson and Jenkin (1968) studying the interaction of mouse macrophages with *Salmonella typhimurium.*

It would be pertinent now to discuss recent and more quantitative experiments concerning this reaction in the invertebrates.

Removal of foreign particles from the circulation of invertebrates

One of the main problems in considering this phenomenon in invertebrates is related to the great diversity of these animals. In any discussion on the present topic this diversity should be borne in mind since it is possible that observations on and conclusions drawn from one group may not necessarily be applicable to others.

Pauley, Krassner and Chapman (1971) followed the removal of five different strains of bacteria from the circulation of the Californian sea hare (*Aplysia californica*). While four of the five strains were removed rapidly from the circulation it was found that *Serratia marcescens* was still present in large numbers after 16 days. Examination of the haemolymph showed that there were agglutinins present for the four strains of bacteria that were removed rapidly but none against *S. marcescence*. Furthermore, concomitant with the removal of bacteria from the circulation, there was a drop in the agglutinin titres. This type of evidence led the workers to suggest that the agglutinins functioned as opsonins for these bacteria.

Other investigations in insects have indicated the possible role of a humoral factor which enables haemocytes to recognize the eggs of the parasite (*Cardiochiles nigriceps*). When eggs from this parasite were implanted into *Heliothis zea*, they were encapsulated, whereas in *H. virescens* they survived and developed normally. Further studies showed that if the eggs were left in *H. zea* for varying periods of time, then cleared of adhering cells and transferred to the susceptible host *H. virescens*, they were encapsulated. These results suggested the possibility that the resistant host possessed recognition factors that are absent in the susceptible host (Salt 1960, 1961).

Recent *in vivo* studies by Tyson and Jenkin (1973) have shown that the rate of elimination of bacteria from the circulation of the freshwater crayfish (*Parachaeraps bicarinatus*) varied with the strain of bacteria injected. These results suggested, by analogy with the vertebrates, that the rate of elimination might be related to the titre of recognition factors circulating in the haemolymph.

In order to test this hypothesis use was made of blockade type experiments. If, in vertebrates that have just eliminated a primary dose of bacteria from the circulation, a second similar dose of the same strain is injected, the latter is removed from the circulation much more slowly. However, if the second dose is pretreated (opsonized) with specific antibody the rate of elimination may be returned to normal. This type of experiment is a very sensitive assay for antibody. Similar experiments to these were performed with crayfish. The data showed that crayfish could be blockaded and this could be reversed by pretreating the second dose with haemolymph taken from normal animals. Prior adsorption of the haemolymph used for opsonization with the specific strain of bacteria prevents the reversal of blockade. Further, it was found that if the primary dose of bacteria was pretreated with haemolymph prior to injection, thus preventing removal of recognition factors when injected, the animal is not blockaded and the second dose is cleared at normal rates. These studies suggested that the recognition of bacteria by haemocytes of the crayfish is mediated by recognition factors circulating in haemolymph.

In vitro studies on phagocytosis in invertebrates

In vivo studies on the phagocytosis of particles whilst important are of limited value in defining the mechanisms involved in recognition. Until recently little research had been carried out *in vitro* on the phagocytosis of foreign particles by phagocytes from invertebrates. This was due in part to the difficulty of preparing suitable cell cultures or monolayers of cells. However, a few papers in this area have appeared in recent years indicating again the involvement of humoral factors in this recognition process.

Tripp (1966) demonstrated that monolayers of amoebocytes from the oyster (*Crassostrea virginica*) would ingest rabbit erythrocytes. Pretreatment of the erythrocytes with haemolymph from the oyster enhanced ingestion although comparable levels of phagocytosis could be obtained if the amoebocytes were incubated with untreated cells but for much longer periods of time.

Stuart (1968) has carried out a similar series of investigations using phagocytic cells from the octopus (*Eledone cirrosa*). Human erythrocytes were ingested by these cells only if they had been pretreated with haemolymph. Specific antibody raised in rabbits to these erythrocytes would not function as an opsonin in this particular system.

The specificity of these factors in invertebrates has received little attention. Using haemocytes from the snail (*Helix aspersa*) Prowse and Tait (1969) found that the ingestion of yeast cells and sheep erythrocytes was dependent on haemolymph factors. Adsorbing the haemolymph with yeast cells removed the opsonic activity against these particles but did not effect the ability of the haemolymph to opsonize sheep erythrocytes. These data indicate a measure of specificity in these reactions.

The recognition of foreignness by cells of the crayfish (*Parachaeraps bicarinatus*) has been examined by McKay and Jenkin (1970b). They found, as did Stuart (1968) working with the octopus, that the uptake of vertebrate erythrocytes was dependent on factors in the haemolymph. In a limited study they showed that the opsonin or recognition factors that enhance the uptake of sheep erythrocytes by crayfish haemocytes are phylum specific. There appeared to be a measure of specificity in this reaction since adsorbing the haemolymph with erythrocytes from one species of vertebrate still left opsonic activity toward the erythrocytes from another species.

In contrast to these observations Scott (1971) demonstrated that the adherence of sheep and chicken erythrocytes to the surface of haemocytes from the cockroach (*Periplanata americana*) is independent apparently of humoral factors. Adherence was reduced considerably by treating the monolayers with 0·2 per cent trypsin although lipase and lecithinase had little effect. It is conceivable that trypsin destroyed a 'receptor' for sheep erythrocytes which was on the surface of the haemocytes. Incubation of the trypsin-treated haemocytes with cockroach haemolymph failed to restore the ability of their cells to take up sheep erythrocytes, which suggested that the receptors, if free and of a cytophilic nature, were not present in the haemolymph to any significant level. The trypsin-treated haemocytes appeared viable as judged by trypan blue or neutral red uptake. Recently, Anderson *et al.* (1973) have found that the haemocytes from the cockroach (*Blaberus cranifer*) are capable of phagocytosing *in vitro* a number of different strains of bacteria. The uptake of bacteria was independent of haemolymph which suggests that recognition is mediated by membrane-associated receptors.

Quantitative studies *in vitro* on the phagocytosis of bacteria by haemocytes from the crayfish (*Parachaeraps bicarinatus*) showed that these cells are capable of taking up bacteria in the absence of haemolymph (Tyson & Jenkin 1974). This appears at first to contradict the previous findings by these same authors who showed that the elimination of bacteria from the circulation of the crayfish was dependent on recognition factors free in the haemolymph (Tyson & Jenkin 1973).

Further studies showed that if the haemocytes were treated with trypsin they were unable to ingest bacteria unless they had been opsonized with crayfish haemolymph. These data suggested that the recognition factors for bacteria were both on the membrane of the phagocyte and free in the haemolymph. This raises the interesting question as to whether they are the same? That is to say do the recognition factors in the haemolymph possess cytophilic properties or are the membrane associated factors an integral part of the cell membrane? In order to answer these questions the following experiments were performed. Monolayers of haemocytes were treated with trypsin and divided into two groups. One group was incubated in tissue culture medium with serum from the crayfish, whilst the other group was incubated in culture medium alone. Following the period of incubation the cells were washed *in situ* and unopsonized bacteria added to the monolayers. Only those monolayers pre-incubated with serum were able to phagocytose bacteria. One could argue that incubation in the presence of serum provided a richer nutritional environment and so the cells were able to resynthesize membrane-associated recognition factors. This seems unlikely since haemocytes incubated in serum that had been previously adsorbed with bacteria were unable to ingest unopsonized bacteria. This would suggest that the recognition factors free in the haemolymph are cytophilic (Tyson & Jenkin 1974).

Whilst the data obtained from studies on the cockroach and crayfish appear to conflict it is not improbable that they have similar recognition mechanisms. In the case of the cockroach the recognition factor may have a much higher affinity for the membrane of the haemocytes such that they may be absent from the haemolymph or present in very low titre.

Previous studies by McKay, Jenkin and Rowley (1969) showed that erythrocytes would not adhere to the haemocytes unless these particles had been pretreated with haemolymph. The results are at variance with those reported for bacteria (Tyson & Jenkin 1974). However, studies in the vertebrates offer an explanation for such observations. Miescher, Spiegelberg and Benacerraf (1963) showed that the amount of specific antibody required to facilitate the uptake of erythrocytes by phagocytes was greater than that required for bacteria due to the differences in surface area between the two particles. It is possible therefore, that the concentration of these molecules on the membrane of the crayfish haemocytes is not sufficient to bind erythrocytes but is sufficient to bind bacteria.

In summary, most *in vitro* studies on the uptake of particles by haemocytes from invertebrates indicate that recognition is facilitated by factors free in the haemolymph. In certain species of invertebrates these recognition factors may be associated with the membrane of the phagocytic cell.

Since some investigators have suggested that the haemagglutinins present in the sera from invertebrates function as the recognition units enabling invertebrate phagocytic cells recognize foreign erythrocytes, it might be pertinent to discuss what is known about the physico-chemical properties of such molecules (Tripp 1966, McKay & Jenkin 1970b).

The physico-chemical properties of haemagglutinins in serum from invertebrates

Extensive studies by Cantacuzène (1923) revealed the presence of haemagglutinins in the sera of invertebrates from various phyla such as the Annelida,

Arthropoda and Mollusca. Furthermore, his data indicated that in some cases these haemagglutinins were inducible by prior immunization with sheep or rabbit erythrocytes (Cantacuzène 1919). Such an observation has not been confirmed by recent research (Tripp 1966, McKay 1970).

The first attempts to purify the haemagglutinins from the haemolymph of invertebrates was carried out by Tyler and Metz (1945a). They found that the haemolymph obtained from the spiny lobster (*Panulirus interruptus*) agglutinated red cells from a number of different vertebrates and spermatozoa from invertebrates. Based on extensive cross adsorption studies with erythrocytes and spermatozoa, there appeared to be 8–10 different haemagglutinins. These haemagglutinins were purified by iso-electric precipitation at pH 4·8–5·0 which separated them from the haemocyanin (Tyler & Scheer 1945). Electrophoresis of this material revealed two components of which the more slowly migrating possessed the haemagglutinating activity. Antibodies raised against purified haemocyanin reacted with the purified haemagglutinins which led the authors to suggest that these proteins cross-reacted. However, it is possible that the haemocyanin preparation used for immunization was contaminated with the haemagglutinins and this resulted in antibodies to both materials.

More recently Marchalonis and Edelman (1968) have purified and characterized the haemagglutinin for horse erythrocytes from the horseshoe crab (*Limulus polyphemus*). Initially, haemocyanin was separated from the serum by ultra-centrifugation at 100,000 *g* for 5 h. The clear supernatant was further purified by zone electrophoresis on starch gel and the eluted fraction containing the haemagglutinating activity run on sephadex G200. The active fraction was used for further analysis. The molecular weight of the purified haemagglutinin was 400,000 and had a sedimentation coefficient of 13·4S. The molecule could be dissociated into sub-units of 67,000 molecular weight at pH 2·0 or pH 9·0. Further dissociation into units of 22,500 molecular weight could be achieved with either 20 per cent acetic acid or 8 M urea. Thus the haemagglutinin appears to be made up of 6 units each composed of three sub-units of 22,500 molecular weight. Electron micrographs of the purified haemagglutinin showed molecules with a very uniform ring-shaped structure. Close examination of the single molecules have indicated that they have a hexagonal shape with a six-fold symmetry which is consistent with the concept that the molecule is composed of six units. Although the haemagglutinin sub-unit has a molecular weight similar to the light chains of immunoglobulin and shows some similarity in amino acid composition (Table 4.1) it appears likely that the Limulus haemagglutinin and the antibodies of vertebrates are unrelated evolutionary developments. This is suggested from the fact that the sub-units are all of the same molecular weight and do not show the heterogeneity on starch gel electrophoresis characteristic of the polypeptide chains of antibody.

Acton *et al.* (1969) isolated and purified the haemagglutinin for sheep

Table 4.1. The amino acid composition of the purified haemagglutinins from various invertebrate species

Amino acids	Amino acid composition (moles per cent)					
	Phyla					
	Mollusca			Arthropoda		Echinodermata
	*Helix pomatia**	*Crassostrea virginica*†	*Velesunio ambiguus*‡	*Limulus polyphemus*§	*L. polyphemus*¶	*Asterias forbesi*¶
Aspartic acid	11·4	17·5	15·1	11·1	10·4	13·4
Threonine	5·9	6·3	6·4	6·6	6·0	8·7
Serine	10·9	3·7	15·3	8·15	6·7	7·9
Glutamic acid	7·6	9·9	8·9	12·1	12·9	13·8
Proline	6·5	3·7	2·2	5·0	3·9	6·0
Glycine	4·7	9·4	10·1	8·3	9·5	8·4
Alanine	5·4	7·9	6·4	4·7	5·3	6·0
Valine	7·3	3·0	6·4	5·0	7·4	7·4
Cysteine	2·9	5·1	0	3·0	2·5	5·2
Methionine	1·5	1·2	0	1·2	1·1	1·9
Isoleucine	6·0	4·1	1·15	4·5	5·0	4·9
Leucine	6·0	7·7	5·1	10·3	9·8	7·4
Tyrosine	4·6	2·1	0	3·7	1·4	1·8
Phenylalanine	2·1	2·8	12·7	3·9	3·8	2·8
Lysine	5·2	0	3·8	5.3	6.8	6.0
Histidine	1·3	11·1	2·6	4·3	5·3	2·2
Arginine	5·9	4·4	3·8	2·6	2·2	4·7
Tryptophane	4·5	Not done	Not done	Not done	Not done	Not done

* Data obtained from Hammerström and Kabat (1967). Expressed originally as residues/100,000 g protein.
† Data obtained from Acton, Bennett, Evans and Schrohenloher (1969). Expressed originally as mole/moles of protein.
‡ Data obtained from Jenkin and Rowley (1970). Expressed originally as g/100 g of protein.
§ Data obtained from Marchalonis and Edelman (1968). Expressed originally as g/100 g of protein.
¶ Data obtained from Finstad, Litman, Finstad and Good (1972). Expressed originally as μmole/mg protein.

erythrocytes from the oyster (*Crassostrea virginica*). The intact molecule had a sedimentation coefficient of 33·4S but could be dissociated into sub-units by acid or alkaline pH. Complete dissociation to a sub-unit of 20,000 mol. wt. could be obtained by dialysis against 5 M-guanidine-HCl at pH 7·5. Haemagglutinating activity was dependent on Ca^{++} ions and was abolished by dialysis against a chelating agent such as sodium citrate.

The haemagglutinin for human A erythrocytes from the snail (*Helix pomatia*) has been extracted from the albumin gland in a highly purified form (Hammarström & Kabat 1969). A single step purification was achieved by the specific adsorption of the snail haemagglutinin on to columns of polyleucine chemically coupled to purified hog mucin containing $A^{+}H$ blood group activities. The haemagglutinin was eluted with N-acetyl-D-galactosamine in physiological saline. The material was pure as judged by gel filtration and ultracentrifugation. The mol. wt. of the haemagglutinin was estimated to be 100,000 as determined from analytical ultra-centrifuge data. Amino acid analysis (Table 4.1) revealed that the molecule contained cysteine and was rich in aspartic acid, glutamic acid, serine, valine and arginine.

More recent work on this haemagglutinin (Hammarström 1973) has established that the intact molecule has a molecular weight of 79,000 as determined by further ultracentrifugation studies. The molecule can be dissociated into six sub-units of 13,000 molecular weight by reduction with excess dithiothreitol in 6 M-guanidine-HCl and alkylation with iodoacetamide. While the haemagglutinin is found in the albumin gland and eggs of snails it is absent from the haemolymph which suggests that it might have an important biological role in the reproductive processes of this animal but not be involved necessarily in the recognition of foreign material by the phagocytic cells from this animal.

Specific haemagglutinins to erythrocytes from various vertebrate species in the serum of the Murray mussel (*Velesunio ambiguus*) have been purified and characterized (Jenkin & Rowley 1970). Initially, whole serum was precipitated with 50 per cent $(NH_4)_2SO_4$ and the pellet containing haemagglutinating activity purified further on a sucrose density gradient. This material gave a symmetrical peak in the ultracentrifuge with a sedimentation coefficient of 28S. Further purification of the haemagglutinin specific for rabbit red cells was carried out on the material obtained from the sucrose density gradient. The haemagglutinin was adsorbed on to stroma prepared from rabbit erythrocytes and eluted with a glycine/HCl buffer at pH 3·0. This purified haemagglutinin was rich in aspartic acid, phenylalanine and glutamic acid (Table 4.1) but had only trace amounts of cysteine, methionine and tyrosine. The haemagglutinin from *V. ambiguus* appears to have a sub-unit structure similar to *Limulus polyphemus* (Marchalonis & Jenkin 1970, unpublished observations).

Recently, Finstad, Litman, Finstad and Good (1972) have described the purification of the haemagglutinins for horse erythrocytes from the horseshoe crab, *Limulus polyphemus* and the sea star, *Asterias forbesi.* Initially, serum from Limulus or coelomic fluid from Asterias were spun at 100,000 ***g*** in the ultracentrifuge to remove the haemocyanin. They were then subjected to zone electrophoresis on agar and finally, in the case of agglutinin from Asterias, run on a sucrose density gradient.

The activities of both agglutinins were completely dependent on Ca^{++} ions and dialysis against ethylenediaminotetra-acetate (EDTA) caused irreversible inactivation. The peptide maps of the tryptic digests of the respective agglutinins were dissimilar in their patterns and also from the patterns of purified light and heavy chains of vertebrate immunoglobulins.

The Limulus agglutinin and Asterias agglutinin were of different molecular size having sedimentation coefficients of 12·6S and 6·5S respectively. Both consisted of sub-units of 25–30,000 mol. wt. as defined by polyacrylamide gel electrophoresis in sodium dodecyl sulphate. The amino acid analysis (Table 4.1) of these agglutinins revealed that they were rich in aspartic and glutamic acid and there were also detectable levels of cysteine.

From these studies it is quite clear that there are considerable differences in the molecular weight of the haemagglutinins purified from various invertebrates, ranging from greater than 1,000,000 to 79,000. However, there are certain interesting similarities. Amino acid analysis indicate that all the haemagglutinins are rich in aspartic and glutamic acid (Table 4.1). These proteins all possess a sub-unit structure and can be dissociated into these sub-units by a series of different chemical treatments which do not destroy disulphide linkages. It would appear also that these sub-units are dissimilar to the purified light and heavy chains of vertebrate immunoglobulins.

Whilst the above indicate structural similarities between the haemagglutinins, they have not been tested, unfortunately, for their biological function factors. Recently, Tyson and Jenkin (unpublished observation) have purified the haemagglutinins and recognition factors for bacteria in crayfish serum. Rabbits were immunized with sheep erythrocytes preopsonized with crayfish serum. The immunoglobulin fraction of the rabbit antiserum was coupled to Biogel A50M for use as an affinity column. Such a column not only removed all the haemagglutinating activity but also the opsonic activity from crayfish serum. Since previous studies had shown that there were opsonins specific for bacteria and also for erythrocytes in the serum, the fact that you could remove all these activities by such a column as the above indicated that these molecules were antigenically related. This was substantiated further by the observation that an affinity column prepared from an antiserum raised in rabbits against opsonized bacteria whilst removing all the opsonizing activity also removed the haemagglutinating activity from crayfish serum.

Further purification of the eluate obtained by affinity chromatography on a calibrated Biogel P-150 column showed that the haemagglutinins and opsonins were molecules with a molecular weight of 81,000 daltons. These molecules could be dissociated into a unit of 52,000 daltons by treating with EDTA. Further studies involving polyacrylamide chromatography in the presence of sodium dodecyl sulphate showed that the molecule could be dissociated finally into sub units having a molecular weight of 13,500 daltons.

These results are interesting since they show for this species of animal that the recognition factors are an antigenically and structurally related group of molecules as are the immunoglobulin molecules of vertebrates and have functions similar to their vertebrate counterparts.

Conclusion

Recent studies on the recognition and phagocytosis of foreign material by phagocytic cells from invertebrates strongly favour the idea that the recognition mechanism is based on a system of serum proteins analogous in function to the immunoglobulin molecules of vertebrates. It would appear that there is no structural relationship between the molecules possessing this biological function in the invertebrates and those in the vertebrate kingdom. However, structural relationships do exist between these molecules within the invertebrates.

Now that this system has been defined there are a number of important questions to be answered, for example, where are these molecules synthesized? Is there any relationship between the cells taking up the foreign material and the cells synthesizing the recognition factors? How specific are these recognition factors? If the molecule has a sub-unit structure, do all the sub-units have similar specificities? One could add more questions to the list but the reader will see from the questions posed that invertebrate immunology is still in its infancy. However, I believe that answers to some of these questions will be forthcoming in the future and providing sufficient phyla are studied, they may well indicate the evolutionary pathway of this ubiquitous system.

References

Ackermann G. (1902) Anatomic und Zwittrigkeit der *Cucumaria laevigata*. *Ztschr. Wiss. Zoo.* **72,** 451.

Acton R.T., Bennett J.C., Evans E.E. & Schrohenloher, R.E. (1969) Physical and chemical characterisation of an oyster haemagglutinin. *J. Biol. Chem.* **244,** 4128.

Anderson R.S., Holmes B. & Good A. (1973) *In vitro* bactericidal capacity of *Blaberus craniifer* haemocytes. *J. Invert. Path.* **22,** 127.

Arvy L. (1953) *Bull. Soc. Zoo. (France)* **78,** 158.

Baumgarten J. (1888) *Ztschr. F. Klein. Med.* **15,** 1.

BENACERRAF B., SEBESTYEN M.M. & SCHLOSSMAN S.A. (1959) A quantitative study of the kinetics of blood clearance of ^{32}P labelled *Escherichia coli* and *Staphylococci* by the reticulo-endothelial system. *J. Exp. Med.* **110,** 27.

BERKEN A. & BENACERRAF B. (1966) Properties of antibodies cytophilic for macrophages. *J. Exp. Med.* **123,** 119.

BIOZZI G. & STIFFEL C. (1962) Role of normal and immune opsonin in the phagocytosis of bacteria and erythrocytes by the reticulo-endothelial cells, pp. 249. In *Mechanism of cell and tissue damage produced by immune reactions.* Benno Schwabe and Co., Basel.

BOYDEN S. (1963) Cellular recognition of foreign matter. *Int. Rev. Exptl Path.* **2,** 311.

CAMERON G.R. (1932) Inflammation in earthworms. *J. Path. Bact.* **35,** 933.

CAMERON G.R. (1934) Inflammation in the caterpillars of Lepidoptera. *J. Path. Bact.* **35,** 933.

CANTACUZÈNE J. (1919) Anticorps normaux et expérimentaux chez quelques invertébrés morins. *Compt. Rend. Soc. Biol.* **82,** 1087.

CANTACUZÈNE J. (1922a) Sur la role agglutenant des urnes chez *Sipunculus nudus. Compt. Rend. Soc. Biol.* **87,** 259.

CANTACUZÈNE J. (1922b) Reactions d'immunitie chez *Sipunculus nudus* vaccine contra un bacterie. *Compt. Rend. Soc. Biol.* **87,** 264.

CANTACUZÈNE J. (1923) Celebre. 75*e Anniv. Fond. Soc. Biol.* **48.**

CLARK H.L. (1899) The Synaptas of the New England Coast. *Bull. U.S. Fish. Com.* **19.**

COHN Z.A. & MORSE S.I. (1959) Interactions between polymorphonuclear leucocytes and staphylococci. *J. Exp. Med.* **110,** 419.

CUENOT L. (1902) Organes agglutinants et organs ciliophagocytaires. *Arch. Zoo. Exp. Gen. Series* **3,** 10.

DURHAM H.E. (1888) On the emigration of amoeboid corpuscles in starfish. *Proc. Roy. Soc. Lond. B.* **43,** 327.

FENN W.O. (1921) The phagocytosis of solid particles. III. Carbon and quartz. *J. Gen. Physiol.* **3,** 575.

FINSTAD C.L., LITMAN G.W., FINSTAD J. & GOOD R.A. (1972) The characterisation of purified erythrocyte agglutinins from two invertebrate species. *J. Immunol.* **108,** 1704.

HAMMERSTRÖM S. & KABAT E.A. (1969) Purification and characterisation of a blood group A reactive haemagglutinin from the snail (*Helix pomatia*) and a study of its binding site. *Biochem.* **8,** 2696.

HAMMERSTRÖM S. (1972) Snail (*Helix pomatia*) agglutinin. In *Methods in Enzymology. XXVIII. Complex Carbohydrates,* Part B. Academic Press, New York.

HARVEY W.R. & WILLIAMS C.M. (1961) The injury metabolism of the Cecropia silkworm. I. Biological amplification of the effects of localized injury. *J. Insect Physiol.* **7,** 81.

HYMAN L.H. (1940) *The Invertebrates,* 1. McGraw-Hill Book Co.

JENKIN C.R. & BENACERRAF B. (1960) *In vitro* studies on the interaction between mouse peritoneal macrophages and strains of *Salmonella* and *Escherichia coli. J. Exp. Med.* **112,** 403.

JENKIN C.R. & ROWLEY D. (1961) The role of opsonins in the clearance of living and inert particles by cells of the reticulo-endothelial system. *J. Exp. Med.* **114,** 363.

JENKIN C.R. & JACKSON G.D.F. (1968) Further studies with artificial antigens and immunity to mouse typhoid. I. Use of O-acetylated galactans in the purification of specific antibody against Antigen 5. *Immunol.* **15,** 789.

JENKIN C.R. & ROWLEY D. (1970) Immunity in invertebrates III. Purification of a haemagglutinin to rat and rabbit erythrocytes from the haemolymph of the Murray Mussel (*Velesunio ambiguus*). *Aust. J. exp. Biol. med. Sci.* **48,** 129.

JEON K.W. & BELL L.G.E. (1965) Pseudopod and food cup formation in *Amoeba proteus. Exptl Cell. Res.* **38,** 536.

LEA M.S. & GILBERT L.I. (1961) Cell division in diapausing silk worm pupae. *Am. Zoo.* **1,** 368.

LISTER J. (1896) Presidential address. *Rep. Brit. Ass. Adv. Sc.* (*Lond.*) p. 26.

MACKANESS G. (1960) The phagocytosis and inactivation of streptococci by macrophages of normal rabbits. *J. Exp. Med.* **112,** 35.

MARCHALONIS J.J. & EDELMAN G.H. (1968) Isolation and characterisation of a haemagglutinin from *Limulus polyphemus. J. Mol. Biol.* **32,** 453.

MAST S.O. & HAHNERT W.F. (1935) Feeding, digestion and starvation in *Amoeba proteus* (Leidy). *Physiol. Zoo.* **8,** 255.

MCKAY D. (1970) The immune response in the fresh water crayfish (*Parachaeraps bicarinatus*). Ph.D. Thesis, Univ. Adelaide, S. Australia.

MCKAY D. & JENKIN C.R. (1970a) Immunity in the invertebrates. The fate and distribution of bacteria in normal and immunised crayfish (*Parachaeraps bicarinatus*). *Aust. J. exp. Biol. med. Sci.* **48,** 599.

MCKAY D. & JENKIN C.R. (1970b) Immunity in the invertebrates. The role of serum factors in phagocytosis of erythrocytes by haemocytes of the fresh water crayfish (*Parachaeraps bicarinatus*). *Aust. J. exp. Biol. med. Sci.* **48,** 139.

MCKAY D., JENKIN C.R. & ROWLEY D. (1969) Immunity in the invertebrates. I. Studies on the naturally occurring haemagglutinins in the fluids from invertebrates. *Aust. J. exp. Biol. med. Sci.* **47,** 125.

METCHNIKOFF E. (1907) *Immunity in Infective Diseases*, Cambridge University Press.

MIESCHER P.A., SPIEGELBERG H. & BENACERRAF B. (1963) Studies on the mechanism of immune phagocytosis of sensitised bacteria and red cells by the reticulo-endothelial system in mice. In *Role du Système Réticulo-Endothélial dans l'immunitié Antibacteriénne et Antitumorale*, Editions du Centre National de la Recherche Scientifique.

MURRAY I.M. (1963) The mechanism of blockade of the reticulo-endothelial system. *J. Exp. Med.* **117,** 139.

NELSON R.A. & LEBRUN J. (1956) The requirement for antibody and complement for *in vitro* phagocytosis of starch granules. *J. Hyg.* **54,** 8.

NORMAN S.J. & BENDITT E.P. (1965) Function of the reticulo-endothelial system. I. A study of the phenomenon of carbon clearance inhibition. *J. Exp. Med.* **122,** 693.

PAULEY G.B., KRASSNER S.M. & CHAPMAN F.A. (1971) Bacterial clearance in the Californian sea hare (*Aplysia californica*). *J. Invert. Path.* **18,** 227.

POTTER E.V. & STOLLERMAN G.H. (1961) The opsonisation of bentonite particles by γ-Globulin. *J. Immunol.* **87,** 110.

PROWSE R.H. & TAIT N.T. (1969) *In vitro* phagocytosis by amoebocytes from the haemolymph of *Helix aspersa. Immunol.* **17,** 437.

READE P. (1968) Phagocytosis in invertebrates. *Aust. J. exp. Biol. med. Sci.* **46,** 219.

READE P. & READE E. (1972) Phagocytosis in invertebrates. II. The clearance of carbon particles by the clam (*Tridacna maxima*). *J. Reticuloendothel. Soc.* **12,** 349.

ROWLEY D. & TURNER K.J. (1966) The number of molecules of antibody required to promote phagocytosis of one bacterium. *Nature* **210,** 496.

ROY D.L. (1951) Agglutination of Bacteria: A feeding method in the soil Ameba Hartmanella sp. *J. Exptl. Zoo.* **118,** 443.

SALT G. (1960) Experimental studies on insect parasitism. XI. The haemocytic reaction of a caterpillar under varied experimental conditions. *Proc. Roy. Soc.* (*Lond.*) *B* **151,** 446.

SALT G. (1961) The haemocytic reaction of insects to foreign bodies, p. 175. In *The Cell and the Organism.* Cambridge University Press.

SCOTT M.T. (1971) Recognition of foreignness in invertebrates. II. *In vitro* studies of cockroach phagocytic haemocytes. *Immunol.* **21,** 817.

SCHULTZ E. (1895) Excretion bei den Holothurien. *Biol. Centralbl.* **15,** 198.

Spiegelberg H.L., Miescher P. & Benacerraf B. (1963) Studies on the role of complement in the immune clearance of *Escherichia coli* and rat erythrocytes by the reticulo endothelial system in mice. *J. Immunol.* **90,** 751.

Stuart A.E. (1968) The reticulo-endothelial apparatus of the lesser octopus (*Eledone cirrosa*). *J. Path. Bact.* **96,** 401.

Theèl H. (1901) Case of hermaphroditism in holothuroids. *Svenska. Vetensk. Acad. Handl.* **27,** No. 6.

Tripp M.R. (1966) Haemagglutinin in the blood of the oyster (*Crassostrea virginica*). *J. Invert. Path.* **8,** 478.

Tyler A. & Metz B. (1945) Natural heteroagglutinins in the serum of the spiny lobster (*Panulirus interruptus*). I. Taxonomic range of activity, electrophoretic and immunising properties. *J. Exp. Zoo.* **110,** 387.

Tyler A. & Scheer B.T. (1945) Natural haemagglutinins in the serum of the spiny lobster (*Panulirus interruptus*). II. Chemical and antigenic relation to blood proteins. *Biol. Bull.* **89,** 193.

Tyson C.J. & Jenkin C.R. (1973) The importance of opsonic factors in the removal of bacteria from the circulation of the crayfish (*Parachaeraps bicarinatus*). *Aust. J. exp. Biol. med. Sci.* **51,** 609.

Tyson C.J. & Jenkin C.R. (1974) Phagocytosis of bacteria *in vitro* by haemocytes from the crayfish (*Parachaeraps bicarinatus*). *Aust. J. exp. Biol. med. Sci.* **52,** 341.

Von-Behring E. (1888) *Centralbl. für Klin. Med.* No. 38.

Von-Behring E. & Kitasato S. (1890) Über das Zustandekommen der Diptheria Immunität und der Tetanus immunität bei tieren. *Dtsch. med. Wschr.* **16,** 1113.

Wigglesworth V.B. (1950) *The Principles of Insect Physiology*, 4th edit. Methuen & Co. Ltd., London.

Wright A. & Douglas S.R. (1903) *Proc. Roy. Soc. (Lond.) B* **72,** 375.

Yonge C.M. (1937) Evolution of and adaptation in the digestive system of the metazoa. *Biol. Rev.* **12,** 87.

Chapter 5. Phylogeny of Cellular Immunity Among Vertebrates*

M. R. Tam, A. L. Reddy, R. D. Karp and W. H. Hildemann

Introduction

Mixed leukocyte cultures (MLC) reactions versus non-specific mitogen responsiveness

Phylogeny of MLC and mitogen responses

Delayed hypersensitivity in vertebrate immunity

Evolution of macrophages and lymphoid tissue

Transplantation and tumour immunity
Fishes
Amphibians
Reptiles
Birds
Mammals

Phylogenetic perspectives

Introduction

Specificity and memory have been generally accepted as the essential attributes of vertebrate or, indeed, any immune responses. Given these two salient characteristics as benchmark criteria, a far-ranging look at molecular, cellular and dynamic components of immune responses, especially in so-called lower vertebrates, is needed to discern differences of phylogenetic importance. In other words, comparisons of immunocompetence at successive phylogenetic levels should take multiple variables into account. However, the main focus of this chapter will be cellular or cell-mediated immunity (CMI). In a more limited sense, CMI has implied those reactions mediated by thymus-derived lymphocytes or T cells. A more generally acceptable view of cellular immunity would include all specific immune responses mediated by living lymphoid or macrophage-type cells and their non-antibody effector molecules. CMI at the mammalian level is primarily associated with the T-cell pathway. The distinctive B-cell pathway, involving bone marrow- or at least non-thymus-derived lymphocytes, is regarded as the source of all immunoglobulin antibody production. These major pathways of cell-mediated and humoral antibody immunity are interconnected or integrated at the mammalian level of

* Aided by NIH grants AI 07970 and CA 15788.

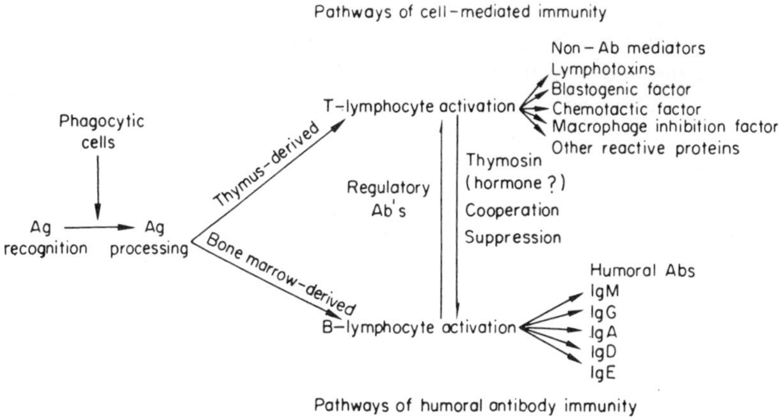

Fig. 5.1. Integrated pathways of cell-mediated and humoral antibody immunity at the mammalian level of immunoevolution. Elaborate and as yet poorly understood regulatory mechanisms are involved (after Hildemann, *Nature*, 1974).

phylogeny (Fig. 5.1). This simplified diagram of present understanding raises many questions and provides few unequivocal answers concerning sources, signals and regulatory mechanisms involved in specific immune responses.

The types of immune reactions usually associated with CMI and the T-cell pathway include mixed leucocyte culture reactions, responsiveness to certain mitogens, delayed-type cutaneous hypersensitivity, transplantation immunity, and tumour immunity. Specific transplantation immunity with concomitant immunologic memory is now known in all classes of the subphylum Vertebrata. This is the most extensively studied area suitable for phylogenetic comparisons. Although we shall deal as best we can with other correlates or manifestations of cellular immunity in this chapter, the reader should bear in mind that decisive data on non-mammalian vertebrates is still quite limited.

Mixed leukocyte culture (MLC) reactions versus non-specific mitogen responsiveness

Since the description of MLC reactivity by Bain and Lowenstein (1964) and by Bach and Hirschorn (1964), this *in vitro* assay is now widely used to measure the strength of histoincompatibility in man and in experimental animals. In a two-way MLC reaction, viable lymphocytes from unrelated individuals of the same species are cultured together *in vitro*; they respond by stimulating each other with rapid proliferation and differentiation into blast cells. The magnitude of response of one specific lymphocyte population is measured by inhibiting DNA synthesis in another stimulating population of lymphocytes subjected to sublethal doses of radiation or mitomycin treatment.

Thymus-derived lymphocytes (T cells) are the main source of cells responding to allogeneic cells. Depletion of T cells by neonatal thymectomy (Wilson *et al.* 1967, Alm & Peterson 1970), anti-θ treatment (El-Armi & Osoba 1973), or congenital T-cell deficiencies (Oppenheim 1972) is found to inhibit positive MLC reactions. Moreover, studies in mice using chromosomal markers and fluorescence techniques indicate a majority of proliferating cells are T cells (Festenstein 1969, Johnson & Wilson 1970). MLC reactions appear to be immunologically specific and analogous *in vivo* to graft-versus-host reactions (Cantor & Mosier 1972, Bloom 1971, El-Armi & Osoba 1973). While positive MLC reactions usually take 4–6 days to mature, accelerated responses in 2–3 days can be produced by priming the responding cells by prior sensitization with histoincompatible stimulatory cells (Adler *et al.* 1970, Andersson & Hayry 1973). The magnitude of the proliferative MLC response is dependent on the genetic disparity in both major and minor histocompatibility antigens identified serologically (SD). Two individuals may appear identical for SD antigens but still give positive MLC reactions which have been attributed to lymphocyte-defined (LD) antigens (Amos & Bach 1968, Yunis & Amos 1971, Dausset *et al.* 1972, Widmar *et al.* 1973). In mice, strong stimulation in MLC may depend on differences in immune response genes rather than SD antigens specified by the *H-2* gene complex (Bach *et al.* 1972).

Mammalian MLC reactions appear to be biphasic in the sense that two functionally different lymphocyte populations are mobilized. Activation of responding cells in the initial phase requires alloantigens associated with living lymphocytes. In the second phase, cytotoxic or killer cells are generated in the responding lymphocyte populations which can destroy target cells syngeneic to the stimulatory cells in a cell-mediated lympholysis assay. But SD differences are needed in addition to LD differences (Bach *et al.* 1973, Alter *et al.* 1973) to generate cytotoxic cells. Absorption of reactive lymphocytes on specific monolayers of allogeneic target cells impairs the production of cytotoxic cells in the second phase (Bach *et al.* 1973). To what extent such maturation of cellular immunity occurs in non-mammalian vertebrates remains to be discovered.

Plant lectins such as phytohaemagglutinins (PHA) and concanavalin A (Con A) contain mitogens which are strong stimulators of mammalian T-cell reactivity. Mitogen responsiveness then, like MLC reactions, can be regarded as an *in vitro* model of cell-mediated immune responses. Although both PHA and Con A in soluble form bind with equal specificity to T and B (non-thymus derived) cells, only T cells are activated to proliferate and differentiate into blast cells (Greaves & Janossy 1972, Andersson *et al.* 1972). At present, the mechanism of selective activation of T cells by PHA and Con A is not understood but evidence suggests that they bind specifically to carbohydrate moieties of glycoproteins on the lymphocyte surface (Kornfield & Kornfield 1970), leading to activation as shown by formation of surface patches, capping and internalization of receptors (Greaves & Janossy 1972).

Although MLC reactions, as well as PHA and Con A reactions, are very sensitive indicators of the presence of T cells, recent studies in rats and humans show disassociation between these reactions indicative of heterogeneity in T-cell populations. For instance, lymphocytes from two patients with congenital thymic dysplasia were found to have the capacity to respond in MLC reactions, but had impaired PHA responsiveness (Meuwissen *et al.* 1968). Similarly, rat thymocytes could be separated on a density gradient into separate MLC- and PHA-responsive cells (Colley *et al.* 1970). Serums from multiparous women were found to specifically block MLC reactions, but not PHA responses (Robert *et al.* 1973). There is also evidence suggesting two distinct cell populations in human fetuses responding to PHA and in MLC (Carr *et al.* 1973). Human fetal liver lymphocytes were found to acquire MLC but not PHA reactivity very early before any identifiable thymus formation. Distinct MLC and PHA responsive cells appeared only after differentiation of the thymus. Similar disassociation of PHA and MLC responses have been reported in mice (Howe & Manziello 1972). Moreover, PHA reactive cells were found to appear earlier than Con A responsive cells in mice (Mosier 1973). Although the proportion of T lymphocytes responding to mitogens has not been quantified with any precision, the kinetics of these responses suggest that the cells reacting in MLC are far less numerous than those activated by mitogens *in vitro*. However, it is not clear whether different lymphocyte populations respond in MLC as opposed to mitogen stimulation or whether the same lymphocytes acquire the ability to respond in these reactions depending on their maturational stage.

Phylogeny of MLC and mitogen responses

Apart from mammals, few studies have been undertaken on the phylogenetic aspects of MLC and mitogen responses. However, lymphoid cells from fishes (Cooper 1969, Olson 1967), amphibians (Goldstein & Cohen 1972), and chickens (Weber 1970) have been investigated. Since MLC, PHA, and Con A responses are specific indicators of the presence of mammalian T cells, it would be interesting to investigate these responses in various primitive vertebrates as well as advanced invertebrates. Recognition of and reaction to foreignness or non-self in MLC-type reactions may be regarded as a primordial manifestation of cell-mediated immunity describable as *quasi-immunorecognition* (Hildemann & Reddy 1973). This property is already exhibited by *invertebrates* ranging from coelenterates to protochordate tunicates in the form of sharply discriminating proliferative responses to allogeneic cells. Hyperplastic stolons and overgrowths at the localized zones of contact in one or both colonies of *Hydractinia* have been observed. Indeed, a hierarchy of hyperplastic potential was found in groups of ten strains of this coelenterate (Ivker 1972). In addition, allograft reactions indicative of primordial cell-mediated immunity (PCMI) with short-term memory have been reported in annelids (Cooper 1970, Duprat 1970) and echinoderms (Hildemann & Dix 1972, Karp & Hildemann, unpublished). Specialized types of leucocytes, notably lymphocytes (haemocytes) and granulocytes, were found to take a major part in the destruction of orthotopic foreign grafts. PCMI is also apparent in immunized oysters (*Crassostrea virginica*) as shown by the specificity of enhanced clearance of T2 bacteriophage (Acton 1970). Extensive haematological studies in protochordates indicate the presence of lymphocytes (Andrew 1962) which are X-ray sensitive (Freeman 1964), a property exhibited by all vertebrate lymphocytes. The responsiveness of these cells in MLC and mitogen stimulation tests have yet to be studied in detail. Such studies should shed some light on the evolution of primordial cell-mediated immunity in T-type lymphocytes and also add information regarding polymorphism of histocompatibility antigens and cell surface receptors. Our preliminary studies of blood cells in the tunicate (*Ciona intestinalis*) and in Pacific hagfish (*Eptatretus stoutii*) show that they do synthesize new DNA and proliferate in response to PHA stimulation. However, a higher concentration of PHA and a longer culture period are required than has previously been reported in mammalian lymphocyte cultures to obtain positive blastogenic responses. Efforts are underway in our laboratory to study MLC reactions and other mitogenic responses in primitive vertebrates and advanced invertebrates. Lymphocytes from *Ciona* and *Eptatretus* do have the capacity to form rosettes with sheep red blood cells which could be regarded as an indication of T-cell function (Reddy & Hildemann, unpublished).

Previously PHA has been reported to stimulate some protozoans to divide (Agrell 1966a,b, Zech 1966), but the capacity to differentiate into blast cells is apparently restricted to the T-type lymphocytes of higher animals. Early in the evolution of immunity, diverse cells apparently possessed not only the ability to bind PHA and divide, but were also capable of recognizing foreign cell surfaces. This allowed *quasi-immunorecognition* as manifested by allogeneic incompatibility reactions already evident in coelenterates. The ability of specialized leucocytes to differentiate into blast cells by PHA stimulation and to show target cell cytolytic activity in the form of primordial cell-mediated immunity appeared later in invertebrate evolution. Even epithelial cells of normal adult human skin have the capacity to bind PHA and then divide (Zech 1966); whether parenchymal cells other than leucocytes from higher vertebrates have retained the cognate capacity of immunorecognition is doubtful. This function may have become restricted during evolution as specialized leucocytes assumed the role of immunosurveillance. Mammalian ontogeny appears to recapitulate phylogeny in the sense that MLC-type reactivity precedes other correlates of cellular immunity. This view is also supported by the biphasic nature of MLC reactions already cited.

Delayed hypersensitivity in vertebrate immunity

The term delayed hypersensitivity (DH) as studied in mammalian species is derived from observations of a delayed set of reactions to certain immunogens. Contact with chemical substances which then combine with body proteins, infection by microbial agents, or transplantation of foreign tissue can result first in sensitization, and then manifestation of either a generalized (systemic) or localized DH reaction, usually after a latent period of about a week. For example, characteristic cutaneous DH lesions may be demonstrated by an intradermal challenge of purified protein derivative (PPD) in an animal previously sensitized to tuberculin. After a few hours an erythematous reaction (redness) develops, confined to the site of inoculation, which is soon followed by induration and thickened skin, warm to the touch. A severe reaction may even lead to an area of necrosis. Histologically, a transient inflammatory response characterized by granulocyte infiltration soon evolves into a response consisting mostly of lymphocytes and macrophages. Sensitivity is a T-cell dependent function, since DH may be transferred only with viable lymphocytes (or extracted 'transfer factor' in certain mammals), and not with serum antibodies. Moreover, neonatal thymectomy will greatly impair the DH-type responses.

Delayed hypersensitivity has been studied extensively in mammals, and to a lesser extent in avian species; there has been little work on DH in the lower vertebrates. In different mammalian species there is a surprisingly great variation of the DH response to tuberculin: man, guinea-pigs, and rabbits exhibit strong responses, while rats and mice display much weaker reactions which may however be improved by the use of adjuvants. Reports of direct demonstrations of DH-type reactions in lower vertebrates (sensitization and challenge with a defined antigen, with time-course studies and histology) are sparse or even non-existent for some classes. Finstad *et al.* (1966) attempted to elicit DH reactions in Atlantic hagfish (*Myxine glutinosa*), lampreys (*Petromyzon marinus*), guitar fish (*Rhinobatos productus*), horn sharks (*Heterodontis francisci*), and paddlefish (*Polyodon spathula*) by intramuscular injections of complete Freund's adjuvant containing *Mycobacterium tuberculosis* (FCA). All horn sharks and guitar fish along with 80 per cent of the lampreys died by 21 days' post-sensitization, exhibiting necrosis of the skin at the site of inoculation. It is not clear whether these animals succumbed to an uncontrolled, necrotizing inflammatory response due to a DH reaction or to an opportunistic microbial invasion, or to toxicity of the mineral oil adjuvant itself. The surviving lampreys were then challenged with old tuberculin (OT) and the paddlefish with FCA. All lampreys and paddlefish developed skin reactions not unlike those described for mammalian recipients. However, control groups which had received OT only for the first time were not included, nor were passive or adoptive transfer experiments performed. Sigel, however, could not produce any adjuvant lesions in lemon sharks (reported in the discussion of Finstad *et al.* 1966). Papermaster *et al.* (1964) observed DH reactions in FCA sensitized OT-challenged lampreys. They additionally reported that *Ascaris* extracts were effective in sensitization of a primitive teleost fish, the bowfin (*Amia calva*); antigen challenge after one month resulted in the development of localized induration within 3 days. In an advanced teleost, the trout (*Salmo gardineri*), Ridgway *et al.* (1966) have described a delayed-type corneal reaction to PPD, reaching its peak in 3–5 days when challenged one month after sensitization with FCA.

Billingham and Silvers (1965) have indicated that the population of mammalian T lymphocytes necessary for adoptive transfer of a DH reaction has not been separated from the population of lymphocytes necessary for adoptive sensitization against allografts. Thus, both functions may reside in the same subpopulation of lymphocytes. Allograft rejection with long-term memory in lower vertebrates (Hildemann & Clem 1972) may also be accompanied by a DH-type reaction. Caution is advisable in extrapolation of these findings because the mechanism of allograft rejection in mammalian systems may be more complicated, having been shown to depend in part on humoral antibodies. Acute allograft rejection has been demonstrated in various birds (Hašek *et al.* 1963), higher anuran amphibians (Cohen 1971) and all advanced teleost fishes so far investigated (Hildemann 1972a). All exhibited primary (first-set) rejection times of less than 21 days, and accelerated secondary (second-set) rejection. When primitive amphibians, the urodeles and apods (Cohen, 1970a), reptiles (Borysenko 1970), cartilaginous fishes (Perey *et al.* 1968, Borysenko & Hildemann 1970), or cyclostomes (Hildemann 1970) were investigated, chronic rejection of primary allografts (>30 days) was found. An explanation advanced to account for the longer interval necessary for graft rejection has postulated limited histocompatibility differences within some species of lower vertebrates (Marchalonis & Cone 1974), and hence less vigorous allograft rejection. However, another possible explanation may be that the interaction of B lymphocytes and helper T lymphocytes to produce a coordinated DH, cellular, and humoral response is less well developed or lacking at lower levels of the immunophylogenetic tree. Moreover, allograft rejection has not yet been found to result in alloantibody formation in primitive fishes (Borysenko & Hildemann 1970). This finding may be correlated with the production of only IgM-type antibody in cyclostomes and elasmobranchs, whereas integrated T- and B-cell function is required for IgG production in mammals and for switchover from specific IgM to IgG production.

Nevertheless, acute rejection of *repeat* allografts is obtainable in primitive fishes, so the inherent capacity for vigorous immune responsiveness must be available for mobilization.

Evolution of macrophages and lymphoid tissue

The amoeba as a 'prototype macrophage' can serve to illustrate that no animals, however simple, can survive for long in a hostile environment without the aid of a system of functioning phagocytic cells. The functions of these phagocytes in invertebrates as well as vertebrates were described in the pioneering work of Metchnikoff (1893), who emphasized the importance of the operation of such a phagocytic defence mechanism in humans. Such phagocytic function in primitive animals is associated with their feeding and nutrition, in addition to protection against potential pathogens. In the course of evolution, animals have apparently become less dependent upon macrophage-derived nutrition. However, the macrophage seems to have retained all other primitive mechanisms of defence, i.e. phagocytosis, pinocytosis, and encapsulation; an important newer role of participation in the immune response has been acquired in advanced invertebrates and vertebrates. Macrophages have been shown to trap, process, and store antigens, and are thus a cell type necessary for the induction of an immune response. Upon 'activation' (stimulation) of macrophages, they can synthesize, store, and ultimately secrete proteolytic enzymes or lymphokine-like substances. Vertebrate macrophages are thought to possess receptors on their surface membranes for immunoglobulin, thus conferring a degree of immune specificity to the activated macrophages by means of cytophilic antibody. Thus, sensitized macrophages have been demonstrated to participate *in vivo* in the immune response to microbial invaders, allografts, and neoplasms, as well as being implicated in the DH reaction.

Exactly where in phylogeny the macrophage acquired its additional complex immunological functions remains to be ascertained. Very few reports exist concerning macrophage functions in the immune reactions of non-mammalian vertebrates. Nelstrop *et al.* (1968) concluded that a second dose of T_1 bacteriophages was cleared more rapidly than a primary dose in shore crabs (*Limulus* sp.), lampreys (*Petromyzon marinus*), and goldfish (*Carassius auratus*), but surprisingly, not by the dogfish shark (*Squalus acanthus*), or a land snail. Since accelerated clearance, presumably involving phagocytosis by 'sensitized' macrophages, occurred in the absence of circulating antibody, they postulated that a more primitive mechanism of immunity (specific macrophage-bound antibody?) was evident. However, small numbers of animals were used, difficulty with animal survival was often encountered, and specificity controls were lacking. Macrophage functions may possibly have become more numerous and complex with the concomitant development of lymphoid organs and diversification of lymphoid cell types. The cell surface membrane receptors which have been shown to exist in even the most primitive animals studied (Humphreys 1970, Campbell & Bibb 1970, Theodor 1970) to distinguish between self and non-self antigens probably have directly evolved into immunorecognition and consequent immunoincompatibility reactions. Fichtelius (1970) has suggested that the first lymphoid cells probably were evolved from epithelium, a prime candidate because of its capacity for rapid cellular division and its present functional association with thymus and bursal lymphoid organs. In an octopus (*Eledone cirossa*), a cephalopod mollusc which branched off the main line of vertebrate evolution early in phylogeny, primitive organs were found consisting of phagocytic-type cells only; no lymphocyte-like cells were observed (Stuart 1968). Immunologic functions have not yet been adequately studied in higher molluscan species.

With compartmentalization of lymphoid cells in discrete organs, the more primitive T-cell type functions probably led to helper T-cells and multiple B-cell types capable of antibody production. The cyclostomes, including the hagfish (*Eptatretus stoutii*), clearly possess both B- and T-cell competence (Hildemann 1970, Hildemann & Thoenes 1969), but appear to have a limited repertoire of responsiveness associated with limited organization of lymphoid tissues. The chondrichthyes or elasmobranchs, the most primitive fish possessing a well-organized thymus, are capable of both early 19S and later 7S IgM responses. Anuran amphibians possess spleen, thymus, liver, and kidney, and, in addition, lymphnode-like structures in the coelom indicative of the increasing complexity of lymphoid tissues found in higher vertebrates (Good & Papermaster 1964). Advanced teleost fish with a well developed spleen and thymus are admirably responsive to diverse antigens and produce antibodies of two or more molecular classes. Cells similar to mammalian plasma cells have been identified in the bowfin, a primitive teleost fish (Finstad & Good 1966), but not at lower levels of phylogeny.

The extent of macrophage participation in specific immune responses of invertebrates and lower vertebrates is unknown. Studies with mammalian lymphoid cells *in vitro* have shown that an adherent cell, presumably a macrophage, is necessary both for prompt and vigorous humoral antibody responses to many antigens and for consummation of cell-mediated (T-cell) killing in target cells. This macrophage participation in specific immune responses may be less well developed in lower vertebrates. More efficient communication between T and B cells mediated by macrophages in higher vertebrates may subserve the need for more elaborate immunorecognition.

Transplantation and tumour immunity

Fishes

Primitive fishes (Agnatha and Chondrichthyes) all reject initial allografts by discriminating but slowly mobilized immune reactions (Hildemann 1970). Hagfish (*Eptatretus stoutii*), for example, possess a very effective short-term memory in the T-cell pathway as shown by accelerated rejection of repeat skin allografts. However, repeat grafts have also led to prolonged survivals. Whether this is due to specific immunoblocking (enhancement) or a negative 'lapse' in memory is unknown. Horn sharks (*Heterodontis francisci*) have shown a gradual, stepwise increase in induced transplantation immunity. Four successive sets of skin allografts showed decreasing median survival times (MSTs) of 41·1, 16·7, 9·3 and 7·4 days, respectively. Thus, by the fourth-set graft, a vigorous acute response was demonstrable. At no time, even with further immunization by direct injection of allogeneic cells, were serum alloantibodies demonstrable (Borysenko & Hildemann 1970). The current picture of transplantation immunity in primitive fishes then is one of specific, highly effective cellular immunity not dependent upon concomitant production of humoral antibodies.

Among primitive bony fishes as exemplified by the paddlefish (Perey *et al.* 1968) and arowana (Borysenko & Hildemann 1969), a transition from slow to rapid elicitation of transplantation immunity is evident. Advanced bony fishes without reported exception all show acute rejection of first-set integumentary allografts and accelerated rejection of second-set grafts with a vigour of cellular immunity at least equal to that of any laboratory mammal (Hildemann 1972a). Since higher fishes also respond vigorously to diverse xenogeneic antigens by abundant antibody production, integrated T- and B-cell pathways have already evolved at this level of phylogeny. However, little or nothing is known about details of such major topics as cell cooperation, specific immunoregulation or memory.

A low incidence of cancer has been recorded among primitive fishes such as sharks, rays and skates (Wellings 1969). We have yet to detect an instance of spontaneous cancer among hundreds of Pacific hagfish kept under aquarium conditions, but unfortunately these animals have rarely survived more than six months in captivity. Almost every tumour type has been reported in advanced bony fishes (Wellings 1969; Dunbar 1969, Andrew 1969).* Efforts to transplant these tumours into members of the same teleost species have generally failed which is not surprising because these tumours carry strong transplantation antigens distinguishing donors from recipients. Attempts to induce cancer, especially in primitive fishes with known tumorigenic agents under laboratory conditions are underway. One of us (RDK) is currently trying to induce tumours in hagfish and sharks by several methods proven efficacious in mammals. The weak histocompatibility barriers characteristic of these species should allow decisive transplantation experiments despite the absence of inbred animals.

* See also Chapter 7 for a discussion of tumours of lower vertebrates.

Amphibians

Understanding of transplantation immunity in all major groups of amphibians—apodans, urodeles, and anurans—is now substantial thanks to the extensive studies of Cooper (1969), Cohen (1971), Volpe (1970), and their colleagues among others. In general, species of apodans and urodeles display weak histocompatibility barriers while stronger disparities are characteristic of the more advanced anurans. To what extent these differences hinge on histocompatibility gene evolution versus inherent immune responsiveness remains unclear. Long-term T-cell memory is not necessarily a function of the presence of strong histoincompatibilities, since urodeles are capable of accelerated rejection of second-set skin allografts placed more than three months after rejection of the initial allografts (Cohen 1970b). However, initial grafts must be in place for more than 10 days before heightened responsiveness to a repeat graft is demonstrable (Cohen 1972). Thymus-derived lymphocytes must play a central role in alloimmunity, since bilateral thymectomy of urodele larvae effectively abolishes subsequent responsiveness. Prompt and vigorous allograft reactions in frogs even during larval development (Hildemann & Haas 1959) reveals cell-mediated immunity at the anuran level as impressive as that found in advanced fishes, birds and mammals. T lymphocytes are again implicated as effector cells because early thymectomy impairs allograft rejection (Cooper & Hildemann 1965, Curtis & Volpe 1971, Horton & Manning 1972). However, thymectomy after development of peripheral lymphoid organs in late larval life did not affect immune capacity. Thymic lymphocytes are ontogenically derived from the thymus primordium of frog embryos and not from circulating stem cells that migrated into the organ (Turpen *et al.* 1973). This was shown by reciprocal transplantation of undifferentiated thymic primordia between diploid and triploid individuals. All lymphocytes in the bone marrow, spleen and kidneys of adult frogs appear to be descendants of the original thymic stem lymphocytes. The thymus then may be regarded as the stem cell source of both T and B cells in advanced amphibians.

Considerable work has been done on the biology of amphibian tumours (Mizell 1969). A spontaneous lymphosarcoma quite possibly of non-viral aetiology in Mexican axolotls (*Ambystoma mexicana*) has been extensively studied by Delanney and Blackler (1969). Susceptible animals could be made immune to this tumour by a regimen of implantation and excision. Strains of axolotls resistant to the tumour became susceptible if they were either thymectomized at an early larval stage or were made tolerant to donor strain tissue. In addition to further demonstrating the T-cell dependence of tumour immunity, the weak histocompatibility barriers characteristic of urodeles evidently constitute no impediment to the mobilization of effective tumor resistance. Attempts to induce neoplasia in urodeles with chemical carcinogens (Breedis 1952, Ingram 1971) yielded only four tumours, all after long latency periods, among some 700 animals tested. Relative resistance to tumorigenesis or to the chemical carcinogens used is suggested, but other approaches invite investigation. Inducible immunity to various tumours in several anuran amphibians has been studied as reported elsewhere in this volume. A spontaneous and virally induced lymphoma in *Xenopus laevis* can be transmitted to xenogeneic newts as well as allogeneic hosts by implantation which leads to transformation of recipient cells by the escaping virus (Ruben 1969). Animals can be made immune to tumorigenesis, yet their tissue will pass the virus to unsensitized recipients and cause tumours. Interestingly, the amount of lymphosarcoma developed at any given time is greater in animals kept at 15°C than in animals kept at 25°C. This almost certainly reflects the greater vigour of the immune response at the higher temperature. In another anuran lymphoid tumour system, Hadji-Azimi and Fischberg (1971) produced a series of identical twins in *X. laevis* toads to allow syngeneic as well as allogeneic tumour transplants. Cancerous hepatic allografts grew progressively, while normal hepatocytes were rejected. Evidently certain tumour cells under given experimental conditions are able to 'sneak through' host defences even across large histocompatibility gaps.

Reptiles

Representatives of the Chelonia (turtles), Squamata (lizards and snakes) and Crocodilia so far studied all have shown chronic rejection of first-set allografts (Borysenko 1970, Terebey 1970) with reactions similar to those found in primitive fishes and lower amphibians. Allograft MSTs at physiologically normal temperatures all fell in a range of 40–90 days. In the garter snake (*Thamnophis Sirtalis*), Terebey (1972) found a heavy infiltration of lymphocytes during early stages of allograft rejection, whereas macrophages predominated later. Newly hatched snapping turtles (*Chelydra serpentina*) injected with adult, allogeneic spleen cells succumbed to acute graft-versus-host (GVH) reactions at 30°C, but chronic GVH reactivity with a lesser incidence of mortality obtained at the more normal temperature of 20°C (Borysenko & Tulipan 1973). Immunologically mature turtles (four-months old) were not affected by spleen inocula and spleen cells from adult xenogeneic donors (*Chrysemys picta*) were ineffective in producing disease in immature snapping turtles.

Although the incidence of naturally occurring cancer appears low in reptiles (Zwart & Harshbarger 1972), evidence concerning experimental cancer induction in this class of vertebrates is lacking. Ziegel and Clark (1971) and Orr *et al.* (1972) both described tumours found in snakes, but no attempts were made to check for transplantability or other malignant traits. Since foreign tissue rejection in snakes is chronic and temperature-dependent, one could determine transplantability even in allogeneic animals. Zwart and Harshbarger (1972) reported a malignant lymphoma in a water lizard. Clark *et al.* (1972) claim to have transformed a lizard cell line (*Gekko gecko*) with SV-40 virus. It would be interesting to see if these cells transformed *in vitro* would grow as a tumour *in vivo*. Understanding the role of cellular immunity in the control of cancer in reptiles will require laboratory induction of cancer and subsequent experiments under controlled conditions.

Birds

Common birds characteristically display prompt and vigorous transplantation immunity indicating both the presence of strong histocompatibility antigens and a well-developed capacity for cell-mediated immunity (Hildemann 1972b). This assertion is supported by extensive studies in turkeys (Healey & Russel 1962), ducks (Hašek *et al.* 1963) and chickens (Gilmour 1963, Hašek *et al.* 1966), but birds from numerous other taxononic orders have yet to be investigated. Allograft immunity in chickens is clearly thymus-dependent (Aspinall *et al.* 1963). Moreover, skin allografts in tolerant chickens are destroyed by adoptive transfer of immune lymphoid cells, but not by immune serum (Hašek *et al.* 1968). Perey and Dupuy (1970) found that bursectomized and X-irradiated chickens still exhibited typical acute allograft reactions. Bubenik *et al.* (1970) found in ducks that immune serum could activate otherwise tolerant lymphocytes to mount cytotoxic reactions against allogeneic target cells. Since the immune serum alone was neither cytotoxic nor complement-fixing, the lymphocytes were apparently armed by cytophilic antibodies. Although cellular immunity in birds clearly involves T lymphocytes, the probable cooperative roles of granulocytes and macrophages remain to be delineated.

Studies of cancer have been directed toward economically-important chickens, turkeys, and ducks, representing only two of the 32 orders of birds. On the genetic side, inbred Pekin ducks display a low incidence of 3-methylcholanthrene-induced tumours, whereas Pekin × Muscovy F1 hybrids show a high incidence (Rigdon 1972). Since ducks appear to have a very low incidence of spontaneous tumours, experimental manipulation promises new insights concerning the bases of effective tumour immunity. Lines of chickens bred for resistance to tumour viruses (Cotter *et al.* 1973) also invite immunological studies. Marek's disease, a fatal lymphoproliferative disease of chickens of viral origin, causes degeneration and necrosis of bursa follicles with concomitant depression of both cellular and humoral immunity (Nazerian 1973). This disease then attacks the very centres that might otherwise provide protection. Immune serum has been found to provide protection for uninfected chickens. Increased cooperation between T- and B-cell pathways appears likely at the phylogenetic level of birds. The corresponding functional dissociation between thymus and bursa of Fabricius provides a tidy anatomical basis for further studies of the relative importance of cellular versus humoral immunity toward well-defined antigens.

Mammals

Elaborate homeostatic regulation, including still poorly understood T- and B-cell cooperation and suppression, is operative in birds and mammals. Integrated pathways of cell-mediated and humoral antibody immunity at the mammalian level of immunoevolution are diagrammed in Fig. 5.1. Important details of immunorecognition, especially tolerance, immunoblocking, memory, and mechanisms of specific cell-mediated immunity, remain controversial or unknown. The cytoarchitecture of the lymphoid system and the molecular diversity of antibodies produced attain progressively higher levels of complexity in the evolution from fishes to mammals. Given the abundant complexity surrounding mammalian immune responses, it is not surprising that much controversy is centred on the nature of the effector cells involved in transplantation and tumour immunity. Most workers report that T lymphocytes are the essential effector cells, but this assertion is clouded by uncertainty about T-cell mediators and how they function. Increasing evidence for T-cell heterogeneity also raises unsettling questions.

Golstein *et al.* (1972) among others claim that T cells are responsible for cytotoxicity against allogeneic target cells *in vitro*. More dramatically, Reed and Manning (1973) report that nude mice which are congenitally athymic accept full-thickness human skin grafts for their lifetime without any immunosuppressive treatment. Typical of earlier findings, Manning and Jutila (1972) report that suppression of humoral antibody production did not alter the course of skin allograft rejection in mice. However, Winn *et al.* (1973) found that thymectomized mice treated with antilymphocyte serum and then grafted with rat skin showed hyperacute rejection of the rat skin upon subsequent injection of mouse anti-rat serum. Many investigators have found that humoral antibodies can decisively influence kidney allograft survival by promoting either cytotoxic (IgM) or specific blocking (IgG) reactions (cf. Hildemann & Mullen 1973). Depending on the test system then, antibodies may either be synergistic with or antagonistic toward effective CMI in mammals.

There is an impressive array of evidence pointing to T lymphocytes as essential for tumour cell destruction. However, macrophages and even cytotoxic antibodies can also be decisive, the latter especially against leukaemias and lymphomas. For example, peritoneal macrophages, peritoneal lymphocytes, and lymph-node cells each had the capability of adoptively inhibiting the growth of tumour cells in irradiated syngeneic recipients (Bennett 1965). The sceptic may well question the probable mixture of cell types involved in such experiments. Macrophages may become specifically armed to kill target tumour cells by a mechanism that apparently does not involve cytotoxic antibodies (Den Otter *et al.* 1972). Rouse *et al.* (1972) found that thymocytes (i.e. T cells) immunized *in vitro* against allogeneic spleen cells and then assayed for ability to reject donor-type tumour cells *in vivo* did so in a ratio as low as 1:1. B-cell cooperation did not appear necessary for this activity. More directly, Freedman *et al.* (1972) reported rejection of DBA/2 tumour cells in irradiated mice reconstituted with immune T cells, but immune spleen cells depleted of T cells did not show this cytotoxic activity. Similar results were obtained for polyoma virus-induced cancer in mice (Allison 1972) with the additional finding that prior thymectomy greatly increased tumour susceptibility. Numerous studies with thymectomized and irradiated mice (Castro 1972, Franks *et al* 1973b), antilymphocyte serum-treated mice (Franks *et al.* 1973a) and congenitally athymic mice (Giovanella *et al.* 1973) have shown that T-cell depleted animals will support the growth of diverse types of foreign tumours. T-cell depletion with increasing age in mammals including man is associated with thymic atrophy and is demonstrable by diminishing cutaneous responses to ubiquitous antigens and reduced responsiveness to mitogenic effects of PHA (Mackay 1972). Such failing T-lymphocyte function could account for impaired immunosurveillance with predisposition to both cancer and infectious disease. The marked effect of lowered body temperature in retarding the rate of ageing in ectothermic vertebrates may operate through immunological mechanisms (Liu & Walford 1972). Even a mild lowering of temperature suppresses both cellular and humoral immune processes in ectotherms.

At several levels of phylogeny, different types of organ allografts have shown strikingly different survival times. This has tended to confuse characterization of underlying immune processes. Kallman (1970) found that fin and scale allografts were always rejected earlier than heart allografts in teleost platyfish. Cohen (1970a) also found that heart allografts survived for longer than skin allografts in urodele amphibians. White and Hildemann (1969), Sorensen *et al.* (1972) and Warren *et al.* (1973) reported prolonged survival of kidney allografts in rats which showed acute rejection of skin from the same donor strain. Warren and his co-workers (1973) found that heart and skin allografts in rats were rejected at the same times when (1) the routes of sensitization were equated by using the same sites for grafting, (2) graft sizes were the same and (3) periods of ischemia were of the same duration. This would argue against organ-specific antigens as the cause of the differential survival times. Rather, a combination of physiological factors and target tissue accessibility are implicated.

Phylogenetic perspectives

Certain major sequential steps in the phylogeny of immunologic reactivity

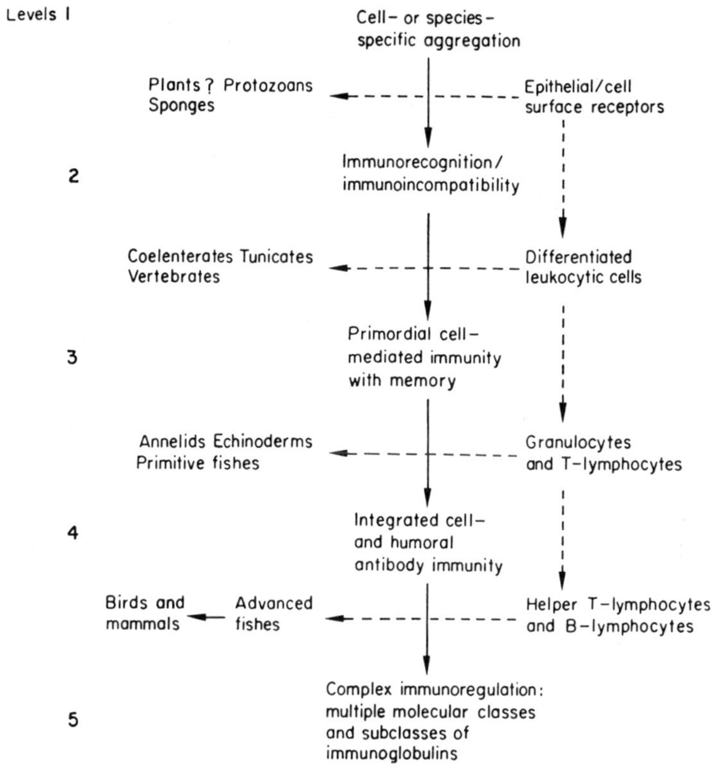

Fig. 5.2. Major steps in phylogeny of immunologic reactivity. Specific cellular immunocompetence is already apparent at the level of Coelenterates, while cell-mediated immunity with memory is first detected in advanced invertebrates. Earlier manifestations of immunoreactivity appear to have been retained during progressive evolution and diversification of immunocyte functions (after Hildemann, *Nature*, 1974).

are suggested as illustrated in Fig. 5.2. An understanding of specific cellular immunity in vertebrates forces one to consider earlier levels of immuno-evolution. Specific immunorecognition/immunoincompatibility is first evident at the invertebrate level of coelenterates, while cell-mediated immunity with at least short-term memory has been detected initially in advanced invertebrates, notably annelids, echinoderms and possibly molluscs. There are many information gaps in invertebrate phylums not yet studied decisively or at all (see also Cooper & Jenkins, Chapters 3 and 4, this volume). Immuno-incompatibility as regularly shown by allogeneic contact reactions appears primitive and has surely persisted as an effective surveillance mechanism throughout metazoan phylogeny. MLC reactivity in modern birds and mammals has properties similar to the allogeneic proliferative antagonism seen in coelenterates and tunicates. Progressively more differentiated leucocytic cells probably assumed this second-level function as adaptive specialization continued during phylogeny. Primordial cell-mediated immunity with memory may be regarded as a third level associated with cooperation of granulocytes (macrophages) and T lymphocytes in allograft-type reactions. This function became well developed in primitive fishes associated increasingly with longer-lived memory. Chronic or slow CMI reactivity to foreign tissue appears to provide as effective immunosurveillance for 'lower' vertebrates as promptly mobilized CMI reactions provide for 'advanced' vertebrates. If anything, lower vertebrates and invertebrates are *less* susceptible to cancer induction in the light of available evidence.

Integrated cell- and humoral antibody immunity may have first evolved in advanced bony fishes. At this vertebrate level helper T cells and B cells capable of producing two or more molecular classes of antibodies are demonstrable. If the thymus is indeed the stem cell source of both T and B lymphocytes in fishes and amphibians, evolution of the bursa of Fabricius as a separate source of B cells may be merely a special adaptation of the reptilian-avian branch of the phylogenetic tree. Complex immunoregulation in birds and mammals involves multiple classes and subclasses of immunoglobulins as well as a thymic hormone in ways just beginning to be understood.

References

Acton R.T. (1970) *Immunological and immunochemical studies of the oyster* (*Crassostrea virginica*). MSS Information Corp., New York, 134 pp.

Adler W.H., Takiguchi T., Marsh B. & Smith R.T. (1970) Cellular recognition by mouse lymphocytes *in vitro*. II. Specific stimulation of mouse lymphocytes by histocompatibility antigens in mixed cell cultures. *J. Immunol.* **105,** 984.

Agrell I.P.S. (1966a) PHA as a mitotic stimulation on free living amoeba. *Exp. Cell. Res.* **42,** 403.

Agrell I.P.S. (1966b) The mitogenic action of phosphate and PHA on free living amoeba. *Exp. Cell. Res.* **43,** 691.

Allison A.C. (1972) Interactions of antibodies and effector cells in immunity against tumours. *Ann. Inst. Pasteur* **122,** 619.

Alm G.V. & Peterson R.D.A. (1970) Effect of thymectomy and bursectomy on the in vitro response of chick spleen cells to PHA, SRBC and allogeneic cells. *Fed. Proc.* **29,** 430.

Alter B.J., Schendel D.J., Bach M.L., Bach F.H., Klein J. & Stimpfling J.H. (1973) Cell mediated lympholysis. Importance of serologically defined H-2 regions. *J. Exp. Med.* **137,** 1303.

Amos D.B. & Bach F.H. (1968) Phenotypic expression of the major histocompatibility locus in man (HL-A): Leukocyte antigens and MLC culture reactivity. *J. Exp. Med.* **128,** 623.

Andersson J., Sjoberg O. & Moller G. (1972) Mitogens as probes for immunocyte activation and cellular cooperation. *Transplant. Rev.* **11,** 137.

Andersson L.C. & Hayry P. (1973) Specific priming of mouse thymus dependent lymphocytes to allogeneic cells in vitro. *Eur. J. Immunol.* **3,** 595.

ANDREW W. (1962) Cells of the blood and coelomic fluids of tunicates and echinoderms. *Amer. Zoologist* **2,** 285.

ANDREW W. (1969) Tumors and aging. *Nat. Can. Inst. Monogr.* **31,** 129.

ASPINALL R.L., MEYER R.K., GRAETZER M.A. & WOLFE H.R. (1963) Effect of thymectomy and bursectomy on the survival of skin homografts in chickens. *J. Immunol.* **90,** 872.

BACH F.H., BACH M.L., SONDEL P.M. & SUNDHARDAS G. (1972) Genetic control of MLC reactivity. *Transplant. Rev.* **12,** 30.

BACH F.H. & HIRSCHORN K. (1964) Lymphocyte interactions: A potential histocompatibility test in vitro. *Science* **143,** 813.

BACH F.H., SEGALL M., STOUBER K.Z. & SONDEL P.M. (1973) Cell-mediated immunity: separation of cells involved in recognitive destructive phases. *Science* **180,** 403.

BAIN B. & LOWENSTEIN L. (1964) Genetic studies on the mixed lymphocyte reaction. *Science* **145,** 1315.

BENNETT B. (1965) Specific suppression of tumor growth by isolated peritoneal macrophages from immunized mice. *J. Immunol.* **95,** 656.

BILLINGHAM R.E. & SILVERS W.K. (1965) Sensitivity to homografts of normal tissues and cells. *Ann. Rev. Microbiol.* **17,** 531.

BLOOM B.R. (1971) *In vitro* approaches to the mechanism of cell-mediated immune reactions. *Advances in Immunology* **13,** 101.

BORYSENKO M. (1970) Transplantation immunity in reptilia. *Transplant. Proc.* **2,** 299.

BORYSENKO M. & HILDEMANN W.H. (1969) Scale (skin) allograft reaction on the primitive teleost, *Osteoglossum bicirrhosum. Transplantation* **8,** 403.

BORYSENKO M. & HILDEMANN W.H. (1970) Reactions to skin allografts in the horn shark, *Heterodontis francisci. Transplantation* **10,** 545.

BORYSENKO M. & TULIPAN P. (1973) The graft-versus-host reaction in the snapping turtle, *Chelydra serpentina. Transplantation* **16,** 496.

BREEDIS C. (1952) Induction of accessory limbs and of sarcoma in the newt (*Triturus viridescens*) with carcinogenic substances. *Cancer Res.* **12,** 861.

BUBENIK J., PERLMAN P. & HASEK M. (1970) Induction of cytotoxicity of lymphocytes from tolerant donors by antibodies to target cell allo-antigens. *Transplantation* **10,** 290.

CAMPBELL R.D. & BIBB C. (1970) Transplantation in coelenterates. *Transplant. Proc.* **2,** 202.

CANTOR H. & MOSIER D.E. (1972) Maturation of reactivity in histocompatibility antigens. *Transplant. Proc.* **4,** 159.

CARR M.C., STITES D.P.L. & FUDENBERG H.H. (1973) Dissociation of response to PHA and adult allogeneic lymphocytes in human foetal lymphoid tissue. *Nature* (*New Biol.*) **241,** 279.

CASTRO J.E. (1972) Human tumours grown in mice. *Nature* (*New Biol.*) **239,** 83.

CLARK H.F., JENSEN F. & DEFENDI V. (1972) SV 40-induced transformation of cells of the lizard *Gekko gecko. Int. J. Cancer* **9,** 599.

COHEN N. (1970a) Tissue transplantation immunity and immunologic memory in urodela and apoda. *Transplant. Proc.* **2,** 275.

COHEN N. (1970b) Immunological memory involving weak histocompatibility barriers in urodela amphibians. *Transplantation* **10,** 382.

COHEN N. (1971) Amphibian transplantation reactions: A review. *Amer. Zoologist* **11,** 193.

COHEN N. (1972) Time relationships in the development of immunity in urodele skin allografts transplanted across weak histocompatibility barriers. *Transplantation* **13,** 514.

COLLEY D.A., SHIH WU A.Y. & WAKSMAN B.H. (1970) Cellular differentiation in the thymus. II. Surface properties of rat thymus and lymph node cells separated on density gradients. *J. Exp. Med.* **132,** 1107.

COOPER A.J. (1969) Ammocete lymphoid cell populations *in vitro*, pp. 137–147. *4th Leukocyte Culture Conference*. Hanover, New Hampshire.

COOPER E.L. (1969) Immunity and tolerance in amphibia, p. 130. In *Biology of Amphibian Tumors*, ed. Mizell M. Springer-Verlag, New York.

COOPER E.L. (1970) Transplantation immunity in helminths and annelids. *Transplant. Proc.* **2,** 216.

COOPER E.L. & HILDEMANN W.H. (1965) Allograft reactions in bullfrog larvae in reaction to thymectomy. *Transplantation* **3,** 446.

COTTER P.F., COLLINS W.M., CORBETT A.C. & DUNLOP W.R. (1973) Regression of Rous sarcomas in two lines of chickens. *J. Poult. Sci.* **52,** 799.

CURTIS S.K. & VOLPE E.P. (1971) Modification of responsiveness to allografts in larvae of the leopard frog by thymectomy. *Develop. Biol.* **25,** 177.

DAUSSET J., LE BRUN A. & SASPORTES M. (1972) The MLC between parents and children of identical HL-A phenotype: hypothesis of a genetical recognition system. *C. R. Acad. Sci. Paris* **275,** 2279.

DELANNEY L.E. & BLACKLER K. (1969) Acceptance and regression of a strain-specific lymphosarcoma in Mexican axolotls, p. 409. In *Biology of Amphibian Tumors*, ed. Mizell M. Springer-Verlag, New York.

DEN OTTER W., EVANS R. & ALEXANDER P. (1972) Cytotoxicity of murine peritoneal macrophages in tumor allograft immunity. *Transplantation* **14,** 220.

DUNBAR C.E. (1969) Lymphosarcoma of possible thymic origin in salmonid fishes. *Nat. Cancer Inst. Monogr.* **31,** 167.

DUPRAT P.C. (1970) Specificity of allograft reactions in *Eisenia foetida*. *Transplant. Proc.* **2,** 222.

EL-ARMI M.O. & OSOBA D. (1973) Physical properties of mouse spleen cells involved in the mixed leukocyte reaction and graft-vs-host disease. *J. Immunol.* **110,** 1476.

FESTENSTEIN H. (1969) Evaluation of the MLC reaction in the mouse model, p. 165. In *Proc. of the Symposium: Transpl. Antigens, Oral Tissue Typing*, eds Elves M.W. & Nisbet.

FICHTELIUS K.E. (1970) Cellular aspects of phylogeny of immunity. *Lymphology* **1,** 50.

FINSTAD J. & GOOD R.A. (1966) Phylogenetic studies of adoptive immune responses in the lower vertebrates, p. 173. In *Phylogeny of Immunity*, eds Smith R.T., Miescher P.A. & Good R.A. Univ. of Florida Press, Gainesville.

FRANKS C.R., CURTIS K. & PERKINS F.T. (1973a) Long-term survival of Hela tumours in mice treated with anti-lymphocyte serum. *Brit. J. Cancer* **27,** 390.

FRANKS C.R., PERKINS F.T. & HOLMES J.T. (1973b) Subcutaneous growth of human tumours in mice. *Nature* **243,** 91.

FREEDMAN L.R., CEROTTINI J.C. & BRUNNER K.T. (1972) In vivo studies of the role of cytotoxic T cells in tumor allograft immunity. *J. Immunol.* **109,** 1371.

FREEMAN G. (1964) The role of blood cells in the process of asexual reproduction in the tunicates *Perophora viridis*. *J. Exp. Zool.* **156,** 157.

GILMOUR D.G. (1963) Strong histocompatibility effects associated with the *B* blood group system of chickens. *Heredity* **18,** 123.

GIOVANELLA B.C., YIM S.O., MORGAN A.C., STEHLIN J.S. & WILLIAMS L.J. Jr (1973) Metastases of human melanomas transplanted in nude mice. *J. Nat. Cancer Inst.* **50,** 1051.

GOLDSTEIN S.J. & COHEN N. (1972) Phylogeny of immunocompetent cells. I. In vitro blastogenesis and mitosis of toad (*Bufo marinus*) splenic lymphocytes in response to PHA and MLC. *J. Immunol.* **108,** 1025.

GOLSTEIN P., WIGZELL H., BLOMGREN H. & SVEDMYR E.A.J. (1972) Cells mediating specific in vitro cytotoxicity. II. Probable autonomy of thymus-processed lymphocytes (T cells) for the killing of allogeneic target cells. *J. Exp. Med.* **135,** 890.

Good R.A. & Papermaster B.W. (1964) Ontogeny and phylogeny of adoptive immunity. *Adv. Immunol.* **4,** 1.

Greaves M. & Janossy G. (1972) Elicitation of selective T and B lymphocyte response by cell surface-binding ligands. *Transplant. Rev.* **11,** 87.

Hadji-Azimi I. & Fischberg M. (1971) Normal and cancerous tissue transplantation in allogeneic and syngeneic *Xenopus laevis. Cancer Res.* **31,** 1594.

Hăsek M., Chutna J., Nouza K., Karakoz F. & Skamene E. (1968) *Advances in Transplantation,* p. 15, eds Dausset J., Hamburger J. & Mathé G. Munksgaard, Copenhagen.

Hăsek M., Hort J., Lengerova A. & Vojtiskova M. (1963) Immunological tolerance in the heterologous system. *Folia Biol. (Praha)* **9,** 1.

Hăsek M., Knizetova F. & Mervartova H. (1966) Syngeneic lines of chickens. I. Inbreeding and selections by means of skin grafts and tests for erythrocyte antigens in C line chickens. *Folia Biol. (Praha)* **12,** 335.

Healey W.V. & Russell P.S. (1962) A skin-grafting analysis of fowl parthenogens: Evidence for a new type of genetic histocompatibility. *Ann. N.Y. Acad. Sci.* **99,** 698.

Hildemann W.H. (1970) Transplantation immunity in fishes: Agnatha, Chondrichthyes, and Osteichthyes. *Transplant. Proc.* **2,** 253.

Hildemann W.H. (1972a) Transplantation reactions of two species of Osteichthyes (Teleostei) from South Pacific coral reefs. *Transplantation* **2,** 261.

Hildemann W.H. (1972b) Phylogeny of transplantation reactivity, Chap. 1. In *Transplantation Antigens—Markers of Biological Individuality,* eds Kahan B.D. & Reisfeld R.A. Academic Press, New York.

Hildemann W.H. (1974) Some new concepts in immunologic phylogeny. *Nature* **250,** 116.

Hildemann W.H. & Clem L.W. (1972) Phylogenetic aspects of immunity. Workshop #33, p. 1305 *Proc. 1st International Congress of Immunology,* ed. Amos D.B. Academic Press, New York and London.

Hildemann W.H. & Dix T.C. (1972) Transplantation reactions of tropical Australian echinoderms. *Transplantation* **15,** 624.

Hildemann W.H. & Haas R. (1959) Homotransplantation immunity and tolerance in the bullfrog. *J. Immunol.* **83,** 478.

Hildemann W.H. & Mullen Y. (1973) The weaker the histoincompatibility, the greater the effectiveness of specific immunoblocking antibodies. *Transplantation* **15,** 231.

Hildemann W.H. & Reddy A.L. (1973) Phylogeny of immune responsiveness: marine invertebrates. *Fed. Proc.* **32,** 2188.

Hildemann W.H. & Thoenes G.H. (1969) Immunological responses of the Pacific hagfish. I. Skin transplantation immunity. *Transplantation* **7,** 506.

Horton J.D. & Manning M.J. (1972) Response to skin allografts in *Xenopus laevis* following thymectomy at early stages of lymphoid organ maturation. *Transplantation* **14,** 141.

Howe M.L. & Manziello B. (1972) Ontogenesis of the in vitro response of murine lymphoid cells to cellular antigens and phytomitogens. *J. Immunol.* **101,** 534.

Humphreys T.D. (1970) Specificity of aggregation in Porifera. *Transplant. Proc.* **2,** 194.

Ingram A.J. (1971) The reactions of carcinogens in the axolotl (*Ambystoma mexicanum*) in relation to the regeneration field control hypothesis. *J. Embryol. Exptl Morphol.* **26,** 425.

Ivker F.B. (1972) A hierarchy of histoincompatibility in *Hydractinia echinata. Biol. Bull.* **143,** 162.

Johnston J.M. & Wilson D.B. (1970) Origins of immunoreactive lymphocytes in rats. *Cellular Immunol.* **1,** 430.

KALLMAN K.D. (1970) Genetics of tissue transplantation in *Teleostei. Transplant. Proc.* **2,** 263.

KORNFIELD R. & KORNFIELD S. (1970) The structure of a phytohemagglutinin receptor site from human erythrocytes. *J. Biol. Chem.* **245,** 2536.

LIU R.K. & WALFORD R.L. (1972) The effect of lowered body temperature on lifespan and immune and non-immune processes. *Gerontologia* **18,** 363.

MACKAY I.R. (1972) Ageing and immunological function in man. *Gerontologia* **18,** 285.

MANNING D.D. & JUTILA J.W. (1972) Effect of anti-immunoglobulin anti-sera on homograft rejection in mice. *Nature (New Biol.)* **237,** 58.

MARCHALONIS J.J. & CONE R.E. (1973) The phylogenetic emergence of vertebrate immunity. *Aust. J. Exp. Biol. Med. Sci.* **51,** 461.

METCHNIKOFF E. (1893) *Lectures on the comparative pathology of inflammation,* 224 pp. Dover. Publications, Inc., N.Y., 1968, republication of 1893 edition.

MEUWISSEN H., BACH J., HONG R. & WOOD R.A. (1968) Lymphocyte studies in congenital thymic dysplasia: the one-way stimulation. *J. Pediat.* **72,** 177.

MIZELL M. (ed.) (1969) *Biology of amphibian tumors.* Springer-Verlag, New York, 484 pp.

MOSIER D. (1973) Transient appearance of PHA reactive thymocytes in the foetal mouse. *Nature (New Biol.)* **242,** 184.

NAZERIAN K. (1973) Marek's disease: A neoplastic disease of chickens caused by a herpesvirus. *Adv. Cancer Res.* **17,** 279.

NELSTROP A.E., TAYLOR G. & COLLARD P. (1968) Studies on phagocytosis. III. Antigen clearance studies in invertebrates and poikilothermic vertebrates. *Immunology* **14,** 347.

OLSON G.B. (1967) Non-specific and specific lymphoid blastogenesis in leukocyte culture from *Polyodon spathula* and *Dasyatis americana. Fed. Proc.* **26,** 357.

OPPENHEIM J.J. (1972) Wherefore the mixed leucocyte reaction, p. 357. In *Transplantation Antigens,* eds Kahan B.D. & Reisfeld R.A., Academic Press, New York.

ORR H.C., HARRIS L.E. JR, BADER A.V., KIRSCHSTEIN R.L. & PROBST, P.G. (1972) Cultivation of cells from a fibroma in a rattlesnake, *Crotalus horridus. J. Nat. Cancer Inst.* **48,** 259.

PAPERMASTER B.W., CONDIE R.M., FINSTAD, J. & GOOD R.A. (1964) Evolution of the immune response. I. The phylogenetic development of adaptive immunologic responsiveness. *J. Exp. Med.* **119,** 105.

PEREY D.Y.E. & DUPUY J.M. (1970) Role of afferent lymphatics and lymph nodes during sensitization and effector mechanisms of cellular immunity in birds and mammals. *Transplant. Proc.* **2,** 321.

PEREY D.Y.E., FINSTAD J., POLLARA B. & GOOD R.A. (1968) Evolution of the immune response. VI. First and second-set homograft rejection in primitive fishes. *Lab. Invest.* **19,** 591.

REED N.D. & MANNING D.D. (1973) Long-term maintenance of normal human skin on congenitally athymic (nude) mice. *Proc. Soc. Exp. Biol. Med.* **143,** 350.

RIDGWAY G.J., HODGINS H.O. & KLONTZ G.W. (1966) The immune response in teleosts, p. 199. In *Phylogeny of Immunity,* eds Smith R.T., Miescher P.A. & Good R.A. Univ. of Florida Press, Gainesville.

RIGDON R.H. (1972) Tumors in the duck (family Anatidae): A Review. *J. Nat. Cancer Inst.* **49,** 467.

ROBERT M., BETUEL H. & REVILLARD J.P. (1973) Inhibition of MLC by sera from multipara. *Tissue Antigens* **3,** 39.

ROUSE B.T., WAGNER H. & HARRIS A.W. (1972) In vivo activity of in vitro immunized lymphocytes. *J. Immunol.* **108,** 1353.

RUBEN L.N. (1969) Possible immunological factors in amphibian lymphosarcoma development, p. 368. In *Biology of Amphibian Tumors*, ed. Mizell M. Springer-Verlag, New York.

SORENSEN S.F., BILDSOE P. & SIMONSEN M. (1972) Mixed lymphocyte culture and graft-versus-host analyses of organ-grafter rats that defy normal rules for rejection. *Transplant Proc.* **4,** 181.

STUART A.E. (1968) The reticulo-endothelial apparatus of the lesser octopus, *Eledone cirrosa. J. Path. Bact.* **96,** 401.

TEREBEY N. (1970) The homograft reaction in the snake. *Anat. Rec.* **166,** 389.

TEREBEY N. (1972) A light microscopic study of the mononuclear cells infiltrating skin homografts in the garter snake, *Thamnophis sirtalis* (Reptilia: colubridae). *J. Morphol.* **137,** 149.

THEODOR J.L. (1970) Distinction between 'self' and 'not-self' in lower invertebrates. *Nature (London)* **227,** 690.

TURPEN J.B., VOLPE E.P. & COHEN N. (1973) Ontogeny and peripheralization of thymic lymphocytes. *Science* **182,** 931.

VOLPE E.P. (1970) Transplantation immunity and tolerance in anurans. *Transplant Proc.* **2,** 286.

WARREN R.P., LOFGREEN J.S. & STEINMULLER D. (1973) Differential survival of heart and skin allografts in inbred rats. *Transplant. Proc.* **5,** 717.

WEBER W.T. (1970) Qualitative and quantitative studies on mixed homologous chicken thymus cell cultures. *Clin. & Exp. Immunol.* **6,** 919.

WELLINGS S.R. (1969) Neoplasia and primitive vertebrate phylogeny: Echinoderms, prevertebrates, and fishes—A Review. *Nat. Cancer Inst. Monogr.* **31,** 59.

WHITE E. & HILDEMANN W.H. (1969) Kidney versus skin allograft reactions in normal adult rats of inbred strains. *Transplant. Proc.* **1,** 395.

WIDMER M.B., ALTER B.J., BACH F.H., BACH M.L. & BAILEY D.W. (1973) Lymphocyte reactivity to serologically undetected components of the major histocompatibility complex. *Nature (New Biol.)* **212,** 239.

WILSON D.B., SILVERS W.K. & NOWELL P.C. (1967) Quantitative studies in the MLC interactions in rats. II. Relationship of the proliferative responses to the immunologic status of the donors. *J. Exp. Med.* **126,** 655.

WINN H.J., BALDAMUS C.A., JOOSTE S.V. & RUSSELL P.S. (1973) Acute destruction by humoral antibody of rat skin grafted to mice: The role of complement and polymorphonuclear leukocytes. *J. Exp. Med.* **137,** 893.

YUNIS E.K. & AMOS D.B. (1971) Three closely linked genetic systems relevant to transplantation. *Proc. Nat. Acad. Sci. (USA)* **68,** 3031.

ZECH L. (1966) The effect of PHA on growth and DNA synthesis of some protozoa. *Exp. Cell. Res.* **44,** 312.

ZIEGEL R.F. & CLARK H.F. (1971) Histologic and electron microscopic observations on a tumor-bearing viper: establishment of a 'C'-type virus producing cell line. *J. Nat. Cancer Inst.* **46,** 309.

ZWART P. & HARSHBARGER J.C. (1972) Hematopoietic neoplasms in lizards: report of a typical case in *Hydrosaurus amboinensis* and a probable case in *Varanus salvador*. *Intl. J. Cancer* **9,** 548.

Chapter 6. The Phylogeny of Cell–Cell Cooperation in Immunity

L. N. Ruben

Introduction

The avian system

The poikilotherm systems

Visualization of immune responses
The effect of immunogen dosage
The effect of immunogen dose on the primary anti-red cell response of the newt, *Triturus viridescens*
Morphological distinctions between 'helper' RFC and antibody producing RFC

Visualization of immune responses *continued*
Measuring 'helper' activity
Measuring antibody-forming cell activity
Anamnesis
The effect of immunogen dose on the primary anti-erythrocyte response of the leopard frog, *Rana pipiens*
A comparison with the rodent and a final speculation
Summary and conclusions

Introduction

Unlike other authors contributing to this volume I lack an extensive literature to review. In fact, only a handful of published papers address themselves to the subject of this chapter. Furthermore, I will be threading a thin line through other chapters. It is, nevertheless, important to establish a separate status for this subject which encompasses so much of the thinking in immunology today. I will also take this occasion to report new information from my own laboratory which sheds some light on the phylogeny of immunity and is, therefore, central to the purpose of this book. Because of the nature of this information it will be necessary to first review literature on immunogen dosage and the nature of receptor sites on collaborating cells in mammals.

In recent years intensive investigation in mammalian systems has been directed at the interaction or cooperation between thymus-dependent (T) and thymus-independent (B) lymphocytes, as humoral specific antibodies are produced in response to certain immunogens, e.g. heterologous erythrocytes. The first indications of this type of cell–cell interaction *in vivo* are attributable to the study of Claman *et al.* (1966). Claman and Chaperon (1969), Miller and Mitchell (1968), Nossal *et al.* (1968), Rajewski *et al.* (1969), and Mitchison *et al.* (1970) have all added significantly to our knowledge but have paid little attention to the phylogenetic aspects of this phenomenon. Recently, the importance of cellular cooperation in humoral immune responses was questioned by Good and Finstad (1971) who argue that such events are most likely unnatural responses to unnatural immunogens. For those of us trained in developmental biology the concept of interaction during the progressive differentiation of cells which generate 'luxury' molecules is paramount in our thinking (see Fleischmajer & Billingham 1968, for example). 'Luxury' molecules are those which are not necessary for cellular survival but which serve to distinguish one cell type from another. They may be visible, e.g. myofibrils, or discernible only by assay of cellular products or enzymes unique for a cellular species. Indeed, this type of interaction between cells as individuals or as populations is and has been the hallmark of experimental embryology for some time. Since Auerbach (1962, 1971a,b) has previously examined an embryological view of differentiation as it applies to immunologic phenomena, it need not be restated here. Rather within the context of this book it is appropriate to suggest an additional possibility; namely, even if it should turn out that cellular cooperation is not a major aspect of immunologic response in organisms presently on the earth, it represents, nevertheless, an important phylogenetic step which should be explored if we are to gain full understanding of immune responses as they occur in ourselves.

Cellular cooperation between thymus-dependent and thymus-independent cells is well documented for mammalian systems *in vitro* (Auerbach 1967, Raff 1970, Kettmann & Dutton 1970, Chan *et al.* 1970, Hirst & Dutton 1970, Kettman & Dutton 1971). The actual mechanism through which this interaction occurs has been the subject of considerable speculation (Bretscher & Cohn 1970, Mitchison 1971, Dutton *et al.* 1971a,b, Feldman & Nossal 1972). Thus it may be of special value that non-mammalian vertebrates be studied in this regard so that these different systems, each offering unique advantages, be utilized in an effort to more clearly define the nature of cell–cell interactions. Their unique features are described in chapters which deal more specifically with the different animal groups used for the study of immunity.

The macrophage, which represents a third sub-population of the lymphoreticular system, has also been implicated as a participant in cell–cell interactions in thymus-dependent antigenic responses (Feldmann & Basten 1972). The necessity for the presence of the macrophage or adherent (A) cell for anti-SRBC responses was first established by Mosier (1967). This finding is in accord with Feldmann and Nossal's view (1972) that the function of the macrophage is to present antigen to the B-cell surface. Recently, Schmidtke and Unanue (1971) showed that B cells bind to the surface of macrophages whereas T cells do not. Further, the macrophage population appears not to be required when T-independent antigens, such as polymerized *Salmonella* flagellin, are used (Diener *et al.* 1970) or when solubilized SRBC antigens are tested with macrophage-depleted spleen populations (Feldmann & Palmer

1971). The demonstration that macrophages possess receptor sites which bind both IgM and IgG (Uhr 1965, Berken & Benacerraf 1966, Lay & Nussenweig 1969) supports the notion that the macrophage presents concentrated and polymerized antigen to the B cell. The macrophage is believed to receive antigen via a complex with immunoglobulin (Feldmann & Nossal, 1972, Feldmann *et al.* 1973) from the T-cell surface (Marchalonis *et al.* 1972a,b, Rieber & Riethmuller 1974). This type of model has been challenged because certain workers (Vitetta *et al.* 1971) failed to isolate immunoglobulin from T cells. However, evidence for such a model was independently reported for rats (Tanaguchi & Tada 1974) and a number of workers have now detected and/or isolated surface immunoglobulin of mammalian T cells (for reviews see Warner 1974, Marchalonis 1975). It should also be noted that Calkins and Golub (1972) were able to show lymphocyte-macrophage cooperation in the absence of physical contact between the two cell types. See also Chapter 2 for a discussion of modes of cooperation between T and B cells.

The reader will find the Proceedings of the Third Sigrid Juselius Symposium of 1971 especially useful in providing varied presentations dealing with these cellular interactions. Extensive reviews by Miller (1970, 1972), Miller *et al.* (1971), Playfair (1971), Roitt *et al.* (1969), and the *Transplantation Reviews Vol. I* are also important since they explore the subject in detail.

The avian system

If it were possible to identify one demonstration which firmly establishes the importance of phylogenetic approaches to immunologic studies it would be, in my opinion, that suggested by Warner *et al.* (1962) and later proved by Cooper *et al.* (1966) which showed that avian immune responses can be dissociated and that two subpopulations of lymphocytes are involved. One population is thymus-dependent and provides for cell-mediated responses, while the other is derived from the bursa of Fabricius and determines humoral antibody capacities. Thus the avian system offers the extraordinary opportunity to study these two sub-populations of lymphocytes which are distinguishable both anatomically and physiologically. Since the ontogeny of the immune system will be considered in detail elsewhere, it would be inappropriate and unnecessary to develop the embryological and immunological evidence for the existence and the behaviour of these two sub-populations of immunocompetent cells here. The issue at hand is not the validity of their existence, but whether the two avian cellular sub-populations will interact in response to certain immunogens, as has been demonstrated in rodents. In establishing whether cellular cooperation takes place, it is necessary to show that when particular immunogens are presented to animals, members of thymus-dependent and thymus-independent sub-populations of lymphoid cells become activated. Alm (1971) showed that such a requirement might exist in the avian system. He combined thymectomy with sublethal X-irradiation of recently hatched white leghorns. Subsequent immunization with sheep red blood cells (SRBC) failed to elicit increased haemagglutinin titres or increases in the numbers of direct (19S-IgM) or indirect (7S-IgG) plaque forming cells (PFC) in the spleen. He proposed several possible explanations of his results while clearly favouring the view that the thymus-dependent cells of the chicken are likely to be behaving as they do in mice, i.e. by responding to heterologous red cells. Moreover, although they may not produce antibody themselves (Davies *et al.* 1967, Falkoff & Kettman 1972), a function relegated to the B-cell population (Mitchell & Miller 1968, Nossal *et al.* 1968), they will respond to the presence of the immunogen by aiding the B cell in its response. The B cell of the mouse would seem then to correspond to the bursa-dependent cell of the chicken. Thymectomy and X-irradiation of these newly-hatched chicks did produce higher 'background' haemagglutinin titres and PFC to SRBC. Therefore, since bursectomy combined with X-irradiation eliminates 'background' levels of anti-SRBC PFC, Alm (1970) suggests that two different lymphoid populations are likely to be involved. In 1971 Dwyer and Warner, using I^{125} labelled monomeric flagellin of *Salmonella adelaide*, showed that both the embryonic chicken thymus and the bursa possess antigen binding cells (ABC), although the bursa contains many more than does the thymus. The nature of these avian antigen-binding cells is unclear. Dwyer *et al.* (1971) demonstrated, however, that this type of assay will label B cells in athymic (nude) mice. The number of ABC within the spleen increases during development. This increase in the spleen is probably due to the migration of lymphoid cells from the bursa. Lymphoid traffic during chicken development has been studied by Hemmingsson and Linna (1972) and Hemmingsson (1972a,b). Van Alten and Meuwissen (1972) demonstrated that bursa cells themselves appear to be capable of both local defence, through antibody production specific for cloacally introduced SRBC, as well as fulfilling their primary task of seeding immunocompetent cells to other sites. The issue of whether cellular cooperation between thymus-dependent and thymus-independent lymphoid populations takes place after heterologous red cell immunization was clarified by Rouse and Warner (1972) who found depression of humoral antibody formation following thymectomy and coincident use of anti-thymocyte serum (ATS). This depression in the level of humoral antibody formation exists after challenge by horse red blood cells (HRBC) and dinitrophenylated bovine serum albumin ($DNP_{20}BSA$). Simultaneous production of humoral antibody against *Brucella abortus* is normal. Rouse and Warner (1972) also suggest that while previous attempts (Warner & Szenberg 1962, Isakovic *et al.* 1963, Cooper *et al.* 1966) to show interaction between thymus-dependent and thymus-independent lymphoid cells in the chicken were unsuccessful, they may have achieved a more effective depletion of the T-cell population by virtue of combining neonatal thymectomy with ATS treatment. It is important to note how recent these discoveries are which deal with cell interactions in non-mammalian organisms.

The poikilotherm systems

Anti-red cell responses can be demonstrated in all modern vertebrate classes including the most primitive living vertebrates, the marine hagfish of the division Agnatha (see Abramoff & LaVia 1970, Du Pasquier 1973 for recent reviews). Further, while thymic tissue is identifiable in all vertebrates except the hagfish (Good *et al.* 1966), little is known about thymus dependence in vertebrates more primitive than amphibia. Both humoral and cell-mediated responses have been noted in all the vertebrate classes, but their relationship to sub-populations of lymphocytes has not been adequately explored. On the other hand, within the amphibia, it is well known that thymectomy depresses cell-mediated immune responses (Cooper & Hildemann 1965, Curtis & Volpe 1971, Horton & Manning 1972, Tournefier 1973). The controls which relate to humoral immune responses, however, have been less thoroughly studied. Cooper *et al.* (1971) suggested that the amphibian thymus may mediate only cellular responses in spite of having reported (Cooper *et al.* 1965) that thymectomy of bullfrog tadpoles (*R. catesbiana*) interferes with humoral responses to goldfish serum emulsified in Freund's incomplete adjuvant. Moticka *et al.* (1973) found thymic immunologic activity when SRBC are used as an antigen, and Manning and Turner (personal communication) found depression of anti-SRBC haemagglutinin formation following larval thymectomy of *Xenopus laevis*, the South African clawed toad. Finally, Du Pasquier (1970) reported depressed anti-SRBC responses in thymectomized *Alytes obstetricans* larvae. A recent developmental study from this laboratory (Kidder *et al.* 1973) using South African clawed toad larvae, showed that while the initiation of the allograft response in young larvae is dependent only on the development of lymphopoiesis in the thymus (Horton 1969, Ruben *et al.* 1972) the development of the anti-erythrocyte response, as measured by the 'rosette' assay (immunocyto-adherence) (Zaalberg 1964, Biozzi *et al.* 1966) depends on the differentiation of lymphocytes within the spleen, an event which occurs one week later at normal environmental temperatures. That is, of course, just what one would expect if cell-mediated responses in amphibia involved only thymus-dependent cells, whereas anti-red cell humoral responses might require two cooperating populations of separate derivation. At the time of this writing, the only paper which relates directly to this question of whether cellular cooperation in humoral immune responses takes place in poikilotherms is a recent report on the newt, *Triturus viridescens* (Ruben *et al.* 1973). The newt or salamander was chosen especially because it is a member of the highest vertebrate order which does not utilize bone marrow for haemapoiesis (Cowden & Dyer 1971). This organism, therefore, allows us to focus on the question of the existence of a thymus-independent cell equivalent in all non-mammalian vertebrates which have neither a bursa nor an active bone marrow.

One method of demonstrating cellular cooperation *in vivo* involves the use of haptens such as trinitrophenyl (TNP) (Rajewski *et al.* 1969, Mitchison *et al.* 1970). Haptens are simple molecules capable of combining with an antibody. However, they must be conjugated with an 'immunogenic' carrier such as red cells (Rittenberg & Pratt 1969, Kettman & Dutton 1970) in order to initiate anti-hapten antibody synthesis. Pre-immunization with the specific red cell to be used later as the carrier enhances the anti-hapten response and suggests that at least two cell populations are involved. One responds specifically to the carrier, the so-called 'helper' population, which is thymus-dependent (Falkoff & Kettman 1972) in mammalian systems and the other produces antibodies specific for both the carrier and the hapten. Hemolytic plaque forming cells (PFC) are normally assayed in agar (Jerne & Nording 1963). In mammalian systems the antibody producing cells are of bone marrow origin (Mitchell & Miller 1968). Control experiments for this carrier-specific enhancement involve pre-immunization with heterologous erythrocytes different from the carrier and/or presentation of the carrier-TNP without pre-immunization. Because pre-immunization with specific carrier does not add to the concentration of TNP available to the system its action can be viewed as cooperative and the degree of enhancement provided serves as a measure of 'helper' activity. In the mouse, 'helper' activity is θ-sensitive and radio-resistant (Kettman & Dutton 1971). The θ antigen is on the surface of thymus-derived lymphocytes (Reif & Allen 1964) and was first used by Raff (1969) as a marker in studying T-cell function in immune responses. Our data clearly show that enhancement of an anti-hapten response can be demonstrated by pre-immunization with the carrier red cell type (chicken red cells, CRBC) but not with a different red cell population (toad, *Bufo marinus*, red cells, TRBC). Carrier specificity of 'helper' activity was established in this way. Consequently, we speculated that anti-erythrocyte humoral responses may never have been direct in evolution, such that one immunogen acted upon one type of cell to produce specific antibody. Yet while cellular cooperation now appears likely to be an early phylogenetic feature of immune responses, without further information we cannot exclude the possibility that parallel evolution may have led to the appearance of cellular cooperation in urodeles, the order to which newts belong (Noble 1931, Romer 1962). If this should prove to be the case, cell–cell interactions of this type may have evolved as an event quite separate from their appearance in birds and mammals. What is more, if we hope to use this system as a model which will allow us insights into the physiology of mammalian cooperation, it is essential to determine which of these alternatives applies.

Visualization of immune responses

The effect of immunogen dosage

Work with mammals has clearly shown that high immunogen doses obviate some of the necessity for cellular cooperation. A 10- to 1000-fold increase in antigen dose is required by neonatally thymectomized mice in order for them to generate a titre of antibody equivalent to that produced by normal mice (Claman & Chaperon 1969, Sinclair & Elliott 1968). More recently, Taylor (1971) confirmed that high doses of immunogen require less 'helper' activity in the stimulation of the humoral response in thymectomized mice. These findings are in accord with those of Mitchison (1964, 1971) who found that T cells are triggered by lower dosages of antigen than are B cells, in spite of the fact that there appear to be fewer antigen receptor sites on the surface of T cells (Raff *et al.* 1970, Roelants 1972, Pernis *et al.* 1971, Bankhurst & Warner 1971, Bankhurst *et al.* 1971, Nossal *et al.* 1972). Mitchison found that the tolerance threshold to bovine serum albumin was between 100 and 1000 times lower for T as compared to B cells. Whether these results suggest either greater affinity of T cells for small amounts of antigen or a greater capacity to be triggered by small amounts of antigen–antibody complex will not concern us here. Mitchison, however, proposed what has become known as the 'local concentration' hypothesis concerning cellular collaboration. Namely, that at least one function of the 'helper' or T cell may be to focus or concentrate low doses of antigen on the surface of the B cell. While the *in vitro* studies of Dutton *et al.* (1971b), which demonstrated that T cells are still required to trigger antibody production, regardless of the antigen concentration, seem to mitigate against such a model, there is additional evidence which can be cited in its favour. For instance, the plant mitogen, phytohaemagglutinin (PHA), normally stimulates lymphoblastosis of T cells *in vitro*, an activity which correlates well with cell-mediated immune activity *in vivo* (Greaves *et al.* 1968, Carr *et al.* 1973). PHA can be polymerized on sepharose beads and, once polymerized, it is capable of stimulating B cells (Andersson *et al.* 1972a,b, Greaves & Bauminger 1972). The lectin Concanavalin A, also normally effects T cells and becomes capable of stimulating B cells when it is used in high concentrations, coupled with some insoluble matrix or presented along with thymus factors (Andersson *et al.* 1972). For the most part, antigens which are known to stimulate the thymus-independent cells directly seem to be polymerized (Miller 1971, Wilson & Feldmann 1972). Coutinho and Möller (1973) found these polymerized T-independent antigens to have active mitogenic properties while T-dependent antigens fail to stimulate B cells. Regardless of whether one thinks of T lymphocytes and/or macrophages as the primary 'helper' cells, concentration *and* polymerization of antigen appear to play a role in B-cell stimulation and the generation of humoral antibody.

While immunoglobulin receptors may engage in the triggering of B-cell proliferation, these receptors may also have a passive role, e.g. functioning to ensure efficient binding between some mitogenic molecule to the B-cell surface when T-independent antigens are presented. T-dependent antigens may function by antigen bridging, thereby assuring intimate association between interacting cells.

Playfair (1971) has also recently reported that low doses of SRBC prime mouse T cells better than they prime B cells. He points out, however, that strain differences must be taken into account, since the New Zealand Black (NZB) hybrid (NZB × Balb/c F1) tends to respond more vigorously to priming at both the T and B cell levels than the C57Bl × Balb/c F1. Greaves and Möller 1970, Greaves *et al.* 1970, Kettman and Dutton 1971, and Falkoff and Kettman 1972 demonstrated that priming of T-cell activity can be quickly established by very low doses of antigen which fail to stimulate antibody production. Several other studies have also been reported which show that small antigen doses with little or no potential to stimulate a detectable primary response nevertheless provide sufficient memory for a substantial secondary response (Salvin & Smith 1964, McDevitt *et al.* 1966, Hanna *et al.* 1967). While high doses of antigen initiate optimum primary responses, subsequent challenges may give poorer secondary responses than can be achieved by low dosage priming (Uhr *et al.* 1962, Sevhag & Mandel 1964a,b, Sterzl 1966).

Low and high antigen doses can stimulate DNA synthesis in lymph node cells *in vitro* (Paul *et al.* 1968). Segal *et al.* (1971) and Nakamura *et al.* (1972) have demonstrated that at least one cell cycle appears to be critical for carrier specific priming and for B-cell production of DNP specific antibody. Marchalonis (1971) using ^{3}H-thymidine incorporation in conjunction with rosette assays of immunized *Bufo marinus* found that the increase in splenic RFC could be largely accounted for by cell division. In addition to the role cellular proliferation might play in T-cell priming, it is suggested that antigen may direct a 'homing' of specific T cells into the spleen (Sprent *et al.* 1971) or the activation of previously inactive T cells (Miller *et al.* 1971). Although T-cell proliferation may be initiated by low antigen doses, Kappler and Hoffman (1973) using vinblastine as an inhibitor of mitosis have shown that while the priming of 'helper' activity precedes the appearance of APC by as much as one day in the mouse, T cells lag behind B cells after the onset of cellular division. They suggest their evidence indicates that T cells, whose activity increases during priming may represent a different cellular population from those which serve to 'help' in the initiation of the primary B-cell response. Later I shall present data which suggests that this does not seem to be true in the newt.

The relative rate of antibody synthesis increases with the antigen dose, at least up to some optimal dose level (Sterzl & Trnka 1957, Winebright &

Fitch 1962, Uhr & Finkelstein 1963, Svehag & Mandel 1964b). Various investigators suggest that the correlation between antigen dose level and the rate of antibody production is due to either an increase in the number of cells producing antibodies during the exponential phase of antibody formation or to an increase in the quantity of antibody generated in each of the antibody-producing cells (APC) (Perkins *et al.* 1961, Bradley & Watson 1963, Urso & Makinodan 1963, Uhr & Finkelstein 1963, Svehag & Mandel 1964b). Wigzell *et al.* (1966) and Campbell and Kind (1969), however, present evidence which provides a choice between these alternatives. In assaying for PFC by the agar plate technique of Jerne and Nordin (1963), they note that while the number of PFC is enhanced, the size of the individual lytic zone around each PFC does not increase. It is therefore possible to state that as higher dose levels are used, capable of initiating earlier and higher levels of PFC activity and serum antibody titres, enhancement is due to an increase in the number of cells producing antibody. Additional mitoses at the antigen-sensitive or the precursor cell level must be taking place, since each PFC appears to generate the same amount of specific antibody regardless of the dose of the antigen utilized. Albright and Evans (1965) employ an *in vivo* transfer system of donor cells into an irradiated host to study the kinetics of haemagglutinating antibody production in mice and find that the latent period is antigen dose-dependent. These findings are similar to those of Uhr *et al.* (1962).

All of the information I have reviewed thus far from experiments which have studied antibody production shows higher antigen doses initiating increases in the amount of antibody, the number of PFC generating that antibody, and an earlier onset of the response. It must be pointed out that haemolytic plaque and haemagglutination assays measure *only* these features of the immune response. The experiments I will soon be presenting with amphibia involve immunocyto-adherence (ICA) assays which have the potential for measuring not only antibody-producing cell activity (thymus-independent in the mammal) but also 'helper' activity (thymus-dependent in the mammal) because they measure the total number of cells which are capable of binding antigen. In addition, the combination of ICA with carrier-hapten immunization provides a formidable tool for visual analyses of collaboration in immune responses.

Sell and Gell (1965) and Sell (1967) clearly point up the presence of immunoglobin on the surface of lymphoid cells, since they are able to stimulate blast transformation of circulating rabbit lymphocytes *in vitro* with anti-allotype serum. Functional immunoglobin associated with the T-cell sub-population in humoral responses is indicated by Greaves *et al.* (1970), Warner *et al.* (1970), Feldman and Diener (1971), Davie *et al.* (1971), Lesley *et al.* (1971), and Rittenberg and Bullock (1972) using anti-IgG or anti-θ antibodies. A similar approach was also used by Mason and Warner (1970) and Reithmuller *et al.* (1971) who suppressed cell-mediated immune responses.

All of these studies entail the use of various anti-sera whose purity may be questionable (Greaves & Raff 1971, Takahashi *et al.* 1971).

Using the ICA technique (rosette assay) Zaalberg *et al.* (1968) found a ten-fold increase in the number of antigen binding cells as compared to the number of antibody-producing cells seen by the plaque method. Rosette forming cells (RFC) may form as a consequence of very small amounts of antibody being present on the surface of lymphoid cells relative to the amount that may be required for detection of haemolytic plaque formation. It does seem to be the case that the optimal SRBC dose (25 per cent) for the primary response as detected by assays for PFC is the same as that which generates optimum RFC numbers (Moav & Harris 1970). The same dosage level (50 per cent) SRBC is also optimum for the secondary response when both assays are used. When mammalian cells are used, rosette formation is an active process at 37°C. Antibody is secreted and multiple layers of red cells may be caused to adhere to the immunized cell surface. At 4°C RFC formation appears to be due to pre-existing antibody on the spleen cell surface (Elson *et al.* 1972). No rosettes will form when protein inhibitors are used. Further, it is found that RFC and PFC appear to come off a density gradient at about the same point; therefore Elson *et al.* (1972) hypothesize that the cell populations are the same. In general then, antigen-binding cells (RFC) outnumber antibody-secreting cells (PFC) at peak response. This difference may be due to the different sensitivities of the two tests, antigen-binding cells being different from antibody-secreting cells. Greaves and Möller (1970) and Greaves, Möller and Möller (1970) suggest that antigen-binding cells, as determined by the rosette assay, include not only differentiated cells actively secreting antibody which can be identified by the multiple layers of red cells adherent on the plasma cell surface, but also antigen-sensitive cells that may be capable of producing or releasing antibody. These non-secreting spleen cells might be either bone marrow derived precursors for future antibody-secreting cells or they might be thymus derived cells which function by helping the B cell generate specific antibody. In general, the evidence that some of the antigen-binding cells observed in immunocyto-adherence assays are thymus-derived cells comes from studies using the θ isoantigen. That anti-θ and serum complement significantly repress the number of antigen-binding cells counted has been reported by Greaves and Möller (1970), Greaves and Hogg (1971) and Raff (1971). Recently, Greaves and Raff (1971) and Takahashi *et al.* (1971) questioned earlier anti-θ studies on grounds that anti-θ sera is usually contaminated with antibodies directed against surface determinants other than θ. At least one of these has been shown to be present on thymus-independent (B) cells. More recently, however, Bach and Dardenne (1972) report visualization of T-cell rosettes; antigen-binding cells which are part of the *in vivo* hydrocortisone resistant pool of thymocytes. They suggest that both T and B cells involved in the anti-sheep RBC immune response will form spontaneous rosettes. As Bach and Dardenne (1972) point out, some 75 per cent of the anti-sheep RFC are θ-positive and sensitive to azathioprine. The ratio of T to B cells among normal mouse spleen anti-sheep RFC appears to be about two-thirds T (θ-positive) cells to one-third B (θ-negative) cells. Their data also confirm the existence of specificity at the level of T cells already suggested by (1) double transfer experiments (Miller & Mitchell 1969), (2) tolerance in the thymus, (3) specificity of mitosis induction in T cells, and (4) specific inactivation of thymus cells by I^{125} labelled antigen (Basten *et al.* 1971). Since Bach and Dardenne have also shown that the totality of thymus-dependent spleen and thymus RFC are inhibited by anti-immunoglobulin serum this suggests that the receptors of T cells share antigens with immunoglobulins. This is also suggested by inhibition studies of thymus antigen-binding cells by Basten *et al.* (1971). Recently, human lymphocyte rosette formation has been inhibited by the use of anti-T cell serum by Wortis *et al.* (1973). Modabber *et al.* (1970) report antigen binding of cells in the normal mouse thymus which is specific and can be inhibited by cross reactive materials. Immunocompetent thymus cells have been reported by Raff (1971) and Leckband and Boyse (1971).

While some antigen-binding cells as assayed by immunocyto-adherence may be formed by the thymus-dependent sub-population of lymphoid cells, there is no question that at least some of them are of B-cell origin. Surgical bursectomy of chicken embryos (Hemmingsson & Alm 1972) will drastically impair both the rosette-forming and plaque-forming cell responses later in life. It appears then that both of these responses, antigen binding and antibody producing, are primarily bursa dependent, *at least in the chicken.* Further, Theis *et al.* (1973) report the absence of RFC in chickens with delayed hypersensitivity agammaglobulinaemia. For a recent review of this issue see Crone *et al.* (1972). In the mouse, Hunter, Munro, and McConnell have recently reported (1972) that they were unable to detect rosette forming cells in 'educated' T-cell populations. Their work, along with the reports of Greaves and Raff (1971) and Takahashi *et al.* (1971) in combination with the situation in chicken as revealed by bursectomy, focuses attention on the question of whether any T cells will form rosettes. The studies of McConnell (1971) and Haskill *et al.* (1972) provide us with impressive proof that the same cells which are capable of forming multilayered rosettes, i.e. secretory RFC (S+), which are separable from non-secreting RFC (S−) by centrifugation are the same cells assayed when one studies plaque-forming cells (PFC). Haskill *et al.* (1972) categorize their RFC in terms of the number of red cells bound to the surface of sensitized spleen cells. After high and low doses of antigen were provided, gluteraldehyde fixation was used to study the rosettes. Gradient separation under gravity was used to show that multilayered RFC separated in the same fraction as those cells which were capable of producing PFC. Like Greaves, Möller and Möller (1970), Haskill *et al.* (1972) also found that the low dose appears to give a relatively stronger T-cell response, that is, in comparison with the B-cell stimulation. Thymus-dependent cells produce RFC which seem to fall into two main classes, one with binding capacities of SRBC of around five and the other with a binding capacity of around nine. Unlike Hunter *et al.* (1972) these authors found that 'educated' thymocytes still display the rather narrow low antigen-binding rates found in normal thymic lymphocytes. By and large the RFC population in normal thymus binds only a few SRBC and appears to be primarily small and medium lymphocyte types. Adult thymectomy was found to reduce the numbers of RFC which had low numbers of red cells adherent on their surface. It is interesting that with the decrease in minimal binding T-cell RFC, there is a concomitant increase in higher binding capacity B RFC, something which has been noted by others following thymectomy (Bach *et al.* 1971, Bach & Dardenne 1972). These morphological distinctions are reinforced by studies utilizing anti-θ which fail to effect the production of multilayered B RFC. Haskill *et al.* (1972) suggest that the reason T RFC are so difficult to identify in the earlier studies is that they are so fragile. Gluteraldehyde fixation will stabilize them however.

Scanning electron microscopy of human T- and B-cell rosettes (Lin *et al.* 1973) would appear to support the contention that T RFC are especially fragile. Gluteraldehyde-fixed RFC from human peripheral blood or tonsils are distinguished as T RFC or B RFC in accordance with the capacity of T cells to bind SRBC and for B cells to form rosettes with complement-coated human red cells. While all of the lymphocytes have multiple microvilli on their surface, those on T RFC are generally smaller, smoother, and fewer in number than on the B RFC. The contact between the SRBC and the T RFC appears to be solely the function of the microvilli. B RFC on the other hand bind red cells to villous and non-villous portions of the RFC surface. Since multilayer (APC) RFC are normally generated at 37°C in mammalian studies, it would not be surprising that the increase in kinetic energies involving binding-site molecules might cause T RFC bindings, already weaker than those of B cells, to be all the more fragile and difficult to visualize without fixation.

The effect of immunogen dose on the primary anti-red cell response of the newt, *Triturus viridescens*

Our initial report on the newt includes data from a preliminary series of experiments in which it is found that the intensity of the primary and secondary immune responses as measured on a single assay date appear to be inversely proportional to the challenge dose of HRBC. Within certain limits this could be because all newt responses are inversely proportional to dose, while another possibility is that response-time courses for different immunogen doses vary such that on a particular assay date and at 23°C one would find antigen-binding levels to be inversely proportional to immunogen dose. Assays performed on other dates, however, might not always fit the case. Because the information that follows is new or has not been presented in detail (Ruben, 1975), let me take the time to quickly describe the quantitative assay technique used. The animals are immunized *in vivo* by intraperitoneal (i.p.) heterologous blood cells such as horse (HRBC), chicken (CRBC), or sheep (SRBC). The immunized newts are kept continuously at 25°C. The red cells are washed, centrifuged, and resuspended in Alsever's solution. The organ to be assayed, the spleen, is mechanically disassociated in seven parts Leibovitz (L-15 GIBCO) to two parts twice glass distilled water after specific periods of post-injection time. Cell suspensions of appropriate concentrations are prepared. Fifty γ ($1\text{–}5 \times 10^5$ spleen cells) aliquots of these cells are then mixed with 10 γ of 1 per cent (about 10^6) of test or control red cells in subsequently covered glass test tubes (10×75 mm) and incubated overnight in the cold at 3–5°C. Antigen binding occurs where specific receptor sites exist on the surface of the previously immunized cells and the adherence is of appropriate red cells (at least three) thereby forming rosettes. Rosette forming cells (RFC) are then counted visually after resuspension of the incubation mixture in Improved Neubauer haemocytometer chambers (American Optical). The data are expressed in terms of RFC per 10^6 (Ruben *et al.* 1973). Since this incubation assay is performed in the cold, it remains a measure of the primary response in spite of the association of the immunized cells with the same type of erythrocytes used for immunization. Data on immunologic memory can be obtained by rechallenging the host before removing the organ to be tested. The rosettes generated by the immunized cells from these cold-blooded animals tend to be relatively stable; and, while care is normally taken to resuspend the incubation mixture gently by rotation before introducing it into the haemocytometer chambers, my tests show that more vigorous agitation of the incubation mixture will only reduce the total number of RFC counted under more gentle resuspension methodology by about 15–20 per cent.

Recently, I explored the issue of what the effect of dosage might be on the anti-erythrocyte response in the newt. The data (Fig. 6.1) clearly show that in the newt there are translocations of the time courses of the primary responses such that the lower the immunogen dose the quicker will be the response. The peak intensity levels of each of the three responses to dilutions of HRBC, however, are in direct proportion to the concentration of immunogen. The intensity peaks are very nearly linear for the three linearly diluted doses. The three doses used to study the primary response are 0·2 ml of 25 per cent, 0·25 per cent, and 0·0025 per cent HRBC. Each data point represents an average of RFC of 16 chambers, eight from each of two different cellular

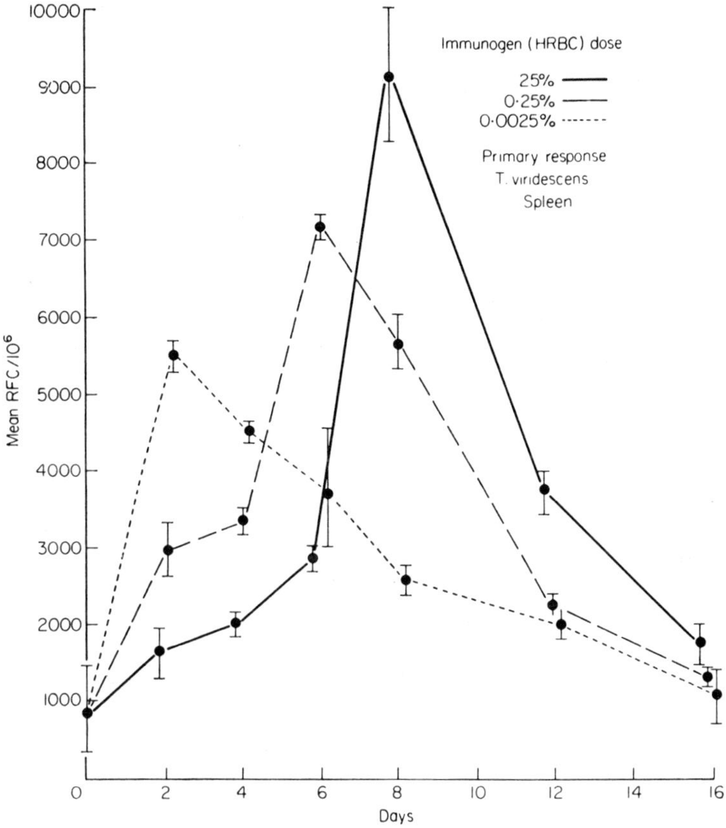

Fig. 6.1. The effect of immunogen (HRBC) dose on the primary immune response in the spleen of the adult newt as assayed by immunocyto-adherence.

pools. Four adult newts are needed to supply each pooled spleen cell population. The standard deviations demonstrate the degree of variation between the average RFC values from the two different cellular pools. These cellular pools are from spleens taken from animals obtained from the same dealer (Mrs L. Babbit, Petersham, Massachusetts, U.S.A.) but approximately 4 months later than when the first group of newts had been challenged and tested. The data which are used to construct these curves appear in Table 6.1. Careful study of these time course curves makes it clear that by assaying at 2, rather than 4-day intervals, as had been done in the original report on the newt, a new 'shoulder' or period of decreasing rate of increase in the number of antigen-binding cells within the spleen appears between days 2 and 4 when the two more concentrated dosages had been used. When all antigen-binding cells generated in these responses are taken into account, the translocations

Table 6.1. The effect of immunogen dosage (percentage HRBC) on the primary immune response of the newt (spleen).

Day	0·0025 per cent HRBC Total RFC/10⁶*	S−†	S+	0·25 per cent HRBC Total RFC/10⁶	S−	S+	25 per cent HRBC Total RFC/10⁶	S−	S+
0 (Background)	877 ± 553	550 ± 314	328 ± 242	877 ± 533	550 ± 314	328 ± 242	877 ± 553	550 ± 314	328 ± 242
2	5521 ± 11	5426 ± 0	96 ± 11	2957 ± 318	2284 ± 55	873 ± 19	1652 ± 311	1610 ± 371	42 ± 59
4	4459 ± 131	3367 ± 440	1103 ± 557	3337 ± 4	2389 ± 82	943 ± 70	1990 ± 35	1518 ± 35	472 ± 22
6	3706 ± 759	3211 ± 1103	496 ± 343	7173 ± 94	6349 ± 466	825 ± 561	2810 ± 138	2438 ± 173	372 ± 35
8	2533 ± 161	1784 ± 171	749 ± 330	5622 ± 335	4301 ± 796	1321 ± 1131	9151 ± 840	5640 ± 943	3512 ± 103
12	1972 ± 234	1396 ± 285	576 ± 285	2172 ± 50	1659 ± 111	513 ± 509	3686 ± 226	3087 ± 527	599 ± 60
16	1031 ± 318	718 ± 45	313 ± 363	1235 ± 26	860 ± 257	375 ± 284	1668 ± 258	1303 ± 431	361 ± 165

* An average of 16 haemacytometer chamber counts from four incubations involving two different cellular pools, each of which is comprised of spleen cells from four newts, is used for all data presented in this table (see text for details).

† S− (non-secretor) refers to RFC with adherent cells attached only to the spleen cell itself, while S+ (secretor) refers to RFC where additional erythrocyte layers have attached to sensitized cells.

in time reflected in the response curves are reversed from what had been found with the antibody-producing cell data of mammalia. That is, rather than finding that higher doses speed up the immune response in the newt spleen, I find that the lower the dose the quicker the response will be. I will assume for the moment that this reversal of time courses of this complex of cellular activities in the newt has to do with the introduction of data concerning 'helper' cell activity. It should be noted at this point that one cannot speak of T-cell rosettes or B-cell rosettes with regard to this data from the newt. Here I will speak of antigen recognizing (ARC) or 'helper' cell activity and antibody producing cell (APC) activity, since neither thymus involvement nor the equivalent of bone marrow originated cells has been yet demonstrated in this species. If the curves obtained with these doses of HRBC are expressions of both 'helper' cell activity and antibody-producing cell activity, then the activity between day 0 and day 2 may involve either the recruitment of 'helper' cells or their mitogenesis, an activity favoured by lower immunogen doses in mammals. The reduction in the rate of increase in the antigen-binding cells involved within the spleen between days 2 and 4 may reflect the period of 'helper' activity itself, when precursors of the APC can be triggered. The reduced slope of the curves may result from some of these 'helper' cells becoming memory cells and entering the circulation. They would therefore escape detection in assays of splenic RFC activity. Finally, the steep increase in cell numbers seen between day 4 and day 8 could represent APC mitogenesis. One should note that neither of these last two activities is detectable when the lowest of the doses, 0·0025 per cent HRBC, is used. It would appear, then, that either the ARC or 'helper' cells remove this small amount of immunogen effectively enough without involvement of an additional cellular population or that disappearance of the 'helper' cell population from the spleen is partially matched by increasing numbers of antibody-producing cells so as to provide for gradual replacement of one type of rosette-forming cell by another. Haskill and Axelrad (1971) visualize this time-dependent progressive shift in the proportion of antigen recognizing cell rosettes to antibody producing cell rosettes in the mammal.

Morphological distinctions between 'helper' RFC and antibody producing RFC

Fig. 6.2 shows the time course curves for the primary anti-HRBC responses in newts after sorting out the numbers of non-secretory rosettes (S − RFC) from secretory rosettes (S + RFC). The same data (see Table 6.1) which is used to generate the time-course curves in Fig. 6.1 is used to affect this separation. When the adherent red cell population is only a single cell layer thick, regardless of their number in excess of three, I consider it to be an S − RFC or ARC RFC. In regard to cellular collaboration, I will soon suggest that these S − RFC reflect 'helper' activity. If two or more layers of red cells

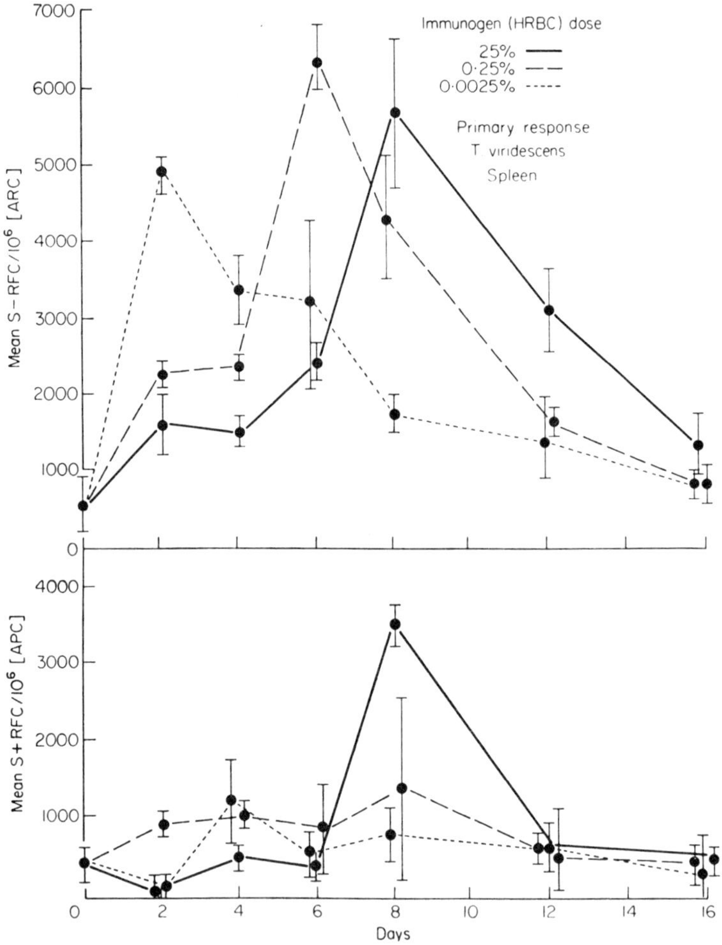

Fig. 6.2. The response curves for ARC (S^-) RFC and APC (S^+) RFC following challenge by three different immunogen (HRBC) doses in the spleen of the newt, *Triturus viridescens.*

adhere to the surface of a spleen cell, regardless of the number in excess of three, it is identified as an S+RFC or antibody producing cell RFC. Not all of the surface has to be occupied by red cells on immunized spleen cells for them to be classified as APC or S+RFC. Fig. 6.3 is a photomicrograph of an RFC bearing tufts of HRBC bound to its surface. Polarization of antigen-binding activity is a common phenomenon and probably reflects localization of receptor sites. The convention I am using for morphological categorization of RFC is that of Greaves, Möller and Möller (1970). Regardless of the number of erythrocytes bound to a surface, it seems reasonable to assume

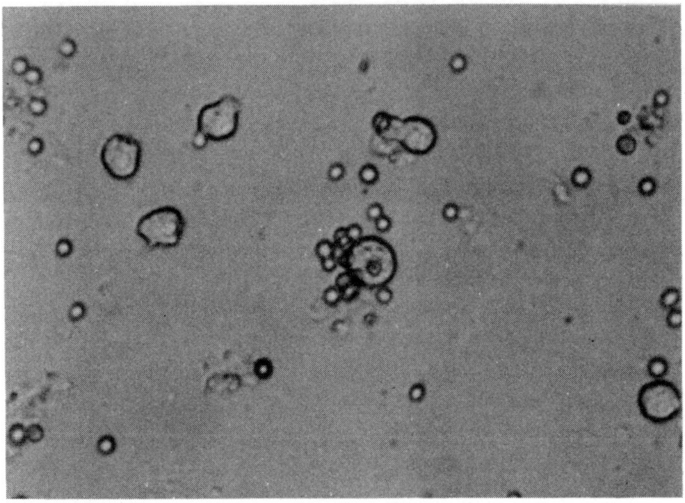

Fig. 6.3. An APC (S^+) RFC from the newt spleen. Binding of multiple layers of red cells (HRBC) may occur locally suggesting a patchy distribution of surface determinants, ×150.

that some secretion of antibody is necessary for a second layer of adherence to develop. The rosettes of the newt are not killed and fixed. Fresh suspensions of the incubation mixtures are introduced into haemocytometer chambers. An advantage of using the amphibian system is the stability of rosettes in the absence of fixation. It turns out that when the numbers of S−RFC alone are curved they correspond closely to those already described for the total RFC responses with two important exceptions. One important difference seems to be that the peak number of ARC or S−RFC of the 25 per cent HRBC dose curve is about 1000 RFC/10^6 less than that seen at the peak response for the next lower (0·25 per cent) dosage. This is in keeping (1) with information from studies discussed earlier with mammalia which show that higher immunogen doses obviate some of the necessity for 'helper' activity while affecting APC turn on, and (2) our own data which shows that the only substantial population of S+RFC appears at this time: at 8 days and only with the highest challenge dose. Another, perhaps more striking difference involves the enhancement of the declining slope of the 2- and 4-day 'shoulders' of the 0·25 per cent and the 25 per cent S−RFC curves. This strongly supports an earlier speculation that either depression of ARC generation, or the migration of memory cells from the spleen might accompany 'helper' activity. The original upward slope on the curves recording total rosette forming cell activity, may then be accounted for in terms of early APC generation. Information about the S+RFC seems far less reliable than the total RFC data, since large standard deviations which represent deviations even between assays using the same populations of pooled cells exist. This unreliability suggests an instability with regard to the outer adherent layer (s). Even minor differences in the shearing force generated during resuspension of the incubation mixtures may be sufficient to loosen these, while those erythrocytes actually adhering to the surface of the sensitized cells would be more firmly held. Moreover, it should be noted that in all likelihood only a fraction of the potential numbers of APC may actually be visualized at low temperatures (3–5°C). The effect of temperature on immune responses *in vivo* has been studied in some detail (Allen & McDaniel 1937, Bisset 1947, Evans & Horton 1961, Kruger & Twedt 1962, for example). A second advantage to using amphibia for rosette assays appears to be the capacity of some RFC to secrete antibody while being incubated in the cold!

Because proper identification of the RFC type is so crucial to the case being presented, two modifications of the technique can be used to be more certain that the curves are actually reflecting a transition from ARC RFC to APC RFC during the progress of immune response. One modification suggested by Marchalonis (personal communication), involved raising the temperature of the mixture of immunized cells with the adhering erythrocytes to 25°C for 2 hours prior to overnight incubation in the cold. This period of prior warming helps to maximize the secretory aspect and allow a more accurate description of the number of secretory rosettes which are usually counted with only cold incubation conditions. The prior warm temperature treatment does not increase the proportion of secretory rosettes at 2 days after challenge but does at 8 days (Table 6.2). This is supportive of the view that during the first week of response there is a very high percentage of ARC or S−RFC which subsequently declines in the face of increasing numbers of secretory or APC RFC. This increase in S+RFC after prewarming is time, but not strongly dose-dependent, although there is a somewhat greater increase in S+RFC with the higher dose at 8 days.

Another modification which is useful entails testing whether cytophilic antibody is playing a role in the generation of false rosettes. Conceivably, rosettes can be created by having a few secretor cells release antibody 'gluing' the red cells to spleen cell surfaces lacking in those specific receptor sites. One might also imagine that S− can become S+RFC in a similar manner. High titre (1:512) newt anti-HRBC serum was incubated with unimmunized spleen cells of the newt for two hours at 25°C. The cells are then washed in fresh Alsever's and incubated as usual in the cold with HRBC. The serum was collected by heart drainage from immunized animals. It was pooled and tested after decomplementation in micro-haemagglutination plates (Cooke Engineering). The serum (not decomplemented) fails to alter the number of spontaneous rosettes which are generated and the proportion of nonsecretory to secretory rosettes remains as before. This serum can also be used with newt spleen cells which are immunized with 0·0025 per cent and 25 per cent HRBC

Table 6.2. Effect of pre-warming* on newt spleen cell multiple layer (S+RFC). Antigen-binding of HRBC (primary response).

	HRBC dosage									
	0·0025 per cent					25 per cent				
	Cold		Warm			Cold		Warm		
Assay day	% S−†	% S+	% S−	% S+	% incr. S+	% S−	%S+	%S−	% S+	% incr. S+
2	91‡	9	90	10	1	91	9	89	11	2
8	75	25	57	33	8	79	21	52	38	19

* Pre-warming entails placing cellular mixtures at 25°C for 2 hours prior to the usual overnight incubation in the cold.

† S− refers to the percentage non-secretory RFC/10^6 spleen cells, % S+ refers to the percentage multilayered or secretory RFC/10^6 spleen cells.

‡ These figures are averages of two different experimental series. They represent 16 chamber counts as described for Table 6.1.

2 and 8 days earlier. Serum incubation does not alter the original data. Following the suggestion of Kapp and Benaceraff (1972) potential cytophilic antibody activity can also be tested, using immunized and unimmunized cells from the spleen of newts, incubated with serum collected at the time of the peaks of the cellular or rosette response. Kapp and Benaceraff (1972) find that cytophilic antibody is especially high at the time of peak cellular activity and one should not then limit cytophilic antibody tests to high titre antisera. These sera also fail to alter the previous RFC data.

The 25°C pre-incubation experiments as well as the cytophilic antibody experiments suggest that the total number of rosettes previously counted represent a number which is not temperature or cytophilic antibody-dependent. Furthermore, the increase in the proportion of S+RFC with higher temperature found at the 8-day assay date but not early in the immune response suggests that if there is an error in terms of the differential counts, then it is an error which favours S−RFC over S+RFC. This supports the view that initially S−RFC predominate only to give way to higher numbers of S+RFC as the immune response progresses.

Measuring 'helper' activity

It is possible to determine levels of 'helper' activity by combining the immuno-cyto-adherence assay with carrier-hapten immunization (Ruben *et al.* 1972). The immunization is affected by an *in vivo* challenge i.p. of 0·2 ml of 10 per cent CRBC-TNP at 2, 4, 6, or 8 days following high (25 per cent) or low (0·0025 per cent) dose pre-immunization with 0·2 ml CRBC. All assays are performed 8 days after the newts receive the CRBC-TNP. The intensity of the response as measured against 1 per cent HRBC-TNP less that generated with 1 per cent HRBC is a measure of the 'helper' activity available to the animals at 2, 4, 6, or 8 days after pre-immunization with the carrier as described below. The use of high and low dose priming affords the opportunity to test the dose dependence as well as the kinetics of 'helper' capacity to a single challenge dose. The RFC/10^6 counted with HRBC assay provide a measure of background anti-HRBC activity as well as the degree of cross-reactivity generated by CRBC priming. This value is subtracted from the number of RFC/10^6 formed in association with HRBC-TNP. The number of RFC/10^6 remaining then is a measure of anti-TNP activity. Since no anti-TNP activity can be demonstrated in the absence of carrier priming, this value can be referred to as response enhancement, i.e. 'helper' activity (Table 6.3). In all cases heavily substituted TNP-red cells are used for challenge, while lightly substituted TNP-red cells are used for assays. These conjugates are prepared according to the methods of Rittenberg and Pratt (1969), as modified by Kettman and Dutton (1970). A control for enhancement by pre-immunization

Table 6.3. Measurement of 'helper' activity in newt spleen cells by varying the time between challenges of carrier (CRBC) and carrier-hapten (CRBC-TNP) and carrier dose (CRBC-TNP = 10 per cent in all cases).

Carrier	Percentage carrier dose	Days between injections	Anti-TNP*RFC/10^6 ('Helper' activity)	Percentage increase in S+RFC
CRBC	0.0025	2	7113±613	79
		4	6642±1775	85
		6	2551±424	95
		8	246±346	100
CRBC	25	2	1636±114	66
		4	1791±1215	69
		6	2404±620	100
		8	0±0	—
SRBC	0·0025	2–8	0±0	—
SRB	25	2–8	0±0	—
—	—	—	0±0	—

* Anti-TNP RFC/10^6 are determined by subtracting the RFC/10^6 assayed with HRBC from the number assayed with HRBC–TNP. All assays were done 8 days after CRBC–TNP injection.
† Control with 10 per cent CRBC–TNP injected at day 0 and assayed 8 days later.

with carrier consists of presentation of only the 0·2 ml of 10 per cent CRBC-TNP by i.p. injection followed by assays with HRBC and HRBC-TNP 8 days later. Carrier specificity is demonstrable by substituting SRBC for CRBC high or low dose priming. Carrier specificity controls are used for each priming dose as well as each of the times tested in the original series. All experimental points shown in the curves (Fig. 6.4) of 'helper' activity following high and

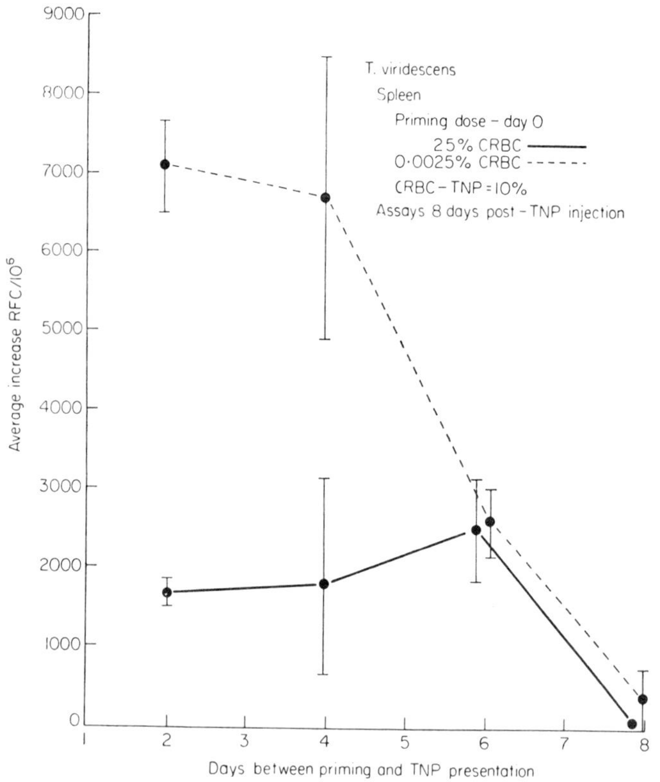

Fig. 6.4. Anti-TNP RFC enhancement, i.e. 'helper' activity is both dose- and time-dependent in the spleen of the newt.

low dose CRBC priming are average values measured from two separate spleen cell pools of four adult newts each. These two sets of experiments were performed several weeks apart from each other. The animals were all collected from Petersham, Massachusetts, U.S.A.

All of the control series show values of less than zero RFC/10^6. Negative values have been obtained routinely in controls using this test system. This seems to suggest that the presence of TNP in the assay interferes with rosette formation. The positive rosette values obtained with carrier-specific priming should therefore be viewed as actually being higher than the counts reported here.

As in the dosage experiments, all assay data is collected in terms of the number of non-secretory and secretory rosettes. These data appear in Table 6.4. The results are especially enlightening in pointing up both the dose and time dependence of available 'helper' activity. They add substance to speculations made earlier that (1) low doses more successfully stimulate 'helper' cells than high immunogen doses (2) one can distinguish 'helper' activity from antibody-producing cell activity in terms of the morphological separation of non-secretory from secretory RFC and finally (3) by using the rosette assay with these newts it is possible to visualize the progressive shift in time during the immune response of non-secretory (helper) to secretory (APC) rosettes. It is important to note that the data show that most of the enhancement of anti-TNP activity exposed by combining the rosette assay with carrier-hapten immunization can be accounted for by secretory rosettes. Anti-hapten activity is expected to be an antibody-producing cell activity and not one of the 'helper' cell population which responds to the carrier. The data firmly support this expectation.

Therefore, 'helper' activity is greatest with low dosage priming between days 2 to 4 pre-challenge and it decreases rapidly thereafter. It is particularly interesting that the degree of difference between 'helper' activity after low and high dose priming is about the same as that noted earlier in the dosage experiments when one compares the proportion of non-secretor rosettes generated by the two extreme immunogen dosages used. The primary significance of the above finding may be that this is the first time antigen-binding, non-secretory RFC have been correlated with a function. Further, contrary to the conclusion drawn by Kappler and Hoffman (1973) that T mitogenesis and 'helper' activity may involve separate sub-populations. It would seem that, in the newt at least, those cells generated or recruited early in the response to low dose priming are likely to be the same cells which provide 'helper' function, unless, of course, 'helper' activity were to be carried on by non-antigen binding cells.

Measuring antibody producing cell activity

It is possible, by maximizing 'helper' activity and varying the time after presentation of hapten for assay, to visualize the kinetics of antibody cell-producing activity. Maximization of 'helper' activity is achieved by using low dosage priming with CRBC followed by CRBC-TNP four days later. Assays of anti-TNP activity through immunocyto-adherence with HRBC and HRBC-TNP at 2-day intervals clearly demonstrate that anti-TNP activity appears 8 days after TNP challenge and is gone from the spleen of the newt two days later (Fig. 6.5). This datum agrees exactly with the

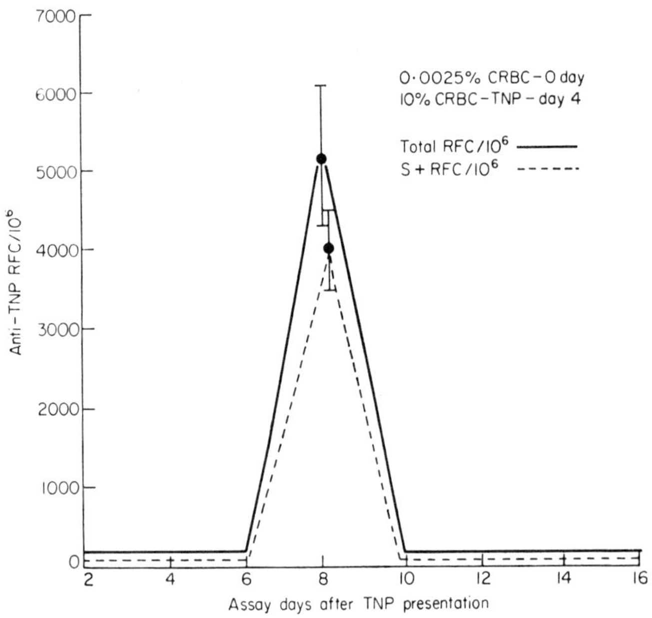

Fig. 6.5. The kinetics of anti-TNP RFC activity in the spleen of the newt.

secretory rosette data obtained with the primary response to HRBC which show a peak of S+RFC at 8 days. It also supports the view that multilayered rosettes are antibody-producing cells, since nearly all of the carrier specific enhancement of the anti-TNP response can be accounted for by increase in this type of RFC.

Use of the carrier-hapten system combined with immunocyto-adherence then provides the investigator with the opportunity to visualize both 'helper' cell activity and antibody producing cell activity during the progressing immune response.

Anamnesis

At the same time that the extensive exploration of the effect of the three antigen dosages on the primary response was being studied, other adults from the same newt population were simultaneously studied with respect to the secondary response. In all instances the second challenge consists of 0·2 ml of 10 per cent HRBC and is administered by i.p. injection 4 days after the priming dose. The curves (Fig. 6.6) compare the respective primary response curve at each priming dose with the secondary response at each point in time. As before the standard deviations refer to variations between two populations of spleen cells drawn from quartets of different test animals. The data used to

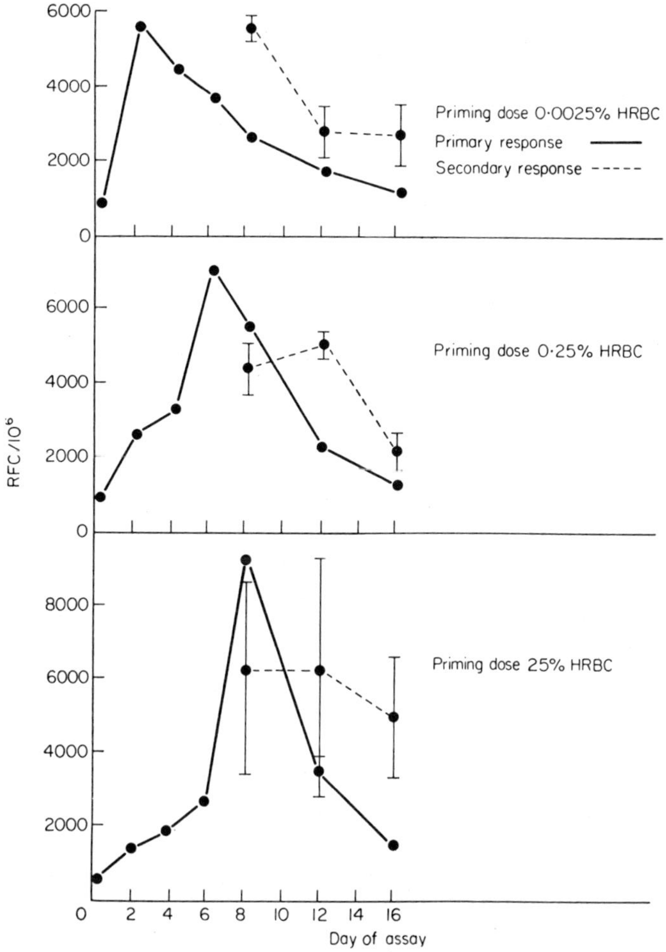

Fig. 6.6. A comparison of both primary and secondary responses with different immunogen (HRBC) doses in the spleen of the newt. The second challenge is 10 per cent in all cases on day 4.

construct these curves appear in Table 6.4. They suggest that while after the first week following the second challenge, the secondary response is usually greater than the comparable primary response to the same *initial* challenge, its value rises more slowly, and it does not exceed the peak primary response regardless of the primary challenge dose! Further low dose priming comes closest to initiating a secondary response which approximates the peak of the primary response. While only preliminary data on the secondary response in this species showing a modest doubling of the comparable primary response has been published (Cohen 1966, 1968, Tournefier *et al.* 1969, Ruben *et al.*

Table 6.4. Effect of varying priming dose (HRBC) on the secondary response in newt spleen cells. (In all cases the second challenge is 10 per cent HRBC, injected 4 days after the primary.)

Assay day	Priming dose 0·0025 per cent Primary	Secondary	0·25 per cent Primary	Secondary	25 per cent Primary	Secondary
8	2533 ± 161	5627 ± 0	5622 ± 335	4381 ± 660	9151 ± 840	6168 ± 2610
12	1972 ± 234	2519 ± 564	2172 ± 50	5260 ± 154	3686 ± 226	6625 ± 3382
16	1031 ± 318	2622 ± 972	1235 ± 972	2011 ± 438	1668 ± 258	4987 ± 1622

1972), have demonstrated anamnesis in allograft rejection in salamanders. However, while Cohen (1970) observed that second-set grafts *may* be rejected more rapidly than first-set grafts, some may survive even longer or break down with first-set timing! Only modest secondary responses have been reported for the South African clawed toad, *Xenopus laevis*, by Yamaguichi *et al.* (1972) and Manning and Turner (1972). Evans *et al.* (1965) in reviewing antibody synthesis in poikilothermic vertebrates report that they failed to obtain higher titres on secondary immunization of the reptiles *D. dorsalis* and *S. obesus* with rabbit γ-globulin or human γ-globulin. They further show that experiments designed to demonstrate immunologic memory in the marine toad *Bufo marinus* using *Salmonella typhosa* H antigen injected three months after the primary injection stimulated antibody titre increase. This titre failed to reach a geometric mean titre as high as that attained in the primary period, however. When the interval between challenges was extended to 240 days the results were still the same. Immunofluorescent studies suggest a two-fold increase in antibody in secondary responses. Similar studies with the guitar fish, *Rhinobatus productos*, a cartilaginous fish and the bowfin, *Amia calva*, fail to reveal substantial secondary responses to Keyhole Limpet haemocyanin. Failure to show anamnesis in the sting ray *Dasyatis say* is also described. In light of this background it seemed worthwhile for us to investigate the secondary anti-red cell response of the newt more thoroughly. Ms Sheryl Swink performed a series of experiments in my laboratory in which she injected 0·2 ml high (25 per cent) or low (0·0025 per cent) dose HRBC priming challenges i.p. and followed these with a secondary challenge (i.p.) of 0·2 ml 10 per cent HRBC 4, 8, and 12 days after primary challenge. The responses were then monitored at 4-day intervals after secondary challenge. Rosette assays were used to visualize the cellular responses, while haemagglutinin assays provide information on serum antibody titre. The immunocyto-adherence data appear in Table 6.5 and the curves of total RFC activity are available in Fig. 6.7. Non-secretory and secretory RFC data after low and high dose priming appear in Fig. 6.8. All of these experiments were done

Table 6.5. Secondary responses of newt spleen cells with variation in the time between injections and priming dose (second challenge = 10 per cent to HRBC in all cases).

	Priming dosage						
	0·0025 per cent HRBC			25 per cent HRBC			
Assay	Days between injections			Days between injections			Parameter
day	4	8	12	4	8	12	measured
8	2109	—	—	1794	—	—	S−RFC/10^6
	4270	—	—	1331	—	—	S+RFC/10^6
	6379	—	—	3125	—	—	Total RFC/10^6
12	868	650	—	1003	896	—	S−RFC/10^6
	87	532	—	617	359	—	S+RFC/10^6
	955	1182	—	1620	1255	—	Total RFC/10^6
16	517	587	496	101	1269	164	S−RFC/10^6
	388	744	0	152	3321	109	S+RFC/10^6
	905	1331	496	253	4590	273	Total RFC/10^6
20	873	581	958	596	1646	427	S−RFC/10^6
	635	1163	479	496	2212	0	S+RFC/10^6
	1508	1744	1437	1092	3858	427	Total RFC/10^6
24	521	2405	1616	80	1425	855	S−RFC/10^6
	608	954	1869	477	2137	2992	S+RFC/10^6
	1129	3359	3485	557	3562	3847	Total RFC/10^6

with a population of adult newts purchased from a different dealer in Massachusetts (U.S.A.). A few interesting conclusions are suggested by these data. First, maximizing 'helper' activity by using low dose priming followed by a challenge 4 days later provides a peak response equal to that determined earlier with carrier-hapten immunization (6379 RFC/10^6 as compared with 7100 RFC/10^6). It is only 15 per cent higher than the peak primary response of 5500 RFC/10^6 with 0·0025 per cent HRBC in the different adult population used earlier. Secondly, there is a dramatic shift in the proportion of non-secretory to secretory RFC when one compares the peak low dose initiated primary response (98 per cent S− : 2 per cent S+) to the peak of the low dose primed secondary response (33 per cent S− : 67 per cent S+). Thirdly, high dose priming which generates little 'helper' activity does not stimulate substantial secondary responses either. The peak secondary response in the cellular assay data is achieved after 8 days, when an 8-day interval separates the primary and secondary challenge. This looks suspiciously like a primary response with regard to the number of S+RFC at 8 days! An 8-day period seems to be required for a high dose primary challenge of HRBC to reach its cellular peak. Most of the data points obtained with these cellular assays are not substantially above background which may mean that many sensitized cells leave the spleen after a secondary challenge. The haemagglutinin data

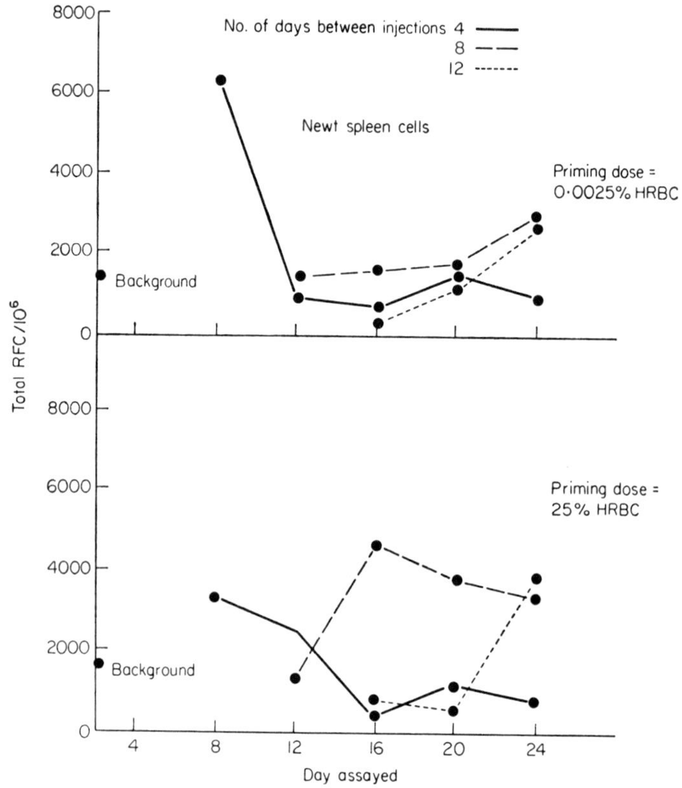

Fig. 6.7. Alterations in secondary responses in the newt spleen when the priming dosage and the time between challenges is varied. The second challenge is 10 per cent HRBC.

(Fig. 6.9, Table 6.6) are especially interesting, since they suggest that with high dose priming, the longer the interval between primary and secondary challenge, the higher will be the serum antibody titre. Blood is withdrawn by cardiac drainage and the serum is decomplemented prior to use. That the antibody titres show progressive increases in their peaks which are not expressed in the cellular data supports the view that many sensitized cells leave the spleen after a secondary challenge but continue to produce antibody elsewhere in the system.

The effect of immunogen dose on the primary anti-erythrocyte response of the leopard frog, *Rana pipiens*

The dosage experiments which I have already described in detail with adult newts have now been repeated with adult *Rana pipiens* by a former student

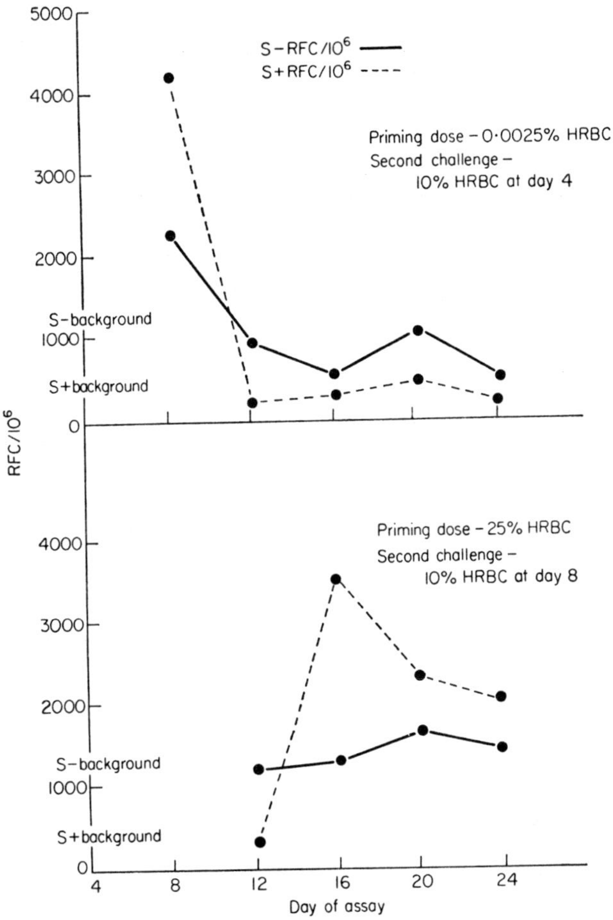

Fig. 6.8. The character of the secondary response with respect to the proportion of S^- to S^+ RFC in the newt spleen when 'helper' activity is maximized at two priming doses.

of mine, Paula R. Levin. She used SRBC as the immunogen rather than HRBC and the volume injected i.p. was increased to 0·5 ml because of the larger volume of these adult frogs. As in all of the experiments I have already described the environmental temperature of immunized animals is maintained at 25°C. The curves of spleen cell activity for the three time courses following challenge with 25 per cent, 0·25 per cent, and 0·0025 per cent SRBC appear in Fig. 6.10. Spleens from four adult frogs were assayed individually for each data point. The standard deviations in these series then are illustrative of individual variation. The curves are clearly very similar to those with the newt. It appears to be the case that in the frog as well, that the lower the

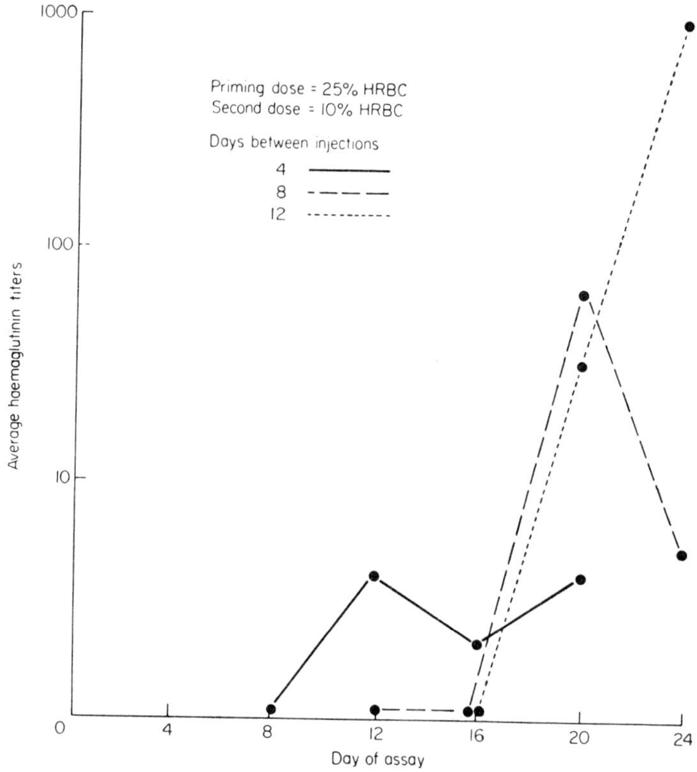

Fig. 6.9. Changes in average haemagglutinin titres as the time between primary and secondary challenges has been varied.

Table 6.6. Average haemagglutinin titres of secondary responses when the time between injections is varied (primary dose = 25 per cent HRBC, the second challenge = 10 per cent HRBC).

Assay day	Days between injections 4	8	12
8	<1:2*	—	—
12	1:4	<1:2	—
16	1:2	<1:2	<1:2
20	1:4	1:65	1:34
24	—	1:5	1:1024

* The titres are determined by the ratio of $1:2^N$ where N = the number of wells with agglutination. The average refers to the average of determinations from two experimental series.

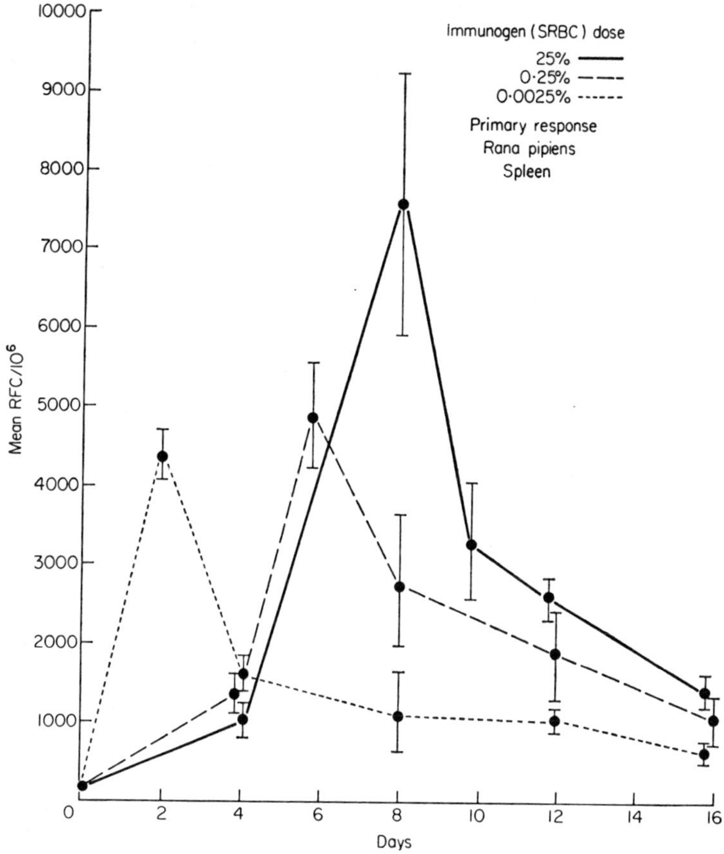

Fig. 6.10. The effect of immunogen (SRBC) dose on the primary immune response in the spleen of the frog, *Rana pipiens*.

dosage the more rapid will be the cellular response, but the higher the dose the more intense the peak of cellular activity. The data appear in Table 6.7.

The frog offers one advantage over the newt in that the thymii of four adults will provide a pool of cells substantial enough for an immunocyto-adherence assay. The curves for frog thymus cell activity in response to these same three SRBC dosages appear in Fig. 6.11. In these curves the standard deviations reflect variation between different cellular pools. Two aspects of the thymus cell results seem to be of special interest. First, since all of the antigen-binding cells of the thymus were of the non-secretory type, this result can be viewed as additionally supportive of the morphological-behavioural distinctions made earlier with regard to non-secretory RFC being recognizable 'helper' cells in the newt. In mammalian systems these 'helper' cells are thymus-dependent cells and in the absence of solid experimental data, it is

Table 6.7. Primary immune response in *Rana pipiens* adults (total RFC/10^6 viable spleen cells counted).

Assay day	0·0025 per cent	HRBC dose 0·25 per cent	25 per cent
2	3875±619*	1790±275	1035±265
4	1552±171	1386±455	1022±282
6	—†	4874±662	3246±156
8	1140±481	2727±822	7550±1737
10	—	—	3246±716
12	1011±112	1925±682	2546±265
16	615±58	944±414	1420±187

* Since individual spleens were assayed, standard deviations refer to variation among individuals (4).
† No assays were performed on these days.

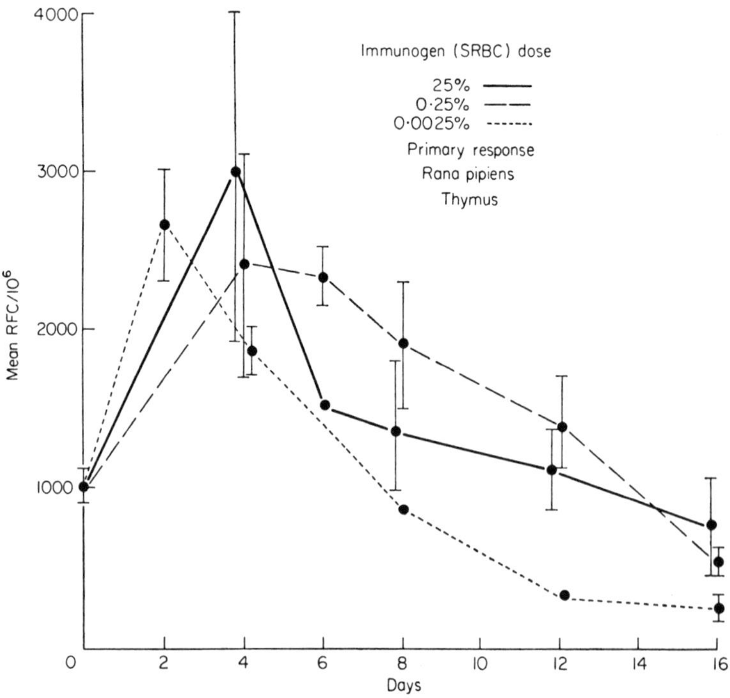

Fig. 6.11. The effect of immunogen (SRBC) dose on antigen binding in the thymus of the frog, *Rana pipiens*.

interesting to suggest that non-secretory RFC may be thymus-dependent in the frog, and perhaps in the newt as well. Secondly, a rapid increase in the number of antigen-binding cells takes place within the thymus after challenge which disappears quickly thereafter. Neither the rise nor the fall appears to be dose-dependent. The data are in Table 6.8.

Table 6.8. Primary immune response in *Rana pipiens* adults (total RFC/10^6 viable thymus cells counted).

Assay day	0.0025 per cent	0.25 per cent	25 per cent
2	2615±624*	2493±121	3016±1092
4	1839±104	2407±786	3120±1088
6	—‡	2344±122	1508†
8	896†	1905±449	1348±476
10	—	—	1250†
12	337†	1425±229	1158±330
16	296†	518±8	775±268

* Since thymic from four individuals were pooled for each assay, standard deviations refer to differences between two different cellular pools.
† These figures are from only one cellular pool of thymocytes.
‡ No assay was performed on these days.

If we now view the totality of the frog and newt data, we arrive at an important conclusion which refers back to a question I posed at the end of the introductory portion of this chapter. Namely, that the similarity found with regard to the immunologic behaviour of the newt and the frog suggests that the newt responses, rather than being unique for urodele adaptive evolution, are in fact representative of a fundamental vertebrate pattern. The salamander, a tailed amphibian, is a member of the Urodele order and is morphologically more primitive than the frog, a member of the most advanced order (Anura, tailless). As I indicated earlier, demonstration of the fundamental nature of these responses is essential if we are to view them as having evolutionary significance with regard to understanding the mammalian immune response. That members of these two disparate modern groups show commonality suggests that 'ancestral' amphibia seem likely to have had these characteristics and that they were in turn passed on to the 'ancestral' reptiles which eventually gave rise to the modern reptiles, birds, and mammals.

It might be worth mentioning that in an evolutionary context, the results with the newt would seem to confirm the obvious. Namely, that selection pressures must be such that vertebrates are caused to respond to those dosages they are most likely to encounter in nature, i.e. low dosages. Nevertheless, they retain, or have developed in parallel, the capacity to contend with relatively enormous amounts of foreign material they would in all probability not be exposed to in the wild.

A comparison with the rodent and a final speculation

This amphibian data becomes even more interesting when we take a look at the situation in the mammal. In Fig. 6.12, I have taken the liberty of curving

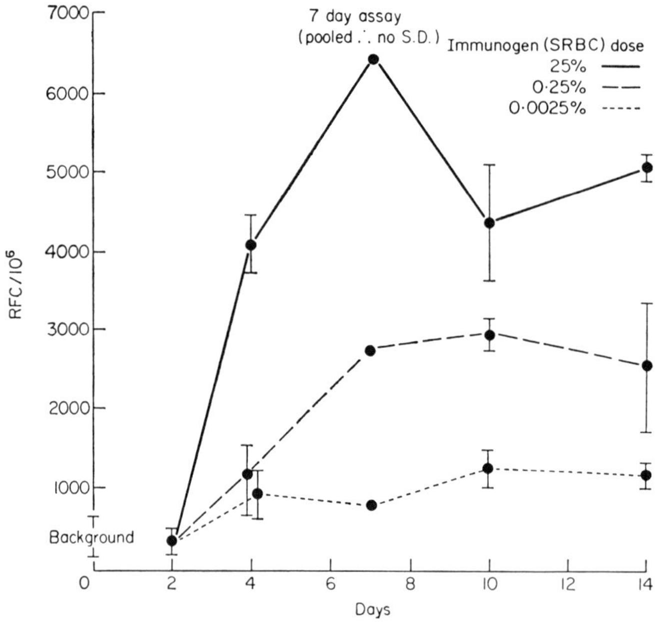

Fig. 6.12. The effect of immunogen (SRBC) dose on the primary immune response of the spleen of the mouse.

data which was presented in tabular form of immunocyto-adherence assays by Greaves, Möller and Möller (1970). They used the three doses of red-cell immunogen I have been dealing with in this report. While the three time-course curves in the mammal are similar to those of the amphibian in that their peak intensities are directly proportional to dose, the rodent curves do not show the translocation of the peaks earlier in time with decreasing dose! In fact, the authors interpret their data to suggest that there was a decrease in the time required to reach peak intensity as the dosage *increased*! One might be tempted to say from these curves, using the standard deviation data presented, that for at least the two lower dosages it is not really clear where the peaks are to be found. One possible interpretation of this apparent difference is that the immune response may develop much more rapidly in the mammal than in amphibia. The total of the mammalian data therefore may represent only that part of the response which occurs after day 10 in the amphibian (Auerbach, personal communication). If this is the case, one might expect that antigen-binding activity prior to 2 days in the rodent might show the dosage translocations I have found in the amphibia.

A somewhat different interpretation of a fundamental distinction between amphibia and mammals has to do with the activity and number of 'helper' cells. It may simply be the case that amphibian 'helper' cells are less efficient than mammalian T cells. More of them may have to be present in order for B cells to be triggered. That the 'helper' cells of the amphibian may be individually less efficient than those of the mammal is suggested by data from a recent report by Du Pasquier *et al.* (1972) who are able to label thymus and thymus-derived splenic cells of the toad *Xenopus laevis* by immunofluorescence. Mammalian T cells appear to have too little immunoglobulin on their surfaces (Raff 1970) for one to use this relatively low resolution assay. It is interesting in this context that Du Pasquier *et al.* find more immunofluorescence (immunoglobulin) associated with the surface of non-thymus-derived than thymus-derived cells. Further, when Weiss *et al.* (1972) studied alterations in immunofluorescent staining after thymectomy of developing larvae, they found increases in the number of the more heavily stained splenic lymphocytes. This shift would be in accord with the compensatory development of B type RFC following thymectomy of mammalia (Bach & Dardenne 1972, Haskill *et al.* 1972). One possibility is that this ability to label the amphibian T cell is a consequence of there being a greater number of binding sites on thymus-dependent cells of the amphibian. This greater number of binding sites might suggest that in fact they are less efficient. That is to say, more binding sites may have to be utilized in order for thymus-dependent cells to elicit 'helper' activity or to engage in cell-mediated immune responses. Lopez *et al.* (1974) have reported that much higher doses of Concanavalin A and Phytohaemagglutinin must be used to initiate T cell mitogenesis in the shark. Their interpretation is that there may be fewer receptor sites but the requirement that more receptor sites be utilized could also explain their results. While it is possible that 'helper' cell activity and allograft cell-mediated immune response activities in amphibia may be separate, it should be pointed out that in general the cell-mediated immune responses which have been shown to be T-dependent are less efficient in amphibia than in the mammalia (Cohen 1971). Perhaps during evolution there has either been (a) an increase in 'helper' cell efficiency or (b) an increased independence on the part of the antibody-producing, B-cell population. In any case, it now seems possible that cellular cooperation is a primitive phenomenon, probably derived from entirely thymus-dependent related responses of the delayed hypersensitivity type. As a consequence of evolution, it may be in process of being phased out in favour of the more efficient condition, that of antibody-producing cells responding directly to an immunogen to yield specific antibody. Polymerized antigens are most likely to serve as natural (bacterial) immunogens for animals and are T-independent (Miller 1971, Feldman & Wilson 1972). This suggests that selective pressures may have been most intense where repeated exposures provided positive adaptive values, thereby encouraging evolutionary change. That is, evolutionary change of a behaviour is liable to be most quickly and efficiently affected when the frequency of the incidence of that behaviour is high!

Summary and conclusions

Anti-erythrocyte responses have been demonstrated in all modern vertebrate groups. By combining carrier-hapten studies with immunocyto-adherence assays, it has been possible to show that cellular cooperation takes place in anti-HRBC responses of the urodele, *Triturus viridescens*. This group of animals is of special interest because it is the most advanced phylogenetically without haemapoeitic bone marrow. While thymii can be found in all but the most primitive modern vertebrates, the hagfish, active bone marrow does not make its appearance until the adult phase of the most advanced amphibia, the Anura (frogs and toads). Cell–cell interactions in immune responses seem likely then to have arisen in evolution before the appearance of a bursa or bone marrow which normally provides the thymus-independent sub-population of lymphocytes in avian and mammalian immunity.

Dosage variation of the red cell immunogen has proved useful in visualizing the immune response in these phylogenetically important groups. Amphibia seem especially useful in using rosette assays, since antigen binding is relatively stable and antibody secretion can occur causing multiple layered rosettes to form even at cold temperatures.

These two characteristics afford the investigator the opportunity to visualize both secretory (antibody-producing cell) rosettes and non-secretory ('helper' cell) rosettes without using a 37°C incubation which would be expected to increase kinetic energies of the molecules involved in binding; perhaps accounting for T-cell rosette instability reported in mammalian systems. Thus two types of RFC are distinguishable on morphological grounds. The non-secretory rosettes appear early in the primary response and are rapidly generated in large numbers after low dose priming of both newts and frogs. Their number is relatively less after high dose priming and in time, as the immune response progresses regardless of dose. The intensity of the maximum response, however, as measured by the number of RFC/10^6 is directly proportional to the concentration of the challenge dose. Priming by high dosage therefore generates a response curve which increases slowly with few non-secretory RFC present initially and which peaks late as a consequence of the generation of large numbers of secretory RFC. Carrier-hapten studies, in which the time of presentation of the hapten after specific carrier challenge is varied are useful to measure 'helper' activity. This activity is clearly both dose- and time-dependent. Low dose priming by carrier (CRBC) will produce a degree of 'helper' enhancement of anti-TNP activity which correlates with the number of non-secretory RFC generated during the primary anti-red cell response. The relatively small degree of 'helper' function found after high dose priming by carrier also correlates with the lower number of non-secretory RFC of the primary HRBC response. The degree of 'helper' function available after both immunogen dosages dissipates rapidly in time. It has therefore been possible for the first time to correlate the number of non-secretory RFC observed visually, with the suspected physiological behaviour of these cells. Variations in the assay time after presentation of hapten clearly demonstrate that when 'helper' activity is maximized, secretory rosette formation in the newt spleen against the TNP hapten begins, peaks, and disappears within the 6–10-day period. The kinetics of anti-TNP activity are found to correspond exactly with those seen when red cells serve as the primary challenge and relate to the time when the only significantly large population of multi-layered (secretory) RFC can be observed. Therefore, both behavioural portions of the progressive immune response, 'helper' activity and antibody-producing cell activity, may be visualized in the spleen of the newt by combining carrier-hapten studies with immunocyto-adherence.

Studies on anamnestic responses using high and low dose priming confirm the results obtained using the carrier-hapten system. That is, low dose priming with the second challenge 4 days later, at a time which maximizes 'helper' activity, initiates a 'relatively' successful secondary cellular response, while high dose priming fails to generate as substantial a secondary cellular response (in proportion to the primary) when 4 days serve to separate the two challenges. It must be noted, however, that the best low dose primed secondary response only exceeds the peak primary response by 15 per cent. It would appear that the newt may be utilizing most of its full *cellular* immunologic capacity in the spleen when it is generating primary responses. Serum antibody titres, however, may be increased by progressively lengthening the interval between high dose priming and the second challenge.

Comparison of these results with information drawn from mammalian experimental material suggests that while there are many similarities which link amphibian responses to those of mammals, there also appear to be a few striking differences. They serve to point up the value of what to some may be 'esoteric' species. For instance, Du Pasquier *et al.*'s (1972) finding that T cells of the South African clawed toad *Xenopus laevis*, and the Bullfrog, *Rana catesbiana*, have so much immunoglobulin on their surface, they can be visualized by immunofluorescence coupled with findings reported here concerning low dose priming and 'helper' activity, suggest that amphibia may serve as ideal systems for analysis of the nature of the kind of receptor sites which have proved to be so elusive in mammalia.

If I have effectively described how little is understood of the intriguing collaboration of cells in immune responses of non-mammalian vertebrates, I have succeeded in at least one part of my stated goal. If I have stimulated others to begin to explore these kinds of questions with model systems which offer unique features and advantages, this would be the greatest satisfaction an author could ask for.

Acknowledgments

I am grateful to the National Science Foundation U.S.A. (GB-38480) and the National Institutes of Health, Bethesda, Md. U.S.A. (AI–12846) for the partial support of my research. The research assistance and support through discussion of Ms Sheryl Swink are also gratefully acknowledged as is the technical assistance of Ms Judith Ruben and the editorial assistance of Ms Cass Hylton. This chapter is dedicated to my father, Dr Samuel Ruben, who by example showed me the excitement scientific investigation could provide.

References

Abramoff P. & La Via M.F. (1970) Development of the immune response, p. 93. In *Biology of the Immune Response*. McGraw-Hill Inc., New York.

Albright J.F. & Evans T.W. (1965) Influence of antigen dose on kinetics of hemagglutinating antibody production. *J. Immunol.* **95,** 368.

Allen F.W. & McDaniel E.C. (1937) A study of the relation of temperature to antibody formation in cold blooded animals. *J. Immunol.* **32,** 142.

Alm G.V. (1970) The *in vivo* spleen response to sheep erythrocytes in bursectomized irradiated chickens. *Acta Path. Microbiol. Scand.* **78,** 641.

Alm G.V. (1971) *In vitro* studies of chicken lymphoid cells. IV. The effect of thymectomy on the antibody response *in vivo* and on the *in vitro* reactivity of spleen cells to sheep erythrocytes, allogenic cells and phytohemagglutinin. *Int. Arch. Allergy* **41,** 345.

Andersson J., Möller G. & Sjoberg O. (1972a) Selective induction of DNA synthesis in T and B lymphocytes. *Cell. Immunol.* **4,** 381.

Andersson J., Möller G. & Sjoberg O. (1972b) B lymphocytes stimulated by concanavalin A in the presence of humoral factors released by T cells. *Eur. J. Immunol.* **2,** 99.

Auerbach R. (1962) Embryological development of the immune system (a round table discussion). *J. Cell. Comp. Phys.* **60,** Suppl. 1, 159.

Auerbach R. (1967) The development of immunocompetent cells. *Devel. Biol.* Suppl. 1, 254.

Auerbach R. (1971a) Towards a developmental theory of antibody formation: the germinal theory of immunity, Vol. 1, p. 23. In *Developmental Aspects of Antibody Formation and Structure*, eds Sterzl J. & Riha I. Academic Press, London and New York.

Auerbach R. (1971b) Towards a developmental theory of immunity: cell interactions,

p. 393. In *Cell Interactions and Receptor Antibodies in Immune Responses*, eds Mäkelä O., Cross A. & Kosunen T.U. Academic Press, London and New York.

Bach J.F. & Dardenne M. (1972) Antigen recognition by T lymphocytes. II. Similar effects of azothioprine, anti-lymphocyte serum and anti-theta serum on rosette-forming lymphocytes in normal and neonatally thymectomized mice. *Cell. Immunol.* **3,** 11.

Bach J.F., Dardenne M. & Davies A.J.S. (1971) Early effect of adult thymectomy. *Nature N.B.* **231,** 110.

Bankhurst A.D. & Warner N.L. (1971) Surface immunoglobulins on mouse lymphoid cells. *J. Immunol.* **107,** 368.

Bankhurst A.D., Warner N.L. & Sprent J. (1971) Surface Ig on thymus and thymus-derived lymphoid cells. *J. Exp. Med.* **134,** 1005.

Basten A., Miller J.F.A.P., Warner N.L. & Pye J. (1971) Specific interaction of thymus-derived (T) and non thymus-derived (B) lymphocytes by I^{125}-labelled antigen. *Nature N.B.* **231,** 104.

Berken A. & Benacerraf B. (1966) Properties of antibodies cytophilic for macrophages. *J. Exp. Med.* **123,** 119.

Biozzi G., Stiffel C., Mouton D., Liacopoulos-Briot M., Decreuspond C. & Bouthillier Y. (1966) Etude du phénomène de l'immuno cyto-adhérence au cours de l'immunisation. *Ann. Inst. Pasteur* **110,** Suppl. 3, 7.

Bisset K.A. (1947) The effect of temperature on immunity in amphibia. *J. Path. Bact.* **59,** 301.

Bisset K.A. (1948) The effect of temperature upon antibody production in coldblooded vertebrates. *J. Path. Bact.* **60,** 87.

Bradley S.C. & Watson D.W. (1963) Production of neutralizing antibody by mice inoculated with actinophage. *J. Immunol.* **90,** 782.

Bretscher P.A. & Cohn M. (1970) A theory of self-nonself discrimination. *Science* **189,** 1042.

Calkins C.E. & Golub E.S. (1972) Direct demonstration of lymphocyte-macrophage cooperation in the absence of physical contact between the two cell types. *Cell. Immunol.* **5,** 579.

Campbell P.A. & Kind P. (1969) Differentiation of antibody-forming cells. II. Effect of antigen dose on proliferation of precursor cells and plaque forming cells. *J. Immunol.* **102,** 1084.

Carr M.C., Stites D.P. & Fundenberg H.H. (1973) Dissociation of responses to phytohemagglutinin and adult allogenic lymphocytes in human foetal tissues. *Nature. N.B.* **241,** 279.

Chan E., Mishell R.I. & Mitchell G.F. (1970) Cell interaction in an *in vitro* immune response: requirement for theta-carrying cells. *Science* **170,** 1215.

Claman H.N. & Chaperon E.A. (1969) Immunological complementation between thymus and marrow cells—a model for the two cell theory of immunocompetence. *Transplant. Rev.* **1,** 92.

Claman H.N., Chaperon E.A. & Triplett R.F. (1966) Thymus-marrow cell combinations —synergism in antibody production. *Proc. Soc. Exp. Biol. Med.* **122,** 1167.

Cohen N. (1966) Tissue transplantation immunity in the adult newt, *Diemictylus viridescens.* II. The rejection phase: first and second-set allograft reactions and lack of sexual dimorphism. *J. Exp. Zool.* **163,** 173.

Cohen N. (1968) Chronic skin graft rejection in the Urodela. I. A comparative study of first- and second-set allograft reactions. *J. Exp. Zool.* **167,** 37.

Cohen N. (1970) Tissue transplantation immunity and immunologic memory in Urodela and Apoda. *Transplant. Proc.* **2,** 275.

Cohen N. (1971) Amphibian transplantation reactions: A review. *Amer. Zool.* **11,** 193.

COOPER E.L., BACULI B.S. & BROWN B.A. (1971) New observations on lymph gland (L.M.I.) and thymus activity in larval bullfrogs, *Rana catesbiana*, p. 1. In *Morphological and Functional Aspects of Immunity*, Plenum Press, N.Y. *Adv. Exp. Med. Biol*, **12,** 1.

COOPER E.L. & HILDEMANN W.H. (1965) Allograft reactions in bullfrog larvae in relation to thymectomy. *Transplant*, **3,** 446.

COOPER M.D., PETERSON R.D., SOUTH M.A. & GOOD R.A. (1966) The functions of the thymus system and bursa system in the chicken. *J. Exp. Med.* **123,** 75.

COUTINHO A. & MÖLLER G. (1973) B cell mitogenic properties of thymus-independent antigens. *Nature N.B.* **245,** 12.

COWDEN R.R. & DYER R.F. (1971) Lymphopoietic tissue and plasma cells in Amphibians. *Amer. Zool.* **11,** 183.

CRONE M., KOCH C. & SIMONSEN M. (1972) The elusive T cell receptor. *Transplant Rev.* **10,** 36.

CURTIS S.H. & VOLPE E.P. (1971) Modification of responsiveness to allografts in larvae of the leopard frog by thymectomy. *Devel. Biol.* **22,** 177.

DAVIE J.M., ROSENTHAL A.S. & PAUL W.E. (1971) Receptor on immunocompetent cells. III. Specificity and nature of receptor on dinitrophenylated guinea pig albumin I^{125}-binding cells of immunized guinea pigs. *J. Exp. Med.* **134,** 517.

DAVIES A.J.S., LEUCHARS S.E., WALLIS V., MARCHANT R. & ELLIOTT E.V. (1967) The failure of thymus derived cells to produce antibody. *Transplant.* **5,** 222.

DIENER E., SHORTMAN K. & RUSSELL P. (1970) Induction of immunity and tolerance in the absence of phagocytic cells. *Nature* (*Lond.*) **225,** 731.

DU PASQUIER L. (1970) L'acquisition de la compétence immunologique chez les Vertébrés. Etude chez la larve des crapaud accoucheur *Alytes obstetricians*. These Doctorat ès Sciences, Université de Bordeaux, No. 290.

DU PASQUIER L. (1973) Ontogeny of the immune response in cold-blooded vertebrates. In *Current Topic In Microbiology and Immunology* **61,** 37. Springer-Verlag, Berlin, Heidelberg and New York.

DU PASQUIER L., WEISS N. & LOOR F. (1972) Direct evidence for immunoglobulins on the surface of thymus lymphocytes of amphibian larvae. *Eur. J. Immunol.* **2,** 366.

DUTTON R.W., CAMPBELL P., CHAN E., HIRST J.A., HOFFMAN M., KETTMAN J., LESLEY J., MCCARTHY M., MISHELL R.I., RAIDT J.D. & VANN D. (1971a) Thymus derived mediator, p. 31. In *Cellular Interactions in the Immune Response. Proc. Second Int. Convoc. Immunol. Buffalo, N.Y.* Karger, Basel.

DUTTON R.W., FALKOFF R., HIRST J.A., HOFFMAN M., KAPPLER J.W., KETTMAN J.R., LESLEY J.F. & VANN D. (1971b) Is there any evidence for a non-antigen specific diffusable chemical mediator from the thymus-derived cell in the initiation of the immune response? Volume I, p. 355. In *Progress in Immunology*, ed. Amos D.B. Academic Press, London and New York.

DWYER J.M., MASON S., WARNER N.L. & MACKAY I.R. (1971) Antigen binding lymphocytes in congenitally athymic (nude) mice. *Nature N.B.* **234,** 252.

DWYER J.M. & WARNER N.L. (1971) Antigen binding cells in embryonic chicken bursa and thymus. *Nature N.B.* **229,** 210.

ELSON C.J., ALLAN D., ELSON J. & DUFFUS W.H.P. (1972) The relationship between the morphology of rosette-forming cells and their mode of rosette formation. *Immunol.* **22,** 291.

EVANS E.E. & HORTON S.L. (1961) Synthesis and electrophoretic distribution of antibodies in the amphibian *Bufo marinus. Proc. Soc. Exp. Biol. Med* **107,** 71.

EVANS E.E., KENT S.P., ATTLEBERGER M.H., SIEBERT C., BRYANT R.E. & BOOTH B. (1965) Antibody synthesis in poikilothermic vertebrates. *Ann. N.Y. Acad. Sci.* **126,** 629.

FALKOFF R. & KETTMAN J. (1972) Differential stimulation of precursor cells and carrier-specific thymic derived cell activity in the *in vivo* response to heterologous erythrocytes in mice. *J. Immunol.* **108,** 54.

FELDMANN M. & BASTEN A. (1972) Specific collaboration between T and B lymphocytes across a cell-impermeable membrane *in vitro. Nature N.B.* **237,** 13.

FELDMANN M. & DIENER E. (1971) Reversible blocking effect of anti-mouse immunoglobulin serum on the induction of immunity and tolerance *in vitro. Nature (Lond.)* **231,** 183.

FELDMANN M. & NOSSAL G.J.V. (1972) Tolerance, enhancement and the regulation of interactions between T cells, B cells and macrophages. *Transplant. Rev.* **13,** 3.

FELDMANN M. & PALMER J. (1971) The requirement for macrophages in the secondary response to antigens of small and large size. *Immunol.* **21,** 685.

FLEISCHMAJER P. & BILLINGHAM R.E. (1968) *Epithelial-Mesenchymal Interactions.* The Williams and Wilkins Co., Baltimore.

GOOD R.A. & FINSTAD J. (1971) Experimental and clinical models of immune deficiency and reconstitution of immunologic capacity, p. 27. In *Cell Interactions and Receptor Antibodies in Immune Responses*, eds Mäkelä O., Cross A. & Kosunen T.U. Academic Press, London and New York.

GOOD R.A., FINSTAD J., POLLARO B. & GABRIELSEN A.E. (1966) Morphologic studies on the evolution of lymphoid tissues among the lower vertebrates, p. 149. In *Phylogeny of Immunity*, eds Smith R.T., Miescher P.A. & Good R.A. University of Florida Press, Gainesville.

GREAVES M.F. (1970) Biological effects of anti-immunoglobulins. Evidence for immunoglobulin receptors on T and B lymphocytes. *Transplant. Rev.* **5,** 45.

GREAVES M.F. & BAUMINGER S. (1972) Activation of T and B lymphocytes by insoluble phytomitogens. *Nature N.B.* **235,** 67.

GREAVES M.F. & HOGG N.M. (1971) Immunoglobulin determinants on the surface of antigen binding T and B lymphocytes in mice. *Progr. Immunol.* **1,** 111.

GREAVES M.F. & MÖLLER E. (1970) Studies on antigen-binding cells. I. The origin of reactive cells. *Cell Immunol.* **1,** 372.

GREAVES M.F., MÖLLER E. & MÖLLER G. (1970) Studies on antigen-binding cells. II. Relationships to antigen-sensitive cells. *Cell. Immunol.* **1,** 386.

GREAVES M.F. & RAFF M.C. (1971) Specificity of anti-θ in cytotoxicity and functional tests on T lymphocytes. *Nature N.B.* **233,** 239.

GREAVES M.F., ROITT I.M. & ROSE M.E. (1968) Effect of bursectomy and thymectomy on the responses of chicken peripheral blood lymphocytes to phytohemagglutinin. *Nature (Lond.)* **220,** 293.

HANNA M.G. JR, MAKINODAN T. & FISHER W.D. (1967) Lymphatic tissue germinal center localization of I^{125}-labelled heterologous and isologous macroglobulins, p. 86. In *Germinal Centers in Immune Response*, eds Cottier H., Odartchenko N., Schindler R. & Congdon C.C. Springer-Verlag, New York.

HASKILL J.S. & AXELRAD M.A. (1971) Altered antigen binding by immunocompetent cells as a reflexion of immunological history. *Nature N.B.* **231,** 219.

HASKILL J.S., ELLIOTT B.E., KERBEL R., AXELRAD M.A. & EIDINGER D. (1972) Classification of thymus-derived and marrow derived lymphocytes by demonstration of their antigen-binding characteristics. *J. exp. Med.* **135,** 1410.

HEMMINGSSON E.J. (1972a) Ontogenetic studies on lymphoid cell traffic in the chicken. II. Cell traffic from the bursa of Fabricius to the thymus and spleen in the embryo. *Int Arch. Allergy* **42,** 764.

HEMMINGSSON E.J. (1972b) Ontogenetic studies on the lymphoid cell traffic in the chicken. III. Cell traffic from the thymus. *Int. Arch. Allergy* **43,** 481.

HEMMINGSSON E.J. & ALM G.V. (1972) The effect of embryonic bursectomy on the rosette-forming cells in the chicken. *Eur. Journ. Immunol.* **2,** 380.

HEMMINGSSON E.J. & LINNA T.J. (1972) Ontogenetic studies on lymphoid cell traffic in the chicken. I. Cell migration from the bursa of Fabricius. *Int. Arch. Allergy* **42,** 693.

HIRST J.A. & DUTTON R.W. (1970) Cell components in the immune response. III. Neonatal thymectomy: Restoration in culture. *Cell. Immunol.* **1,** 190.

HORTON J.D. (1969) Ontogeny of the immune response to skin allografts in relation to lymphoid organ development in the amphibian *Xenopus laevis* Daudin. *J. Exp. Zool.* **170,** 449.

HORTON J.D. & MANNING M.J. (1972) Response to skin allograft in *Xenopus laevis* following thymectomy at early stages of lymphoid maturation. *Transplant.* **14,** 141.

HUNTER P., MUNRO A. & MCCONNELL I. (1972) Properties of educated T cells for rosette formation and cooperation with B cells. *Nature N.B.* **236,** 52.

ISAKOVIC K., JANKOVIC B.D., POPESKOVIC L. & MILOSEVIC D. (1963) Effect of neonatal thymectomy, bursectomy and thymo-bursectomy on hemagglutinin production in chickens. *Nature* (*Lond.*) **200,** 273,

JERNE N.K. & NORDIN A.A. (1963) Plaque formation in agar by single antibody producing cells. *Science* **140,** 405.

KAPP J. & BENACERRAF B. (1972) The rosette cell response of several mouse strains to immunization with both sheep and pigeon erythrocytes; magnitude of errors caused by cytophilic antibody. *Eur. J. Immunol.* **2,** 467.

KAPPLER J.W. & HOFFMAN M. (1973) Regulation of the immune response. III. Kinetic differences between thymus and bone marrow derived lymphocytes in the proliferative response to heterologous erythrocytes. *J. Exp. Med.* (in press).

KETTMAN J. & DUTTON R.W. (1970) An *in vitro* primary immune response to 2,4,6-trinitrophenyl substituted erythrocytes: Response of carrier and hapten. *J. Immunol.* **104,** 1558.

KETTMAN J. & DUTTON R.W. (1971) An *in vitro* primary immune response to 2,4,6-trinitrophenyl substituted erythrocytes: The radioresistance of the enhancing of cells from carrier immunized mice. *Proc. Nat. Acad. Sci. U.S.A.* **68,** 699.

KIDDER G.M., RUBEN L.N. & STEVENS J.M. (1973) Cytodynamics and ontogeny of the immune response of *Xenopus laevis* against sheep erythrocytes. *J. Embryol. Exp. Morph.* **29,** 73.

KRUEGER R.G. & TWEDT R.M. (1962) Cellular demonstration of antibody production in *Rana pipiens. Bact. Proc.* **1,** 73.

LAY W. & NUSSENZWEIG V. (1969) Ca^{++}-dependent binding of antigen–19S antibody complexes to macrophages. *J. Immunol.* **102,** 1172.

LECKBAND E. & BOYSE E.A. (1971) Immunocompetent cells among mouse thymocytes: a minor population. *Science* **172,** 1258.

LESLEY J., KETTMAN J.R. & DUTTON R.W. (1971) Immunoglobulins on the surface of thymus-derived cells engaged in the initiation of a humoral response. *J. Exp. Med.* **134,** 618.

LIN S.P., COOPER A.G. & WORTIS H.H. (1973) Scanning electron microscopy of human T-cell and B-cell rosettes. *New England J. Med.* **289,** 548.

LOPEZ D.M., SIGEL M.M. & LEE J.C. (1974) Phylogenetic studies on T cells. I. Lymphocytes of the shark with differential response to phytohemagglutinin and con-canavalin A. *Cell. Immunol.* **10,** 287.

MANNING M.J. & TURNER R.J. (1972) Some responses of the clawed toad, *Xenopus laevis* to soluble antigens administered in adjuvant. *Camp. Biochem. Physiol.* **42,** 735.

MARCHALONIS J.J. (1971) Immunoglobulins and antibody production in amphibians. *Amer. Zool.* **11,** 171.

MARCHALONIS J.J. (1975) Lymphocyte surface immunoglobulin. *Science* **190,** 20.

MARCHALONIS J.J., ATWELL J.L. & CONE R.E. (1972a) Isolation of surface immunoglobulin from lymphocytes from human and murine thymus. *Nature N.B.* **235,** 240.

MARCHALONIS J.J., CONE R.E. & ATWELL J.L. (1972b) Isolation and partial characterization of lymphocyte surface immunoglobulins. *J. Exp. Med.* **135,** 956.

MASON S. & WARNER N.L. (1970) The immunoglobulin nature of the antigen recognition site on cells mediating transplantation immunity and delayed hypersensitivity. *J. Immunol.* **104,** 762.

MCCONNELL I. (1971) Antigen receptors on the surface of antibody secreting cells. *Nature N.B.* **233,** 177.

MCDEVITT H., ASKONAS B.A., HUMPHREY J.H., SCHECTER I. & SELA M. (1966) The localization of antigen in relation to specific antibody-producing cells. Use of a synthetic polypeptide (T-G-A-L) labelled with iodine-125. *Immunol.* **11,** 337.

MILLER J.F.A.P. (1970) Cellular basis of the immune response, p. 3. In *New Concepts in Allergy and Clinical Immunology. Proc. VII Int. Cong. Allergology.*

MILLER J.F.A.P. (1971) Interaction between thymus-dependent (T) cells and bone marrow-derived (B) cells in antibody responses, p. 293. In *Cell Interactions and Receptor Antibodies in Immune Responses,* eds Mäkelä O., Cross A. & Kosunen T.U. Academic Press, London and New York.

MILLER J.F.A.P. (1972) Lymphocyte interactions in antibody responses. *Int. Rev. Cytol.* **33,** 77.

MILLER J.F.A.P., BASTEN A., SPRENT J. & CHEERS C. (1971) Interaction between lymphocyte in immune responses. *Cell. Immunol.* **2,** 469.

MILLER J.F.A.P. & MITCHELL G.F. (1968) Cell to cell interaction in the immune response. I. Hemolysin-forming cells in neonatally thymectomized mice reconstituted with thymus or thoracic duct lymphocytes. *J. Exp. Med.* **128,** 801.

MILLER J.F.A.P. & MITCHELL G.F. (1969) Thymus and antigen reactive cells. *Trans. Rev.* **1,** 3.

MILLER J.F.A.P., SPRENT J., BASTEN A., WARNER N., BREITER J., ROWLAND G., HAMILTON J., SILVER H. & MARTIN W. (1971) Cell to cell interaction in the immune response. VII. Requirement for differentiation of thymus derived cells. *J. Exp. Med.* **134,** 1266.

MITCHELL G.F. & MILLER J.F.A.P. (1968) Cell to cell interaction in the immune response. II. The source of hemolysin-forming cells in irradiated mice given bone marrow and thymus or thoracic duct lymphocytes. *J. Exp. Med.* **128,** 821.

MITCHISON N.A. (1964) Induction of immunological paralysis in two zones of dosage. *Proc. Roy. Soc.* (*Biol.*) **161,** 225.

MITCHISON N.A. (1971) The relative ability of T and B lymphocytes to see protein antigen, p. 149. In *Cell Interactions and Receptor Antibodies in Immune Responses,* eds Mäkelä O., Cross A. & Kosunen T.U. Academic Press, London and New York.

MITCHISON N.A., TAYLOR R. & RAJEWSKI K. (1970) Cooperation of antigenic determinants in the induction of antibodies, p. 547. In *Developmental Aspects of Antibody Formation and Structure,* ed. Sterzl J. Publ. House Czech. Acad. Sci., Prague.

MOAV N. & HARRIS T.N. (1970) Rosette formation in relation to active synthesis of antibody. *J. Immunol.* **105,** 1501.

MODABBER F., MORIKAWA S. & COONS A.H. (1970) Antigen-binding cells in normal mouse thymus. *Science* **170,** 1102.

MOSIER D. (1967) A requirement for two cell types of antibody formation *in vitro. Science* **158,** 1573.

MOTICKA E.J., BROWN B.A. & COOPER E.L. (1973) Immunoglobulin synthesis in bull frog larvae. *J. Immunol.* **110,** 855.

NAKAMURA I., SEGAL S., GLOBERSON A. & FELDMAN M. (1972) DNA replication as a prerequisite for the induction of primary antibody response. *Cell. Immunol.* **4,** 351.

NOBLE G.K. (1931) *The Biology of Amphibia*. Dover Publications, New York.

NOSSAL G.J.V., CUNNINGHAM A., MITCHELL G.F. & MILLER J.F.A.P. (1968) Cell to cell interaction in the immune response. III. Chromosomal marker analysis of single antibody forming cells in reconstituted, irradiated or thymectomized mice. *J. Exp. Med.* **128,** 839.

NOSSAL G.J.V., WARNER N.L., LEWIS H. & SPRENT J. (1972) Quantitative features of a sandwich radioimmuno-labelling technique for lymphocyte surface receptors. *J. Exp. Med.* **135,** 405.

PAUL W.E., SISKIND G.W. & BENACERRAF B. (1968) Specificity of cellular immune responses. *J. Exp. Med.* **127,** 25.

PERKINS E.H., ROBINSON M.A. & MAKINODAN T. (1961) Agglutinin response, a function of cell number. *J. Immunol.* **86,** 533.

PERNIS B., FORNI L. & AMANTE L. (1971) Immunoglobulins as cell receptors. *Ann. N.Y. Acad. Sci.* **190,** 420.

PLAYFAIR J.H.L. (1971) Cell cooperation in the immune response. *Clin. Exp. Immunol.* **8,** 839.

PLAYFAIR J.H.L. (1972) Response to mouse T and B lymphocytes to sheep erythrocytes. *Nature N.B.* **235,** 115.

RAFF M.C. (1969) Theta isoantigen as a marker of thymus derived lymphocytes in mice. *Nature (Lond.)* **224,** 378.

RAFF M.C. (1970) Role of thymus-derived lymphocytes in the secondary humoral response in mice. *Nature (Lond.)* **226,** 1257.

RAFF M.C. (1971) Evidence for a subpopulation of mature lymphocytes within mouse thymus. *Nature N.B.* **229,** 182.

RAFF M.C. (1971) Surface antigenic markers for distinguishing T and B lymphocytes in mice. *Transplant. Rev.* **6,** 52.

RAJEWSKI K., SCHIRRMACHER V., NASE S. & JERNE N.K. (1969) The requirement of more than one antigenic determinant for immunogenicity. *J. Exp. Med.* **129,** 1131.

RIEF A.E. & ALLEN J.M.V. (1964) The AKR thymic antigen and its distribution in leukemias and nervous tissue. *J. Exp. Med.* **120,** 413.

RIEBER E.P. & RIETHMÜLLER G. (1974) Surface immunoglobulin on thymus cells. I. Increased immunogenicity of heterologous anti-Ig bound to thymus cells. *Z. Immunitaets forsch.* **147,** 262.

RIETHMULLER G., RIEBER E.P. & SEEGER I. (1971) Suppression of graft versus host reaction by univalent anti-immunoglobulin antibody. *Nature (Lond.)* **230,** 248.

RITTENBERG M.B. & BULLOCK W.W. (1972) *In vitro* initiated secondary anti-hapten response. III. Separable roles of hapten and carrier in immune paralysis. *Immunochemistry* **9,** 491.

RITTENBERG M.B. & PRATT K.L. (1969) Antitrinitrophenyl (TNP) plaque assay. Primary response of Balb/c mice to soluble and particulate immunogen. *Proc. Soc. Exp. Biol. Med.* **132,** 575.

ROITT J.M., GREAVES M.F., TORRIGIONNI G., BROSTOFF J. & PLAYFAIR J.H.L. (1969) The cellular basis of the immunological responses. *Lancet* **ii,** 367.

ROMER A.S. (1962) *The Vertebrate Body*. W. B. Saunders Co., Philadelphia and London.

ROUSE B.T. & WARNER N.L. (1972) Depression of humoral antibody formation in the chicken by thymectomy and anti-lymphocyte serum. *Nature N.B.* **236,** 79.

RUBEN L.N. (1975) Ontogeny, phylogeny and cellular cooperation. In *Ontogeny of Immunity*, ed. Cooper E.L. *Amer. Zool.* **15,** 93.

RUBEN L.N., STEVENS J.M. & KIDDER G.M. (1972) Suppression of the allograft response by implants of mature lymphoid tissues in larval *Xenopus laevis*. *J. Morph.* **138,** 457.

RUBEN L.N., VAN DER HOVEN A. & DUTTON R.W. (1973) Cellular cooperation in hapten-carrier responses in the newt (*Triturus viridescens*). *Cell. Immunol.* **6,** 300.

SALVIN S.B. & SMITH R.F. (1964) The specificity of allergic reactions. VII. Immunologic unresponsiveness, delayed hyper-sensitivity and circulating antibody and hapten-protein conjugates in adult guinea pigs. *J. Exp. Med.* **119,** 851.

SCHMIDTKE J. & UNANUE E. (1971) Interaction of macrophages and lymphocytes with surface immunoglobulins. *Nature N.B.* **237,** 15.

SEGAL S., GLOBERSON A. & FELDMAN M. (1971) A bicellular mechanism in the immune response to chemically defined antigens. *Cell. Immunol.* **2,** 205.

SELL S. (1967) Studies on rabbit lymphocytes *in vitro*. V. The induction of blast transformation with sheep anti-sera to rabbit immunoglobulin subunits. *J. Exp. Med.* **125,** 289.

SELL S. & GELL P.G.H. (1965) Studies on rabbit lymphocytes *in vitro*. I. Simulation of blast transformation with anti-allotype serum. *J. Exp. Med.* **222,** 423.

SINCLAIR N.R. & ELLIOT E.V. (1968) Neonatal thymectomy and the decrease in antigen sensitivity of the primary response and immunological 'memory' systems. *Immunol.* **15,** 325.

SPRENT J., MILLER J.F.A.P. & MITCHELL G.F. (1971) Antigen-induced selective recruitment of circulating lymphocytes. *Cell. Immunol.* **2,** 171.

STERZL J. (1966) Immunological tolerance as the result of terminal differentiation of immunologically competent cells. *Nature* (*Lond.*) **209,** 416.

STERZL J. & TRNKA Z. (1957) Effect of very large doses of bacterial antigen on antibody production in newborn rabbits. *Nature* (*Lond.*) **179,** 918.

SVEHAG S. & MANDEL B. (1964a) The formation and properties of poliovirus-neutralizing antibody. I. 19S and 7S antibody formation: differences in kinetics and antigen dose requirements for induction. *J. Exp. Med.* **119,** 1.

SVEHAG S. & MANDEL B. (1964b) The formation and properties of poliovirus-neutralizing antibody. II. 19S and 7S antibody formation: differences in antigen dose requirement for sustained synthesis, anamnesis and sensitivity to X-irradiation. *J. Exp. Med.* **119,** 21.

TAKAHASHI T., OLD L.J., MCINTIRE, K.R. & BOYSE E.A. (1971) Immunoglobulin and other surface antigens of the immune system. *J. Exp. Med.* **134,** 815.

TANIGUCHI M. & TADA T. (1974) Regulation of homocytotropic antibody formation in the rat. X. IgT-like molecule for the induction of homocytotropic antibody response. *J. Immunol.* **113,** 1757.

TAYLOR R.B. (1971) Antigen dose and the avidity of antibody from thymectomized mice, p. 325. In *Cell Interactions and Receptor Antibodies*, eds Mäkelä O, Cross A. & Kosunen T.U. Academic Press, New York.

THEIS G.A., WEINBAUM A.I., THORBECKE G.J. (1973) Absence of RFC in delayed hypersensitive agammaglobulinemic chickens. *J. Immunol.* **111,** 457.

TOURNEFIER A. (1973) Développment des organes lymphoides chez l'amphibien urodele *Triturus alpestris* Laur.; tolérance des allogreffes après la thymectomie larvaire. *J. Embryol. Exp. Morph.* **29,** 383.

TOURNEFIER A., CHARLEMAGNE J. & HOUILLON C. (1969) Èvolution des homogreffes cutanées chez l'amphibien urodèle *Pleurodeles waltlii* Michah: Résponses immunitairés primaire et secondaire. *Compt. Rend* **268,** 1456.

UHR J. (1965) Passive sensitization of lymphocytes and macrophages by antigen-antibody complexes. *Proc. Nat. Acad. Sci.* (*U.S.A.*) **54,** 1599.

UHR J. & FINKELSTEIN M.S. (1963) Antibody formation. IV. Formation of rapidly and slowly sedimenting antibodies and immunological memory to bacteriophage ØX 174. *J. Exp. Med.* **117,** 457.

UHR J.W., FINKELSTEIN M.S. & BAUMAN J.B. (1962) Antibody formation. III. The primary and secondary antibody response to bacteriophage ØX 174 in guinea pigs. *J. Exp. Med.* **115,** 655.

URSO P. & MAKINODAN T. (1963) The roles of cellular division and maturation in the formation of precipitating antibody. *J. Immunol.* **90,** 897.

VAN ALTEN P.J. & MEUWISSEN H.J. (1972) Production of specific antibody by lymphocytes of the bursa of Fabricius. *Science* **176,** 45.

VITETTA E.S., BAUR S. & UHR J.W. (1971) Isolation and characterization of Ig from mouse spleen lymphocytes. *J. Exp. Med.* **134,** 242.

WARNER N.L. (1974) Membrane immunoglobulins and antigen receptors on B and T lymphocytes. *Adv. Immunol.* **19,** 67.

WARNER N.L., BYRT P. & ADA G.L. (1970) Blocking of the lymphocyte antigen receptor site with anti-immunoglobulin serum, *in vitro. Nature (Lond.)* **226,** 942.

WARNER N.L. & SZENBERG A. (1962) Effect of neonatal thymectomy on the immune response in the chicken. *Nature (Lond.)* **196,** 784.

WARNER N.L., SZENBERG A. & BURNET F.M. (1962) The immunological role of different lymphoid organs in the chicken. I. Dissociation of immunological responsiveness. *Austr. J. Exp. Biol. Med. Sci.* **40,** 373.

WEISS N., HORTON J.D. & DU PASQUIER L. (1972) The effect of thymectomy on cell surface associated and serum immunoglobulin in the toad, *Xenopus laevis* (Daudin): A possible inhibitory role of the thymus on the expression of immunoglobulins. *Colloque La Soc. Française d'Immunol.* 165.

WIGZELL H., MÖLLER G. & ANDERSSON B. (1966) Studies at the cellular level of the 19S immune response. *Acta. Path. et Microbiol. Scand.* **66,** 530.

WILSON J.D. & FELDMANN M. (1972) Dynamic aspects of antigen binding to B cells in immune induction. *Nature N.B.* **237,** 3.

WINEBRIGHT J. & FITCH F.W. (1962) Antibody formation in the rat. I. Agglutinin response to particulate flagella from *Salmonella typhosa. J. Immunol.* **89,** 891.

WORTIS H.H., COOPER A.G. & BROWN M.C. (1973) Inhibition of human lymphocyte rosetting by anti-T sera. *Nature N.B.* **243,** 109.

YAMAGUCHI N., KURASHIGE S. & MITSUHASHI S. (1973) Immune response in *Xenopus laevis* and immunochemical properties of the serum antibodies. *Immunol.* **24,** 109.

ZAALBERG O.B. (1964) A simple method for detecting single antibody forming cells. *Nature (Lond.)* **202,** 1231.

ZAALBERG O.B., VAN DER MEUL V.A. & VAN TWISK M.J. (1968) Antibody production by isolated spleen cells: a study of the cluster and plaque techniques. *J. Immunol.* **100,** 451.

Chapter 7. Phylogeny of Neoplasia and Immune Reactions to Tumours

Michael Balls and Laurens N. Ruben

Introduction

Malignant tumours: definition, characterization and classification

Malignant cell populations in invertebrates
A controversial issue
Features of invertebrates which might affect tumour development
The value of research on tumour incidence in invertebrates
The occurrence of neoplasia in invertebrates

Malignant cell populations in lower vertebrates
Potential significance
Relevant features of vertebrates
Occurrence of tumours in the lower vertebrates

Major points to emerge from a review of tumours in the invertebrates and lower vertebrates
Occurrence of tumours
Distribution of cases
Chemical carcinogens and the lower animals
Viruses and tumours in the lower animals
Epidemiological studies
Distribution, frequency and importance of haemopoietic neoplasms

Major points to emerge from a review of tumours in the invertebrates and lower vertebrates *continued*
Amphibian tumours and limb regeneration

Control mechanisms and cancer

The immune response and malignancy
Tumour-specific transplantation antigens or tumour autoantigens
Immunological deficiency and malignancy
Immunosuppression and malignancy
Immunological tolerance
Immune surveillance and malignancy
Humoral antibodies and malignancy
The immune system and the stimulation of tumour growth
Immunotherapy and malignancy
Immunity and malignancy—some conclusions

Immunity and malignancy in the lower vertebrates
Lymphoreticular tumours in *Xenopus*
Lymphosarcoma in the Mexican axolotl (*Ambystoma mexicanum*)
The renal adenocarcinoma of *Rana pipiens*

Conclusions

Introduction

'The apparent importance of the immunologic mechanism in tumor surveillance raises interesting phylogenetic and evolutionary questions. The capacity to mount an immunologic defense against foreign or altered cells arises in evolution at or about the stage of the hagfish, a primitive cyclostome. Curiously, it is the general consensus that neoplasms, in the true sense of the word as used in mammalian pathology, are rare or absent in animals of the lower end of the phylogenetic scale.'

Statements such as that above (Prehn 1969) are very common in the literature, and frequently serve as a prelude to a unifying hypothesis of neoplastic transformation and tumour development. The purpose of this chapter is to discuss the issues raised by such statements, including the following:

(1) Do 'true' neoplasms occur in the invertebrates and lower vertebrates?
(2) Do immune surveillance mechanisms exist in vertebrates, which normally protect them from the aberrant behaviour of their own cells?
(3) Do similar mechanisms exist in invertebrates? If not, how are invertebrates protected from the aberrant behaviour of their own cells?
(4) What can research on tumours in the invertebrates and lower vertebrates contribute to our understanding of neoplasia, and, in particular, to studies on the mechanisms that control (or fail to control) the development of malignant cell populations?

The importance of a comparative approach to the cancer problem has long been recognized by some but a particularly significant step was taken in 1965, when the U.S. National Cancer Institute and the Smithsonian Institution set up the Registry of Tumors in the Lower Animals (RTLA). Under the supervision of its director, Dr J. C. Harshbarger, the RTLA collects and analyses specimens of tumours and related disorders in poikilothermic vertebrates and invertebrates, and publishes annual reports of its activities (Harshbarger 1969). More recently, the UICC Committee on Epidemiology set up a sub-committee on comparative oncology (Dawe 1970a). Thus, we can hope for a more efficient analysis and exchange of information in the future—and that the prevailing opinion will come to be based on knowledge and not, as is all too often the case at present, on ignorance.

Our discussion will be mainly limited to the lower vertebrates and invertebrates. The enormous scope of the subject we have been asked to consider precludes adequate discussion of all topics so, where necessary, we have referred to recent review articles.

Malignant tumours: definition, characterization and classification

One of the major problems in human pathology is the distinction between tumours and other abnormal proliferative conditions. This problem is magnified when considering tumours in the lower animals, since our knowledge of normal histology, tumours and other proliferative diseases is much more limited, and since many authors have used words such as 'tumour' and 'neoplasm' to describe all kinds of unusual lumps or cell aggregations. We shall use 'tumour' and 'neoplasm' interchangeably, but strictly according to the *definition* of Willis (1960): ' A tumour is an abnormal mass of tissue, the growth of which exceeds and is uncoordinated with that of normal tissue, and persists in the same excessive manner after cessation of the stimuli which evoked the change.'

The tumours of any given cell type may show a wide range of rates of growth and degrees of danger to the host. At one extreme of the range are *benign* or *innocent* tumours, which grow only slowly, remain quite local, do not invade neighbouring tissues, and do no harm, except by virtue of their position, accidental complications or the production of excessive quantities of hormones or other products. At the other extreme are *malignant* tumours, which grow rapidly, invade and spread, and usually prove fatal. Between these two extremes are many intermediate conditions, and Willis (1960) argued that the commonly-put question, 'Is this tumour innocent or malignant?' should properly be, 'How innocent or malignant is this tumour?'

The relationship between tumour and host is dynamic and progressive. This must be taken into account when the characteristic features of malignancy are looked for in a particular case. These *characteristic features* (see also Tarin 1972) are:

Increased rate of cell proliferation. The ability to proliferate is one of the most essential pre-requisites for the transformation of a normal cell into a malignant cell (see Oehlert 1973). Eighty per cent of spontaneously-arising tumours in man occur in tissues which continuously change their cell populations and which are in direct contact with the external environment (the tracheobronchial, gastrointestinal and urogenital tracts, and the skin).

Cellular pleomorphism, or morphological variation between cells of similar origin, varies in degree between tumours and in different parts of the same tumour. Carter (1968) suggested that this cell variation might be the basis of the breakdown of controls of cell movement and cell proliferation.

Disturbance of tissue architecture and of cell–cell relationships. Interactions between cells are important in *morphogenesis* (the development of form), are also involved in *morphostasis* (the maintenance of form), and may be important in neoplastic development (Tarin 1972).

Invasion of adjacent tissues occurs in normal processes, such as the growth of the hair follicle and of the mammary duct, and in the implantation of the blastocyst in the uterus. However, the invasiveness of malignant cells is comparatively random and unrestrained.

Metastasis, the major clinical problem in human cancer, is the spread of tumour cells or fragments from the primary site to other parts of the body, where they grow, invade and destroy normal tissues.

Aberrant synthetic activity—many tumours show an alteration in the rate of synthesis and in the range of proteins, hormones and other products normally synthesized by their tissue of origin, often producing substances normally found in other tissues and/or at other stages of development.

Killing the host. Malignant tumours normally progress until they kill the host, though spontaneous regression sometimes occurs.

It is obvious that malignant tumours are more easily distinguished from other hyperproliferative conditions than are benign tumours. Willis (1960) argued that hyperplasia and inflammatory reactions are normally 'useful' to the host, but this argument is not tenable when autoimmune diseases and harmful allergic reactions are considered. Malformations are anatomical abnormalities arising during development, and their growth is coordinated with that of the rest of the body. Teratomas are both malformations and neoplasms. Thus, although the value of the treatment given is dependent on a correct diagnosis, the distinction between tumours and other conditions is frequently very difficult. The diagnosis problem is even greater in animals and has undoubtedly been the greatest single handicap to progress in comparative oncology (see discussions by Harshbarger & Taylor 1968, Pauley 1969).

Linked to the problems of definition and characterization are the problems of *classification* and *nomenclature.* Willis (1960) argued that groupings should be simple and basic, and that nomenclature should be simple and precise. He considered that *histogenic classification* (organization according to tissue or origin) is correctly the fundamental basis of tumour classification in man, though metaplasia in some tumours, which come to look unlike their tissues of origin, leads to difficulties. He opposed *regional classification* as misleading, since, for example, carcinoma of the intestine has more in common with carcinoma of the lung than with myoma of the intestine. He also opposed *aetiological classification*, since carcinomas of the skin are produced by a variety of factors, whereas a single chemical carcinogen or oncogenic virus can produce a whole range of tumours. The most useful basic classification scheme is as follows:

Tumours of epithelial tissues—more benign tumours are known as epitheliomas, papillomas or adenomas; more malignant tumours are known as carcinomas.

Tumours of non-haemopoietic mesenchymal tissues—more benign tumours are called fibroma, osteoma, chondroma, etc.; more malignant tumours are called fibrosarcoma, osteosarcoma, chondrosarcoma, etc.

Tumours of haemopoietic tissues—usually considered separately from other mesenchymal tissues, since cells produced by haemopoietic tissues are normally freely mobile, circulating cells.

Tumours of neural tissues—a diverse group, including ganglioneuroma and glioma.

Pigment cell tumours—including melanoma and melanosarcoma.

Embryonic tumours of the viscera—including nephroblastoma and hepatoblastoma.

Teratomas—tumours composed of multiple tissues foreign to the parts in which they arise.

It is encouraging that comparative pathologists have tended to use the basic terminology and classification systems of human pathology (usually because they *were* pathologists of humans or showed their material to them). This is justifiable because of tissue-type specificity. Comparison of the cells of corresponding tissues in very different species, vertebrate and invertebrate, reveals marked similarities—for example, muscle cells from different animals have much in common, as do nervous, secretory and epithelial cells. Of course, there are major differences between vertebrates and invertebrates, but these are due more to the arrangement of tissues into functional units (organs) than to differences between the cells themselves. Special classification schemes for particular animal groups, such as that proposed by Barry and Yevich (1972), are unnecessary. What *is* essential, is that as much information as possible about each case should be recorded and, in the case of the lower animals, deposited (along with specimens) with the RTLA at the Smithsonian Institution in Washington, D.C. Dawe (1969a) listed the heading under which such information should be sought and recorded.

Malignant cell populations in invertebrates

A controversial issue

Whether or not malignant cell populations comparable with those in vertebrates occur in invertebrates is a controversial question. Good and Finstad (1969) proposed that the capacity for malignant development appeared in close temporal association with the development of the lymphoid system and of adaptive immunity—in the lower vertebrates. They further proposed that malignancies 'identifiable to the human oncologist or mammalian oncologist' should be found among all vertebrates, but not in the invertebrates. Dawe (1969a) considered that the apparently low incidence of neoplasia could be because:

(1) the lower animals have low rates of incidence of aberrant cell populations;
(2) they have a rate of incidence of aberrant cell populations equal to that in vertebrates, but counteracting mechanisms that suppress incipient neoplasms do so more efficiently than do the immune systems of vertebrates;
(3) they have variable rates of incipient neoplasia, but are protected by a combination of 'palaeoprotective' and 'neoprotective' mechanisms.

Dawe's third point is very important, as it suggests that there are features of the various invertebrate phyla which might influence the development of malignant cell populations and which are therefore worth investigating.

Features of invertebrates which might affect tumour development

A brief consideration of the major features of the invertebrate phyla suggests a number of reasons why malignant cell populations would be expected rarely, not at all, or at rates comparable with those found in vertebrates. These features include:

Regenerative capacity. The power of regeneration (the ability to restore body form by tissue replacement and reorganization) appears to be inversely proportional to the degree of tissue differentiation (A. Needham 1952). Waddington (1935) predicted that species with greater regeneration capacities would have a lower tumour incidence—an idea which was developed by J. Needham (1942) and which was discussed more recently by Seilern-Aspang and Kratochwil (1962) and Prehn (1971). Needham (1952) discussed the taxonomic distribution of regeneration capacity, and stressed that the ability to restore lost parts varies *within* phyla, as well as *between* phyla. Small fragments of some *Protozoa*, *Coelenterata*, *Platyhelminthes*, *Annelida* and *Echinodermata* can develop into intact organisms, but within these groups are species with much more limited regeneration capacities. Holothurian echinoderms can eject their viscera and then replace them. Although normally a defence mechanism against predators, the ability to shed and replace parts may also be of value in dealing with aberrant self. Autectomy certainly occurs in platyhelminths (see Dawe 1969a), where damaged or abnormal parts are shed and replaced. Of the arthropods, adult *Crustacea*, *Myriapoda*, *Arachnida* and larval *Insecta* can regenerate legs, but regenerative capacity is much more restricted in adult *Insccta*. The invertebrate chordates regenerate well, but little or no regeneration occurs in *Nematoda*, *Rotifera*, *Acanthocephala* and *Nemertina*, and regeneration capacity is comparatively restricted in the *Mollusca*.

Asexual reproduction is also a feature of many invertebrate groups, but does not occur in vertebrates. The capacity to reproduce asexually parallels regenerative ability on the whole, but is lost where tissue specialization is highly developed. Regeneration often follows asexual reproduction—for example, when parts break off members of ophiuroid echinoderm colonies. However, arthropods regenerate well but do not reproduce asexually, whereas the platyhelminth *Dendrocoelum lacteum* can reproduce asexually but has limited regenerative capacity.

Determinate or indeterminate growth. Indeterminate growth is that which continues after sexual maturity and approaches a limit only very late in life. It is characteristic of most invertebrate phyla, but determinate growth, where no somatic cells are capable of further proliferation once development is complete, is shown by *Nematoda*, *Rotifera*, *Acanthocephala*, *Temnocephala* and *Insecta*. In general, indeterminate growth is a feature of animals which retain regenerative capacity, but molluscs show indeterminate growth whilst possessing relatively limited regenerative ability.

Size. There appears to be a negative correlation between large size and the retention of regenerative capacity, and a positive correlation between large size and the development of a high degree of tissue differentiation and multiple organ systems.

Longevity. The life-span of the mature individual must also be taken into account. Some adult insects live for only a few hours, which, along with restricted somatic cell proliferation, makes it unlikely that comparative pathologists would find 'true' neoplasms in them. Life-spans vary considerably within invertebrate phyla, most of which contain individual species with recorded life-spans of months or years.

A more detailed consideration of these questions is beyond the scope of this chapter, but these points are all discussed in two books by A. Needham, published in 1952 and 1964. These books should be compulsory reading for all who feel tempted to speculate about the reasons for the apparent low incidence of malignant cell populations in the invertebrates. It seems clear that the invertebrates most likely to develop neoplasia are those which live for long periods as mature adults, show indeterminate growth, do not reproduce asexually as adults, and have a comparatively limited capacity for regeneration. On these grounds, the phylum *Mollusca* is most likely to contain tumour-bearing individuals, but tumours are unlikely to be found in many phyla, particularly those whose adult stages lack somatic cells capable of proliferation.

The value of research on tumour incidence in invertebrates

In addition to providing information on basic aspects of malignancy and requirements for susceptibility to tumour development, there are more direct reasons for believing that invertebrate oncology is important (see Harshbarger 1973):

(1) previously unrecognized carcinogens might be identified;
(2) invertebrates might concentrate chemicals, including carcinogens, which occur in the environment at low levels;
(3) invertebrates might act as reservoirs and/or vectors for viruses oncogenic in higher animals;
(4) special mechanisms for controlling malignant cell populations might be found, such as natural resistance or anti-tumour substances (e.g. mercenene, Schmeer 1966).

The occurrence of neoplasia in invertebrates (see also Dawe & Harshbarger 1969)

The status of invertebrate tumours is very confused at present and a detailed review is beyond the scope of this chapter. Cantwell *et al.* (1968) published a bibliography of more than 400 literature references to invertebrate 'tumours', but it is doubtful whether many of the reports listed concerned neoplasms as defined and discussed earlier in this chapter. As far as we know, no clearly established tumours have yet been found in the *Protozoa*, *Porifera*, *Coelenterata*, *Platyhelminthes* (Martelli & Chandebois 1973), *Nematoda*, *Annelida*, *Rotifera*, *Arthropoda* other than *Insecta*, *Acanthocephala*, *Temnocephala* or invertebrate *Chordata*. Pigmented lesions with mitotic figures and which invaded normal tissues were described in the ophiuroid echinoderm, *Ophiocomina nigra*, by Fontaine (1969).There is now good evidence that malignant tumours exist in the *Insecta* and *Mollusca*.

Harshbarger and Taylor (1968) reviewed the literature on insect 'neoplasms', and considered spontaneous lesions, lesions induced by nerve severance, by salivary duct ligation and severance, by chemicals, radiation and viruses. They concluded that the vast majority of the reported 'tumours' could be explained by processes other than neoplastic transformation, such as wound healing, parasitic infection, inflammatory reactions, and that none of the reports satisfied the criteria for malignant cell populations. Since that review, Gateff and Schneidermann (1969) have described three tumours in *Drosophila melanogaster* which seem to satisfy these criteria. The first, an invasive neuroblastoma of the larval brain, has been transferred from fly to fly for 45 transfer generations. The tumours are invasive and lethal, and are controlled by a specific recessive gene. The same mutant gene is responsible for a second neoplasm, which is also transplantable and lethal, but is not invasive. It occurs in the imaginal discs of the mutant larva. The third tumour arose spontaneously in imaginal eye-antennal discs cultured *in vivo* in the abdomens of adult flies (Hadorn 1969). These tumours are of great interest, as they provide an opportunity for studying the genetics of susceptibility to tumour development—in a species whose genetic material has been more completely mapped than that of any other animal. Gateff and Schniedermann (1969) also discussed previous reports of tumours in insects, and the reasons why they think it unlikely that malignant cell populations occur frequently in adult insects. The three cases mentioned all occurred in pre-adult stages.

Reports of tumours in molluscs were reviewed by Pauley (1969) and by Pauley and Sayce (1972), and are summarized in Table 7.1. Pauley (1969) listed the criteria of neoplasia on which his literature survey was based, and which included uncontrolled growth, infiltration, invasion and mitotic figures. He concluded that most of the earlier reports of tumours concerned hyperplasia rather than neoplasia. Mitosis is rarely observed in mollusc

Table 7.1. Reports of tumours in molluscs

Type of tumour	Species	Common name	Diagnosis	Reference
Epithelial	*Crassostrea commercialis*	Sydney rock oyster	Papillary epithelioma	Wolf (1969, 1972)
	C. gigas	Pacific oyster	Epithelioma	Pauley & Sayce (1972)
	Limax flavus	Yellow slug	Epithelial tumour	Szabo & Szabo (1935)
	Achatina fulica	Giant African snail	Epithelial tumour	Michelson (1972)
Mesenchymal	*Mytilus edulis*	Blue mussel	Sarcomatoid neoplasm	Farley (1969b)
	Crassostrea virginica	American oyster	Sarcomatoid neoplasm	Newman (1972)
	Ostrea lurida	Olympia oyster	Sarcomatoid neoplasm	Farley & Sparks (1970)
	Crassostrea virginica	American oyster	Mesenchymal tumour	Couch (1969)
	C. gigas	Pacific oyster	Mesenchymal tumour	Pauley & Sparks*
	C. gigas	Pacific oyster	Mesenchymal tumour	Sparks†
Haemopoietic	*C. virginica*	American oyster	Haemopoietic neoplasm	Farley (1969a)
	C. gigas	Pacific oyster	Haemopoietic neoplasm	Farley (1969a)
	Mytilus edulis	Blue mussel	Lymphoma	Farley‡
	Ostrea lurida	Olympia oyster	Haemopoietic neoplasm	Farley‡
Neural	*Crassostrea gigas*	Pacific oyster	Ganglioneuroma	Pauley, Sparks & Sayce (1968)
Embryonic	*Mercenaria mercenaria*	Quahaug	Germ cell tumours	Barry & Yevich (1972)
Other	*Ampullarius australis*	La Plata apple snail	Undifferentiated neoplasm	Krieg§

* RTLA accession number 135.
† RTLA accession number 153.
‡ See Dawe and Berard (1971).
§ RTLA accession number 269.

somatic tissues (Hillman 1963), so Pauley felt that mitotic figures were a particularly useful indication of abnormality. He found no reported cases of metastasis. Invasive neoplasms arising from the mantle epithelium have been found in the Sydney rock oyster, *Crassostrea commercialis* (Wolf 1969, 1971) and in the Pacific oyster, *Crassostrea gigas* (Pauley & Sayce 1972). Farley found invasive sarcomatoid tumours with atypical mitotic figures in ten of 100 Blue mussels (*Mytilus edulus*). Epizootic undifferentiated sarcomas are also known in *Ostrea lurida* (Farley & Sparks 1970). Individual cases of mesenchymal tumours were described in *Crassostrea virginica* by Newman (1972)—an invasive tumour in one of 1400 oysters examined, and by Couch (1969)—a tumour resembling a mouse reticulum cell sarcoma in one of 5000 oysters. Farley (1969a,b, also Dawe & Berard 1971) has identified haemopoietic tumours in four mollusc species, and further study may well show that some of the other mesenchymal tumours were in fact tumours of haemopoietic tissues.

Pauley and Sparks (1968) found a ganglioneuroma in *C. gigas*. The tumour was composed of collagen and nervous tissue, and had replaced much of the normal tissue. Barry and Yevich (1972) found ovarian tumours in 12 of 316 Quahaugs (*Mercenaria mercenaria*) and testicular tumours in two of 223 males. One of the ovarian tumours was invasive, but none of the testicular tumours had invaded normal tissues. The Quahaug tumours were considered to be of germ cell origin.

On the basis of this evidence and in the knowledge that at least 15 other mollusc tumours are currently being investigated (Harshbarger 1973), there seems no doubt that tumours comparable with those in vertebrates occur in molluscs.

Krieg (1972) presented a survey of 57 epithelial tumours induced with methylcholanthrene in *Ampullarius australis*, many of which were considered malignant. Krieg discussed the suitability of gastropod molluscs for experimental carcinogenesis, and made a point which seems a fitting conclusion to this section of our chapter: 'Observations so far suggest that not all invertebrate species are capable of developing neoplastic processes. However, the line of determination for the neoplastic process is not, as was thought earlier, between the vertebrates and invertebrates, but within the latter group of animals.'

Malignant cell populations in the lower vertebrates

Potential significance

A comparative study of vertebrate tumours is justifiable for many reasons, including:

(1) the need for a clearer understanding of all features of malignancy and neoplastic development;
(2) the search for factors which increase or reduce susceptibility to tumour formation;
(3) the detection of new oncogenic agents, which might cause tumours in mammals, including man;
(4) the increasing deposition in the environment of industrial, agricultural and domestic chemicals, which might themselves be carcinogenic or co-carcinogenic (an increase in tumours in lower animals should be taken as a warning signal);
(5) the lower vertebrates might act as reservoirs for oncogenic viruses, or might store, and even concentrate, harmful chemicals (this would be especially serious if food species were involved);
(6) lower vertebrates might be suitable for experimental techniques which cannot be used with birds or mammals.

Relevant features of vertebrates

Vertebrates differ from invertebrates in many ways. The vertebral column and endoskeleton permit growth to sizes not attainable in the invertebrates, but cells at the external surface are more directly exposed to the external environment than are those of invertebrates which possess an exoskeleton. No vertebrates show asexual reproduction or determinate growth. Indeterminate growth is typical of fish, amphibians and reptiles, but birds and mammals develop to a maximum body size comparatively quickly, then maintain their tissues by a balanced system of cell loss and replacement. The rate of cell production/loss varies greatly in different tissues and it is those tissues which have the fastest rates of cell turnover that are most susceptible to neoplastic transformation. Since the rate of cell turnover is affected by tissue damage, it is logical to consider the possibility that neoplastic development is an abnormal form of wound healing (Haddow 1972). Regenerative capacity is more restricted than in the invertebrates, but varies between and within classes. Fish can replace fins and scales, and can heal minor wounds. Reptiles can regenerate tails but not limbs. Mammals and birds do not regenerate lost parts in the strict sense of the term. They can heal superficial wounds and can replace parts of some visceral organs, such as liver, by cell proliferation. However, such repair is best considered an extension of the cell turnover system, and does not involve tissue reorganization into organs on the scale of, say, limb regeneration in the amphibians, whose powers of regeneration are exceptional for vertebrates. Urodele amphibians can regenerate limbs, tail, gills, lens, iris and retina, and can replace parts of some visceral organs. Anuran amphibians are less regeneration-competent as adults, but some can regenerate the lens from cornea, iris or retina (which indicates the possibility of tissue reorganization into alternative structures). Regeneration-competence is also influenced in amphibians by age and size—younger individuals from smaller species regenerate better than older individuals of the same species or individuals of the same age of larger species.

There are a number of other trends in the vertebrates. The higher vertebrates become progressively less dependent on water for respiration, movement and breeding; the individual zygote becomes progressively more important for the survival of the species; the higher vertebrates are more independent of environmental temperature. The lower vertebrates have a less sophisticated immune system than do birds and mammals, but they also seem to be less seriously affected by bacterial and parasitic infections which are very common in them. Reichenbach-Klinke and Elkan (1965) suggested that poikilotherms have a high natural resistance to bacterial infection and only succumb to the bacteria within and around them when they are weakened by other factors, such as poor living conditions or dietary deficiencies. The vertebrates are also, in general, long-lived by comparison with the invertebrates.

Occurrence of tumours in the lower vertebrates

Neoplasms in the lower vertebrates are better documented and more easily compared with tumours in birds or mammals than are those in invertebrates. This is largely because, in spite of our comments on tissue-type specificity, tissue organization is very similar throughout the vertebrates. Tumours in the poikilotherms were reviewed by Schlumberger and Lucké (1948), Lucké and Schlumberger (1949), Reichenbach-Klinke and Elkan (1965), and Scarpelli (1969). Table 7.2 gives a summary of the main types of tumour reported.

Super-class *Pisces* contains three classes, the *Agnatha* (hagfishes and lampreys), the *Chondrichthyes* (cartilaginous fish) and the *Osteichthyes* (bony fish). The incidence of tumours in fish was also reviewed by Wellings (1969) and by Mawdesley-Thomas (1971), who also (1969) produced a bibliography of 458 references on fish neoplasia. The *Agnatha* are considered very important by comparative immunologists, since they are the lowest vertebrates known to possess a thymus gland (Good & Papermaster 1964, Good *et al.* 1966). One tumour has been reported in an agnathan—multiple cutaneous and subcutaneous lesions in an adult sea lamprey, *Petromyzon marinus*, which resembled neurilemmomas in mammals (RTLA accession number 89, Dawe 1969a). The summary in Table 7.2 of the reports listed by Wellings (1969) makes it clear that the cartilaginous and bony fish are susceptible to a range of tumours comparable with those in higher vertebrates.

Spontaneous tumours in *Amphibia* have been reviewed by Balls (1962) and by Balls and Clothier (1974). Table 7.2 clearly shows that both anuran

Table 7.2. Reports of tumours in cold-blooded vertebrates

Type of tumour	Numbers of species with reported tumours Fish* Agnatha	 Fish* Chondrichthyes	 Fish* Osteichthyes	 Amphibia† Anura	 Amphibia† Urodela	 Reptilia‡ Chelonia	 Reptilia‡ Squamata
Epithelial	0	3	122	9	8	3	20
Mesenchymal	0	5	114	9	6	1	15
Haemopoietic	0	1§	16	4	2	0	12
Neural	1¶	0	13	1	1	0	0
Pigment cell	0	3	26	4	3	0	4
Embryonic	0	0	0	2	1	0	0
Teratoma	0	0	2	2	1	0	0

* Data from Wellings (1969).
† Data from Balls and Clothier (1974).
‡ Data from RTLA reports (up to 1972), Dawe and Berard (1971), Kast (1967), Cowan (1968) and Table 7.3.
§ RTLA accession 523 (see Harshbarger 1972).
¶ RTLA accession 89 (see Dawe 1969a).

and urodele amphibians are subject to a wide range of tumours, in spite of their regenerative ability. Balls (1962) listed 42 reports for anurans and 15 reports for urodeles, but the comparable figures in the 1974 review were 66 and 34, respectively. This suggests that the number of tumours found is mainly a reflection of the interest of research workers. The 1960s certainly saw a dramatic growth in interest in amphibian tumours, and included a symposium on amphibian tumour biology (Mizell 1969).

The renal adenocarcinoma of the American leopard frog, *Rana pipiens*, is undoubtedly the most studied and, to date, the most significant tumour in the lower vertebrates. Lucké (1938) suggested a viral aetiology for the tumours, and virus particles in the tumour cells were first identified in the electron microscope by Fawcett (1956). As Rafferty (1973) pointed out, early experiments on frog renal tumours served as important forerunners of current investigations on the possible relationship between herpes-type viruses and tumours in man (Nahmias *et al.* 1972). Rafferty (1973) has proposed a life-cycle for the frog viruses; Tweedell, Michalski and Morek (1972) have developed a bioassay for the virus; McKinnell and Ellis (1972) discussed the epidemiology of the frog renal tumours (McKinnell 1973).

The only other amphibian tumours subjected to extensive experimental studies are the lymphoreticular tumours (Balls & Ruben 1968, and later sections of this chapter).

Table 7.2 does not list all the tumours reported in the *Reptilia*, but is intended to give an indication of the *range* of cases reported in the literature.

Table 7.3. Reports of tumours of the haemopoietic system in lower vertebrates

Group	Species	Common name	Diagnosis	Reference
Reptilia	*Spilotes pallatus*	Tiger rat-snake	Reticulum cell sarcoma	See Kast (1967)
	Naja naja	Egyptian cobra	Lymphosarcoma	Cowan (1968)
	Heterodon platyrhinus	Hognose snake	Lymphosarcoma	Cowan (1968)
	Bitis nasicornis	Rhinoceros viper	Lymphosarcoma	Cowan (1968)
	Eunectes murinus	Anaconda	Lymphosarcoma	Frank & Schepky (1969)
	Crotalus horridus horridus	Timber rattlesnake	Lymphoid leukaemia	Griner*
	Bitis nasicornis	Rhinoceros viper	Lymphosarcoma	See Harshbarger (1972)
	B. nasicornis	Rhinoceros viper	Granulocytic leukaemia	See Harshbarger (1972)
	Varanus salvator	Malayan monitor	Lymphosarcoma	Zwart & Harshbarger (1972)
	Hydrosaurus amboinensis	East Indian water lizard	Lymphoblastic lymphoma	Zwart & Harshbarger (1972)
	Acanthopsis antarticus	Death adder	Reticulum cell sarcoma	Griner*
	Heterodon platyrhinus	Hognose snake	Reticulum cell sarcoma	Snyder*
Amphibia	*Xenopus fraseri*	Clawed toad	Reticulum cell sarcoma	Balls (1962)
	X. laevis laevis	Clawed toad	Reticulum cell sarcoma	Balls (1962)
	X. l. laevis × *X. l. victorianus*	Clawed toad (hybrid)	Reticulum cell sarcoma	Balls (1962)
	X. l. laevis	Clawed toad	Lymphosarcoma	Ruben *et al.* (1968)
	Rana pipiens	Leopard frog	Lymphosarcoma	Duryee (1965)
	R. pipiens	Leopard frog	Plasmacytoma	Schochet & Lampert (1969)
	Cynops pyrrhogaster	Firebellied newt	Lymphosarcoma	Inoue (1954)
	Ambystoma mexicanum	Mexican axolotl	Lymphosarcoma	DeLanney & Blackler (1969)
Pisces†	*Carcharhinus milberti*	Brown shark	Reticulum cell sarcoma	Oliviero & O'Gara*
	Esox lucius	Northern pike	Lymphosarcoma	Mulcahy *et al.* (1970)
	E. masquinongy	Muskellunge	Malignant lymphoma	Sonstegard*
	Salvelinus fontinalis	Brook trout	Malignant lymphoma	Herman*
	Salmo clarki	Cut-throat trout	Malignant lymphoma	Smith*

* See Dawe and Berard (1971).
† Not a complete list—see also Dawe (1969b).
See Dawe and Berard (1971) for reports of haemopoietic neoplasms in birds and mammals, and Table 7.2 for reports in molluscs.

Two recent kinds of report are of some interest. First, tumours of haemopoietic tissues have recently been found in a number of reptile species (see Table 7.3). Secondly, Zeigel and Clark (1969, 1971) found C-type virus particles in a cell line isolated from the spleen of a Russell's viper (*Viperia russelli*) which had a myxofibroma. C-type viruses have been implicated as oncogenic agents in chickens, mice and rats.

Major points to emerge from a review of tumours in the invertebrates and lower vertebrates

Occurrence of tumours

Malignant cell populations comparable with those in man, other mammals and birds occur in the lower vertebrates (fish, amphibians and reptiles) and in molluscs. A brief survey of the lower animals suggests that various factors (such as life-span, growth characteristics, regeneration capacity, degree of tissue and organ differentiation, cell proliferation in the adult, and importance of the individual for survival of the species) must be taken into account in assessing the likelihood that a particular group will develop neoplasia. Variations should be expected (and exploited for experimental purposes) within as well as between animal groups. In general, the lower vertebrates and molluscs have more characteristics consistent with neoplastic development than do other invertebrate groups, such as echinoderms, annelids, arthropods, coelenterates, sponges and the invertebrate chordates.

Distribution of cases

Most of the reported tumours in amphibians and reptiles were found in animals kept in zoological gardens or in laboratories. This is clearly mainly because animals kept in captivity are observed more closely than are members of the same species in the wild, but the influence of crowding, unusual feeding, increased longevity and the stress of captivity may also contribute to a higher tumour incidence than occurs in the wild. Conversely, many of the tumours in fish and those in molluscs occurred in natural populations, which are regularly monitored because of their food or sporting value. Although all reports of tumours in lower animals are of value in providing background information, tumours used in experimental work are more useful than are mere discussions of histopathology. Tumours available on a regular basis are particularly useful—a number of such tumours are listed in the RTLA reports (Harshbarger 1972), and include haemopoietic neoplasms in molluscs (Farley & Sparks 1970), various fish tumours, including lymphoreticular tumours in the Northern pike (Mulcahy *et al.* 1970), and renal tumours in the leopard frog (McKinnell 1973).

Chemical carcinogens and the lower animals

It has long been known that barnacles (Zechmeister & Koe 1952) and oysters (Cahnmann & Kuratsume 1957) accumulate polynuclear hydrocarbons, and mussels accumulate the radioactive isotopes of heavy metals from sea water (Pentreath 1973). Chemical carcinogens induce tumours in lower animals, e.g. dimethylnitrosamine induces hepatomas in fish (Stanton 1965, Ashley & Halver 1968) and amphibians (Ingram 1972). The carcinogenicity of the aflatoxins was discovered by fisheries biologists following a hepatoma epidemic in hatchery-reared Rainbow trout (Wales 1970). The significance of liver tumours in animals was discussed by Mawdesley-Thomas (1970). Much less is known about the effects of chemical carcinogens on invertebrates (Harshbarger 1967, Harshbarger *et al.* 1970).

Viruses and tumours in the lower animals

The link between herpes-type viruses and frog renal adenocarcinoma has already been mentioned. A herpes-type virus infection, the first to be found in an invertebrate, was reported in the oyster, *Crassostrea virginica*, by Farley *et al.* (1972). The virus particles were strikingly similar in fine structure to those found in the frog kidney tumours. Virus inclusions were more prevalent in oysters kept at elevated water temperatures (28–30°C) than at normal ambient temperatures (18–20°C), and were associated with a lethal disease, which was possibly a haemoproliferative disease.

There is evidence that arthropods can be vectors for tumour viruses. Shope fibroma virus and squirrel fibroma virus can be transmitted by the bites of mosquitoes and fleas (WHO 1965), and the distribution in the body of soft tissues sarcomas in the Afghan is correlated with the distribution of arthropod bites (Sobin 1968). Mosquitoes can also transmit a hamster reticulum cell sarcoma by the transfer of cells (Banfield *et al.* 1966). The distribution of Burkitt's lymphoma in man in Africa suggested an insect vector, and herpes-type viruses have been suggested as the aetiological agents for this lymphoma (Rafferty 1973).

Epidemiological studies

Very few epidemiological surveys have been carried out with lower vertebrates or invertebrates, but certain studies give cause for concern. Brown *et al.* (1973) compared tumour incidence in 17 fish species, and found that 4·38 per cent of 2121 fish from polluted waters had tumours, compared with 1·03 per cent of 4639 fish from unpolluted waters. Farley (1969b) found sarcomatoid neoplasms in ten of 100 mussels (*Mytilus edulis*) from a wild population, and there are indications that other mollusc tumours may have a distribution which varies according to location. After extensive studies over many years, McKinnell and Ellis (1972) concluded that renal tumours in *Rana pipiens* are more frequent where frogs are more abundant. This situation is not dissimilar to that found with leukaemia in cattle, where herd size is directly correlated with leukaemia frequency.

Distribution, frequency and importance of haemopoietic neoplasms

Proliferative disorders morphologically comparable with the leukaemias and lymphomas in man have now been identified in all the major vertebrate groups and in molluscs (Table 7.1, Table 7.3, Dawe & Berard 1971). Since leukaemias are abnormal, progressive, unrestrained, probably autonomous, invasive and disseminated cellular proliferations, most investigators agree that they are neoplastic (Rappaport 1966). Other important features include immaturity and imperfect differentiation of the proliferating cells, abnormal nuclear forms, asynchrony of cellular and nuclear maturation, and abnormal mitotic figures. Neoplasia of haemopoietic tissues may be attributed to multifocal origin or to spread from a single focus. Many inflammatory and reactive disorders of lymphoid tissues may produce cell populations that resemble malignancy (Rappaport 1966).

Within the last few years, a number of tumours of the lymphoreticular system have been found in *reptiles* (Table 7.3), but we know of no experimental studies on them. The neoplastic nature of the cases reported in *amphibians* has been the subject of some controversy. Dawe (1969a,b, 1970b) has repeatedly stated his opinion that the *Xenopus* and *Cynops pyrrhogaster* tumours were granulomata-induced by mycobacteria and were not comparable with tumours in mammals. Balls and Ruben (1968) considered the bacteria to be secondary residents rather than a prime cause of the lesions in *Xenopus*, particularly as the tumours were transmissible by cell-free filtrates. Ruben and Stevens (1970) suggested that the lymphoreticular tumours were histologically distinguishable from mycobacterial granulomata in *Xenopus* and in *Notophthalmus viridescens*. Clothier and Balls (1973a,b) showed that *Xenopus* granulomata (induced by *Mycobacterium marinum*) and lymphoreticular tumours differed in histology, development, distribution of mitotic figures and cells in S-phase, involvement of small lymphocytes, aetiology, and means of transmission. However, Clothier and Balls agreed with Dawe that the lesions induced by acid-fast bacteria (but not by cell-free filtrates) in *Cynops pyrrhogaster* and other species by Inoue and Singer (1970) should be classed as granulomata and not as lymphoreticular tumours. The lymphosarcoma of *Ambystoma mexicanum* (DeLanney & Blackler 1969) is transplantable only within the C^h histocompatibility strain or to thymectomised hosts of incompatible strains, and cannot be transferred by subcellular fractions. The amphibian lymphoreticular tumours have been used in a number of experiments on the relationship between the immune response and neoplasia. These experiments will be discussed later.

Many more cases of *fish* haemopoietic neoplasms have been reported than are listed in Table 7.3 (Wellings 1969; Dawe 1970b). Most of the fish tumours were classed as lymphosarcomas, and they were frequently associated with leukaemia.

Dawe and Berard (1971) formed the impression that 'in descending the evolutionary pathways' haemopoietic neoplasms tended to become non-specialized or undifferentiated. They suggested that this was because the varieties of specialized normal blood cell types are more limited in lower vertebrates, and that they may all be capable of reversion to lymphoid stem cells or haemocytoblasts.

Farley has now found haemopoietic neoplasms in four mollusc species (Table 7.1). Two main aspects of mollusc blood cell tumours are likely to be important—their epizootiology and epidemiology (especially in relation to environmental pollution). In addition to its respiratory and trophic functions, the presence of blood in connective tissue spaces serves as a fluid skeleton to give temporary rigidity to certain parts of the body. The haemocytes in molluscs also play a role in excretion and, by phagocytosis, in non-localized intracellular digestion and in lime transport (Morton 1958).

Jones (1969) discussed haemocytes and the problem of insect tumours. Insects contain no erythrocyte-equivalent or respiratory pigment and, like molluscs, have an open circulatory system. Haemocytes divide and mature in the circulating blood and are therefore exceptions to the principle of determinate growth in adult insects. Haemopoietic organs have not been verified beyond doubt. Codreanu (1939) studied a highly proliferative blood cell disease in mayfly nymphs (*Heptaginia* and *Rhithrogena*) parasitized by chironomids. The blood cells were larger than normal, nests of tumour cells grew in various tissues, and normal and abnormal mitotic figures were seen. Insect haemocytes play an important role in defence against infection, both by phagocytosis and by encapsulating infected areas (Matz *et al.* 1971).

An intensification of the comparative approach to haemopoietic neoplasia would probably be very rewarding, because:

(1) investigations of the relationship between the immune system and neoplasia suggest that this relationship is particularly important in haemopoietic tumours;
(2) viruses induce haemopoietic tumours in mammals and in birds, and there is indirect evidence for a viral aetiology for lymphoid tumours in the Northern pike (Mulcahy 1970), in *Xenopus* (Balls & Ruben 1968) and in man. This is not surprising, because lymphoreticular cells are probably particularly liable to viral infection as a result of their role in defence

against infection; cell proliferation is an integral part of lymphoreticular tissue function, and cells in division are likely to be most susceptible to environmental insults capable of altering transcriptional and translational controls;

(3) radiation-induced haemopoietic tumours occur in mammals and in man, though there is no information as yet on radiation carcinogenesis and lymphoreticular tumours in lower animals.

Amphibian tumours and limb regeneration

As mentioned earlier, Waddington (1935) and Needham (1942) suggested that cells would be less susceptible to neoplastic transformation if they were part of an 'individuation field'—a somatic region capable of exerting morphogenetic controls on the cells within it, so that it tended to form a whole organism or whole part of an organism, such as an organ. Their ideas actually contained two separate hypotheses: the first applies to oncogenesis—the development of tumours; the second applies to already-formed tumours placed in an individuation field. By definition, the regeneration-competent amphibian limb represents a persistent individuation field in a post-embryonic vertebrate.

The absence of spontaneous tumours in regeneration-competent amphibian limbs favours the first of the Waddington-Needham hypotheses, though it is still not clear whether this is due to lack of tumours or to lack of observations. Another point to be considered is that not all amphibians can regenerate limbs, and that in species that can, the ability to do so falls off with age. Tumours of limb tissues are not frequent in these situations either. The situation regarding experimental demonstration of the first hypothesis is even more confused. Seilern-Aspang and Kratochwil (1962, 1963, 1965) reported the selective conversion of chemically-induced epithelial tumour cells to normal cells in regeneration-competent areas, but not in other parts of *Triturus cristatus*. Ruben and Stevens (1963) showed that foreign implants induced a regeneration blastema in urodele limbs in the absence of amputation, resulting in the formation of a supernumerary limb. We later found that histologically-normal kidney allografts to *Xenopus* forelimbs induced not only lymphosarcomas but also accessory cartilage nodules (Balls & Ruben 1964). Implants of *Rana pipiens* kidney and *Triturus cristatus* kidney also induced lymphosarcomas in the forelimbs of *Xenopus* (Ruben & Balls 1964a). We concluded that both phenomena, lymphosarcoma formation from lymphoid tissue and accessory limb structures from limb tissues, were reponses to the same initiation events, and we noted that the greater the genetic disparity between donor and host, the stronger was the observed response (Ruben & Balls 1964c). Other experiments (Ruben & Balls 1964b, Ruben *et al.* 1966) showed that methylcholanthrene crystals also induced tumours of lymphoid tissue and *normal* but accessory limb structures in *Xenopus* and *Triturus* forelimbs. This was in line with the earlier experiments of Breedis (1952), who found far more cases of induced accessory limb structures than of tumours, when he injected chemical carcinogens into newt limbs. Further, Pizarello and Wolsky (1966), who were unable to initiate tumours in *Triturus cristatus* regenerating tail, viewed regeneration and oncogenesis as antagonistic phenomena.

Thus, while it appears that forces in the limb field directed limb tissues toward the formation of normal limb structures, no control was exerted on precursor cells of lymphoid tumours or on already established lymphoid tumours. These observations may be relevant to the problem of metastasis in tumours—the local controls which may control the primary tumour to some extent may be absent in other parts of the body.

Experimental support for the second aspect of the Waddington-Needham hypotheses, namely, that a regenerating system might impose controls on previously transformed neoplastic cells is, if it is possible, even less clear. Negative evidence has been offered by Ruben (1963), studying the frog renal tumour in urodele limbs, Balls and Ruben (1964a,b) with the *Xenopus* lymphosarcoma in *Xenopus* limbs, and Sheremetieva (1965) using an axolotl melanoma in the axolotl regnerating tail. Additional failures to observe neoplastic transformation back to normal tissue by a regenerating system were reported by Breedis (1954), Peredelsky (1941), Schevtchenko (see Sheremetieva, 1965) and Ciaccio (1941) with urodele amphibians and Erwin and Gordon (1955) with fish. Results supporting the control of neoplastic cells introduced into a regenerating system have been reported by Rose and Wallingford (1948) and Mizell (1960, 1961, 1965, 1966), who used the renal adenocarcinoma of *Rana pipiens*.

The experiments of Seilern-Aspang and Kratochwil (1965) actually bridge both concepts, for they were concerned not only with the generation of neoplasia within regeneration competent regions in the triclad platyhelminth, *Dendrocoelum lacteum*, and the newt, *Triturus cristatus*, but also the fate of a tumour, should it form elsewhere in the body, when regeneration was initiated. Their studies support both of the Waddington-Needham hypotheses, but we feel constrained to note our concern with regard to the classification of the tumours they have studied as 'true neoplasms' in the light of the criteria listed earlier in this chapter.

Control mechanisms and cancer

As developmental biologists, we are naturally attracted by the concept of 'neoplasia as a *developmental process* akin to normal development in some respects, but differing from it in important particulars that are not well-defined' (Foulds 1969). There are many similarities between neoplasia and normal development, including the following:

(1) Although experimental analysis has provided an alarming mass of information about both processes, we *understand* very little about either.
(2) Both processes are concerned with *relationships*—between the cells of a population, and between populations of cells. In other words, both are ultimately about organization at the cellular level, and not merely about molecular control mechanisms in single cells—see the attacks of Smithers (1962) on the cytologist approach to cancer, and of Weiss (1973) on the cytologist approach to differentiation.
(3) Both processes are affected and controlled by *many factors*, including the nature and quality of the genetic information, nuclear–cytoplasmic interactions, cell–cell interactions (Tarin 1972), hormones, cell proliferation and loss kinetics, growth factors, humoral factors (Metcalf 1971), systems-control mechanisms (Dawe 1969a), age of the host, environmental factors (including chemicals, radiation and viruses), disease in other parts of the host, etc. (to include all the other factors we have omitted).
(4) The *interaction* of factors influencing both processes should be anticipated. We should not search for *the* controlling factor (see the network concept of biological organization and control postulated by Weiss (1973) and discussed in Foulds, 1969).
(5) The fourth dimension, *time*, is a vital factor in both processes, since both are progressive. Waddington's concept of stages of precompetence, competence, determination and overt differentiation are equally applicable to both processes (though terms such as predisposition, transformation and latency are more familiar in discussions of neoplastic development).
(6) *Stability* is a feature of both processes, but arguments about absolute irreversibility are sterile in considerations of either process (Dustin 1972).

This short section is included solely to put into perspective our discussion of the relationship between the immune system and neoplasia. Such a relationship is only a part of the complex interactions that occur between malignant cell populations and their hosts. After all, Foulds (1969) managed to write a very thought-provoking book on neoplastic development, but included only a brief reference to the immune system in a section on the historical aspects of tumour transplantation.

The immune response and malignancy

The proposition that malignant tumours encounter immunological resistance in the host is long-established, and the immunological aspects of neoplasia have now come to dominate the cancer research literature, just as papers on chemical carcinogenesis were dominant a few years ago. This surge of interest is partly a reflection of the growing general interest in immunology (what disease does *not* have its immunological aspects, and what modern biological research does not require serological procedures or radioimmunoassays?). In addition, two major events stimulated interest in the immunological aspects of malignancy—the discovery of tumour-specific antigens (Prehn & Main 1957) and the immune surveillance hypothesis (Thomas 1958, Burnet 1970). This is a subject where the current popular view changes almost daily and the cliché that research is out of date before the manuscript reaches the editorial office really is applicable. We shall attempt to summarize the major evidence that a relationship does exist between the immune system and malignant cell populations (Vaeth 1972).

Tumour-specific transplantation antigens or tumour autoantigens

Wherever they can be effectively studied in experimental animals, malignant tumours have been found to show tumour-specific transplantation antigens (Tillack 1972). Tumour-associated antigens have also been detected in most of the human neoplasms investigated (Hellström & Hellström 1973). Anderson and Coggin (1972) argued that the term *tumour autoantigen* (TA) is preferable, since it cannot be said that the antigens are specific to the tumours concerned unless all gene products at all stages of development have been checked. In virus-induced tumours, the TAs are characteristic of the virus, and all cells transformed by a particular virus bear the same TA. Immunization with the virus prevents the subsequent induction of tumours with that virus. Chemically-induced tumours also have TAs but, unfortunately, each tumour has its own individual antigen, even when the same carcinogen produces two different primary tumours in the same individual.

Much attention in recent years has been paid to the formation by neoplastic cells of proteins normally present during a limited period of fetal development. The carcino-embryonic antigens are an indication of retrogenesis—the mixed expression of adult and embryonic genes (Anderson & Coggin 1972). They are found in carcinomas of the gastro-intestinal tract (Gold & Freedman 1965) and in hepatomas (Abelev *et al.* 1963), but, although the presence of fetal antigens may eventually help in the early diagnosis of tumours, their presence in the adult is not specific to malignant cells (Burtin *et al.* 1972). Studies on virus-induced rodent tumours indicate a cross-reaction between fetal antigens and tumour cell antigens (Anderson & Coggin 1972), and LeMevel and Wells (1973) have experimental data which strongly suggest that fetal antigens cross-react with the TAs of chemically-induced tumours.

Immunological deficiency and malignancy

Good (1972) has collected a considerable amount of evidence which suggests that a higher incidence of malignancy, as well as a greater susceptibility to infection, accompanies primary immunodeficiencies (Weigle 1972). Most, but not all, the malignancies were neoplasia of the lymphoreticular system. This evidence may not necessarily support the immune surveillance hypothesis, but may indicate that genetic deficiency in a tissue predisposes to malignancy. It could also be that a negative feedback mechanism operates, which stimulates proliferation in precursor cells because of a deficiency of normally-functioning mature cells.

Immunosuppression and malignancy

It appears that immunosuppressive regimes in animals increase the *de novo* incidence of tumours, increase the occurrence and establishment of metastases (Klein 1969), and also lead to an increased incidence, increased growth rate and decreased latent period for virus-induced tumours. The situation regarding chemically-induced tumours is less clear (Bolton 1973a,b), but Bolton (1973c) obtained results with cyclophosphamide which suggested that the effect of immunosuppression may depend on the stage of progression of the tumour at the time of administration of the drug.

Penn and Starzl (1972) discussed the incidence of tumours in immunosuppressed organ transplant recipients. Up to 31 December 1971, 75 of 7760 patients receiving organ grafts had developed tumours *de novo* some time after the transplantation operation. Penn and Starzl concluded that this tumour incidence was about 80 times greater than in the average population in a comparable age range. Forty-four of the patients had epithelial tumours, and 31 had lesions of mesenchymal origin, 28 of which were lymphoreticular tumours. Apart from the obvious conclusion that organ transplantation clearly involves risks other than an increased incidence of infection and graft rejection, this information has a bearing on tumour-immune system relationships. Good (1972) argued that such cases support the immune surveillance hypothesis, but other explanations are also possible. For example, immunosuppression could increase the chance of infection and transformation by oncogenic viruses or allow latent infections to be expressed (after all, the evidence for a viral aetiology for human tumours is as good as that for the existence of an immune surveillance mechanism). In the case of the lymphoreticular tumours, it could be that immunosuppressive drugs are themselves carcinogenic for lymphoreticular cells, either directly or by interference with normal feedback control mechanisms. This leads to two further points:

(1) What is known of the side-effects of immunosuppressive regimes?
(2) What is known of the long-term effects of drugs given for other purposes

but which are also immunosuppressive (e.g. steroid hormones, including oral contraceptives, Irvine 1973). There is also the risk of an effect on the fetus which may not be expressed until some time after birth (e.g. the effect of diethylstilboestrol).

Immunological tolerance

Research on rodent and chicken virus tumours shows that if viruses are introduced while the capacity to develop an immune response is still immature, virus-induced tumours are more likely to develop if inoculation with that virus occurs later in life. The passage of viruses via the placenta or milk (as in mouse mammary carcinoma) is of possible significance in humans, and the vertical transmission of oncogenic agents is also important, at least theoretically, in the lower animals, as will be discussed later in this chapter.

Immune surveillance and malignancy

In 1958 Thomas made the comment that the allograft response might have arisen as a primary mechanism for defence of the host against neoplasia. This idea was popularized as 'immune surveillance' by Burnet (1970). In *Genes, Dreams and Realities* (1972), Burnet suggests that when a tumour has reached a size at which it can be detected, the spontaneous immune response against it has been overcome. It is difficult to see how direct evidence can be found for a mechanism which can only be detected when it has failed. Good has emerged as the main proponent of the immune surveillance hypothesis, and Prehn as its most forceful critic (Smith & Landy 1970). Allison (Smith & Landy 1970) considered that a surveillance mechanism was decisive in determining whether or not an animal would be infected as a result of natural exposure to a virus. Natural exposure to polyoma virus does not normally lead to *any* tumours in mice, but *all* mice developed tumours when infected with polyoma virus after immunosuppression. Weston (1973) discussed the relationship between the thymus and immune surveillance.

Humoral antibodies and malignancy

Although Good argues that, right or wrong, the immune surveillance hypothesis has stimulated interest in the relationship between the immune system and malignancy, it has tended to divert attention from the role of humoral antibodies. Morton (1972) discussed the correlation between long survival and elevated antibody titre in sarcoma and melanoma patients, and pointed out that the decline of antisarcoma antibody in some patients was specific, and not due to a non-specific decline in the ability to form antibodies against antigens in general.

Hellström and Hellström (1970, 1973) carried out *in vitro* experiments which suggested that blocking antibodies protect tumour cells from T lymphocytes, which would have destroyed them, and considered that there was a parallel blocking *in vivo* (Feldman 1972). Sjögren *et al.* (1971) suggested that blocking antibody might be an antigen–antibody complex. Tumours may flood the blood system with antigen which combines with cytotoxic antibody before it gets to the tumour. This hypothesis fits with the observation that blocking antibody converts to cytotoxic antibody when a tumour is removed. Morton (1972) doubted the *in vivo* significance of blocking antibody. Thompson and Linna (1973) carried out thymectomy and bursectomy in chickens. Their data from thymectomy experiments fitted well with the concept of thymic surveillance in viral oncogenesis, but their bursectomy results did not support a tumour-protecting (enhancement) role for humoral immunity *in vivo*, but suggested that humoral antibodies were involved in *host* protection. Lamon *et al.* (1973) found that anti-tumour activity *in vitro* was dependent on B lymphocytes.

The immune system and the stimulation of tumour growth

Prehn (1972) proposed that the normal immune reaction may have a dual function in relation to neoplasia: (a) stimulation of tumour growth early in the course of the disease or when the immune response is minimal; (b) inhibition of tumour growth at other times. Prehn's evidence was obtained from the subcutaneous inoculation into thymectomised, X-irradiated mice of various numbers of spleen cells from specifically-immunized mice mixed with constant numbers of target tumour cells. Small numbers of admixed immune spleen cells produced a statistically significant, reproducible, acceleration of tumour cell growth in the inoculum, as compared with controls of either non-immune spleen cells or spleen cells from animals immunized against a different, non-cross-reacting tumour. Larger numbers of specifically immune spleen cells resulted in inhibition of tumour cell growth. Slemmer (1972) has found that premalignant mammary gland tissues may be protected by a basement membrane which prevents the expression of their new antigens—thereby affording protection from the host immune response until, having become overtly malignant, the cells break through the basement membrane and thus through the immunological barrier.

Hirsch *et al.* (1972, 1973) found that leukaemia viruses in mice were activated by graft-versus-host responses and by mixed lymphocyte reactions *in vitro*, and that viruses were activated following skin transplantation on to immunosuppressed mice. In 1964, we suggested that a latent lymphoreticular agent in *Xenopus* might be activated by the presence of a skin allograft, and that the stimulation was more marked the greater the genetic disparity between host and graft (Ruben & Balls 1964c).

Immunotherapy and malignancy

One of the main reasons for current interest in the immune response and malignancy is the hope that the immune system might be used to help cancer patients (Mathé 1971, McKhann & Jagarlamoody 1972, Alexander, in Vaeth 1972, Woodruff 1973). Two main kinds of immunotherapy seem possible:

(1) *specific active immunotherapy*, the mounting of specific immune reactions against tumour autoantigens;
(2) *non-specific active immunotherapy*, the general stimulation of the host's immune system by adjuvants of immunity (such as *Corynebacterium parvum*, Woodruff 1973).

Any such methods are more likely to be useful if used in association with other methods of treatment—e.g. for dealing with any cells released into the circulation during surgery—rather than in a direct attack on a solid tumour. Mathé stresses the point that immune methods may not kill many cells, but that they could kill the *last* cell.

The main problem with active immunotherapy and malignancy is that not enough is yet known about the relationship between the immune system and malignancy (though the lack of fundamental understanding did not prevent earlier dramatic advances in immunization against disease).

Immunity and malignancy—some conclusions

At present, it seems reasonable to conclude (with Morton, 1972) that both cellular and humoral immunity are important in controlling the growth of malignant cell populations, and that it is the interaction of the two that is most important. We must also think *quantitatively* about the relationship between tumours and the immune system. Deckers *et al.* (1973) suggest that tumour-specific immunity is effective when tumours are small, but not when they are large. McKhann and Jagarlamoody (1972) wrote of a *balance* between the immune response and the amount of tumour, which could be fitted to Prehn's suggestion of a biphasic effect of the immune system on tumour growth. We must also recognize and consider other contributory factors which affect the immune response and tumour growth. For example, an individual may be able to control incipient malignant cell populations up to a certain size, but the balance may be tipped in favour of progression to clinical disease by:

(1) advancing age, which involves a decrease in immune competence (it also involves a decline in many other capacities, such as wound healing, so age-tumour relationships must not be assumed to be evidence in favour of immune surveillance);

(2) immunosuppressive experiences, whether they be planned in connection with transplant surgery, the incidental side-effects of drugs taken for other purposes, or the result of accidental or necessary irradiation;
(3) the after-effects or co-effects of infectious disease or other disease.

One thing can be said firmly—the control of tumour development by the immune system is only a part of the total network of control (otherwise one would have expected multiple tumours in many tissues in more of the patients on long-term immunosuppressive regimes). Arguments can also be made in support of many other factors, so the most rational opinion at present is that a multiple system of control of cell behaviour operates for the good of the host. Some of the complexity in this regard is apparent in the discussion concerning neoplasia in 'nude' athymic mice (Custer *et al.* 1973). If T-cell immunosurveillance is a primary control mechanism in the control of neoplasia, one might expect athymic mice to generate many spontaneous neoplasms. They do not, but does this necessarily prove that immunostimulation is a requirement for tumour development. As the authors point out, a compensatory development of the humoral immune response could also play a role, and the normally short life-span of athymic mice might also mitigate against tumour development. It may be of interest to point out that evidence concerning the control of *Xenopus* lymphoid tumour development, which we shall discuss shortly, led Ruben and Stevens (1971) to speculate that primitive amphibians may rely on humoral rather than cell-mediated immunity in surveillance, because cell-mediated immunity is relatively weak in urodele amphibians and in *Xenopus* when compared to their capacity to respond with serum antibody.

Immunity and malignancy in the lower vertebrates

It is too early to discuss the question of a relationship between the immune response and malignancy in invertebrates, because it is not yet clear whether invertebrates have an immune response which shows the specificity and memory which characterize the vertebrate immune response, or whether invertebrates contain malignant cell populations comparable with neoplasia in vertebrates. These questions are discussed in other chapters in this book and in earlier parts of this chapter. On the other hand, there are a number of good reasons for investigating the relationship between the immune system and malignancy in the lower vertebrates:

(1) the lymphoreticular system becomes progressively more elaborate in the vertebrates—in terms of the amount and dispersion of lymphoreticular tissue, degree of differentiation of the lymphoreticular tissue, and the variety of leucocytes in the circulating blood;

(2) the variety and degree of specialization of tissues in general is progressively increased in the vertebrates; defence of the organism from infection by foreign organisms is progressively transferred to a particular tissue, and the natural resistance and tolerance of infections noted by Reichenbach-Klinke and Elkan (1965) in all three main groups of poikilotherms is reduced in the homoithermal birds and mammals;
(3) the lower vertebrates offer some advantages over the higher vertebrates as experimental material: for example, the rate of development, allograft response and other processes can be slowed down or speeded up by changing the environmental temperature; free-living embryonic and larval stages permit ontogenic studies which are much more difficult in higher vertebrates;
(4) not only are the lymphoreticular tissues less differentiated and less dispersed, but the number of cells involved is much smaller in poikilotherms than in homoitherms.

In spite of these obvious advantages and of the range of tumours described, relatively little work has been carried out on the immunological aspects of malignancy in the lower vertebrates. We know of no significant experiments with reptile tumours, and very few experiments have been carried out with fish. Mulcahy (1970) reported that 21 per cent of lymphosarcoma-bearing Northern pike had thymus tumours, but she did not consider that the thymus was a primary site or was important in tumour development. Dunbar (1969) described three lymphoid tumours in the salmonid fish, *Salvelinus fontinalis*, two of which apparently arose in the thymus. The third involved the thymus as well as the kidney. By contrast, a number of amphibian tumours have been used in studies on the immunological aspects of neoplasia. These will be briefly discussed in turn.

Lymphoreticular tumours in *Xenopus*

Tumours of the lymphoreticular system in *Xenopus laevis* (the South African clawed toad) were first described by Balls (1962). Early experimental studies, including transmission by cell-free filtrates, were reviewed by Balls and Ruben (1968). Although no virus has yet been isolated from tumour tissue and no virus particles have yet been seen in tumour cells in the electron microscope, the balance of evidence favours a viral aetiology for *Xenopus* lymphoid tumours (Clothier & Balls 1973a). The controversy over the secondary presence of mycobacteria has already been referred to, and was discussed in detail by Clothier and Balls (1973a,b).

Ruben (1969) reported that, regardless of the method of transmission (implants or cell-free filtrates), multiple foci developed in the viscera of the host, then underwent non-caseating, focal necrosis, which in turn was followed by a recurrence of focus formation and growth. The timing of the cycle of growth, necrosis and regrowth was affected by heredity, temperature and agent titre, but was entirely predictable for a given set of conditions. Ruben suggested that immunological factors might play a role in the growth-necrosis cycling, but that the timing and character of the necrosis suggested humoral antibody involvement rather than a cell-mediated response. The necrotic period was delayed by prior injection of 3-methylcholanthrene crystals, lowering the environmental temperature, and injection of tumour homogenate prior to the expected onset of necrosis. Ruben suggested that this delay could have been a result of interference with the immune response.

Ruben (1970) showed that necrosis does not occur in tumour implants in immunologically unresponsive larvae and that such larvae are not themselves susceptible to tumour development. Both the tumour tissue and normal tissue grew well in the tadpole tail, so it appears that necrosis is not a feature of the tumour cells themselves, but is imposed by the host, if it is immune-competent.

Ruben and Stevens (1971) showed that the organismally-imposed necrosis was effectively suppressed by the implantation of allo-tumour grafts, but not by normal tissue allografts. The formation of new tumour foci following necrosis appeared to depend on the acquisition of new tumour cells rather than on cloning by survivors of necrosis in the primary foci. No *Xenopus* which was developing the disease mounted an allograft response against either normal liver or kidney or against normal liver associated with neoplastic foci. This suggests that tumour-bearing *Xenopus* have a deficient cell-mediated immune response, as is the case in Hodgkin's disease in man (Aisenberg 1966). *In vitro* studies (Auerbach & Ruben 1970) showed that tumour-bearing spleens also gave a reduced haemagglutination activity against sheep red blood cells. The reduction in immune competence in tumour-bearing *Xenopus* could explain the secondary involvement of mycobacteria in the tumour tissue—an altered immune response might change the relationship between the toadlet and the bacteria which are ubiquitous in any aquatic environment.

Ruben (1969) was able to immunize *Xenopus* toadlets against tumour induction by injecting low dilutions of low infectivity-titre cell-free tumour filtrates. Splenic fragments, but not liver fragments, from a toadlet which had survived a previous challenge with neoplastic tissue homogenate suppressed tumour growth when implanted into a tumour implant-bearing immune-incompetent toadlet (Ruben & Stevens 1971).

Hadji-Azimi (1969) found differences in the serum proteins of normal and tumour-bearing *Xenopus*. The serum of tumour-bearing animals showed an increased percentage of gammaglobulin and a decreased percentage of albumin. A diffuse increase in immunoglobulin levels follows hepatic parenchymal disease in man and experimentally-induced liver injuries in rats, but an increased synthesis of one of the immunoglobulin classes occurs in multiple myeloma in man and plasmacytoma in mice. It was not shown whether the increase in gammaglobulin in the tumour-bearing *Xenopus* was diffuse or specific to one class of immunoglobulin.

Hadji-Azimi and Fischberg (1971) produced syngeneic *Xenopus* by nuclear transplantation, then studied the immune response to syngeneic and allogeneic grafts of normal liver and of lymphoid-tumour-bearing liver. Normal hepatic tissue allografts were rejected two to three weeks after implantation, while normal hepatic syngeneic grafts, and cancerous hepatic grafts from allogeneic and syngeneic donors were tolerated.

Lymphosarcoma in the Mexican axolotl (*Ambystoma mexicanum*)

DeLanney and Blackler (1969) described a lymphosarcoma which appeared spontaneously and which could be passed only by means of cellular grafts and only to members of the C^h histocompatibility strain. They found that adult histoincompatible hosts did not visibly proliferate tumour or pass it unless they were thymectomised at early larval stages or were made tolerant to the C^h strain prior to tumour transfer. One C^h sub-strain allowed the tumour to proliferate and then it regressed. Just as young animals mature in their capacity to reject skin allografts, histoincompatible strains mature in their ability to regress a tumour. C^h strain animals that invariably die from single tumour transfers could be made immune by a regime of tumour transplantation and excision. DeLanney and Blackler noted that the circumstances associated with the origin of the *Ambystoma* tumour were not inconsistent with the hypothesis of Tyler (1962)—namely that the onset of the tumour may have been associated with immune stress (Schwartz & Beldotti 1965).

The renal adenocarcinoma of *Rana pipiens*

Although some early transplantation experiments were carried out, research on the *Rana pipiens* renal tumour has mainly been concentrated on the viral aetiology of the tumour. Rafferty (1973) has proposed a life cycle for the herpes-type virus which is thought to be the agent involved. He proposed that the virus infects eggs or tadpoles, and that renal tumours then develop in the third or fourth summer. No virus particles are seen in summer-phase tumours, and it appears that a period of prolonged cold is necessary for the production of the mature virus. Virus particles are thought to build up during the winter hibernation period in those frogs which survive the summer, accumulate in the urine, to be shed into the water in the spring. Thus, the next generation of embryos and tadpoles is infected. This is a reasonable suggestion, which is in line with present knowledge. Tweedell (1969) showed that cell-free tumour extracts give rise to tumours in young frogs, if injected into oocytes or embryos. The question of vertical or horizontal transmission of the disease has been discussed in detail by McKinnell (1973). In addition to being important because this was the first example of an oncogenic herpes-type virus (Biggs *et al.* 1972), this work raises two important points. First, animals with embryonic and larval stages which are free-living before they are immune-competent are liable to become infected with, and tolerant to, micro-organisms in their external environment. Horton (1969) and Ruben *et al.* (1972) found allograft response capacity as early as one week of free-living existence in *Xenopus* (12 days from fertilization) and Horton and Manning (1972) showed this response to be thymus-dependent, as is the case in birds and mammals. Kidder *et al.* (1973) have shown that the capacity to generate a humoral response to heterologous red cells correlates with lymphocyte differentiation in the spleen, one week after thymocyte differentiation takes place. Secondly, since free-living stages survive several days whilst immune-incompetent, they must have a considerable natural resistance to infection. This may be the basis of the greater tolerance noted by Reichenbach-Klinke and Elkan (1965) in their survey of disease in fish and amphibians, and of the comparatively greater sensitivity shown by birds and mammals, where early development takes place in an environment which protects early developmental stages from infections.

Kirkwood *et al.* (1969) showed that rabbit antiserum against the frog renal tumour herpes-type virus also precipitated Epstein-Barr virus (which was originally isolated from Burkitt's lymphoma cells), and Fink, King and Mizell (1969) found that sera from frogs cross-reacted with herpes-virus antigen from a Burkitt's lymphoma cell line. Klein (1971) interpreted this as being due to the presence of common group antigens on different herpes viruses, but further research might reveal a closer relationship.

Conclusions

After surveying a very large number of papers concerning a wide variety of animals, we are more than ever convinced that a comparative approach to neoplastic development and its control is not only advisable, but necessary. We have also gained a number of impressions, which suggest to us that research effort would be more profitably spent if some of the lessons to be derived from the past were heeded.

There has been too great a tendency to enter into lengthy discussions on the histopathology of individual cases. The most meaningful types of tumour are those which are available with sufficient regularity for experimental study to be possible. The success of the RTLA will ultimately be judged not on the number of accessions in its collection, but on its ability to stimulate good thinking and good experimental work which leads to the acquisition of useful results.

It is also clear that too many generalizations have been based on lack of information. The clearest case of this phenomenon is the widely-held impression that neoplastic development is confined to the vertebrates. This idea stems partly from the confusion caused by invertebrate pathologists, who have tended to call every unusual lump a tumour, and partly from those vertebrate pathologists who have used this impression so that a vertebrate-restricted cause of neoplastic development could be postulated. Many authors seem eager to base their arguments on divergent evolution, whilst apparently being unaware of convergent evolution. It is ironical that the occurrence of neoplasms in molluscs does not necessarily preclude Good and Finstad's (1969) idea of a phylogenetic relationship between the immune response and the capacity for neoplastic development. The cephalopod molluscs evolved eyes which are anatomically and developmentally similar to those of vertebrates, so why should not the capacity for tumour development arise at different times by convergent evolution, and why was it necessary to predict that 'true neoplasms' would only occur in vertebrates?

The Waddington-Needham suggestion of a negative correlation between regenerative ability and neoplastic development has also frequently been misused. What should have been taken as an intriguing basis for experimental studies has too often been used as a factual point for citation in an argument. There seems to be a danger that the immune surveillance hypothesis may be generally accepted because of its intellectual appeal rather than because there is sound evidence in favour of it.

More effort should be made to take into account and make use of the special features of particular groups of organisms. Our present knowledge of genetics and developmental biology is largely based on the ingenuity of experimental biologists in profiting from the variety of living organisms. Comparative oncologists would do well to try to emulate this. The lack of tumours in nematodes may be because they lack adult somatic cells capable of proliferation, rather than because they lack a lymphoid system. While field biologists should be congratulated on their discovery of a number of significant tumours in molluscs, the group of invertebrates which we feel are most likely to be of value in cancer research in the short-term, what is now needed is laboratory-based research on the effects of chemical carcinogens and viruses under controlled conditions. Another group with a special feature which deserves exploitation are the neotenic amphibians. Studies of the effects of chemical carcinogens on sexually-mature, pre-metamorphic and post-metamorphic axolotls should prove very interesting. We should also be more aware and make more use of the differences that exist *within* animal phyla.

If we consider that the molluscs are the invertebrate group most likely to give useful results following intensive studies, then the amphibians are the equivalent group in the lower vertebrates. Their advantages include:

(1) the ontogeny of immunity can be studied more easily than in reptiles, birds and mammals (du Pasquier 1973);
(2) skin grafting is easier than in fish or reptiles, which have scales;
(3) the immune response can be manipulated by altering the environmental temperature (Simnett 1965);
(4) early thymectomy is possible several days before the thymus becomes lymphoid (Horton & Manning 1972);
(5) early thymectomy does not lead to runting (Manning 1972);
(6) the thymus appears to be the *single* source for all lymphocyte sub-populations in developing *Rana pipiens* (Turpen, Volpe & Cohen 1973); therefore it should be possible one day to study early decision-making on the part of cells whose eventual fate may be anti-tumour surveillance;
(7) neotenic species are available;
(8) species with varying degrees of regenerative capacity are available;
(9) adult tissues, including immune competent tissues, survive and function normally in long-term organ culture (Monnickendam & Balls 1973).

We close this discussion with a comment by A. E. Needham (1962): 'We are impressed and appalled by the frequency of cancer in human populations today but in view of the number of possible hazards and of the number of already known carcinogens it would be reasonable to marvel at the relative rarity of the phenomenon. This is very relevant to the solution of the problems of neoplasia, and indeed of normal growth. As an antidote to any feeling of pessimism about an early solution to the problem of cancer, it is important to recognize that its solution may simultaneously solve the wider problem of the mechanism of growth in general.'

Acknowledgment

We are particularly grateful to Dr J. C. Harshbarger, Director of the RTLA, for the help he so willingly gave us in obtaining the information on which our survey of tumours in the lower vertebrates and invertebrates was based.

References

Abeley G.I., Perova S.D., Khramkova N.I., Postnikova Z.A. & Irlin I.S. (1963) Production of embryonic α-globulin by transplantable mouse hepatomas. *Transplantation* **1**, 174–80.

Aisenberg A.C. (1966) Manifestations of immunologic unresponsiveness in Hodgkin's disease. *Cancer Research* **26**, 1152–60.

Anderson N.G. & Coggin J.H. (1972) Embryonic antigens in virally transformed cells, p. 217. In *Membranes and Viruses in Immunopathology*, ed. Day S.B. & Good R.A. Academic Press, New York and London.

ASHLEY L.M. & HALVER J.E. (1968) Dimethylnitrosamine-induced hepatic cell carcinomas in Rainbow trout. *Journal of the National Cancer Institute* **41,** 531–52.

AUERBACH R. & RUBEN L.N. (1970) Studies of antibody formation in *Xenopus laevis. Journal of Immunology* **104,** 1242–6.

BALLS M. (1962) Spontaneous neoplasms in Amphibia: a review and descriptions of six new cases. *Cancer Research* **22,** 1142–54.

BALLS M. & CLOTHIER R.H. (1974) Spontaneous tumours in Amphibia: a review. *Oncology* **29,** 501–19.

BALLS M. & RUBEN L.N. (1964) Variation in the response of *Xenopus laevis* to normal tissue homografts. *Developmental Biology* **10,** 92–104.

BALLS M. & RUBEN L.N. (1968) Lymphoid tumors in Amphibia: a review. *Progress in Experimental Tumor Research* **10,** 238–60.

BANFIELD W.G., WOKE P.A. & MACKAY C.M. (1966) Mosquito transmission of lymphomas. *Cancer* **19,** 1333–6.

BARRY M.M. & YEVICH P.P. (1972) Incidence of gonadal cancer in the Quahaug, *Mercenaria mercenaria. Oncology* **26,** 87–96.

BIGGS P.M., DE-THÉ G. & PAYNE L.N. (eds) (1972) *Oncogenesis and Herpesviruses.* International Agency for Research and Cancer, Lyon.

BOLTON P.M. (1973a) The effects of immune depression on chemical carcinogenesis in the rat. I. Regional lymphadenectomy. *Oncology* **27,** 430–6.

BOLTON P.M. (1973b) The effects of immune depression on chemical carcinogenesis in the rat. II. Antilymphocyte serum. *Oncology* **27,** 520–4.

BOLTON P.M. (1973c) The effects of immune depression on chemical carcinogenesis in the rat. III. Cyclophosphamide. *Oncology* **27,** 525–32.

BREEDIS C. (1952) Induction of accessory limbs and of sarcoma in the newt, *Triturus viridescens,* with carcinogenic substances. *Cancer Research* **12,** 861–6.

BREEDIS C. (1954) Effects of temperature on a neoplasm-regenerate complex in the newt, (*Triturus viridescens*). *Federation Proceedings* **13,** abstr. 1390.

BROWN E.R., HAZDRA J.J., KEITH L., GREENSPAN I., KWAPINSKI J.B.G. & BEAMER P. (1973) Frequency of fish tumors found in polluted waters as compared to nonpolluted Canadian waters. *Cancer Research* **33,** 189–97.

BURNET F.M. (1970) The concept of immunological surveillance. *Progress in Experimental Tumor Research* **13,** 1–27.

BURNET F.M. (1972) *Genes, Dreams and Realities.* Penguin Books Ltd., Harmondsworth, Middlesex, 250 pp.

BURTIN P., MARTIN E., SABINE M.C. & VON KLEIST S. (1972) Immunological study of polyps of the colon. *Journal of the National Cancer Institute* **48,** 25–32.

CAHNMANN H.J. & KURATSUNE M. (1957) Determination of polycyclic hydrocarbons in oysters collected in polluted waters. *Analytical Chemistry* **29,** 1312–17.

CANTWELL G.E., HARSHBARGER J.C., TAYLOR R.L., KENTON C., SLATICK M.S. & DAWE C.J. (1968) A bibliography of the literature on neoplasms of invertebrate animals. *Gann Monograph* **5,** 57–84.

CARTER S.B. (1968) Tissue homeostasis and the biological basis of cancer. *Nature, London* **220,** 970–4.

CIACCIO G. (1941) Prime ricerche sulla rigenerazione degli arti in tritoni sottoposti ad inienzioni di idrocarburi cancerigeni. *Atti Reale Istituto Veneto Ssci. Let. ed. arti* (Cl. Sc. Matem. e Nat.) **100,** 653–60.

CLOTHIER R.H. & BALLS M. (1973a) Mycobacteria and lymphoreticular tumours in *Xenopus laevis,* the South African clawed toad. I. Isolation, characterization and pathogenicity for *Xenopus* of *M. marinum* isolated from lymphoreticular tumour cells. *Oncology* **28,** 445–57.

Clothier R.H. & Balls M. (1973b) Mycobacteria and lymphoreticular tumours in *Xenopus laevis*, the South African clawed toad. II. Have mycobacteria a rôle in tumour initiation and development? *Oncology* **28,** 458–80.

Codreanu R. (1939) Recherches biologiques sur un chironomide *Symbiocladius rhithrogene* (Zavr.). Ectoparasite 'cancérigène' des Ephémères torrenticoles. *Archives de Zoologie expérimentale et générale* **81,** 1–283.

Couch J.A. (1969) An unusual lesion in the mantle of the American oyster, *Crassostrea virginica. National Cancer Institute Monograph* **31,** 557–62.

Cowan D.F. (1968) Diseases of captive reptiles. *Journal of the American Veterinary Association* **153,** 848–59.

Custer R.P., Outzen H.C., Eaton G.J. & Prehn R.T. (1973) Does the absence of immunological surveillance affect the tumor incidence in 'nude' mice? First recorded spontaneous lymphoma in a 'nude' mouse. *Journal of the National Cancer Institute* **51,** 707–11.

Dawe C.J. (1969a) Phylogeny and oncogeny. *National Cancer Institute Monograph* **31,** 1–40.

Dawe C.J. (1969b) Neoplasms of blood cell origin in poikilothermic animals—a review. *National Cancer Institute Monograph* **32,** 7–28.

Dawe C.J. (1970a) Comparative oncology and environmental carcinogenesis. UICC *Bulletin sur le Cancer* **8,** 2–3.

Dawe C.J. (1970b) Neoplasms of blood cell origin in poikilothermic animals, p. 634. In *Comparative Leukemia Research* 1969, ed. Dutcher R.M. Karker, Basel and New York.

Dawe C.J. & Berard C.W. (1971) Workshop on comparative pathology of hematopoietic and lymphoreticular neoplasms. *Journal of the National Cancer Institute* **47,** 1365–70.

Dawe C.J. & Harshbarger J.C. (eds.) (1969) A symposium on neoplasms and related disorders of invertebrate and lower vertebrate animals. *National Cancer Institute Monograph* **31,** 772 pp.

Deckers P.J., Davis R.C., Parker G.A. & Mannick J.A. (1973) The effect of tumor size on concomitant tumor immunity. *Cancer Research* **33,** 33–9.

DeLanney L.E. & Blackler K. (1969) Acceptance and regression of a strain-specific lymphosarcoma in Mexican axolotls, p. 399. In *Biology of Amphibian Tumors*, ed. Mizell M. Springer-Verlag, New York, Heidelberg and Berlin.

Dunbar C.E. (1969) Lymphosarcomas of possible thymic origin in salmonid fishes. *National Cancer Institute Monograph* **31,** 167–71.

Du Pasquier L. (1973) Ontogeny of the immune response in cold-blooded vertebrates. *Current Topics in Microbiology and Immunology* **61,** 38–88.

Duryee W.R. (1965) Factors influencing development of tumors in frogs. *Annals of the New York Academy of Sciences* **126,** 59–84.

Dustin P. (1972) Cell differentiation and carcinogenesis: a critical review. *Cell and Tissue Kinetics* **5,** 519–33.

Erwin R. & Gordon M. (1955) Regeneration of melanomas in fish. *Zoologica* **40,** 53–84.

Farley C.A. (1969a) Probable neoplastic disease of the hematopoietic system in oysters, *Crassostrea virginica* and *Crassostrea gigas. National Cancer Institute Monograph* **31,** 541–55.

Farley C.A. (1969b) Sarcomatoid proliferative disease in a wild population of Blue mussels (*Mytilus edulis*). *Journal of the National Cancer Institute* **43,** 509–16.

Farley C.A., Banfield W.G., Kasnic G. & Foster W.S. (1972) Oyster herpes-type virus. *Science, New York* **178,** 759–60.

Farley C.A. & Sparks A.K. (1970) Proliferative diseases of hemocytes, endothelial cells and connective tissue cells in molluscs, p. 610. In *Comparative Leukemia Research* 1969, ed. Dutcher R.M. Karker, Basel and New York.

Fawcett D.W. (1956) Electron microscope observations on intercellular virus-like particles associated with the cells of the Lucké renal adenocarcinoma. *Journal of Biophysical and Biochemical Cytology* **2,** 725–42.

FELDMAN J.D. (1972) Immunological enhancement: a study of blocking antibody. *Advances in Immunology* **15,** 167–214.

FINK M.A., KING G.S. & MIZELL M. (1969) Reactivity of serum from frogs and other species with a herpesvirus antigen extracted from a Burkitt lymphoma cultured cell line, p. 358. In *Biology of Amphibian Tumors*, ed. Mizell M. Springer-Verlag, New York, Heidelberg and Berlin.

FONTAINE A.R. (1969) Pigmented tumor-like lesions in an ophiuroid echinoderm. *National Cancer Institute Monograph* **31,** 255–61.

FOULDS L. (1969) *Neoplastic Development.* Vol. 1. Academic Press, London and New York, 439 pp.

FRANK W. & SCHEPKY A. (1969) Metastasierendes Lymphosarkom bei einer Riesenschlange *Eunectes marinus* (Linnaeus, 1758). *Pathologia Veterinaria* **6,** 437–43.

GATEFF E. & SCHNEIDERMANN H.A. (1969) Neoplasms in mutant and cultured wild-type tissues of *Drosophila. National Cancer Institute Monograph* **31,** 365–97.

GOLD P. & FREEDMAN S.O. (1965) Specific carcinoembryonic antigens of the human digestive system. *Journal of Experimental Medicine* **122,** 467–81.

GOOD R.A. (1972) Relations between immunity and malignancy. *Proceedings of the National Academy of Sciences of the U.S.A.* **69,** 1026–32.

GOOD R.A. & FINSTAD J. (1969) Essential relationship between the lymphoid system, immunity and malignancy. *National Cancer Institute Monograph* **31,** 41–58.

GOOD R.A., FINSTAD J., POLLARO B. & GABRIELSON A.E. (1966) Morphologic studies on the evolution of lymphoid tissues among the lower vertebrates, p. 149. In *Phylogeny of Immunity*, ed. Smith R.T., Miescher P.A. & Good R.A. University of Florida Press, Gainesville.

GOOD R.A. & PAPERMASTER B.W. (1964) Ontogeny and phylogeny of adaptive immunity. *Advances in Immunology* **4,** 1–115.

HADDOW A. (1972) Molecular repair, wound healing and carcinogenesis: tumour production a possible overhealing? *Advances in Cancer Research* **16,** 181–234.

HADJI-AZIMI I. (1969) Electrophoretic study of the serum proteins of normal and 'lymphoid tumour'-bearing *Xenopus. Nature, London* **221,** 264–5.

HADJI-AZIMI I. & FISCHBERG M. (1971) Normal and cancerous tissue transplantation in allogeneic and syngeneic *Xenopus laevis. Cancer Research* **31,** 1594–9.

HADORN E. (1969) Proliferation and dynamics of cell heredity in blastema cultures of *Drosophila. National Cancer Institute Monograph* **31,** 351–64.

HARSHBARGER J.C. (1967) Responses of invertebrates to vertebrate carcinogens. *Federation Proceedings* **26,** 1693–7.

HARSHBARGER J.C. (1969) The Registry of Tumors in Lower Animals. *National Cancer Institute Monograph* **31,** XI–XVI.

HARSHBARGER J.C. (1972) *Activities Report RTLA* 1 *February* 1971–10 *February* 1972. Museum of Natural History, Smithsonian Institution, Washington.

HARSHBARGER J.C. (1973) Invertebrate animals—what can they contribute to cancer research? *Federation Proceedings* **32,** 2224–6.

HARSHBARGER J.C., CANTWELL G.E. & STANTON M.F. (1970) Effects of N-nitrosodimethylamine on the crayfish, *Procambarus clarkii*, p. 425. In *Proceedings of the IVth International Colloquium on Insect Pathology.*

HARSHBARGER J.C. & TAYLOR R.L. (1968) Neoplasms of Insects. *Annual Review of Entomology* **13,** 159–90.

HELLSTRÖM K.E. & HELLSTRÖM I. (1970) Immunological enhancement as studies by cell culture techniques. *Annual Review of Microbiology* **24,** 373–98.

Hellström I. & Hellström K.E. (1973) Some recent studies on cellular immunity to human melanomas. *Federation Proceedings* **32,** 156–9.

Hillman R.E. (1963) An observation on the occurrence of mitosis in regenerating mantle epithelium of the Eastern oyster, *Crassostrea virginica. Chesapeake Science* **4,** 172–4.

Hirsch M.S., Ellis D.A., Black P.H., Monaco A.P. & Wood M.L. (1973) Leukemia virus activation during homograft rejection. *Science, New York* **180,** 500–2.

Hirsch M.S., Phillips S.M., Solnik C., Black P.H., Schwartz, R.S. & Carpenter C.B. (1972) Activation of leukemia viruses by graft-versus-host mixed lymphocyte reactions *in vitro. Proceedings of the National Academy of Sciences of the U.S.A.* **69,** 1069–72.

Horton J.D. (1969) Ontogeny of the immune response to skin allografts in relation to lymphoid organ development in the amphibian, *Xenopus laevis* Daudin. *Journal of Experimental Zoology* **170,** 449–66.

Horton J.D. & Manning M.J. (1972) Response to skin allografts in *Xenopus laevis* following thymectomy at early stages of lymphoid organ maturation. *Transplantation* **14,** 141–54.

Ingram A.J. (1972) The lethal and hepatocarcinogenic effects of dimethylnitrosamine injection in the newt, *Triturus helveticus. British Journal of Cancer* **26,** 206–15.

Inoue S. (1954) On the transplantable spontaneous visceral tumour in the newt, *Triturus pyrrhogaster. Science Reports of Tohoku Imperial University* **20,** 226–36.

Inoue S. & Singer M. (1970) Experiments on a spontaneously originated visceral tumour in the newt, *Triturus pyrrhogaster. Annals of the New York Academy of Sciences* **174,** 729–64.

Irvine W.J. (1973) Immunological function and the pill. *Research in Reproduction* **5,** 5, 3.

Jones J.C. (1969) Hemocytes and the problem of tumors in insects. *National Cancer Institute Monograph* **31,** 481–5.

Kast A. (1967) Malignes Adenoameloblastom des Gaumes bei einer Tigerpython. *Frankfurter Zeitschrift für Pathologie* **77,** 135–40.

Kidder G.M., Ruben L.N. & Stevens J. (1973) Cytodynamics and ontogeny of the immune response of *Xenopus laevis* against sheep erythrocytes. *Journal of Embryology and Experimental Morphology* **29,** 73–85.

Kirkwood J.M., Geering G., Old L.J., Mizell M. & Wallace J. (1969) A Preliminary report on the serology of Lucké and Burkitt herpes-type viruses, p. 365. In *Biology of Amphibian Tumors,* ed. Mizell M. Springer-Verlag, New York, Heidelberg, and Berlin.

Klein G. (1969) Experimental studies in tumor immunology. *Federation Proceedings* **28,** 1739–53.

Klein G. (1971) Immunological aspects of Burkitt's lymphoma. *Advances in Immunology* **14,** 187–250.

Krieg K. (1972) *Ampullarius australis* d'Orbigny (Mollusca, Gastropoda) as experimental animal in oncological research. A contribution to the study of cancerogenesis in invertebrates. *Neoplasma* **19,** 41–9.

Lamon E.W., Wigzell H., Andersson B. & Klein E. (1973) Antitumour activity *in vitro* dependent on immune B lymphocytes. *Nature New Biology* **244,** 209–11.

LeMevel B.P. & Wells S.A. (1973) Foetal antigens cross-reactive with tumour-specific transplantation antigens. *Nature New Biology* **244,** 183–4.

Lucké B. (1938) Carcinoma in the Leopard frog: its probable causation by a virus. *Journal of Experimental Medicine* **68,** 457–68.

Lucké B. & Schlumberger H.G. (1949) Neoplasia in cold-blooded vertebrates. *Physiological Reviews* **29,** 91–126.

Manning M.J. (1971) The effects of early thymectomy on histogenesis of the lymphoid organs in *Xenopus laevis. Journal of Embryology and Experimental Morphology* **26,** 219–29.

MARTELLI M. & CHANDEBOIS R. (1973) Functions of the type 1 cell system and the problem of oncogenesis in planarians. *Oncology* **28,** 274–88.

MATHÉ G. (1971) Active immunotherapy. *Advances in Cancer Research* **14,** 1–36.

MATZ G., MOSSIER Y. & VAGO C. (1971) Une réaction de défense cellulaire chez les insectes: l'enkystement épithélial. *Bulletin de la Société Zoologique de France* **96,** 209–15.

MAWDESLEY-THOMAS L.E. (1969) Neoplasia in fish—a bibliography. *Journal of Fish Biology* **1,** 187–207.

MAWDESLEY-THOMAS L.E. (1970) Significance of liver tumour induction in animals, p. 481. In *Metabolic Aspects of Food Safety*, ed. Roe F.J.C. Blackwell Scientific Publications, Oxford.

MAWDESLEY-THOMAS L.E. (1971) Neoplasia in fish—a review. *Current Topics in Comparative Pathology* **1,** 87–167.

McKHANN C.F. & JAGARLAMOODY S.M. (1972) Manipulation of the immune response towards immunotherapy of cancer, p. 577. In *Membranes and Viruses in Immunopathology*, ed. Day S.B. & Good R.A. Academic Press, New York and London.

McKINNELL R.G. (1973) The Lucké frog kidney tumor and its herpes viruses. *American Zoologist* **13,** 97–114.

McKINNELL R.G. & ELLIS V.L. (1972) Epidemiology of the frog renal tumor and the significance of tumor nuclear transplantation studies to a viral aetiology of the tumor: a review, p. 183. In *Oncogenesis and Herpesviruses*, ed. Biggs P.M., de-Thé G. & Payne L.N. International Agency for Cancer Research, Lyon.

METCALF D. (1971) Humoral regulators in the development and progression of leukaemia. *Advances in Cancer Research* **14,** 181–230.

MICHELSON E.H. (1972) A neoplasm in the giant African snail, *Achatina fulica*. *Journal of Invertebrate Pathology* **20,** 264–7.

MIZELL M. (1960) Anuran (Lucké) tumor breakdown in regenerating anuran tadpole tails. *Anatomical Record* **137,** 382–3.

MIZELL M. (1961) Regression of tumor cells in blastema tissue, p. 65. In *Proceedings of Frog Kidney Adenocarcinoma Conference*, ed. Duryee W.R. & Warner L. National Cancer Institute, Bethesda.

MIZELL M. (1965) Effects of tadpole tail regeneration on the Lucké tumor: recovery of tritium-tagged normal cells from tritium-tagged tumor implants. *American Zoologist* **5,** 215.

MIZELL M. (1966) The effects of a regenerating anuran appendage on an anuran tumor. The apparent unmasking of a latent differentiation of a diploid tumor. *Proceedings of the 9th International Cancer Congress, Tokyo* 34.

MIZELL M. (ed.) (1969) *Biology of Amphibian Tumors*. Springer-Verlag, New York Heidelberg and Berlin, 484 pp.

MONNICKENDAM M.A. & BALLS M. (1973) Amphibian organ culture. *Experientia* **29,** 1–17.

MORTON D.L. (1972) Humoral tumor immunity in man: possible role in host defense against cancer, p. 553. In *Membranes and Viruses in Immunopathology*, ed. Day S.B. & Good R.A. Academic Press, New York and London.

MORTON J.E. (1963) *Molluscs*, 2nd edition. Hutchinson, London, 232 pp.

MULCAHY M. (1970) Hemic neoplasms in cold-blooded animals: lymphosarcoma in the pike, *Esox lucius*, p. 644. In *Comparative Leukemia Research* 1969, ed. Dutcher R.M. Karger, Basel and New York.

MULCAHY M.F., WINQVIST G. & DAWE C.J. (1970) The neoplastic cell type in lymphoreticular neoplasms of the Northern pike, *Esox lucius* L. *Cancer Research* **30,** 2712–17.

NAHMIAS A.J., CHANG G.C.H. & FRITZ M.E. (1972) Herpesvirus as infectious and oncogenic agents in man and other vertebrates, p. 293. In *Membranes and Viruses in Immunopathology*, ed. Day S.B. & Good R.A. Academic Press, New York and London.

NEEDHAM A.E. (1952) *Regeneration and Wound Healing.* Methuen, London and Wiley, New York.

NEEDHAM A.E. (1964) *The Growth Process in Animals.* Pitmans, London, 522 pp.

NEEDHAM J. (1942) *Biochemistry and Morphogenesis.* Cambridge University Press, Cambridge, 787 pp.

NEWMAN M.W. (1972) An oyster neoplasm of apparent mesenchymal origin. *Journal of the National Cancer Institute* **48,** 237–43.

OEHLERT W. (1973) Cellular proliferation in carcinogenesis. *Cell and Tissue Kinetics* **6,** 325–5.

PAULEY G.B. (1969) A critical review of neoplasia and tumor-like lesions in mollusks. *National Cancer Institute Monograph* **31,** 509–39.

PAULEY G.B. & SAYCE C.S. (1972) An invasive epithelial neoplasm in a Pacific oyster, *Crassostrea gigas. Journal of the National Cancer Institute* **49,** 897–902.

PAULEY G.B., SPARKS A.K. & SAYCE C.S. (1968) An unusual internal growth associated with multiple watery cysts in a Pacific oyster (*Crassostrea gigas*). *Journal of Invertebrate Pathology* **11,** 398–405.

PENN I. & STARZL T.E. (1972) Malignant tumors arising *de novo* in immunosuppressed organ transplant recipients. *Transplantation* **14,** 407–17.

PEREDELSKY A.A. (1941) The regenerative and tumour growths are not identical, but they are not antagonistic either. *Compte rendus de l'Académie des sciences de l'U.R.S.S.* **32,** 448–50.

PENTREATH R.J. (1973) The accumulation from water of ^{65}Zn, ^{54}Mn, ^{58}Co and ^{59}Fe by the mussel, *Mytilus edulis. Journal of the Marine Biological Association of the United Kingdom* **53,** 127–43.

PIZARELLO D.J. & WOLSKY A. (1966) Carcinogenesis and regeneration in newts. *Experientia* **22,** 387.

PREHN R.T. (1969) The relationship of immunology to carcinogenesis. *Annals of the New York Academy of Sciences* **164,** 449–57.

PREHN R.T. (1971) Immunosurveillance, regeneration and oncogenesis. *Progress in Experimental Tumor Research* **14,** 1–24.

PREHN R.T. (1972) The immune reaction as a stimulator of tumor growth. *Science, New York* **176,** 170–1.

PREHN R.T. & MAIN J.M. (1957) Immunity to methylcholanthrene-induced sarcomas. *Journal of the National Cancer Institute* **18,** 769–78.

RAFFERTY K.A. (1973) Herpes viruses and cancer. *Scientific American* **229, 4:** 26–33.

RAPPAPORT H. (1966) Tumors of the Hematopoietic System. *Armed Forces Institute of Pathology, Washington,* 442 pp.

REICHENBACH-KLINKE H. & ELKAN E. (1965) *The Principal Diseases of Lower Vertebrates.* Academic Press, New York and London, 600 pp.

ROSE S.M. & WALLINGFORD H.M. (1948) Transformation of renal tumors of frogs to normal tissues in regenerating limbs of salamanders. *Science, New York* **107,** 457.

RUBEN L.N. (1963) Lucké carcinoma implants in regenerating and regressing urodele limbs. *Revue suisse de Zoologie* **70,** 224–36.

RUBEN L.N. (1969) Possible immunological factors in amphibian lymphosarcoma development, p. 368. In *Biology of Amphibian Tumors,* ed. Mizell M. Springer-Verlag, New York, Heidelberg and Berlin.

RUBEN L.N. (1970) Immunological maturation and lymphoreticular cancer transformation in larval *Xenopus laevis,* the South African clawed toad. *Developmental Biology* **22,** 43–58.

RUBEN L.N. & BALLS M. (1964a) The implantation of lymphosarcoma of *Xenopus laevis* into regenerating and non-regenerating forelimbs of that species. *Journal of Morphology* **115,** 225–38.

Ruben L.N. & Balls M. (1964b) The implantation of methylcholanthrene crystals into regenerating and non-regenerating forelimbs of *Xenopus laevis. Journal of Morphology* **115,** 238–54.

Ruben L.N. & Balls M. (1964c) Genetic disparity and cancer induction by normal tissue implants in Amphibia. *Science, New York* **146,** 1321–2.

Ruben L.N., Balls M. & Stevens J. (1966) Cancer and super-regeneration in *Triturus viridescens* limbs. *Experientia* **22,** 260–1.

Ruben L.N., Balls M., Stevens J. & Rafferty N.S. (1969) A new transmissible disease in the South African clawed toad, *Xenopus laevis. Oncology* **23,** 228–37.

Ruben L.N. & Stevens J. (1963) Post-embryonic induction in urodele limbs. *Journal of Morphology* **112,** 279–301.

Ruben L.N. & Stevens J.M. (1970) A comparison between granulomatosis and lymphoreticular neoplasia in *Diemictylus viridescens* and *Xenopus laevis. Cancer Research* **30,** 2613–19.

Ruben L.N. & Stevens J.M. (1971) Lymphoreticular neoplasia and immunity in Amphibia. *American Zoologist* **11,** 229–37.

Ruben, L.N., Stevens J. & Kidder G.M. (1972) Suppression of the allograft response by implants of mature lymphoid tissues in larval *Xenopus laevis. Journal of Morphology* **138,** 457–66.

Scarpelli D.G. (1969) Survey of some spontaneous and experimental disease processes of lower vertebrates and invertebrates. *Federation Proceedings* **28,** 1825–33.

Schlumberger H.G. & Lucké B. (1948) Tumors of fishes, amphibians and reptiles. *Cancer Research* **8,** 657–754.

Schmeer A.C. (1969) Mercenene: an antineoplastic agent extracted from the marine clam, *Mercenaria mercenaria. National Cancer Institute Monograph* **31,** 581–91.

Schochet S.S. & Lampert P.W. (1969) Plasmacytoma in *Rana pipiens,* p. 204. In *Biology of Amphibian Tumors,* ed. Mizell M. Springer-Verlag, New York, Heidelberg and Berlin.

Schwartz R.S. & Beldotti L. (1965) Malignant lymphomas following allogenic disease: transition from an immunological to a neoplastic disease. *Science, New York* **149,** 1511–14.

Seilern-Aspang F. & Kratochwil K. (1962) Induction and differentiation of an epithelial tumour in the newt, *Triturus cristatus. Journal of Embryology and Experimental Morphology* **10,** 337–56.

Seilern-Aspang F. & Kratochwil K. (1963) Die experimentelle Aktivierung der Differenzierungspotenzen entarter Zellen. *Wiener Klinisches Wochenschrift* **75,** 337–46.

Seilern-Aspang F. & Kratochwil K. (1965) Relation between regeneration and tumor growth, p. 452. In *Regeneration in Animals and Related Problems,* ed. Kiortsis V. & Trampusch H.A.L. North-Holland, Amsterdam.

Sheremetieva E.A. (1965) Spontaneous melanoma in regenerating tails of axolotls. *Journal of Experimental Zoology* **158,** 101–22.

Simnett J.D. (1965) Prolongation of homograft survival time in the Platanna, *Xenopus laevis* (Daudin), by exposure to low environmental temperature. *Journal of Cellular and Comparative Physiology* **65,** 293–8.

Sjögren H.O., Hellström I., Bansal S.C. & Hellström K.E. (1971) Suggestive evidence that 'blocking antibodies' of tumor-bearing individuals may be antigen-antibody complexes. *Proceedings of the National Academy of Sciences of the U.S.A.* **68,** 1372–5.

Slemmer G. (1972) Host response to premalignant mammary tissue. *National Cancer Institute Monograph* **35,** 57–71.

SMITH R.T. & LANDY M. (eds) (1970) *Immune Surveillance*. Academic Press, New York and London, 536 pp.

SMITHERS D.W. (1962) Cancer—an attack on cytologism. *Lancet* **i,** 493–9.

SOBIN L.H. (1968) Sarcomas in Afghanistan. *Nature, London* **217,** 1072–3.

STANTON M.F. (1965) Dimethylnitrosamine-induced hepatic degeneration and neoplasia in the aquarium fish, *Brachydanio rerio*. *Journal of the National Cancer Institute* **34,** 117–30.

SZABO I. & SZABO M. (1935) Epitheliale Geschwulstbildung bei einem wirbellosen Tier, *Limax flavus* L. *Zeitschrift für Krebsforschung* **40,** 540–5.

TARIN D. (ed.) (1972) *Tissue Interactions in Carcinogenesis*. Academic Press, London and New York, 483 pp.

THOMAS L. (1959) Discussion, p. 529. In *Cellular and Humoral Aspects of Hypersensitive States*, ed. Lawrence H.S. Hoeber-Harper, New York.

THOMPSON K.D. & LINNA T.I. (1973) Bursa-dependent and thymus-dependent 'surveillance' of a virus-induced tumour in the chicken. *Nature New Biology* **245,** 10–12.

TILLACK T.W. (1972) Significance and properties of tumor-specific antigens, p. 145. In *Membranes and Viruses in Immunopathology*, ed. Day S.B. & Good R.A. Academic Press, New York and London.

TURPEN J.B., VOLPE E.P. & COHEN N. (1973) Ontogeny and peripheralization of thymic lymphocytes. *Science, New York* **182,** 931.

TWEEDELL K.S. (1969) Simulated transmission of renal tumors in oocytes and embryos of *Rana pipiens*, p. 229. In *Biology of Amphibian Tumors*, ed. Mizell M. Springer-Verlag, New York, Heidelberg and Berlin.

TWEEDELL K.S., MICHALSKI F.J. & MOREK D.M. (1972) Bioassay of frog renal tumor viruses, p. 198. In *Oncogenesis and Herpesviruses*, ed. Biggs P.M., de-Thé G. & Payne L.N. International Agency for Research on Cancer, Lyon.

TYLER A. (1962) A developmental immunogenetic analysis of cancer, p. 533. In *Henry Ford Hospital International Symposium: Interactions in Normal and Malignant Growth*. Little, Brown & Co., Boston.

VAETH J.M. (ed.) (1972) *The Interrelationship of the Immune Response and Cancer*. Karger, Basel and New York, 222 pp.

W.H.O. (1965) *Technical Report Service*, Number 295, p. 16. World Health Organization, Geneva.

WADDINGTON C.H. (1935) Cancer and the theory of organizers. *Nature, London* **135,** 606–8.

WALES J.J. (1970) Hepatoma in Rainbow trout, p. 351. In *A Symposium on Diseases of Fishes and Shellfishes*, ed. Snieszko S.F. American Fish Society Special Publication Number 5, Washington.

WEIGLE W.O. (1973) Immunological unresponsiveness. *Advances in Immunology* **16,** 61–122.

WEISS P.A. (1973) Differentiation and its three facets: facts, terms and meaning. *Differentiation* **1,** 3–10.

WELLINGS S.R. (1969) Neoplasia and primitive vertebrate phylogeny: echinoderms, prevertebrates and fishes—a review. *National Cancer Institute Monograph* **31,** 59–128.

WESTON B.J. (1973) The thymus and immune surveillance, p. 237. In *Thymus Dependency*, ed. Davies, A.J.S. & Carter R.L. Plenum Press, New York and London.

WILLIS R.A. (1960) *The Pathology of Tumours*, 3rd edition. Butterworths, London, 1058 pp.

WOLF P.H. (1969) Neoplastic growth in two Sydney rock oysters, *Crassostrea commercialis* (Iredale and Roughley). *National Cancer Institute Monograph* **31,** 563–73.

WOLF P.H. (1971) Unusually large tumor in a Sydney rock oyster. *Journal of the National Cancer Institute* **46,** 1078–84.

WOODRUFF M. (1973) Cancer—the elusive enemy. *Proceedings of the Royal Society of London, Series B* **183,** 87–104.

ZECHMEISTER L. & KOE B.K. (1952) The isolation of carcinogenic and other polycyclic aromatic hydrocarbons from barnacles. *Archives of Biochemistry and Biophysics* **35,** 1–11.

ZEIGEL R.F. & CLARK H.F. (1969) Electron microscopic observations on a 'C'-type virus in cell cultures derived from a tumor-bearing viper. *Journal of the National Cancer Institute* **43,** 1097–102.

ZEIGEL R.F. & CLARK H.F. (1971) Histologic and electron microscopic observations on a tumor-bearing viper: establishment of a 'C'-type virus-producing cell line. *Journal of the National Cancer Institute* **46,** 309–21.

ZWART P. & HARSHBARGER J.C. (1972) Hematopoietic neoplasms in lizards: report of a typical case in *Hydrosaurus amboinensis* and of a probable case in *Varanus salvator*. *International Journal of Cancer* **9,** 548–53.

Chapter 8. Immunologic Diversity within the Class Amphibia

Nicholas Cohen

Introduction

Evolution and taxonomy of modern amphibians

Immunoglobulin diversity

Evolution and taxonomy of modern amphibians *continued*

A major histocompatibility complex?

Diversity of lymphoid organs

Conclusion

Introduction

> Most amphibians are abhorrent because of their cold body, pale colour, cartilaginous skeleton, filthy skin, fierce aspect, calculating eye, offensive smell, harsh voice, squalid habituation, and terrible venom; and so their Creator has not exerted his powers to make many of them.
>
> Linnaeus, *Systema Naturae* (1758)

An astonishingly large body of phenomenologic and analytic data has been accumulated by many curious scientists during the past 15 years that clearly delineates many facets of immunity of Linnaeus' loathsome amphibians. One key distillate from the more than 350 publications that constitute this data bank of amphibian immunity is that like all studied representatives of all other vertebrate classes, the amphibians have serum immunoglobulins; possess lymphoid cells with a genetic repertoire that allows them to synthesize specific antibodies in response to their recognition of antigen; reject transplants of allogeneic tissues immunologically; and display at least some form of immunologic memory. A second more surprising and perhaps more significant generalization to be derived from perusing this wealth of data is that there are striking immunologic differences among the Amphibia that are referable to the taxonomic ordering of these vertebrates. 'Representative' salamanders (Urodela or Caudata) differ from 'representative' frogs and toads (Anura) with respect to no fewer than three of the major parameters used to judge 'immunologic sophistication'. These are (1) the number of immunoglobulin classes; (2) the presence of a major histocompatibility complex; and (3) the anatomical and functional diversity of lymphoid tissues. My single purpose in writing this brief chapter is to detail these differences and then use them as a framework for present and future speculation as to their phylogenetic and immunologic implications. In doing so I will not attempt to systematically review all existing data on each facet of amphibian immunity. Such a labour of love would be superfluous since not only do several other chapters in this book derive their essence from amphibian models, but sufficient numbers of well-referenced reviews already cover the recent literature. I refer the reader interested in more facts to the following review articles and chapters which deal with humoral immunity and immunoglobulin structure (Marchalonis 1971, Marchalonis & Cone 1973, Clem 1969, Kubo *et al.* 1973); lymphoid tissues and the cellular basis of immunity (Cooper 1973, Cohen 1975, 1976); transplantation immunity (Cohen 1971, Hildemann 1972); developmental immunity (Du Pasquier 1973); and tumour immunity (Mizell 1968, Rubens & Stevens 1971, Balls & Ruben 1968).

Evolution and taxonomy of modern amphibians

In order to place the following sections in their proper phylogenetic perspective I will first briefly discuss the evolution and classification of the four modern orders that constitute the class, Amphibia (Goin & Goin 1970). Modern amphibians were originally derived from the lobe-finned Crossopterygii which flourished 350 million years ago during the Devonian period (Fig. 8.1). Very early in their evolutionary history, these stock amphibians split into several groups. One gave rise to the amphibian ancestors of the reptiles and higher tetrapods. It is not known whether it also gave rise to any or all of the groups of modern amphibians, for the position of modern amphibian orders is still actively being debated by palaeontologists. Some feel that all recent forms evolved from a single Palaeozoic stock and should, therefore, be grouped in a single subclass (Lissamphibia). Others feel that the modern orders, Caudata or Urodela (salamanders), Trachystomata (sirens), and Gymnophiona or Apoda (caecelians) constitute one super order, Lepospondyli, while the order, Anura (frogs and toads) form their own super order, Salientia. Although I have adopted this latter alternative in this chapter, this issue can only be resolved if and when critical gaps in the fossil records between the earliest known members of these modern orders and the lepospondyls of the Palaeozoic are filled in.

Anurans can be traced back farther than any other amphibians to the early Mesozoic or late Permian around 200 million years ago. Ancestors of

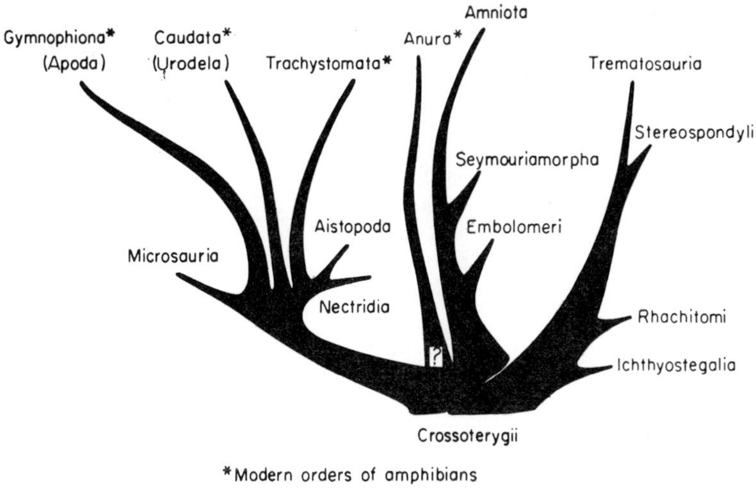

Fig. 8.1. Phylogeny of modern amphibian orders (after Goin **&** **Goin** 1970).

living representatives of the anuran families, Discoglossidae and Pipidae (Table 8.1, Fig. 8.1), can be traced back to the Jurassic; families such as the Ranidae and the Bufonidae have evolved more recently.

Fossil records of modern salamanders date back only as far as the late Jurassic of 150 million years past; those of the apodans go back only a million years. Fossils of now extinct Trachystomata have been dated back 120 million years to the Cretaceous period. Although many authors classify living members of this order, Trachystomata, in the Caudata, these sirens differ so strikingly from known salamanders that others place them in a separate order (Goin & Goin 1970).

All living families and orders of Amphibia are listed in Table 8.1 along with the footnote indicating which families have provided immunologists with their experimental models. This very small list is humbling. It brings home the lesson that those of us who refer to our experimental animal as a 'representative amphibian', are guilty of biologic oversimplification. As an immunologist I find it understandable that immunologic generalizations about an order or class of vertebrates have been (and will be) made from observations on a remarkably restricted phylogenetic sample. As a biologist intrigued by evolution, I worry that the phylogenetic as well as immunologic generalizations we make may eventually prove misleading if not spurious.

Immunoglobulin diversity

The diversity of immunoglobulin classes has apparently increased during the course of evolution. Primitive cartilaginous and bony fishes are generally

Table 8.1. Classification of living amphibians

SUPER-ORDER: LEPOSPONDYLI		
Order		Trachystomata ~ 3 species
	Family	Sirenidae
Order		Gymnophiona (apoda) ~ 158 species
	Families	Ichthyophiidae
		Caecilidae
		Typhlonectidae (t*)
		Scolecomorphidae
Order		Caudata (Urodela) ~ 300 species
	Families	Hynobiidae
		Cryptobranchidae
		Ambystomatidae (t, l, i, d)
		Salamandridae (t, l, i, d)
		Amphiumidae
		Plethodontidae (t, l)
		Proteidae (t, l, i)
SUPER-ORDER: SALIENTIA		
Order		Anura ~ 1900 species
	Suborder	Amphicoela
	Family	Ascaphidae
	Suborder	Aglossa
	Family	Pipidae (t, l, i, d)
	Suborder	Opisthocoela
	Families	Discoglossidae (t, l, i, d)
		Rhinophrynidae
	Suborder	Anomocoela
	Family	Pelobatidae
	Suborder	Diplasiocoela
	Families	Ranidae (t, l, i, d)
		Rhacophoridae
		Microhylidae
		Phrynomeridae
	Suborder	Procoela
	Families	Bufonidae (t, l, i, d)
		Atelopodidae
		Hylidae (t, d)
		Ceratophyridae
		Pseudidae
		Centrolenidae

* Letters in parentheses indicate that certain immunologic studies were performed on at least one species in that family: t = transplantation; l = lymphoid tissues; i = immunoglobulins and antibody responsiveness; d = developmental immunity.

thought to have only a single class of immunoglobulin which corresponds to the IgM class of mammals (Marchalonis & Edelman 1965, Clem & Small 1967, Clem 1971). In contrast, adult anuran amphibians as represented by ranid frogs (Coe & Peel 1970, Marchalonis & Edelman 1966, Geczy *et al.* 1973), bufid toads (Acton *et al.* 1969, Diener & Marchalonis 1970, Lin *et al.* 1971), and pipid toads (Marchalonis *et al.* 1970, Lykakis 1969, Hadji-Azimi 1971, Yamaguchi *et al.* 1973) resemble mammals in that they can synthesize at least two antigenically distinct classes of antibodies. Based on sedimentation coefficients, molecular weights, and migration patterns in immunoelectrophoresis, these 19S and 7S molecules have been tentatively classified as IgM and IgG, respectively. Although the class of heavy molecules seems related phylogenetically to the IgM of more primitive and more advanced vertebrates, confirmation of this relationship awaits further physicochemical analyses of anuran antibodies. The low molecular weight immunoglobulins of frogs have been assigned to the IgG class primarily because of similarities between the molecular weights of their heavy chains and those of the mammalian γ-chains (Marchalonis & Edelman 1966, Marchalonis *et al.* 1970, Acton *et al.* 1972). Recently, however, Geczy *et al.* (1973) and Hadji-Azimi (1971) subjected the heavy chains from *Rana catesbeiana* and *Xenopus laevis*, respectively, to polyacrylamide gel electrophoresis in sodium dodecyl sulphate and noted that they migrated to a position between that occupied by the mammalian γ- and μ-chains. Regardless of whether these variations in mobility reflect actual differences in molecular weight or are a function of factors other than the size of the polypeptide chain (Tung & Knight 1971, Segrest *et al.* 1971), they do suggest that there are some significant structural differences between these phylogenetically disparate subunits (see Chapter 11).

Hadji-Azimi (1973) reported that unlike mammals, the 7S immunoglobulin represents only a minor component of the serums from unimmunized *Xenopus*. Immunization results in a continued increase in 19S immunoglobulin followed only much later by an increase in the lighter molecules. Marchalonis (1971) found only an IgM response to *Salmonella* flagella in *Bufo marinus*, even though antibody activity to this antigen appears in two immunoglobulin classes in mammals. These all too limited observations imply that IgM may be more important than IgG for the survival of an anuran. They also highlight our ignorance of the survival value of having at least two immunoglobulin classes. There are isolated reports indicating (1) that the heavy immunoglobulin of the bullfrog seems more efficient as a haemagglutin than as a precipitating antibody (Coe & Peel 1970) and (2) that immunization of *Xenopus* with the protozoan, *Tetrahymena*, elicits precipitating antibody activity in the 'IgG' class and agglutinating, immobilizing, and lytic activity in both classes (Lykakis & Cox 1968). In other words, we still have much to learn about the relative efficacy of each immunoglobulin class in the frog in such biologically significant functions as antibody-mediated cytotoxicity and enhancement, antigen binding, opsonization, complement-mediated lysis, agglutination, etc. that might relate to the very survival of a species.

The often published generalization that Amphibia have two classes of immunoglobulins has been based on knowledge of immunoglobulins of the Anura and on ignorance of the molecular profiles of immunoglobulins from representatives of the three other amphibian orders. We now know that unlike anurans, only a single class of antibodies can be identified in serum from normal and immune salamanders such as newts (Ambrosius *et al.* 1970), axolotls (Ching & Wedgwood 1967, Houdayer & Fougereau 1972), and mudpuppies (Marchalonis & Cohen 1972). In this regard, it is noteworthy that IgM heavy chains from the mudpuppy, *Necturus*, show a greater antigenic similarity to the μ-chains of the more primitive anuran, *Xenopus*, than they do to the μ-chains from an advanced bufid (Marchalonis & Cohen 1972). These comparative data sharply delimit the phylogenetic history of distinct immunoglobulins to some point(s) in the divergence and/or evolution of amphibian lines. They also imply that γ-like heavy chains of advanced amphibians may be a visible result of gene duplication independent of that which was responsible for the emergence of γ-heavy chains of mammals. However, before we should really accept that urodeles lack the genetic information for the synthesis of heavy chains other than those of the μ type, we should analyse serums and secretions from the most advanced urodeles (i.e. the plethodontids). Indeed, comparative analyses of serum immunoglobulins from representatives of the two totally ignored amphibian orders (Trachystomata and Gymnophiona) might offer us a more complete picture of immunoglobulin evolution.

A major histocompatibility complex?

The ability of anurans and urodeles to reject transplants of histoincompatible tissues has been known for many years but it is only recently that immunologists have begun to study and appreciate the immunologic and immunogenetic bases of these reactions. At this time, it appears that the rapidity with which any amphibian rejects a skin allograft is predictably related to its taxonomic position (Cohen & Borysenko 1970) and to the presence or absence of a major histocompatibility complex (Bach *et al.* 1972). Many comparative studies by several investigators reveal that urodele and apodan amphibians routinely reject skin allografts chronically. At least some primitive anurans reject comparable transplants more rapidly in a subacute fashion while advanced frogs mount the most vigorous and rapid rejection responses comparable to those manifested by outbred birds and mammals (reviews, Cohen 1971, Hildemann 1972).

As in birds and mammals, the rapidity of graft rejection in the Amphibia appears to be related to: (1) the number and immunogenic properties or 'strengths' of the transplantation alloantigens possessed by the donor but not by the recipient and (2) by the genetically-controlled immune response capacity of a recipient towards a given panel of alloantigenic disparities (Cohen & Hildemann 1968, Cohen 1973). A compelling body of published and unpublished data derived from survival times of first-set, second-set, and third-party test grafts exchanged within and between newts from various natural populations is consistent with the hypothesis that urodele amphibians lack a major histocompatibility locus comparable to the *H-2* of mice or the *HL-A* of man. Thus, chronic rejection in urodeles (Cohen 1968) appears to be the outcome of only weak histoincompatibility interactions (Graff & Bailey 1973). My unpublished observations also suggest that at least for the newt, increased chronicity of the rejection reaction is referable to an increase in the extent to which that particular donor and host share effective histocompatibility alloantigens.

In striking contrast to the chronicity of the rejection characteristic of urodeles, acute rejection of all skin allografts during the first few weeks post-transplantation is the typical outcome of experimentation with immunocompetent larvae and adults from many different ranid species (Hildemann & Haas 1959, 1961, Baculi & Cooper 1970, Bovbjerg 1966, Volpe 1964, Macela & Romanovsky 1969). Consistent with what appears to be strong histoincompatibilities between advanced frogs of the same species (but quite different from what is routinely observed with salamanders), are several observations that frogs reject a variety of organ transplants as rapidly as they do skin (Cohen 1971).

As I have already intimated, the rates of graft rejection are of major phylogenetic interest in that they may well reflect a species' histocompatibility antigens and/or immune response capacities. Thus, the different rejection rates of advanced anurans and primitive urodeles may reflect the gradual acquisition during amphibian evolution of new and qualitatively different alloantigenic specificities and/or the association of several weaker specificities in such a way that their cumulative interaction implements corporate strong immunogenicity (i.e. acute rejection). There is some suggestive evidence that such changes may have occurred during anuran evolution itself as well as (or instead of) at the point where ancestors of the urodeles and anurans diverged. In other words, the acquisition of a major histocompatibility complex of anurans may have been relatively recent. These speculations are based on the fact that transplantation studies with several primitive discoglossids including *Alytes* (Delsol & Flatin 1967, 1969), *Bombina* (Cohen & Richards, unpublished observations), and *Discoglossus* (Dupuy 1964) reveal subacute rather than acute rejection patterns. Although *Xenopus* is a well-studied representative of the primitive Pipidae, different conflicting publications specify a rather wide range of skin allograft survival times (Cohen 1971, Horton 1970). Interpretation of such data is difficult because the genetic backgrounds of the experimental *Xenopus* used are not always defined and because some investigators selected their recipients when they were in the perimetamorphic period, a time which has been recently postulated to be associated with the generation of self tolerance (Chardonnens & Du Pasquier 1973). Thus, many phylogenetic insights may still be forthcoming from relatively 'old-fashioned' skin grafting studies in phylogenetically disparate species.

When lymphocytes from two individuals of an outbred mammalian species are mixed *in vitro*, a two-way reaction occurs which has been thought by many to be an *in vitro* correlate of the recognition and effector events of the *in vivo* allograft reaction (Häyry *et al.* 1971, Cohen & Howe 1973). Recently, however, Ling (1973) hypothesized that mixed lymphocyte culture (MLC) reactivities are indicative of a surveillance system directed against abnormal lymphocytes that may be independent of allograft immunity. Regardless of their biological significance, we now appreciate that at least in man and mouse, MLC reactivity appears to be under the genetic control of a locus (MLR) which is separate from but closely linked to those *H-2* genes of mice or to the *HL-A* genes of man which code for serologically definable H-alloantigens. Although MLC reactivity of mammalian cells is either undetectable or comparatively weak when the donors of allogeneic lymphocytes are histoincompatible only at that species' minor H-loci (Colley & De Witt 1969, Mangi & Mardiney 1971), additional MLR loci associated with non-*H-2* loci are also probable (Festenstein 1973). Consistent with this close chromosomal association between *H-2* and MLR, and in accord with the hypothesis that chronically rejecting urodeles lack a major H-locus as it was defined five years ago, while advanced anurans do not, is the reasonable hypothesis that MLC reactivity should be negative for sharks (Borysenko & Hildemann 1970) and for salamanders (Cohen 1968) which reject chronically, and positive for lymphocytes harvested from teleosts (Hildemann 1970, 1972) and anurans which reject grafts acutely (Hildemann & Haas 1961). Thus far, substantial albeit preliminary data have supported this hypothesis. Allogeneic mixes of spleen cells from the anurans, *Xenopus laevis* (Weiss & Du Pasquier 1973, Du Pasquier & Miggiano 1973), *Bufo marinus* (Goldshein & Cohen 1972), and *Rana pipiens* (Collins, Goldstine & Cohen, unpublished data) do give highly significant stimulation indexes. At least in *Xenopus*, MLC reactivity appears to be under the control of a single genetic region (Du Pasquier & Miggiano 1973). Parenthetically, lymphocytes from *Rana* and *Bufo* respond quite well to the mitogens, Con A, PHA, and LPS, when the culture conditions are appropriate (Goldstine *et al.* 1976). Although some recent publications (Sigel *et al.* 1973, Lopez *et al.* 1974) indicate that lymphocyte–lymphocyte interactions do not lead to a detectable proliferative response in the snapper (a teleost), the studies of Etlinger (1975) show excellent reactivity of trout lymphocytes in MLC as well as in response to several mitogens. MLC positive reactions have *not* been detected for sharks (Lopez *et al.* 1974, Sigel *et al.* 1973). In view of the fact that my original hypothesis can only be substantiated by negative data, it is comforting to note that MLC negative or minimal reactions of urodeles have been reported for four species by at least two groups (Collins *et al.* 1976; DeLanney *et al.* 1976; Du Pasquier, private communication) who have used culture conditions which support excellent proliferative responses of anuran lymphocytes. Nevertheless, since lymphocytes from salamanders do not respond as well to Con A and PHA as *Rana* cells (Collins *et al.* 1976), we must consider possible explanations of MLC negativity in salamanders other than the lack of an MLR locus or lack of the proper culture conditions. These include cell to cell inhibition, antigenic similarities of MLR products, lack of or limited numbers of cells carrying appropriate receptors and limited distribution of appropriate receptors on lymphoid cells. At this time, however, I feel that chronic rejection plus the lack of an obvious MLC reaction do support the hypothesis that urodele amphibians lack a major histocompatibility complex. The emergence of a major histocompatibility complex homologous with that of mammals during phylogeny (Cohen & Borysenko 1970) may bear directly on oncogenesis, antibody responsiveness and indeed, on the very survival of a species. For discussions of the possible adaptive significance of such genetic polymorphism I refer the reader to the provocative essays of Snell (1968), Lengerova (1969) and Haughton (1969).

Diversity of lymphoid organs

Amphibia represent a living bridgepoint in the evolution of the lymphoid complex. On the one hand, the simple lymphoid system of the urodele is fundamentally equivalent to that first seen in modern Chondrichthyes (Cohen 1976). Salamanders are characterized by their organized thymuses and spleens (Cowden & Dyer 1971, Hightower & St Pierre 1971). In addition, some of the species examined have limited foci of lymphocytes in the intertubular tissue (Cowden & Dyer 1971), buccal areas (Kingsbury 1912, Klug 1967), and perhaps perihepatic tissues (Ruben *et al.* 1973). On the other hand, the lymphoid complex of anurans is more similar to that of endotherms than it is to that of the urodeles or the primitive fishes. The primitive pipid, *Xenopus*, possesses not only a thymus, spleen, and scattered foci of lymphocytes (Turner & Manning 1973) but a lymphopoietic bone marrow and gut-associated lymphoid tissues or GALT (Goldstine *et al.* 1975). Its lymphoid system, however, is still less complex than that of advanced ranid and bufid anurans. These animals have multiple lymph node-like structures in their necks and axillae (Baculi *et al.* 1970, Horton 1971, Kent *et al.* 1964, Diener & Nossal 1966) which filter blood and lymph and contain antigen trapping (Diener & Nossal 1966), and antibody-forming cells (Diener & Marchalonis 1970). Their well-organized GALT (Figs. 8.2, 8.3) is even more extensive than

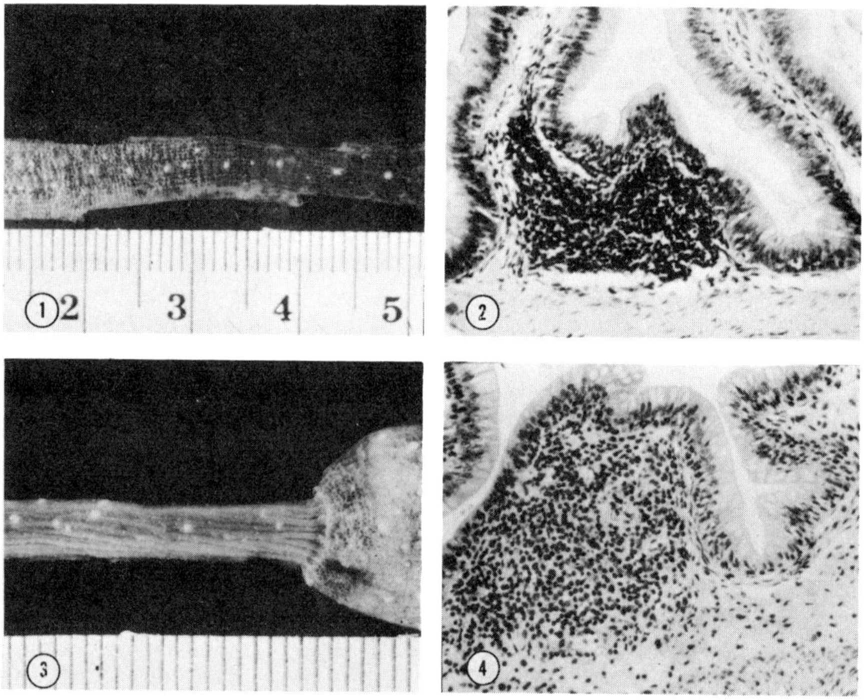

Fig. 8.2. GALT of *Xenopus laevis* (1 and 2): and *Rana pipiens* (3 and 4). (1) After acetic acid treatment (Cornes 1965, Goldstine *et al.* 1975), a characteristic single row of nodules can be seen in the ileum of *X. laevis*. (2) These nodules are collections of small and large lymphocytes (×195). (3) Acetic acid treatment of the small and large intestine of *R. pipiens* reveals that both regions are rich in lymphoid nodules. (4) The overlying epithelium of a nodule in the large intestine is infiltrated with lymphocytes. Scale divisions are millimetres.

that of *Xenopus* (Goldstine *et al.* 1975). These advanced anurans also have lymphoid nodules in the proximal cloaca near its junction with the large intestine (Fig. 8.3). Nodules are also found in orifices of the Wolffian ducts, oviducts, and bladder; in the medial neck of the bladder; along the attachment of the bladder to the large intestine; and around the opening of the bladder duct that leads to the bladder itself (Fig. 8.3, Goldstine *et al.* 1975). Direct macroscopic visualization of these gut- and urogenital-associated lymphoid structures is relatively recent and has been dependent on our technical modifications of the Corne's technique (1965) of acetic acid fixation.

Although the afore-mentioned studies were performed only with a few favourite species, and in spite of our limited knowledge concerning all the detailed functions of the amphibian lymphoid complex, we can still speculate as to the implications of such radical differences between the lymphoid

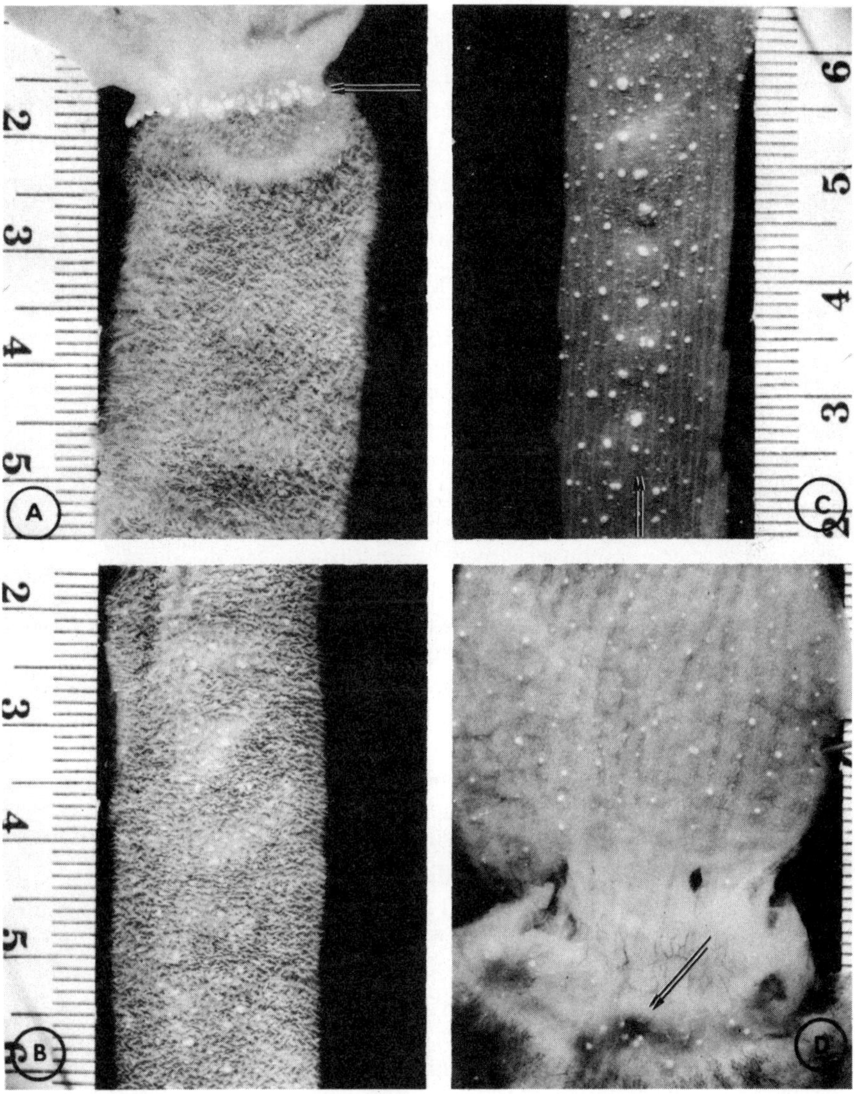

Fig. 8.3. GALT of one *Bufo marinus* (acetic acid-treated tissue). (A) A ring of papillary nodules is present at the junction of the stomach and duodenum (arrow). The adjacent duodenum lacks significant numbers of nodules. (B) In the middle duodenum, a diffuse pattern of small nodules is evident. (C) The ileum shows a longitudinal row of large nodules (arrow) with many smaller nodules located laterally. (D) In the cloacal region (lower portion of this picture) nodules are located proximal to the pigmented cloacal opening. Note that some of these structures appear as papillary projections in the orifice of the bladder duct (arrow). The large intestine above the cloaca has a diffuse pattern of nodules. Scale divisions are millimetres.

systems of anuran and urodele amphibians. Such speculations are facilitated by an awareness of certain of their functional similarities. For example, regardless of their taxonomic location, the thymus of amphibians seems to play a major role in the maturation of immunocompetence (Cooper 1973, Cohen 1975, 1976, Du Pasquier 1973). Thymectomy performed during early larval life impairs alloimmune responsiveness to transplantation alloantigens, xenogeneic erythrocytes, and serum proteins. Recently, thymectomized *Xenopus* have been shown to be impaired in their abilities to localize antigen in their spleens (Horton & Manning 1974). Studies delineating the roles of the thymus and of thymus-derived cells in helper activity, mitotic responses to histocompatibility (MLR) alloantigens, production of lymphokines, and responses to diverse mitogens have either been published (Ruben *et al.* 1973, Chapter 6; Du Pasquier & Horton 1976; Goldstine *et al.* 1976) or are in progress in my laboratory as well as in those of my colleagues. In contrast to this backdrop of what appears to be (at least in mammalian terms) a well-developed T-cell system are two additional intriguing observations. First, thymectomy performed at a developmental stage when it impairs a gamut of *in vivo* immune responses fails to dramatically alter the development of the lymphoid complex of *Xenopus* (Manning 1971), and fails to cause runting disease of early onset (Cantrell & Jutila 1970) in *Xenopus* or other anurans and urodeles (Du Pasquier 1973). Secondly, anuran and urodele larvae exist as free-swimming animals in an antigenically hostile environment long before investigators can detect the onset of immunocompetence by classic laboratory procedures (Du Pasquier 1973). These two observations suggest several mutually inclusive theoretical explanations. First, there may well be an elaborate reticuloendothelial system (RES) that enables the amphibian to survive in nature without total dependence on the T-cell immune system characteristic of endotherms. With the exception of Turner's description of the ontogeny of the RES (1969) and his report that RES blockage actually enhances antibody formation to sheep erythrocytes (1970), we lack a true appreciation of the possible role of the RES in the survival and evolution of amphibians. Perhaps the amphibian RES is a critical link between prime defence systems of invertebrates and higher vertebrates. Second, there may well be a variety of organisms that are normally pathogenic for amphibians (Clothier & Balls 1973, Gloriosa *et al.* 1972) which, antigenically speaking, are thymus-independent. Although the recent studies of Turpen *et al.* (1973, 1975) indicate that those lymphocytes in the peripheral lymphoid tissues which synthesize and secrete antibodies or proliferate in response to lipopolysaccharide—a B-cell mitogen in mammals—are all derived from the thymus during ontogeny, we know nothing about the phylogenetic precursors of the avian bursa of Fabricius. *In vivo* and *in vitro* functional studies with GALT and with the other nodular tissues of the cloaca and bladder could shed some light on the B-cell system of amphibians. The fact that anurans possess GALT and urogenital-associated lymphoid tissues while urodeles do not, raises fundamental questions about the adaptive survival values of these structures. For example, do these tissues play any role in coping with ingested, stored, and excreted materials that are potentially antigenic and pathogenic? In mammals, secretory IgA is involved in such localized immunity and GALT is involved in its production (Craig & Cebra 1971). The fact that we find GALT in the Anura raises significant questions regarding the phylogenetic and ontogenetic origins of secretory IgA (Wang & Fudenberg 1974), its function in immunity, and the types of tissues and cells involved in its production.

Conclusion

Two themes have been developed in each section of this chapter. The first is that there are differences in immunity relative to the taxonomic position of the amphibian studied. I have concentrated only on major differences. Although others such as the lack of significant numbers of plasma cells in salamanders but not in frogs (Cowden & Dyer 1971, Charlemagne, personal communication) or the apparently slower kinetics of antibody formation in salamanders (Ching & Wedgwood 1967), offer some insight into the evolution of the differentiation pathways of antibody forming cells, they are as yet too unsubstantiated to discuss at length. So, too, are apparent differences in the incidence of spontaneous or inducible tumours (Mizell 1968). The second theme is made obvious by the number of times I have taken the liberty of speculation. It is simply that the more we learn about immunity of diverse amphibians, the more we need to know. Fundamental to both themes are the critical questions dealing with how animals with such diverse immune responsiveness continue to survive, flourish, and evolve in an apparent equilibrium with their environment. The continuing search for these answers leaves no doubt that frogs and salamanders will hold their own in research laboratories (as well as in the pockets of small children).

Acknowledgments

I would like to express my appreciation to my collaborators Nancy Collins, Steven Goldstine, Barbara Hrapchak, V. Manickavel, Elsje Schotman, and Delma Thomas for their significant technical and intellectual contributions to much of the unpublished and recently published research cited from my laboratory. This research was supported by research grants AI-08784-05 and HD-07901-06, and a training grant 2T-01-DE00003-16 from the USPHS, by an institutional grant IN-18 from the ACS and by a USPHS Research Career Development Award 1 K04 AI-70736 from the NIAID.

References

ACTON R.I., EVANS E.E., WEINHEIMER P.F., NIEDERMEIER W. & BENNET J.C. (1970) Purification and characterization of two classes of immunoglobulins from the marine toad, *Bufo marinus. Biochemistry* **11,** 2751.

AMBROSIUS H., HEMMERLING J., RICHTER R. & SCHIMKE R. (1970) Immunoglobulins and the dynamics of antibody formation in poikilothermic vertebrates (Pisces, Urodela, Reptilia), pp. 727–44. In *Developmental Aspects of Antibody Formation and Structure*, eds. Sterzl J. & Riha I., vol. 2. Academic Press, New York.

BACH F.H., BACH M.L., SONDEL P.M. & SUNDHARADAS G. (1972) Genetic control of mixed leukocyte culture reactivity. *Transplant Rev.* **12,** 30.

BACULI B.S. & COOPER E.L. (1970) Histopathology of skin allograft rejection in larval *Rana catesbeiana. J. Exptl Zool.* **173,** 329.

BACULI B.S., COOPER E.L. & BROWN B.A. (1970) Lymphomyeloid organs of amphibians. V. Comparative histology in diverse anuran species. *J. Morph.* **131,** 315.

BALLS M. & RUBEN L.N. (1968) Lymphoid tumors in Amphibia: A review. *Prog. Exp. Tumor Res.* **10,** 238.

BORYSENKO M. & HILDEMANN W.H. (1970) Reactions to skin allografts in the horn shark, *Heterodontis francisci. Transplantation* **10,** 545.

BOVBJERG A.M. (1966) Rejection of skin homografts in larvae of *Rana pipiens. J. Exptl Zool.* **161,** 69.

CANTRELL J.C. & JUTILA J.W. (1970) Bacteriologic studies on wasting disease induced by neonatal thymectomy. *J. Immunol.* **104,** 79.

CHARDONNENS X. & DU PASQUIER L. (1973) Induction of skin allograft tolerance during metamorphosis of the toad *Xenopus laevis*: A possible model for studying generation of self tolerance to histocompatibility antigens. *Eur. J. Immunol.* **3,** 569.

CHING Y. & WEDGWOOD R.J. (1967) Immunologic responses in the axolotl, *Siredon mexicanum. J. Immunol.* **99,** 191.

CLEM L.W. (1971) Phylogeny of immunoglobulin structure and function. IV. Immunoglobulins of the giant grouper, *Epinephelus itaira. J. Biol. Chem.* **246,** 9.

CLEM L.W. & LESLIE G.A. (1969) Phylogeny of immunoglobulin structure and function, pp. 62–88. In *Immunity and Development*, ed. Adinolfi M. Spastics International Medical Publications, London.

CLEM L.W. & SMALL P.A. (1967) Phylogeny of immunoglobulin structure and function. I. Immunoglobulins of the lemon shark. *J. Exp. Med.* **125,** 893.

CLOTHIER R.H. & BALLS M. (1973) Mycobacteria and lymphoreticular tumours in *Xenopus laevis*, the South African clawed toad. I. Isolation, characterization and pathogenicity for *Xenopus. Oncology* **28,** 445.

COE J.E. & PEEL L.F. (1970) Antibody production in the bullfrog (*Rana catesbeiana*). *Immunology* **19,** 539.

COHEN L. & HOWE M.L. (1973) Synergism between subpopulations of thymus-derived cells mediating the proliferative and effector phases of the mixed lymphocyte reaction. *Proc. Nat. Acad. Sci. (USA)* **70,** 2707.

COHEN N. (1968) Chronic skin graft rejection in the Urodela. I. A comparative study of first- and second-set allograft reactions. *J. Exptl Zool.* **167,** 37.

COHEN N. (1971) Amphibian transplantation reactions: A review. *Amer. Zool.* **11,** 193.

COHEN N. (1973) Predictable variability in the response of two newt subspecies (*D.v. viridescens* and *D.v. dorsalis*) to first-set allografts. *Folia Biol.* **19,** 169.

COHEN N. (1975) Phylogeny of lymphocyte structure and function. *Amer. Zool.* **15,** 119.

COHEN N. (1976) Phylogenetic emergence of lymphoid tissues and cells. In *The Lymphocyte: Structure and Function*, ed. Marchalonis J.J. Marcel Dekker, New York (in press).

Cohen N. & Borysenko M. (1970) Acute and chronic rejection: Possible phylogeny of transplantation antigens. *Transplant. Proc.* **2,** 333.

Cohen N. & Hildemann W.H. (1968) Population studies of allograft rejection in the newt, *Diemictylus viridescens. Transplantation* **6,** 208.

Colley D.G. & De Witt C.W. (1969) Mixed lymphocyte blastogenesis in response to multiple histocompatibility antigens. *J. Immunol.* **102,** 107.

Collins N.H., Manickavel V. & Cohen N. (1975) *In vitro* responses of urodele Lymphoid cells: Mitogenic and mixed lymphocyte reactivities. *Adv. Exp. Med. Biol.* **64,** 305.

Cooper E.L. (1973) The thymus and lymphomyeloid systems in poikilothermic vertebrates, pp. 13–38. In *Contemporary Topics in Immunology*, eds Davies A.J.S. & Carter R.L. vol. 2. Plenum Press, New York.

Cornes J.S. (1965) Number, size and distribution of Peyer's patches in the human small intestine. I. The development of Peyer's patches. *Gut* **6,** 225.

Cowden R.R. & Dyer R.F. (1971) Lymphopoietic tissue and plasma cells in amphibians. *Amer. Zool.* **11,** 183.

Craig S.W. & Cebra J.J. (1971) Peyer's patches: An enriched source of precursors for IgA-producing immunocytes in the rabbit. *J. Exptl Med.* **134,** 188.

DeLanney L.E., Collins N.H., Cohen N. & Reid R. (1975) Transplantation immunogenetics and MLC reactivities of partially inbred strains of salamanders (*A. mexicanum*): Preliminary studies. *Adv. Exp. Med. Biol.* **64,** 315.

Delsol M. & Flatin J. (1967) Premières observations d'ensemble sur les homogreffes réalisée chez le têtard *l'Alytes obstetricans* Laur. *Compte Rend. Assoc. Anat.* **138,** 398.

Delsol M. & Flatin J. (1969) Métamorphose experimentale de la peau de queue du têtard *d'Alytes obstetricans* Laur. normalement destinée à dégenérer. *Experientia* **25,** 392.

Diener E. & Marchalonis J.J. (1970) Cellular and humoral aspects of the primary response of the toad, *Bufo marinus. Immunology* **18,** 279.

Diener E. & Nossal G.J.V. (1966) Localization of antigens and immune responses in the toad *Bufo marinus. Immunology* **10,** 535.

Du Pasquier L. (1973) Ontogeny of the immune response in cold-blooded vertebrates. *Curr. Topics Microbiol. Immunol.* **61,** 37.

Du Pasquier L. & Miggiano V. (1973) The mixed leukocyte reaction in the toad *Xenopus laevis*: A family study. *Transplant. Proc.* **5,** 1457.

Du Pasquier L., Chardonnens X. & Miggiano V.C. (1975) A major histocompatibility complex in the toad, *Xenopus laevis. Immunogenetics* **1,** 482.

Dupuy G. (1964) Les autogreffes, les homogreffes et les hétérogreffes de peau chez les têtards de *Discoglossus pictus* et *Alytes obstetricans.* Thèse Doctorat en Biologie animale, Bordeaux, France.

Etlinger H.M. (1975) Function and structure of rainbow trout leucocytes. *Doctoral dissertation*, University of Washington, Seattle, Washington.

Festenstein H. (1973) Immunogenetic and biological aspects of *in vitro* lymphocyte allotransformation (MLR) in the mouse. *Transplant. Rev.* **15,** 62.

Geczy C.L., Green P.C. & Steiner L.A. (1973) Immunoglobulins in the developing amphibian, *Rana catesbeiana. J. Immunol.* **111,** 1261.

Glorioso J.C., Amborski R.L., Larkin J.M., Amborski G.F. & Culley D.C. (1974) Laboratory identification of bacterial pathogens of aquatic animals. *Am. J. Vet. Res.* **35,** 447.

Goin C.J. & Goin O.B. (1970) *Introduction to Herpetology*, 2nd ed. W. H. Freeman & Co. San Francisco, 353 pp.

Goldshein S.J. & Cohen N. (1972) Phylogeny of immunocompetent cells. I. *In vitro* blastogenesis and mitosis of toad (*Bufo marinus*) splenic lymphocytes in response to phytohemagglutinin and in mixed lymphocyte cultures. *J. Immunol.* **108,** 1025.

GOLDSTINE S.N., COLLINS N.H. & COHEN N. (1975) Mitogens as probes of lymphocyte heterogeneity in anuran amphibians. *Adv. Exp. Med. Biol.* **64,** 343.

GOLDSTINE S.N., MANICKAVEL V. & COHEN N. (1974) Phylogeny of gut-associated lymphoid tissue. *Amer. Zool.* **15,** 107.

GRAFF R.J. & BAILEY D.W. (1973) The non-*H*-2 histocompatibility loci and their antigens. *Transplant. Rev.* **15,** 26.

HADJI-AZIMI I. (1971) Serum immunoglobulin content in normal and lymphoid tumor-bearing *Xenopus laevis. Cancer Res.* **33,** 1177.

HADJI-AZIMI I. (1971) Studies on *Xenopus laevis* immunoglobulins. *Immunology* **21,** 463.

HAUGHTON G. (1969) Isoantigenic complexity: A speculative essay. *Folia Biol.* (*Praha*) **15,** 239.

HAYRY P., VIROLAINEN M. & DEFENDI V. (1971) Allograft immunity *in vitro*. IV. Proliferative responses and effector mechanisms in mixed cultures of mouse blood lymphocytes. *Transplant. Proc.* **3,** 876.

HIGHTOWER J.A. & ST PIERRE R.L. (1971) Hemopoietic tissue in the adult newt, *Notopthalmus viridescens. J. Morphol.* **135,** 299.

HILDEMANN W.H. (1970) Transplantation immunity in fishes: Agnatha, Chondrichthyes, and Osteichthyes. *Transplant. Proc.* **2,** 253.

HILDEMANN W.H. (1972) Phylogeny of transplantation reactions, pp. 3–73. In *Markers of Biologic Individuality: The Transplantation Antigens*, ed. Reisfeld R.A. Academic Press, New York.

HILDEMANN W.H. & HAAS R. (1959) Homotransplantation immunity and tolerance in the bullfrog. *J. Immunol.* **83,** 478.

HILDEMANN W.H. & HAAS R. (1961) Histocompatibility genetics of bullfrog populations. *Evolution* **15,** 267.

HORTON J.D. (1970) Phylogenetic status of immune systems in *Xenopus. Transplant. Proc.* **2,** 282.

HORTON J.D. (1971) Ontogenesis of the immune system in amphibians. *Amer. Zool.* **11,** 219.

HORTON J.D. & MANNING M.J. (1974) Effect of early thymectomy on the cellular changes occurring in the spleen of the clawed toad following administration of soluble antigen. *Immunology* **26,** 797.

HOUDAYER M. & FOUGEREAU M. (1972) Phylogénie des immunoglobulines: La réaction immunitaire de l'axolotl *Ambystoma mexicanum* cinétique de la réponse immunitaire et caractérisation des anticorps. *Ann. L'Inst Pasteur* **123,** 3.

KENT S.P., EVANS E.E. & ATTLEBERGER M.H. (1964) Comparative immunology: Lymph nodes in the amphibian, *Bufo marinus. Proc. Soc. Exp. Biol. Med.* **116,** 456.

KINGSBURY B.F. (1912) Amphibian tonsils. *Anat. Anz.* **42,** 593.

KLUG H.H. (1967) Submikroskopische Zytologie des Thymus von *Ambystoma mexicanum. Z. Zellforsch* **78,** 388.

KUBO R.T., ZIMMERMAN B. & GREY H.M. (1973) Phylogeny of immunoglobulin, pp. 417–77. In *The Antigens. I*, ed. Sela M. Academic Press, New York.

LENGEROVA A. (1969) Some comments on Haughton's speculative essay on isoantigenic complexity. *Folia Biol.* (*Praha*) **15,** 245.

LIN H.H., CAYWOOD B.E. & ROWLANDS D.T. JR (1971) Primary and secondary immune responses of the marine toad (*Bufo marinus*) to bacteriophage f_2. *Immunology* **20,** 373.

LING N.R. (1973) Immune surveillance of lymphoid tissue. A biological role for the mixed lymphocyte reaction. *Immunol. Commun.* **2,** 119.

LOPEZ D.M., SIGEL M.M. & LEE J.C. (1974) Phylogenetic studies of T-cells. I. Lymphocytes of the shark with differential responses of phytohemagglutinin and Concanavalin A. *Cell. Immunol.* **10,** 287.

LYKAKIS J.J. (1969) The production of two molecular classes of antibody in the toad,

Xenopus laevis homologous with mammalian γM (19S) and γG (7S) immunoglobulins. *Immunology* **16,** 91.

Lykakis J.J. & Cox F.E.G. (1968) Immunological responses of the toad, *Xenopus laevis*, to the antigens of the ciliate, *Tetrahymena pyriformis. Immunol.* **15,** 429.

Macela A. & Romanovsky A. (1969) The role of temperature in separate stages of the immune reactions in anurans. *Folia Biol.* (*Praha*) **15,** 157.

Mangi R.J. & Mardiney M.R. Jr. (1971) The mixed lymphocyte reaction. Detection of single histocompatibility loci and the correlation to skin graft survival in mice. *Transplantation* **11,** 369.

Manning M.J. (1971) The effect of early thymectomy on histogenesis of the lymphoid organs in *Xenopus laevis. J. Embryol. Exp. Morph.* **26,** 219.

Marchalonis J.J. (1971) Immunoglobulins and antibody production in amphibians. *Amer. Zool.* **11,** 171.

Marchalonis J.J., Allen R.B. & Saarni E.S. (1970). Immunoglobulin classes of the clawed toad, *Xenopus laevis. Comp. Biochem. Physiol.* **35,** 49.

Marchalonis J.J. & Cohen N. (1973) Isolation and partial characterization of immunoglobulin from a urodele amphibian (*Necturus maculosus*). *Immunology* **24,** 395.

Marchalonis J.J. & Cone R.E. (1973) The phylogenetic emergence of vertebrate immunity. *Aust. J. Exp. Biol. Med. Sci.* **51,** 461.

Marchalonis J.J. & Edelman G.M. (1965) Phylogenetic origins of antibody structure. I. Multichain structure of immunoglobulins in the smooth dog fish (*Mustelus canis*). *J. Exp. Med.* **122,** 601.

Marchalonis J. & Edelman G.M. (1966) Phylogenetic origins of antibody structure. II. Immunoglobulins of the primary response of the bullfrog, *Rana catesbeiana. J. Exp. Med.* **124,** 901.

Mizell M. (1969) ed. *Biology of Amphibian Tumors.* Recent Results in Cancer Research. Springer-Verlag, New York.

Ruben L.N., v.d. Hoven A. & Dutton R.W. (1973) Cellular cooperation in hapten-carrier responses in the newt, *Triturus viridescens. Cell. Immunol.* **6,** 300.

Ruben L.N. & Stevens J.M. (1971) Lymphoreticular neoplasia and immunity in Amphibia. *Amer. Zool.* **11,** 229.

Segrest J.P., Jackson R.L., Andrews E.P. & Marchesi V.T. (1971) Human erythrocyte membrane glycoprotein: A re-evaluation of the molecular weight as determined by SDS polyacrylamide gel electrophoresis. *Biochem. Biophys. Res. Commun.* **44,** 390.

Sigel M.M., Ortiz-Muniz G., Lee J.C. & Lopez D.M. (1973) Immunobiological reactivities at the cellular level in the nurse shark. *Proc. Symp. Phylogenetic and Ontogenetic Study of the Immune Response and its Contribution to the Immunological Theory.* INSERM (Paris) 113.

Snell G.D. (1968) The *H-2* locus of the mouse: Observations and speculations concerning its comparative genetics and its polymorphism. *Folia Biol.* (*Praha*) **14,** 335.

Tung J.S. & Knight C.A. (1971) Effect of change on the determination of molecular weight of proteins by gel electrophoresis in SDS. *Biochem. Biophys. Res. Commun.* **42,** 1117.

Turner R.J. (1969) The functional development of the reticuloendothelial system in the toad, *Xenopus laevis* (Dandin). *J. Exptl. Zool.* **170,** 467.

Turner R.J. (1970) The influence of colloidal carbon on hemagglutinin production in the toad, *Xenopus laevis. J. Retic. Soc.* **8,** 434.

Turner R.J. (1973) Response of the toad, *Xenopus laevis*, to circulating antigens. II. Responses after splenectomy. *J. Exp. Zool.* **183,** 35.

Turner R.J. & Manning M.J. (1973) Response of the toad, *Xenopus laevis*, to circulating antigens. I. Cellular changes in the spleen. *J. Exp. Zool* **183,** 21.

TURPEN J.B., VOLPE R.P. & COHEN N. (1973) Ontogeny and peripheralization of thymic lymphocytes. *Science* **182,** 931.

TURPEN J.B., VOLPE E.P. & COHEN N. (1975) On the origin of thymic lymphocytes. *Amer. Zool.* **15,** 51.

VOLPE E.P. (1964) Fate of neural crest homotransplants in pattern mutants of the leopard frog. *J. Exp. Zool.* **157,** 179.

WANG A. & FUDENBERG H.H. (1974) IgA and evolution of immunoglobulins. *J. Immunogen.* **1,** 3.

WEISS N. & DU PASQUIER L. (1973) Factors affecting the reactivity of amphibian lymphocytes in a miniaturized technique of the mixed lymphocyte culture. *J. Immunol. Meth.* **3,** 273.

YAMAGUCHI N., KURASHIGE S. & MITSUHASHI S. (1973) Immune response in *Xenopus laevis* and immunochemical properties of the serum antibodies. *Immunology* **24,** 109.

Chapter 9. Regulatory Effects of Temperature upon Immunity in Ectothermic Vertebrates

R. R. Avtalion, E. Weiss and T. Moalem

Introduction

Temperature effect on immunity in lower vertebrates

Temperature effect on antibody production in carp immunized against non-microbial antigens

Antibody production to BSA

Temperature effect on antibody production to BSA

Immunization to hapten-carrier conjugates

Temperature effect on antibody production to carrier-hapten conjugates

Discussion

Introduction

The problem of immunity in ectothermic vertebrates and the influence of environmental temperature, attracted attention of investigators even before the beginning of this century. The early investigators were essentially interested in the immunopathological problems since the influence of seasonal temperatures on the occurrence of fish diseases was evident and had great economic importance. Many representatives of lower vertebrates were tested for their ability to manifest humoral and cell-mediated immunity. These animals, which belonged to a broad range of lower vertebrate species living in various climates, were subjected to various immunization schedules, essentially with microbial antigens and red blood cells, at various temperatures. The results obtained by many investigators were not concordant in many cases. On the basis of our studies on carp injected with bovine serum albumin, we suggested that the natural propagation of some antigens in the immediate environment of poikilothermic animals as well as their climatic adaptation, could have a great influence on their ability to react at low temperature. Natural antibodies to many antigens were found in these animals due, at least partially, to unknown antigenic stimulations. The mechanism by which the temperature affects the antibody production is still unclear. An attempt to explain the regulatory effect of temperature upon immunity in cold-blooded animals was done by Bisset (1946–9). He suggested that the stage of release of antibodies rather than their synthesis is the more affected stage at low temperature. This suggestion was not supported by us, since we could demonstrate that both release and synthesis of antibodies could occur, if the fish were immunized and kept for a short period of time at a high temperature before they were transferred to a low temperature.

In this paper we present a summary of the principal investigation regarding the influence of environmental temperature on the immune response in lower vertebrates. This subject will also be discussed on the basis of our recent findings on the immune response of carp to a hapten-carrier conjugates. This finally leads to a conclusion regarding the nature of the temperature-dependent stages.

Temperature effect on immunity in lower vertebrates

The depressive effect of low environmental temperatures on the immune response was investigated for the first time by Ernst (1890). He reported that frogs infected by the 'red leg' disease were more resistant at high temperatures. Widal and Sicard (1897) immunized frogs of three species (*Rana esculenta*, *R. usca*, *Hyla viridis*), against typhoid bacterium and kept them in various ambient temperatures that ranged between 12°C and 37°C. They came to the conclusion that more rapid antibody production occurred at the higher temperatures rather than at the lower. After them, Metchnikoff (1901) tested the influence of the environmental temperature on the formation of antibodies against diphtheria toxin in alligators (*Alligator mississipiensis*), turtles (*Emus obicularis*) and frogs (*Rana esculenta*). He found that alligators reacted by forming antitoxin in a surrounding temperature of 32–37°C whereas at 28°C they did not react at all, turtles were not immunized at all at a temperature of 20–37°C and the toxin remained in their blood for many months and frogs showed great sensitivity to the toxin and a high mortality rate. No antitoxin activity was detected in their blood.

From the above-mentioned historical works it could be concluded that low ambient temperatures depress the antibody production in these representatives of lower vertebrates, completely or partially, and that the level of temperature seems to be specific for the species. Similar findings were pointed out by temporary investigators who studied this subject more carefully. Inhibition of the antibody production at low temperatures was evident. It resulted in longer latent periods and low titres of slowly-rising antibodies or in complete inhibition of their synthesis. Lower titres of agglutinins to *Pseudomonas punctata* were obtained in carp kept at 12–12·5°C while those kept at 18–20°C showed higher titres, 1 : 10240 (Pliszka 1939a,b). Similar findings were reported by Snieszko (1953), also in carp immunized against the same bacterium. The latent period was found to be longer (15 days) in goldfish and carp, which were immunized against the sperm of the sea-urchin (*Strongylocentrotus purpuratus*) and then kept at 14°C, than those kept at 28°C (7–11 days) (Cushing 1942). Evans and Cowles (1959) showed that no antibodies or few (1:10) were obtained in the desert iguana (*Dipsosaurus dorsalis*) immunized with a formalin-treated Salmonella typhosa antigen and kept at the ambient temperature of 25°C. When the animals were kept at 25–35°C the titres were highest (1:80 to 1:640) and demonstrable after a comparatively shorter period of immunization. Krantz *et al.* (1963) succeeded in immunizing trout at 11°C, but the first detectable antibodies appear one month after the antigenic stimulus, and the peak was reached after 3 months. Ambrosius and Lehmann (1965) obtained better immune response at 18–20°C than at 11°C in the fish *Ictalurus nebulosus.*

What seems to be a complete inhibition of antibody production at low temperatures was demonstrated by other investigators, who immunized many representatives of lower vertebrates, against microbial antigens, red blood cells and soluble antigens, Nybelin (1935) found that eels (*Anguilla anguilla*) which were immunized against Vibrio and kept at 8–9°C, showed no immunization, as opposed to those fish that were kept at 17–18°C, and which showed titres of agglutinins. Bisset (1946–9) investigated the influence of ambient temperature on resistance to pathogens by fish (goldfish) and antibody production by frogs (*Rana temporaria*). He found that frogs kept at 8°C did not produce any antibodies as long as they were kept at that temperature, whereas when they were moved to 20°C agglutinins appeared in their blood. Barrow (1955) found that fish (perch and goldfish) kept at 5, 10 and 15°C did not eliminate infecting trypanosomes, whereas when they were moved to 20°C they eliminated the trypanosomes and produced lytic and agglutinating antibodies. Maung (1963) showed that tortoises (*Testudo ibera*) immunized with *Brucella abortus* antigen, did not produce antibodies at all when kept at 7–10°C. He also found that this animal responded to immunization more quickly and more effectively at 18–30°C (summer) than at 15–25°C (winter). Although in the above-mentioned works investigators did not succeed in immunizing fish at temperatures of about 10°C, other workers were able to demonstrate the existence or acquired immunity at temperatures lower than 10°C. Smith (1940) immunized carp, rainbow trout (*Salmo gardneri*) and brown trout (*Salmo trutta*) with a heat-killed vaccine of *Bacterium salmonicida* which was injected over a period of several weeks, and obtained specific agglutinins to this bacterium in the fish kept at a water temperature of 10°C. But he also reported that while some of the fish did not respond other fish showed agglutinin titres ranging from 1:20 to 1:640. Smith explained that these animals have been exposed to trout furunculosis throughout most of their several years of life. Since a number of trout that were not vaccinated showed agglutinin titres up to 1:80, he assumed that it is very possible that the antibody has been developed in response to this natural exposure of the trout to infections. Papermaster *et al.* (1962) reported that circulating neutralizing antibodies to T_2-phage were detected in the blood of the bullhead (*Ameiurus melas*), kept at 10°C, at the fourteenth day after the phage injection, and the phage particles were cleared from the blood at the fourth day, at this low temperature. However, they did not succeed in demonstrating immunization in the California hagfish, kept at 10°C, to various antigens. They failed to obtain clearance of phage particles or antibodies to the phage in samples of blood taken 4 and 7 days after injection in this animal even when kept at 20°C.

Ridgway (1962) investigated the immune response of sablefish (*Anaplopoma fimbria*) which grow and spend most of their lives in temperatures below 10°C, in the North Pacific. Haemagglutinins were detected at about the 27th day after the first antigenic stimulation, in fish kept at 5–8°C, and their titres increased over periods of five months during which time they were kept at 6–9°C.

The threshold of the low inhibiting temperature is somewhat higher when non-microbial antigens, soluble proteins or red blood cells, were considered. Fijan and Cvetnic (1964, 1966) reported that most of the carp (18 in 20) which were immunized against total calf serum and kept at 13–15°C did not display antibody responses, and none of them reacted when kept at 10–12°C, when immunized against this soluble antigen or against bacteria (*Brucella bovis*, W99). We reported similar findings on carp and frogs (Avtalion *et al.* 1969a,b,c, 1973) which were immunized against BSA. Ridgway *et al.* (1966) reported that rainbow trout which were immunized with chicken erythrocytes and with heat-killed bacteria (agent of the 'red mouth' disease) and then kept at 15°C, showed better immunity to the bacteria. They found that only one fish in twenty, which were immunized against chicken red blood cells, reacted, had very low saline agglutinin titre of 1:4. (Nine of them had antibodies detectable at 1:4 after addition of anti-rainbow trout globulin.) However, 12 in 20 fish, which were injected with heat-killed bacteria showed agglutinin titres of 1:4–1:8. All the 20 had antibodies which were detectable with the anti-rainbow trout globulin. The question which arises here is why fish immunized against bacterial antigens react better at low temperature than those injected with other antigens.

The greater part of known work treating the subject of temperature effect on antibody production in lower vertebrates was carried out using essentially microbial pathogenic and non-pathogenic antigens or red blood cells. Pre-existing 'natural' antibodies to these antigens were reported to occur in fish by many investigators. Since these antigens are universally propagated, and essentially in the surrounding environment of fish, polluted water and slime, we suggest that in such cases the pre-existing antibodies or at least the stage of priming could arise from unknown antigenic stimulus. Krantz *et al.* (1964)

reported that trout having endemic asymptomatic furunculosis have low titres of antibodies to *Aeromonas salmonicida*. Luklyanenko (1965) found antibodies to *Aeromonas punctata* and to *Pseudomonas fluorescens* in sera of ten species of fishes. Bullock and McDaniel (1968) found antibodies to myxobacteria in salmonid fishes associated with gill disease. Sigel *et al.* (1968) found that sera from normal nurse sharks (*Ginglymostoma cirratum*) displayed a broad natural spectrum of antibody-like activity on many antigens tested (influenza and Rous sarcoma viruses, *E. coli*, human cancer cells (KB) and red blood cells from 10 different animal species). Snieszko (1970) assumed that the presence in fish sera of low titres of antibodies to some of the bacteria pathogenic to fish may be considered as evidence that these fish had or have asymptomatic infections. In our laboratory we tested many sera of normal carp against red blood cells of various Forsman positive and negative species. In all cases we obtained natural titres of haemolysins and haemagglutinins (Avtalion *et al.* 1973a).

Temperature effect on antibody production in carp immunized against non-microbial antigens

Antibody production to BSA

In preliminary work done in our laboratory we found that bovine serum albumin (BSA) is an excellent antigen for carp when injected with or without adjuvants. Furthermore, contrary to what occurred in the case of microbial antigens, we could not detect pre-existing antibodies due to innate immunity to this antigen in many carp tested by passive haemagglutination. Thus we assume that the acquired immune response we obtained in this case began in most cases by a real primary response after the first antigenic stimulation. The length of the latent period was determined to be approximately nine days; maximal titres were obtained between the 25th and 35th days; the decrease of antibodies was calculated as having a half life of 12·5 days. The secondary response obtained in other groups of carp was typical of the known anamnestic response in mammals which is characterized by a shorter latent period (4 days) and higher antibody titres. Better results were obtained when the antigen was introduced in emulsion with Freund's complete adjuvant. No significant variations in titres were obtained with doses ranging from 5 mg to 0·1 mg. Soluble BSA was found more immunogenic than insolubilized BSA when injected intraperitoneally in small doses (0·1 and 1 mg). In high doses (20 and 50 mg), however, the insoluble form gave a relatively high antigenic stimulation while the soluble was found to be partially tolerogenic. These results differ from those reported by Draper and Hirrata (1968) in rabbits. They showed that a much smaller amount of insoluble, than soluble,

BSA was needed in order to induce a primary immune response. When higher doses of both forms of BSA were injected into rabbits higher antibody titres were obtained in animals immunized with the soluble form, than in those injected with the insoluble. This result was confirmed by us in rabbits using the same antigens as for carp (Avtalion *et al.*, unpublished).

Temperature effect on antibody production to BSA

The influence of environmental temperature on antibody production in fish immunized with soluble non-microbial antigen was investigated by Fijan and Cvetnic (1964, 1966), Avtalion (1969a,b,c) and Avtalion *et al.* (1970, 1973b). Fijan and Cvetnic reported that partial inhibition of antibody production occurred in carp which were immunized against total calf serum and were kept at temperatures ranging between 11 and 15°C. They came to the conclusion that the maximum limit for the completely inhibiting temperature is situated between 10 and 12°C. In the first experiments done by us on this subject we immunized groups of carp with 10 mg of BSA in emulsion with Freund's complete adjuvant (FCA) and kept them continuously for periods of several days at high (25°C$\pm$1) or at low (14°C) temperature. The fish kept at high temperature served as control groups, and displayed normal primary and secondary responses as described above. In those kept continuously at the low temperature we could not detect any antibody titres, by passive haemagglutination, as long as they were kept at this temperature. Other fish were kept for 8 days after the antigenic stimulation (BSA in CFA) at high temperature and then transferred to low temperature, before the appearance of the first circulating antibodies. Contrary to what was expected, according to Bisset's hypothesis (Bisset 1946–9), these carp developed rising titres of antibodies at this low inhibiting temperature. The fish kept at low temperature were moved to the high temperature after 15, 35, and 70 days. In those carp moved after both 35 and 70 days, the latent period was shortened by three days. Antibodies began to appear in their blood, between the sixth and seventh days after the transfer to hot water, but at relatively low rates, even after receiving a booster dose. Other groups of carp were immunized with small doses of soluble BSA (0·2–0·5 mg/kg body weight) and kept for various periods of time (40–90 days) at low temperature (12–13°C). On the 63rd day after they were moved to high temperature each fish received a booster dose of 0·1 mg BSA. The fish displayed a specific immune tolerance (Avtalion *et al.* 1973a).

Immunization to carrier-hapten conjugate

Groups of carp, 300–50 g in weight, were each injected intramuscularly with 2 mg of penicilloyl-BSA conjugate (pen-BSA) in emulsion with Complete Freund's Adjuvant (CFA). Six weeks later each fish was pre-immunized with

1 mg of Rabbit Gamma Globulin (RGG) in CFA or injected with an equal quantity of a saline emulsion of CFA. Three weeks later all carp received an injection of 2 mg of pen-RGG. The fish were bled one day before this last injection and eight days later. Anti-penicillin antibodies were detected by passive haemagglutination, using penicillin-coated red blood cells. Results showed that the fish which were pre-immunized with RGG displayed an average of about eight-fold antibodies greater than before the secondary stimulation (stimulation factor-8) (Fig. 9.1,Aa). In contrast the group which received saline developed a stimulation factor of less than 2 (Fig. 9.1, Ab).

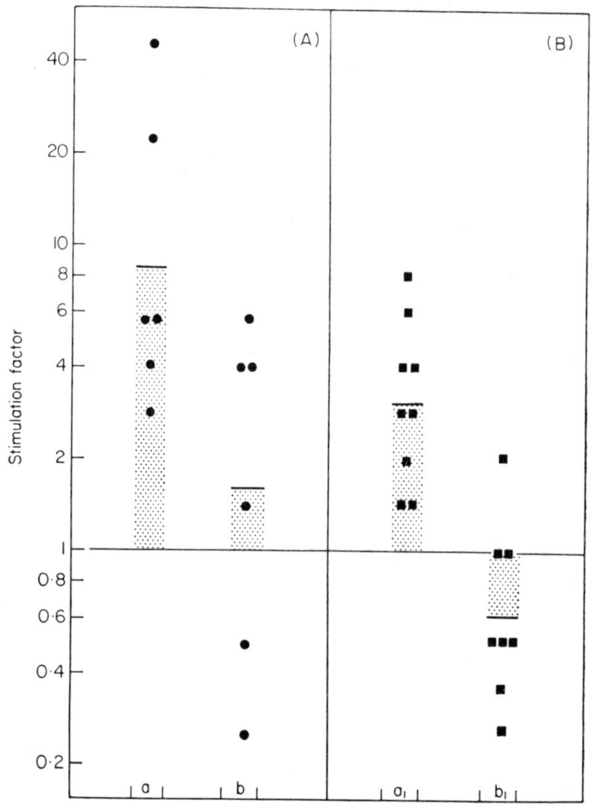

Fig. 9.1. Carrier enhancement in carp and temperature effect. Groups a and a_1 were injected with RGG, following injection of pen-BSA. Groups b and b_1 were injected with saline, following injection of pen-BSA. Groups a_1 and b_1 were transferred to 13°C 3 weeks after RGG or saline. Three days later all groups were injected with pen-RGG. The fish were bled one day before the final injection and 8 days later. Circle, individual stimulation factor (titre after pen-RGG injection/titre before) in groups kept at 25°; square, individual stimulation-factor in groups kept at 13°C; column, geometric mean of individual stimulation-factors.

Temperature effect on antibody production to carrier-hapten conjugates

Groups of carp, kept at 25°C ± 1, were immunized to pen-BSA conjugate as described above. They were moved to a low temperature (13°C ± 1) at various intervals of time (0, 1, 3, 4 days). They were bled every week and their sera were tested for anti-penicillin antibodies by passive haemagglutination. The results obtained were identical to those previously reported by us (Avtalion *et al.* 1973b) in carp immunized with BSA or with bacteria. The anti-penicillin antibodies appeared only in the group that was kept for more than 3 days at high temperature. The other groups did not display antibody titres at low temperature (Table 9.1).

Table 9.1. Antibody titres obtained in carp immunized with pen-BSA and kept at a high temperature (25°C) for 0, 1, 3, and 4 days before they were moved to a low temperature (13°C)

Number of days after transfer to low temperature (13°C)	Number of days in which the fish were kept at high temperature (25°C)								
	0	1	3	4					
14	< 3*	< 3*	< 3*	< 3;†	< 3;	< 3;	< 3;	< 3;	< 3;†
19	< 3	< 3	< 3	< 3;	4;	3;	< 3;	< 3;	< 3;
29	< 3	< 3	< 3	3;	4;	5;	< 3;	< 3;	< 3;
43	< 3	< 3	< 3	7;	6;	8;	< 3;	5;	4;
56	< 3	< 3	3	6;	7;	9;	< 3;	5;	4;

* Mean titre (Log_2) of four or five fish.
† Individual titre (Log_2).

In another experiment two other groups of carp, kept at 25°C, were injected with 2 mg of pen-BSA in emulsion with CFA. Six weeks later one group was pre-immunized with 1 mg of RGG in emulsion with CFA. After three weeks all fish were moved to a low temperature (13°C) and 3 days later they received a booster dose of 2 mg pen-RGG. The fish were bled 1 day before the final injection and 8 days later. The sera were tested for anti-penicillin antibodies by passive haemagglutination. Results showed that all fish which were pre-immunized with RGG, even when kept in the cold, displayed a significant increase in mean antibody titre whereas a decrease in mean titre was obtained in the control group which was injected with saline-CFA emulsion (Fig. 9.1, B).

Discussion

An hypothesis on the regulatory effect of environmental temperature upon immunity in cold-blooded animals was suggested by Bisset (1946–9). He concluded that *the stage of acquisition of the potential for antibody production is distinct and separable from that of production of antibodies and their release into the circulation. This second stage is the more affected by temperature in cold-blooded animals; therefore it is possible for cold-blooded animals to acquire immunity at low temperatures, although it is not manifested until the temperature is raised.* This hypothesis is not concordant with our previously reported findings, since we could demonstrate the occurrence of synthesis and release of antibody in cold temperature in cases where the fish were exposed to the antigen at high temperature.

Lin and Rowlands (1973), working on toads (*Bufo marinus*) immunized against bacteriophage f2, reported that their results were in conflict with those of Bisset. Their animals, which were transferred to a low temperature (15°C) 2 weeks after primary immunization, continued to produce increasing titres of antibodies. This temperature seems to seriously affect the immune response although not completely. Cone and Marchalonis (1972), working on the same animals immunized against horse erythrocytes, came to the conclusion that the immune response to this antigen was separated into two phases by the variation of temperature. A similar conclusion could be reflected from the experiments mentioned above. We obtained rising antibody titres in the cold in fish that were kept for more than 3 days at high temperature. On the other hand, the latent period was shortened by 3 days in fish that were moved to a high temperature after being primed and kept for 35 or 70 days in the cold. Thus we came to the conclusion that the temperature-sensitive event must be situated between the 3rd and 4th days after primary stimulation, and that some early events are not temperature-sensitive; at least phagocytosis and antigen metabolization were not found to be significantly inhibited *in vitro* and *in vivo* (data to be published). The last stages, namely the rising synthesis of antibody and their release into the blood, were also not inhibited. This result was schematized in a sketch (Avtalion *et al.* 1973a) suggesting that priming of immunocompetent cells and cells that are involved in tolerance could occur at low temperatures while the temperature-sensitive event relates to cellular interactions and/or cellular differentiation. There is enough evidence in the recent literature that direct or indirect cellular interactions which regard thymus-derived cells (T), bone marrow-derived cells (B), and macrophages, are involved in the production of antibodies. The carrier-enhancing effect was related to the cooperation between T and B cells. The injection of the carrier alone before a primary, or particularly a secondary stimulation, to the hapten was found to enhance the antibody synthesis to the hapten in mammals (Mitchison 1967, Mitchison *et al*, 1970) and in the newt (*Triturus viridescens*) (Ruben *et al.* 1973). On the basis of the results we reported above (Fig. 9.1, A) it is clear that a secondary carrier-enhancing effect does exist in fish. It follows from this finding that the immune response in fish, and probably in other ectothermic vertebrates, depends (as is the case in mammals) upon interaction between (T) carrier-dependent cells and (B) antibody-forming cells.

In our other experiment (Fig. 9.1, B) we showed that temperature affects the antibody production to the hapten-carrier conjugate. However, the group of fish which were injected with the carrier, before their transfer to low temperature, were able to produce higher titres of anti-hapten antibodies following a secondary stimulation with the hapten-carrier molecule in the cold. In contrast, the fish which received an emulsion of CFA in saline instead of the carrier showed a decrease in their antibody titres. This result implies that the helper-cells which are known as carrier-dependent are involved in the regulatory effect of temperature. Cone and Marchalonis (1972) showed that a population of rosette forming cells (RFC) was developed in toads immunized and kept at low temperature. These RFC were supposed to be of T cells origin. Recent findings in carp immunized with pen-BSA seem to support this point of view (Moalem & Avtalion, in preparation). Thus we suggest that, at low temperature, the primed T cells undergo a certain degree of proliferation but their activation to helper-cells is inhibited. Since it was found that carp immunized with soluble BSA and kept at low temperature become tolerant to BSA (Avtalion *et al.* 1973a), it is possible that in this case, T cells, instead of being activated to helper cells, become suppressor cells.

Acknowledgments

This work was supported by grant number 19(b)E from the Israel Commission for Basic Sciences and by grant number 0–1–210 from Bar-Ilan University, Ramat-Gan, Israel.

We wish to express our gratitude to Professor K. Stern (Bar-Ilan University) for his advice.

References

AMBROSIUS H. & LEHMANN R. (1965) Beiträge zur Immunobiologie poikilothermer Wirbeltiere. III. Der Einflus von Adjuvanten auf die antikorper-Production. *Acta. biol. med. German.* **14,** 830.

AVTALION R.R. (1969a) Influence de la temperature ambiante sur la production des anticorps chez la carp. *Verh. Internat. Verein. Limnol.* **17,** 630.

AVTALION R.R. (1969b) Temperature effect on antibody production and immunological memory in carp (*Cyprinus carpio*) immunized against bovine serum albumin (BSA). *Immunology* **17,** 927.

AVTALION R.R. (1969c) Secondary response and immunological memory in carp (*Cyprinus carpio*) immunized against bovine serum albumin. *Israel J. med. Sci.* **5,** 441.

AVTALION R.R., MALIK Z., LEFLER E. & KATZ E. (1970) Temperature effect on immune resistance of fish to pathogens. *Bamidge, Bull. Fish. Cult. Israel* **22,** 33.

AVTALION R.R., WOJDANI A. & DUCZYMINER M. (1973a) Antibody production in carp (*Cyprinus carpio*) temperature effect and mechanism. Phylogenic and Ontogenic Study of the Immune Response and its Contribution to the Immunological Theory. pp. 75–86, Inserm Editions, Paris.

AVTALION R.R., WOJDANI A., MALIK Z., SHAHRABANI R. & DUCZYMINER M. (1973b) Influence of environmental temperature on the immune response in fish. *Current Topics in Microbiology and Immunology* **61,** 1.

BARROW J.J. JR (1955) Social behavior in fresh-water fish and its effect on resistance to trypanosomes. *Proc. nat. Acad. Sci.* (*Wash.*) **41,** 676.

BISSET K.A. (1946) The effect of temperature on non-specific infections of fish. *J. Path. Bact.*. **58,** 251.

BISSET K.A. (1947a) Bacterial infection and immunity in lower vertebrates and invertebrates. *J. Hyg.* (*Lond.*) **45,** 128.

BISSET K.A. (1947b) The effect of temperature on immunity in amphibia. *J. Path. Bact.* **59,** 301.

BISSET K.A. (1947c) Natural and acquired immunity in frogs and fish. *Path. Bact.* **59,** 679.

BISSET K.A. (1948) The effect of temperature upon antibody production in cold-blooded vertebrates. *J. Path. Bact.* **60,** 87.

BISSET K.A. (1949) The influence of adrenal cortical hormones upon immunity in cold-blooded vertebrates. *J. Endocr.* **6,** 99.

BULLOCK G.L. & MCDANIEL D.W. (1968) Bacterial diseases. *U.S. Fish and Wild. Ser., Prog. in Sport Fish. Res., Resource Publ.* **64,** 18.

CONE R.R. & MARCHALONIS J.J. (1972) Cellular and humoral aspects of the influence of environmental temperature on the immune response of poikilothermic vertebrates. *J. Immunol.* **108,** 952.

CUSHING J.E. (1942) An effect of temperature upon antibody production in fish. *J. Immunol.* **45,** 123.

DRAPER L.R. & HIRATA A.A. (1968) Antibody response in rabbits to soluble and particulate forms of bovine serum-albumin. *Immunol.* **15,** 23.

ERNST P. (1959) *Brit. J. Path.* **8,** 203 (1890) (cited by Bisset 1948).

EVANS E.E. & COWLES R.B. (1959) Effect of temperature on antibody synthesis in the reptile *Dipsosaurus dorsalis. Proc. Soc. exp. Biol.* (*N.Y.*) **101,** 482.

FIJAN N. & CVETNIC S. (1964) Immunitetna reactivost sarana. I. Reativnost jednogodisnjih sarana kod 13–15° C u akvarijskim uslovima. *Vet. Arh.* (*Zagreb*) **1–2,** 17.

FIJAN N. & CVETNIC S. (1966) Immunitetna reativnost sarana. II. Reativnost tokom godine kod drzanja u ribnjacima. *Vet. Arch.* (*Zagreb*) **3–4,** 100.

KRANTZ G.E., REDDECLIFF J.M. & HEIST C.E. (1963) Development of antibodies against *Aeromonas salmonicida* in trout. *J. Immunol.* **91,** 757.

KRANTZ G.E., REDDECLIFF J.M. & HEIST C.E. (1964) Immune response of trout to *Aeromonas salmonicida.* I. Development of agglutinating antibodies and protective immunity. *Prog. Fish. Cult.* **26,** 3.

LIN H.H. & ROWLANDS JR D.T. (1973) Thermal regulation of the immune response in South American Toads (Bufo marinus). *Immunol.* **24,** 129.

LUKLYANENKO V.I. (1965) Natural antibodies in fish. *Zool. Zh.* **44,** 300.

MAUNG R.T. (1963) Immunity in the tortoise *Testudo ibera. J. Path. Bact.* **85,** 51.

METCHNIKOFF E. (1901) *L'immunité dans les maladies infectieuses,* p. 349. Masson & Cie, Paris.

MITCHISON N.A. (1967) Antigen recognition responsible for the induction in vitro of the secondary response. *Cold. Spring. Harbor. Symp. Quant. Biol.* **32,** 431.

MITCHISON N.A., RAJEWSKY K. & TAYLOR R.B. (1970) Cooperation of antigenic determinants and of cells in the induction of antibodies, p. 547. In *Developmental Aspects of*

Antibody Formation and Structure, ed. Sterzl J. & Riha I. Academic Press, New York.

NYBELIN O. (1935) Uber Agglutininbildung bei Fischen. *Z. Immun.-Forsch.* **84,** 74.

PAPERMASTER B.W., CONDIE R.M. & GOOD R.A. (1962) Immune response in the California hagfish. *Nature* (*Lond.*) **196,** 355.

PLISZKA F. (1939a) Untersuchungen über die Agglutinine bei Kappfen. *Zbl. Bakt.* **143,** 262.

PLISZKA F. (1939b) Weitere Untersuchungen uber Immunitatsreaktionen und uber Phagozytose bei Karpfen. *Zbl. Bakt.* **143,** 451.

RIDGWAY G.J. (1962) The application of some special immunological methods to marine population problems. *Amer. Naturalist* **96,** 219.

RIDGWAY G.J., HODGINS H.O. & KLONTZ G.W. (1966) The immune response in teleosts, p. 199. In *Phylogeny of immunity*, ed. Smith, R.T., Miescher P.A. & Good R.A. University Press, Florida.

RUBEN L.N., HOVEN A.V.D. & DUTTON R.W. (1973) Cellular cooperation in hapten-carrier responses in Newt, *Triturus viridesceus. Cell. Immunol.* **6,** 300.

SIGEL M., RUSSELL W.J., JENSEN J.A. & BEASLEY A.R. (1968) Natural immunity in marine fishes. *Bull. off. Int. Epiz.* **69,** 1349.

SMITH W.W. (1940) Production of anti-bacterial agglutinins by carp and trout at 10°C. *Proc. Soc. exp. Biol.* (*N.Y.*) **45,** 726.

SNIESZKO S.F. (1953) Therapy of bacterial fish diseases. *Trans. Amer. Fish. Soc.* **83,** 313.

SNIESZKO S.F. (1970) Immunization of fish: a review. *J. Wildl. Dis.* **6,** 24.

WIDAL F. & SICARD A. (1897) *C.R. Soc. Biol.* (Paris) **49,** 1047 (cited by Bisset 1948).

Chapter 10. Physical Properties of Immunoglobulins of Lower Species: A Comparison with Immunoglobulins of Mammals

Gary W. Litman

Introduction

Classification of immunoglobulins in lower vertebrates

Immunoglobulins of ostrachoderm-derived vertebrates

Immunoglobulins of placoderm-derived vertebrates
Subunit structure (reduction-derived subunits)
Subunit structure (enzymatically-derived subunits)
Interchain and intrachain disulphides
Interchain noncovalent bonding
J chain

Immunoglobulins of placoderm-derived vertebrates *continued*
Carbohydrate composition

Immunoglobulin conformation

Immunoglobulin primary structure
Electrophoretic heterogeneity
Amino acid and peptide composition
Amino acid sequence

Antibody active sites
Combining sites of antibody
Natural antibody

Summary

Introduction

The analysis of protein structure from a phylogenetic perspective has proven one of the most useful approaches for the evaluation of both structure and function within this class of macromolecule. The phylogenetic approach has afforded us the opportunity to evaluate different yet related forms of the same molecule engaged in similar physiological roles and frequently has elucidated basic molecular mechanisms (intermolecular and intramolecular cooperativity, modulation of intermolecular heterogeneity, active site function) which may have been obscured during the passage of evolutionary time. Fundamental questions concerning their genetic control, diffuse molecular heterogeneity and antigen-binding specificity have made immunoglobulins a particularly interesting class of protein for phylogenetic comparison, and, in recent years, a great deal of detailed information regarding lower vertebrate immunoglobulin structure has become available. This chapter will attempt to summarize this data and to interpret it within the framework of our current understanding of mammalian immunoglobulin structure. It is hoped that a clear picture will emerge as to the critical structural events in the functional evolution of the immunoglobulins.

Classification of immunoglobulin in lower vertebrates

The classification of mammalian immunoglobulin has closely paralleled our comprehension of its molecular nature and solution state properties. Initially the electrophoretic mobility and ultracentrifugal behaviour of immunoglobulin provided the basis for class assignment; more recently, primary structure has been employed in both class and subclass distinction. As our analysis of lower vertebrate immunoglobulin structure is not as complete as that of the mammalian counterpart, it follows that our frame of reference for its classification does not differ from that in the initial stages of characterization of the mammalian immunoglobulin.

Marchalonis and Edelman (1965), in the first definitive characterization of an immunoglobulin from a lower vertebrate, classified the HMW (high molecular weight) and LMW (low molecular weight) immunoglobulins of the dogfish shark, *Mustelus canis*, as IgM-based on intersubunit covalent bonding, subunit mass, carbohydrate composition and amino acid composition. The two-size classes of immunoglobulin appeared only to represent a polymer state difference and did not serve as the basis for further class distinction. Using the criteria of intersubunit covalent linkages, subunit mass, amino acid composition and carbohydrate composition, it is possible to detect IgM-like immunoglobulin in virtually all vertebrate species derived from the primitive placoderms. As will be illustrated below, other serologically distinct classes of immunoglobulin differing from the IgM-like molecules in terms of subunit mass and composition of carbohydrates, amino acids and peptides have been detected in the serum of lower vertebrates. Although it is tempting to speculate that some of these molecules represent stages in the expansion of immunoglobulin class diversity, our judgement regarding their relationship to the various classes of mammalian immunoglobulin should be reserved until more definitive molecular analyses such as amino acid sequencing of class determinant regions are available. For the sake of comparison, our laboratory as well as several others has adopted the approach of classifying lower vertebrate immunoglobulin on the basis of size and intraspecies antigenic relationship.

Immunoglobulins of ostrachoderm-derived vertebrates

As the hagfishes and lampreys are the only surviving descendants of the primitive Ostrachoderms, physicochemical characterization of their immunoglobulins is of particular importance in evaluating the phylogenetic development of antibody structure. Although the Cyclostomes are somewhat limited in their capacity to mount a humoral response to both particulate and soluble antigens (Good & Papermaster 1964), the Pacific hagfish, *Eptatretus stoutii*, responds to immunization with keyhole limpet haemocyanin and sheep red blood cells (Thoenes & Hildemann 1970, Linthicum & Hildemann 1970); the sea lamprey, *Petromyzon marinus*, produces antibody to *Brucella abortus*, human 'O' erythrocytes (Pollara *et al.* 1970b) and f-2 bacteriophage (Marchalonis & Edelman 1968b).

The hagfish immunoglobulin is not yet fully characterized, although preliminary studies indicate it to be of a high molecular weight class and stable to heating at 56°C for 30 minutes; this latter point is important as it serves to functionally distinguish inducible hagfish antibody from the naturally-occurring agglutinins also found in these species (Linthicum & Hildemann 1970). In addition, hagfish immunoglobulin exhibits an $S_{20,w}$ of 23·8, is of anodal electrophoretic mobility and contains approximately 3·4 per cent hexose by weight. Further work is currently in progress to characterize the subunit nature of the molecule (Hildemann, personal communication).[1]

Marchalonis and Edelman (1968) performed comprehensive physicochemical characterization of sea lamprey immunoglobulin and found antibody activity to be associated with ~14S and ~7S serum fractions. The purified LMW immunoglobulin exhibited an anodal electrophoretic migration and a sedimentation velocity of 6·6. Unlike other lower vertebrate immunoglobulins, the molecule lacked intersubunit disulphide bonds which may explain the labile nature of the antibody. Molecular weights of the dissociable heavy and light subunits were ~70,000 and ~25,000 respectively. A complicated dissociation of the purified immunoglobulin during centrifugation precluded the precise assignment of a molecular weight. The recent molecular weight estimate of 188,000 (Marchalonis & Cone 1973) is partially substantiated by the measurements of intact molecule and subunit molecular weights.

Our laboratory has analysed the immune response and physicochemical properties of sea lamprey antibody to the human group O erythrocyte (Pollara *et al.* 1970b, Litman *et al.* 1970a). The sea lamprey produces a single, 9S class of antibody directed at the H surface antigen of the red blood cell. The isolated immunoglobulin exhibited an anodal electrophoretic migration and a molecular weight of ~320,000. The molecule was comprised of four identical, ~75,000 molecular weight subunits which were noncovalently bonded and dissociated without reducing agents under mild denaturing conditions or upon storage at 4°C. Complete reduction and alkylation of the 9S immunoglobulin followed by gel filtration in guanidine-HCl liberated an additional low molecular weight (~5,000) fragment. The secondary structure of the 9S immunoglobulin contained significant portions of α helix (>45 per

[1] Superscript figures refer to footnotes appended at end of Chapter.

cent) in contrast to the lack of detectable α-helix in other higher and lower vertebrate immunoglobulins (Litman *et al.* 1971d).

Although the above studies are in agreement concerning the labile nature of the purified lamprey immunoglobulin, disagreement exists regarding subunit composition. One of the more likely explanations for this difference is the nature of the antigen(s) employed in immunization. The immunoglobulin(s) characterized by Marchalonis and Edelman (1968) may reflect the humoral immune response to viral antigens, while the 9S immunoglobulin purified by our group may be the principle inducible class of antibody to cell surface carbohydrate antigens. Based primarily on the 9S immunoglobulin's lack of classic heavy and light chain structure, intersubunit disulphides and solution stability, we postulated a relationship between the molecule and invertebrate agglutinating glycoproteins (Litman *et al.* 1970a). Certain physicochemical properties of the 9S immunoglobulin suggest another possible phylogenetic relationship to the recently described fructosan reactive protein found in the serum of normal nurse sharks (Harisdangkul *et al.* 1972b).[2] Lamprey 9S immunoglobulin may represent a specific, inducible carbohydrate binding protein which, in latter stages of phylogenetic development, exists in a non-inducible form. Primary structure analysis will be required to establish the possible relationships between invertebrate agglutins, lamprey immunoglobulin and higher vertebrate naturally-occurring carbohydrate reactive proteins and immunoglobulins.

Immunoglobulins of placoderm-derived vertebrates

Subunit structure (reduction-derived subunits)

As previously mentioned, one of the principle means for classifying higher and lower vertebrate immunoglobulins involves molecular weight determination of the intact molecule and its structural subunits. Table 10.1 summarizes these mass relationships in the various classes of immunoglobulin derived from twenty-two vertebrate species. Although definitive classifications of single immunoglobulin classes in other species have been made, the studies selected for presentation here attempted identification of more than one size class of immunoglobulin. The carbohydrate content of the immunoglobulins is also presented in the table and will be discussed below. In viewing the data, the reader is encouraged to consult the original sources for details concerning disulphide reduction, chain separation and molecular weight estimation, all of which can significantly influence the actual outcome and interpretation of a given experiment. Fig. 10.1 is a schematic representation of mammalian IgG and IgM which will aid in evaluating subunit structure in both higher and lower vertebrate immunoglobulin.

The following conclusions regarding the immunoglobulins of species phylogenetically distal to the dipnoid fishes can be drawn from the table:

(1) All Elasmobranchean, Chondrostean, Holostean and Teleostean species listed possess no more than two size classes of immunoglobulin; three of the species, the long nose gar, the goldfish and the carp, possess only one detectable immunoglobulin class;
(2) the HMW immunoglobulin class can be either a pentamer, tetramer or dimer; the LMW class is by definition monomeric;
(3) the physicochemical data is most consistent with the major subunits of the polymers and the native monomers containing two heavy chains and two light chains joined by interchain disulphides;
(4) while the heavy chains of the HMW immunoglobulins consistently exhibit molecular weights of ~70,000, the LMW immunoglobulin heavy chains are N38,000–70,000 molecular weight;
(5) there appears to be some variation in the mass of lower vertebrate immunoglobulin light chains which has also been observed in analyses of light chains isolated from higher vertebrate homogeneous (myeloma protein) immunoglobulin (Edelman & Gall 1969).

Further characterization of these immunoglobulins utilizing techniques such as antigenic identity, amino acid composition, peptide mapping, etc., indicates that they bear structural resemblance to higher vertebrate IgM. Although the heavy chain mass of several LMW immunoglobulins is less than 70,000, it is generally felt that these molecules merely represent mass deletions and not new classes of immunoglobulin. The absence of LMW immunoglobulins in several species (gar, goldfish, carp) is also of note, and in the case of the gar immunoglobulin, has been confirmed in several laboratories including our own (Bradshaw *et al.* 1971, Acton *et al.* 1971, Litman, unpublished).

The other, more phylogenetically advanced species categorized in the table each possess a HMW immunoglobulin with the same basic physicochemical properties of the HMW immunoglobulins listed above. All of these are pentamers except for one hexameric form described in the clawed toad, *Xenopus laevis*. LMW, IgM-like immunoglobulins have been conclusively demonstrated in the serum of several species of mammal; in addition, their serum concentration is elevated during the course of infection by malarial parasites. Fig. 10.2 summarizes our concept of the evolution of IgM-like immunoglobulins.

A distinct LMW immunoglobulin class can be detected in the serum of all species found along the evolutionary line of the Sarcopterygii; an exception is found in the apparent single, HMW immunoglobulin class of a Urodele amphibian, the mudpuppy. From Table 10.1, the following conclusions

Table 10.1. Physicochemical properties of immunoglobulins

Class	Animal	Immuno-globulin class	Intact immunoglobulin	Heavy chain	Light chain	Polymer state	Carbo-hydrate	Reference
Chondrichthyes	Horned Shark	HMW	900,000 CN	68,500 CG	23,000 CG	Petamer	9·3	Frommel *et al.*
Elasmobranchii	*Heterodontus francisci*	LMW	180,000 CN	68,500 CG	23,000 CG	Monomer	11.9	(1971b)
	Smooth Dogfish	HMW	982,000 UN	71,600 UA	20,100 UA	Pentamer	8·7	Marchelonis &
	Mustelus canis	LMW	198,000 UN	73,400 UA	20,500 UA	Monomer	7·6	Edelman (1966b)
	Lemon Shark	HMW	900,000–800,000	71,000 CG	23,000–	Pentamer	ND	Clem & Small
	Negaprion brevirostris		UN		22,000 CG			(1967)
		LMW	160,000 UN	71,000 CG	23,000–	Monomer	ND	
					22,000 CG			
	Sting Ray	HMW	950,000 CN	ND	ND	Pentamer (?)	ND	Marchalonis &
	Daysatis centroura	LMW	355,000 CN	72,100 PA	21,900 PA	Dimer	ND	Schonfeld (1970)
Osteichthyes	Paddlefish	HMW	870,000 UN	75,300 UG	23,500 UG	Pentamer	9·0[1]	Pollara *et al.* (1968)
Chondrostei	*Polyodon spathula*		[662,000] UN	[58,100] UG	[21,000] UG	[Tetramer]	[6·8]	
		LMW	180,000 CN	75,300 CG	23,500 CG	Monomer	8·1	[Acton *et al.*
			[ND]	[—]	[—]	[—]	[—]	(1971b)]
Holostei	Bowfin	HMW	(13·6S) UN	70,000 CG	24,000 CG	Tetramer	10·7	Litman *et al.*
	Amia calva	LMW	(6·3S) UN	52,000 CG	24,000 CG	Monomer	9·1	(1971b,c)
	Gar	HMW	610,000 UN	70,000 CG	23,000 CG	Tetramer	4·9	Acton *et al.* (1971a)
	Lepisosteus osseus	LMW	Not present	—	—	—	—	
Teleostei	Giant Grouper	HMW	693,000 UN	70,000 CG	22,000 CG	Tetramer	ND	Clem (1971)
	Epinephelus itaria	LMW	119,000 UN	40,000 CG	22,000 CG	Monomer	> 3·6[2]	
	Goldfish	HMW	ND	72,600 PA	23,300 PA	(?)	ND	Marchalonis (1971)
	Carassius auratus	LMW	Not present	—	—	—	—	
	Carp	HMW	720,000[3]	71,400 PA	24,000 PA	Tetramer	ND	Marchalonis (1971),
	Cyprinus carpio	LMW	Not present	—	—	—	—	Shelton & Smith (1970)

Dipnoi	Australian Lungfish	HMW	(19·4S) UN	70,280 PA	23,140 PA	Pentamer	ND	Marchalonis (1969)
	Neoceratodus forsteri	LMW	(5·9S) UN	37,950 PA	23,010 PA	Monomer	ND	
	African Lungfish	HMW	870,000 CN	70,000 CG	22,500 CG	Pentamer	ND	Litman *et al.* (1971e
	Protopterus aethiopicus	IMW	180,000 CN	70,000 CG	22,500 CG	Monomer	ND	and unpublished)
		LMW	122,000 CN	38,000 CG	22,500 CG	Monomer	5·0	
Amphibia	Mud Puppy	HMW	950,000 CN	69,400 CA	23,000 CA	Pentamer	ND	Marchalonis &
	Necturus maculosus	LMW	Not present	—	—	—	ND	Cohen (1973)
	Clawed Toad	HMW	ND	71,500 PA	23,700 PA	Hexamer	ND	Marchalonis *et al.*
	Xenopus laevis			[74,440] PS	[26,700] PS			(1970), Parkhouse
		LMW	ND	52,700 PA	21,600 PA	—	ND	*et al.* (1970)
				[64,480] PS	[26,700] PS			[Hadji-Azimi (1971)]
	Marine Toad	HMW	880,000 UN	67,000 CG	22,500 CG	Pentamer	7·6	Acton *et al.* (1972a)
	Bufo marinus	LMW	160,000 UN	53,000 CG	22,500 CG	Monomer	4·2	Diener & Marchalonis (1970)
	Bullfrog	HMW	920,000[3] UN	72,100 UA	20,000 UA	Pentamer	10·8	Marchalonis &
	Rana catesbiana	LMW	150,000 UN	53,600 UA	22,000 UA	Monomer	2·1	Edelman (1966a), Marchalonis & Cone (1973)
Reptilia	Snapping Turtle	HMW	900,000 CN	70,000 CG	22,500 CG	Pentamer	ND	Chartrand *et al.*
	Chelydra serpentina	LMW	120,000 CN	38,000 CG	22,500 CG	Monomer	0·9	(1971)
	Turtle	HMW	850,000 UN	70,000 CA	22,500 CA	Pentamer	7[2]	Leslie & Clem
	Pseudamys scripta	IMW	180,000 CN	67,500 CA	22,500 CA	Monomer	ND	(1972)
		LMW	120,000 CN	35,000 CA	22,500 CA	Monomer	ND	
Aves	Domestic Chicken	HMW	823,000 UU	70,000 CG	22,000 CG	Pentamer	7·2[1]	Leslie & Clem
	Gallus domesticus	IMW[4]	170,000 UN	67,000 CG	22,000 CG	Monomer	4·1	(1969a)
	Peking Duck	HMW	ND	—	—	—	—	Zimmerman *et al.*
	Chordapa aves	IMW	178,000 UN	62,000 CUr	23,000 CUr	Monomer	5·4	(1971)
		LMW	118,000 UN	35,000 CUr	23,000 CUr	Monomer	0·6	

Table 10.1. *(contd.)*

Class	Animal	Immuno-globulin class	Intact immunoglobulin	Heavy chain	Light chain	Polymer state	Carbo-hydrate	Reference
Mammalia	Echidna	HMW	950,000 CN	69,000 CUr	22,500 CUr	Pentamer	6·4	Atwell *et al.* (1973)
	Tachyglossus aculeatus	LMW	150,000 CN	49,000 CUr	22,500 CUr	Monomer	1·5	
	Human	IgM	950,000	70,000	22,500	Pentamer	11·8	Edelman & Gall
	Homo sapiens	IgG	150,000	53,000	22,500	Monomer	2·9	(1969)
		IgA	180,000–500,000	64,000	22,500	Monomer-. . .	7·5	
		IgD*	180,000	69,700	22,500	Monomer	12·7	* Leslie *et al.* (1971)
		IgE	196,000	75,000	22,500	Monomer	10·7	

* Data from cited references is supplemented by: (1) Frommel *et al.* (1971a), (2) Acton *et al.* (1972b), (3) Marchalonis and Cone (1973) and (4) The 170,000 molecular weight chicken immunoglobulin is classified as IMW rather than LMW based on its structural similarity to the IMW immunoglobulins of reptilian and avian species. Alternative data and corresponding sources are enclosed in [ ]. Molecular weights are estimated by: C, column chromatography; P, polyacrylamide gel electrophoresis in urea or sodium dodecyl sulphate or U, ultracentrifugation. Solvents or denaturants are: A, acid; G, guanidine-HCl; N, neutral aqueous buffer; Ur, urea or S, sodium dodecyl sulphate (e.g. CG, column chromatography in guanidine-HCl). Polymer state refers to the most probable arrangement of major subunits. Carbohydrate content is total carbohydrate in g/100 g of purified protein. To conform with accepted practice, the commonly employed designates of subclass, superorder and order are included for the fishes (Romer 1970). ND, not determined.

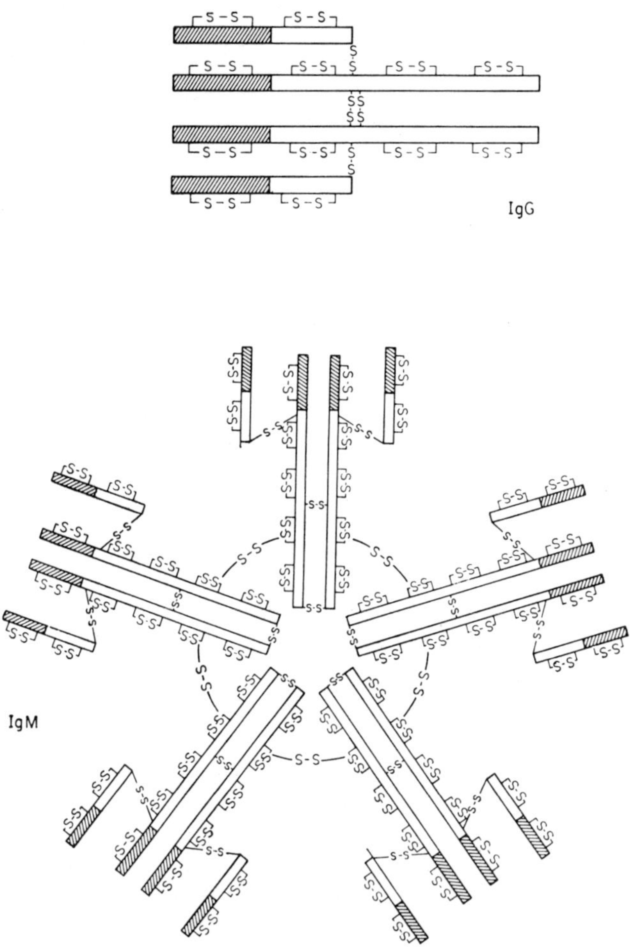

Fig. 10.1. Schematic representation of IgM and IgG molecules. IgG molecule is Eu (IgG_1, κ) constructed from data contained in Edelman and Gall (1969). IgM molecule is Ou (IgM, κ) constructed from data contained in Putnam *et al.* (1973). Bond angles are exaggerated to reflect exact primary structure location of 1/2 cystine residues. Variable regions of heavy or light chains are indicated by shading.

regarding the molecular nature of these LMW immunoglobulins can be drawn:

(1) all LMW immunoglobulins are monomers consisting of two heavy chains and two light chains bonded by intersubunit disulphides;
(2) the heavy chains vary in mass from approximately 35,000–67,000 daltons;

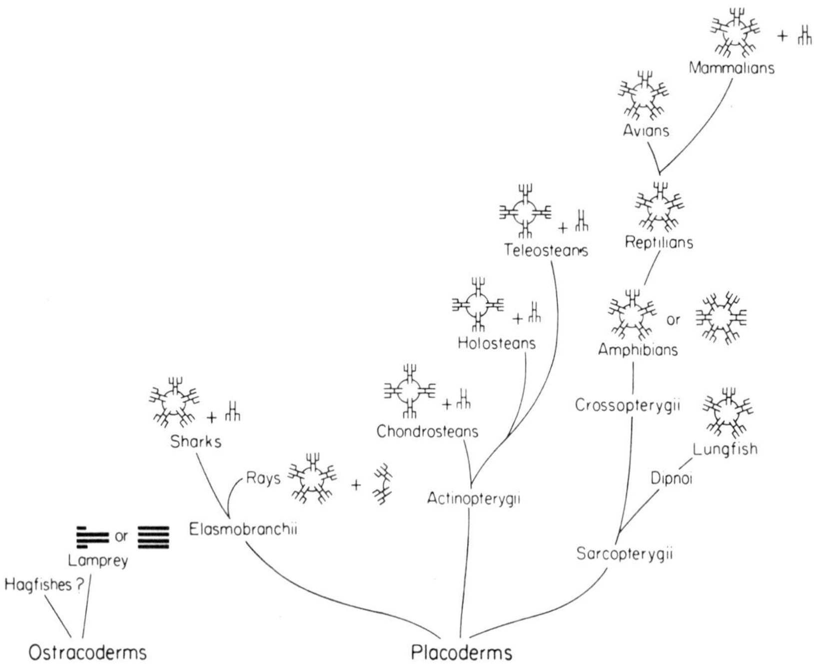

Fig. 10.2. Depicts the IgM-like immunoglobulins found in species representing the principal lines of vertebrate phylogenetic development. The IgM-like molecules associated with the members of a given class are designated and no provision is made for the apparent restrictions of certain Teleostean and Holostean species to a single HMW immunoglobulin class. The length of the heavy chain is not intended to indicate heavy chain mass; deleted 'μ-like' heavy chains have been detected in several phylogenetically critical species. Interchain and intersubunit disulphides are indicated by lines connecting the heavy and light chains. Interchain disulphides are not present in either model of the lamprey immunoglobulin, and its relationship to IgM and other recognition proteins is discussed.

based on this data as well as the dissimilarities in antigenic relationship, amino acid composition, carbohydrate contents and peptide composition relative to the heavy chains of the HMW immunoglobulin, the LMW immunoglobulins are felt to reflect a distinct immunoglobulin class;

(3) the light chains seem identical to those of HMW immunoglobulin;

(4) the interspecies mass differences in heavy chains involve multiples of approximately 10,000–12,000 daltons, the approximate size of an immunoglobulin variable or constant region (Edelman & Gall 1969).

It should be noted that similar mass deficiencies have been demonstrated conclusively in the LMW immunoglobulins of at least two other lower vertebrate species, the bowfin and the grouper. As mentioned above, these deficiencies are generally felt not to represent distinct heavy chain classes, but rather to reflect variable forms of the heavy chain class associated with the HMW, IgM-like immunoglobulins. More detailed examination of these molecules, particularly with the aid of primary structure analysis, will be required before this interpretation can be conclusively established as a legitimate class distinction.

The designation IMW (intermediate molecular weight) is used to categorize a third immunoglobulin class demonstrable in the serum of a dipnoid fish, African lungfish and several reptilian and avian species. From Table 10.1 and information cited in the original texts, the following conclusions can be drawn regarding the physicochemical properties of IMW immunoglobulins:

(1) The molecules are monomers consisting of two heavy and two light chains joined by interchain disulphide linkages;
(2) the heavy chains vary in mass between 62,000 and 70,000 daltons;
(3) the IMW molecules are noticeably absent from the amphibian species so far studied.[3]

Heavy chains of the IMW protein are felt to represent elongated forms (two additional 12,000 molecular weight mass units) of LMW heavy chains. It is not certain whether this difference is a true reflection of the genetic material governing the synthesis of these molecules or represents an enzymatic breakdown product of the IMW to the LMW protein.

The relationships of IMW to HMW and LMW immunoglobulins are not completely clear:

(1) carbohydrate composition—turtle and duck IMW immunoglobulins contain significantly greater amounts of carbohydrate than do the LMW immunoglobulins (Leslie & Clem 1972, Acton *et al.* 1972b, Zimmerman *et al.* 1971);
(2) amino acid composition—duck IMW and LMW immunoglobulins are similar (Zimmerman *et al.* 1971);
(3) antigenic relationships—turtle and duck IMW heavy chains are antigenically related to their LMW counterparts (Leslie & Clem 1972, Zimmerman 1971), turtle IMW heavy chains are not related to their HMW heavy chains; similar analyses have not been performed with duck HMW and IMW heavy chains.

The IMW (IgY) immunoglobulins of the chicken resemble both duck and turtle IMW proteins and, in fact, are antigenically related to duck IMW immunoglobulin (Zimmerman *et al.* 1971).

Two additional classes of immunoglobulin from the chicken have been described. However, insufficient physicochemical data concerning their structures have precluded their inclusion in this table. An IgA-like protein has been detected in both the serum and secretions of chickens (Lebacq-Verheyden *et al.* 1972, Leslie & Martin 1973; Bienenstock *et al.* 1973). The molecule exhibits a molecular weight of ~180,000 in the serum and ~360,000 in the secretions.[4] Both heavy (~70,000 molecular weight) and light chains are found in these proteins. Choi and Good (1971) described an ~300,000 molecular weight immunoglobulin comprised exclusively of heavy chains in the serum of bursectomized and irradiated chickens.

These avian and reptilian immunoglobulin systems best illustrate the complexity of immunoglobulin classification in lower vertebrate species and emphasize the need for more precise definition of terms such as HMW, IMW and LMW before they are employed as meaningful nomenclature.

Subunit structure (enzymatically-derived subunits)

Enzymatic proteolysis has proven one of the most useful probes in elucidating the structure-function relationships of mammalian immunoglobin (Porter 1959, Edelman & Gall 1969). As the ability of proteolytic enzymes to effect modifications in polypeptide chains is dependent upon the primary structure and folding configuration at the site of enzyme action, proteolysis could provide a useful means for making structural comparisons of higher and lower vertebrate immunoglobulins. Klapper *et al.* (1971) digested lemon shark LMW immunoglobulin with papain or trypsin and obtained a 6S fragment consisting of two covalently bonded Fab′ subunits, $F(ab\mu')_2$. The fragment, structurally related to those derived from human IgM under similar conditions, expressed the bacterial agglutinating activity of the parent molecule. Unlike mammalian IgM, however, partial reduction of lemon shark LMW immunoglobulin followed by papain digestion resulted in a breakdown of the molecule to small peptides. Zimmerman *et al.* (1971) digested both IMW and LMW duck immunoglobulin with papain and found only the IMW protein to yield counterparts of Fab and Fc as judged by electrophoretic mobility in starch gel and antigenic relationships of the purified fragments. The LMW immunoglobulin was digested to an Fab-like fragment and small peptides; an Fc equivalent could not be recovered. Leslie and Clem (1972) found turtle IMW immunoglobulin and chicken IgY (IMW chicken immunoglobulin, see Table 10.1) to be degraded by pepsin to 146,000 and 62,500 and 135,000 and 49,500 molecular weight fragments respectively. These authors noted that the turtle LMW immunoglobulin was not susceptible to the action of pepsin under the conditions employed. Litman *et al.* (unpublished) employed trypsin to digest African lungfish LMW immunoglobulin to 43,000 and 34,000 molecular weight subunits. Analysis of antigenic relationships and electrophoretic mobility suggested these fragments to be counterparts of the Fab and Fc subunits of mammalian immunoglobulins. Although certain of these studies suggest common sites for the action of proteolytic enzymes in higher and lower vertebrate immunoglobulin, definite conclusions regarding the enzyme susceptible regions are difficult to form.

Interchain and intrachain disulphides

With the exception of the sea lamprey immunoglobulin(s), interchain disulphide bonding has been qualitatively demonstrated in all studies of lower vertebrate immunoglobulin (Grey 1969, Marchalonis & Cone 1973); however, relatively little quantitative information regarding disulphide bond formation and location is currently available.[5] Acton *et al.* (1971c) used reduction in the presence and absence of increasing concentrations of guanidine-HCl to estimate the number of disulphides in the tetrameric macroglobulins of the paddlefish, gar and catfish. The paddlefish macroglobulin contained 70 disulphides/molecule and the gar macroglobulin contained 82 disulphides capable of reduction at the maximum concentration of guanidine-HCl employed (Acton *et al.* 1971a). Seventeen of the gar immunoglobulin disulphides could be cleaved in the absence of guanidine-HCl. The catfish macroglobulin possessed 74 disulphides capable of titration, as was the case with gar macroglobulin; maximum cleavage in the presence of guanidine-HCl was effected in 1 hour versus the 6 hours necessary to reduce the 90 disulphides of human IgM (Hall *et al.* 1973, Acton *et al.* 1971a).

Zimmerman *et al.* (1971) used partial and total reduction with 2-mercaptoethanol and alkylation with iodoacetamide to analyse interchain disulphides in the LMW duck immunoglobulin. By comparing carboxymethyl cysteine composition in heavy chains, light chains and Fab under the two sets of conditions, the authors concluded that the partial reducing conditions employed were effectively reducing intrachain disulphides in the Fd and possibly in the light chains. At present, we have little information regarding the location of interchain disulphides, although limited proteolytic digestion of lemon shark LMW immunoglobulin (Klapper *et al.* 1971) duck IMW and LMW immunoglobulin (Zimmerman *et al.* 1971) and African lungfish LMW immunoglobulin (Litman *et al.*, unpublished) suggest Light↔Heavy and Heavy↔Heavy interchain disulphide bonding patterns homologous to those of mammalian immunoglobulin. Inter-heavy chain disulphide linkages in the turtle, duck and African lungfish LMW immunoglobulins are more susceptible to reduction than are the inter-Heavy↔Light chain disulphides. Taken collectively, these results tend to suggest that interchain disulphide bonding patterns of higher and lower vertebrate immunoglobulins are similar.

Mammalian immunoglobulins contain one intrachain disulphide linkage/110 amino acids. The intrachain disulphide draws the chain into a series of ~60 amino acid residue loops which represent a conformationally significant feature (Litman *et al.* 1970b) of the variable or constant region domain (Edelman & Gall 1969). With the exception of the studies of Grant *et al.*

(1971) who provided convincing evidence for homology between the regions containing the intrachain 1/2 cystines in chicken, turkey and mammalian light chains, relatively little is known of intrachain disulphide location or formation in the immunoglobulins of lower vertebrates.[6] Evidence regarding the quantity of carboxymethyl cysteine (CMCYS) in the fully reduced and alkylated heavy and light chains, the yield of heavy and light chains following partial reduction and the quantity of CMCYS in the partially reduced immunoglobulins is, however, consistent with one intrachain disulphide per 110–20 amino acids. More definitive statements regarding intrachain disulphides in lower vertebrate immunoglobulin must await isolation and characterization of their cystine-containing peptides. The general method for detection and primary structure location of 1/2 cystine containing peptides proposed by Grant *et al.* (1971) will be useful in such studies.

Interchain noncovalent bonding

The nature and extent of interchain non-covalent bonding in immunoglobulins are more difficult to quantitate as compared to interchain covalent bonding. Part of this difficulty is related to the variety of non-covalent interactions which can exist, e.g. hydrophobic, electrostatic, hydrogen bond, van der Waals, etc., and the complexity involved in independently assessing each force. Furthermore, evaluation of several of these interactions require full knowledge of three-dimensional polypeptide folding; only recently a limited amount of such information has been made available for mammalian immunoglobulins. The majority of statements regarding non-covalent bonding in both higher and lower vertebrate immunoglobulins are based on studies of polypeptide chain dissociation in various solvents. In most studies, interchain disulphides are first reduced and alkylated, the preparation is dialysed against dissociating media such as weak organic acids, and the dialysed preparation subjected to gel filtration chromatography in the dissociating solvent. The ability of a given solvent to allow quantitative resolution of heavy and light chains is taken as an index of the extent of interchain non-covalent bonding. In the studies discussed below, conclusions regarding the relative degree of non-covalent bonding should be viewed with caution, as gel filtration media ordinarily do not discriminate between aggregated and unseparated heavy and light chains. A weak organic acid may be capable of dissociating heavy and light chains; however, once dissociated, the chains may aggregate and be confused with unseparated chains. This tendency to undergo aggregation is related to, but does not reflect, non-covalent bonding between polypeptide chains.

Marchalonis and Edelman (1965) noted that a greater degree of interchain non-covalent bonding existed in dogfish shark HMW immunoglobulin than in mammalian IgM. While rabbit or human IgG and IgM can be reduced and alkylated and separated into heavy and light chains in 1 N acetic or propionic acid, Elasmobranch immunoglobulins require varying concentrations of hydrogen bond donors (urea or guanidine-HCl) to effect quantitative separation of heavy and light chains (Clem & Small 1967; Frommel *et al.* 1971b). Studies of chain dissociation in other lower vertebrate immunoglobulins do not reveal any unifying phylogenetic trends in non-covalent bonding. The heavy and light chains of paddlefish immunoglobulin require the presence of concentrated guanidine-HCl for chain separation (Pollara *et al.* 1968), (Acton *et al.* 1971b), while those of the holosteans, *bowfin* (Litman *et al.* 1971c) and gar (Bradshaw *et al.* 1971) can be quantitatively resolved in 1 N propionic acid. The immunoglobulins of several more phylogenetically distal teleost species require concentrated urea or guanidine for effective separation of chains (Marchalonis 1971) (Hall *et al.* 1973). The chicken LMW immunoglobulin possesses such weak non-covalent interchain bonding that neutral aqueous buffers can support dissociation into heavy and light chains (Dreesman & Benedict 1965). The LMW immunoglobulin of the turtle does not readily dissociate into heavy and light chains in the presence of weak acid alone and requires chromatography in 4–6 M guanidine-HCl for resolution of chains (Chartrand *et al.* 1971). Cleavage of the inter-heavy chain disulphide(s) of the turtle LMW immunoglobulin results in the production of half molecules in neutral aqueous buffer, indicating a weak degree of inter-heavy chain non-covalent bonding and rather intense inter-heavy-light chain non-covalent bonding (Leslie & Clem 1972).

Zimmerman and Grey (1972) proposed a novel technique for quantifying immunoglobulin interchain non-covalent bonding. The authors reduced and alkylated immunoglobulin and separated the component chains by starch gel electrophoresis in varying concentrations of urea. Plots of the light chain dissociated versus urea concentration reflected the degree of non-covalent interchain bonding. Using this technique, the HMW immunoglobulin of the grouper and a species of shark were shown to possess a greater degree of inter-heavy-light chain disulphide bonding than did human IgM.

If interchain hydrogen bonding significantly contributes to the relative proportions of α-helix/β-sheet/randon coil in a multi-subunit protein, circular dichroism may be employed to study this specific form of interchain non-covalent bonding (Litman 1973b) (see discussion below of circular dichroism). The circular dichroic spectra of bowfin immunoglobulin and its heavy and light chains were determined and the latter two spectra were summed in a 1:1 ratio (Litman *et al.* 1971c). The summation spectra could be superimposed on to the spectra of intact bowfin HMW or LMW immunoglobulin, indicating that the degree of hydrogen bonding (interchain β-sheet between heavy and light chains) was minimal.

Variability in a gradation in intensity of interchain non-covalent bonding exists in the immunoglobulins of Placoderm-derived vertebrates. No correlations can be drawn between the level of phylogenetic development of a given species and the degree of interchain noncovalent bonding. The variation in bonding intensity is without a doubt an important function to consider in evaluating structure-function relationships of these molecules.

J chain

In addition to heavy and light chains, a third polypeptide chain generally referred to as 'J' (joining) chain has been detected in rabbit IgA and human IgA (Halpern & Koshland 1970) and IgM polymers. J chain can be cleaved from the heavy chain by reduction and alkylation *and by virtue of its high negative charge* can be separated from heavy and light chains at alkaline pH. Isolated J chain exhibits a molecular weight of approximately 15,000 and is rich in 1/2 cystine residues (7–8/molecule of human IgA J chain [Wilde & Koshland 1973]).

The role of J chain in immunoglobulin structure is unclear at present; it may be involved in inducing disulphide bonding between monomers of polymeric immunoglobulins or may provide the backbone to which the monomers bind. A structure exhibiting the electrophoretic mobility of J chain in alkaline urea gels has been detected in the HMW immunoglobulins of catfish, marine toad and pheasant and was absent in the HMW immunoglobin of both the longnose gar and nurse shark (Weinheimer *et al.* 1971).[7] Klaus *et al.* (1971a) detected the J chain in the HMW immunoglobulin of the leopard shark and found it absent in the LMW immunoglobulin of this species. Pollara *et al.* (1970a) enzymatically cleaved a fragment from paddlefish HMW immunoglobulin which may have represented C terminal portions of heavy chain linked by a J chain. The J chain has not yet been evaluated in other lower vertebrate polymeric immunoglobulins, although such studies would be valuable for the evaluation of its functional significance from a phylogenetic perspective.

Carbohydrate composition

The association of carbohydrate with all classes of mammalian immunoglobulin is well documented (Edelman & Gall 1969). Ordinarily associated with the Fc portion of the heavy chain, carbohydrate has also been demonstrated in lesser quantities on light chains (Abel *et al.* 1968). Alternative theories as to its functional significance involve the direct influences on local conformation within the Fc portion of the molecule or suggest carbohydrate attachment as a pre-requisite to secretion of immunoglobulin from plasma cells. Due to differences in carbohydrate composition of the various mammalian immunoglobulin classes (Table 10.2), total carbohydrate content became one of the parameters first employed in making class assignments in lower vertebrate antibody molecules (Marchalonis & Edelman 1966a,b).

Frommel *et al.* (1971a) compared the hexose, hexosamine, fucose and sialic acid composition of purified lower vertebrate immunoglobulins. Carbohydrate compositions of 8–10 per cent were encountered in the immunoglobulins isolated from vertebrate species below the phylogenetic level of the dipnoid fishes; above this level, where an immunoglobulin class distinct from the IgM like proteins is encountered (Marchalonis 1968, Litman *et al.* 1971e), markedly reduced levels of carbohydrate were detected in the LMW immunoglobulins. This reduced carbohydrate content and the ~38,000 molecular weight of the LMW turtle and duck immunoglobulin heavy chains may reflect the absence of a lower vertebrate homologue of the mammalian immunoglobulin heavy chain constant region where carbohydrate is attached by a glycosidic linkage. This contention is substantiated in part by the findings of Zimmerman *et al.* (1971) who concluded that the carbohydrate of duck low molecular weight immunoglobulin is attached to the Fab rather than the 'abbreviated' Fc region of the molecule. Acton *et al.* (1972b) expanded these earlier studies and analysed the carbohydrate compositions of heavy and light chains derived from the immunoglobulins of species representing the major vertebrate classes. They concluded that:

(1) most carbohydrate was associated with the heavy chains and that the minimal amounts of light chain-associated carbohydrate might be due to contamination by J chain;
(2) duck and catfish HMW immunoglobulins did not contain fucose and
(3) the mannose/galactose ratio was greater than one above, and on the order of one below, the level of the Aves.

Thus, significant differences in carbohydrate composition of higher and lower vertebrate immunoglobulins have been demonstrated, and although a useful structural marker, the functional significance of carbohydrate is not evident at present.

Immunoglobulin conformation

During the past few years our knowledge of immunoglobulin solution conformation has grown significantly. Employing techniques such as circular dichroism (CD), solvent perturbation and fluorescence polarization, it has been possible to compare the conformations of higher and lower vertebrate immunoglobulins. The most useful of the techniques adopted has been CD in the far UV spectral range. This method provides an estimate of the contributions made by α-helix, β-sheet and random coil conformations to the overall secondary structure of a protein molecule when reference is made to amino acid homopolymers stabilized in each of the folding configurations

Table 10.2. N-terminal amino acid sequence

Species	Chain	N-terminal residues 0	1	2	3	4	5	6	7	8	9	10	11	12	Reference
Leopard Shark	light		Asp	Ile	Val	Leu	Thr	Glx	Pro	Gly	Ser	Val			Klaus *et al.*
				Pro	Ile	Met				Pro					(1971b)
						Val									
Paddlefish	light		Asp	Ile	Val	Ile	Thr								Pollara *et al.*
						Leu									(1968)
African Lungfish	light		Asp	—	—	Leu	Thr	Glx	Asx	Ala	Ser	Met	*	Val	Litman *et al.*
															(1971e)
Chicken	light		—	—	Ala	Leu	Thr	Gln	Pro	Ala	—	Ala	Val	Gly	Kubo *et al.* (1970)
Rabbit	light (κ)	Ala	Asp	Ile	Val	Met	Thr	Glx	Thr	Pro	Ser	Ser	Val	Ser	Hood *et al.* (1970)
			Ala	Val	Glx	Val					Ala			Thr	
				Phe		Leu								Glx	
Pig	light (κ)	Ala	—	Ile	Val	Leu	Thr	Glx	Ser	Pro	Ser	Leu	Leu	Ala	Novotony *et al.*
					Glx	Asx	Ser				Thr		Ala	Pro	(1970)
							Glx				Leu		Gly	Ser	
Human	light (λ)		PCA	Ser	Val	Leu	Thr	Gln	Pro	Pro	Ser	Val	Ser	Gly	Dayhoff (1973)
				Tyr	Ala		Ala			Ala	Ala	Ala		Val	
					Glu										
Human	light (κ)		Asp	Ile	Val	Met	Thr	Gln	Ser	Pro	Ser	Ser	Leu	Ser	Dayhoff (1973)
			Glu	Val	Gln	Leu			Thr		Thr	Thr		Pro	
				Met	Leu						Leu	Phe			
											Gly				
											Ala				
											Asx				

Leopard Shark	heavy (HS1)	PCA	Val	Pro	Gly	—	Gln							Klaus *et al.* (1971b)
	(HS2)	PCA	Asp	Leu	Pro	Thr	Pro							
	(UB)	Glu	Ile Val	Val	Leu	Thr	Glx	Pro	Glx	Ala	Glx			
Paddlefish	heavy	Asp	Ile	Val	Ile Leu	Thr								Pollara *et al.* (1968)
Gar	heavy	Asp	Val Ala Leu	Ile Val Leu	Val									Acton *et al.* (1971a)
Chicken	heavy (anti-DNP)	Ala	Val	Thr	Leu	Asp	Glu	Ser	Gly	Gly	Gly	Leu	Gln	Kubo *et al.* (1971)
Human	heavy (V_{H_I})	PCA	Val	Gln His	Leu Val	Val Thr	Glu Gln	Ser	Gly Ser	Ala	Glu Asp Gly	Leu Val	Lys Val	Wang *et al.* (1970) Köhler *et al.* (1970)
	heavy ($V_{H_{II}}$)	PCA	Val	Thr	Leu	Arg Lys Thr	Glu	Ser Asn	Gly	Pro	Ala Thr	Leu	Val	
	heavy ($V_{H_{III}}$)	Glu	Val Ile	Gln	Leu	Val Leu	Glu	Ser	Gly	Gly	Gly Ala	Leu	Val Ile	

Table 10.2 is constructed from the data contained in the cited references following the general suggestions of Litman *et al.* (1971e) regarding alternative amino acids at a single position, qualitative versus quantitative identification of residues and sources of immunoglobulins. Deletions are indicated by (—) and are based on proposed homology with N-terminal sequences of human κ chains.

* No predominant amino acid; Gly, Ala, Ser and Thr are detected in low quantity.

(Beychok 1968, Greenfield & Fasman 1969). While the precise content of the various secondary structures is frequently difficult to estimate due to compensating optical phenomena arising within the polypeptide foldings or through aromatic or disulphide influences, CD has nevertheless proven invaluable in estimating secondary and certain aspects of tertiary structure in a variety of proteins.

With the singular exception of the sea lamprey immunoglobulin, the CD spectra of lower vertebrate immunoglobulins are remarkably similar to each other and to the CD spectra of purified mammalian immunoglobulins (Litman *et al.* 1971d). The spectra exhibit similar contents of β-sheet structure and fail to indicate significant amounts of α-helix, conformation. HMW and LMW immunoglobulins isolated from horned sharks, paddlefish and bowfins had identical CD spectra which were similar to the spectra of human IgM and its reduction derived monomer, 7S IgM. Some interspecies differences in the immunoglobulin CD profiles were noted in the 235 nm spectral region. Although these transitions are though to arise in the Fc portion of mammalian immunoglobulin (Litman *et al.* 1970b, 1973b) there is no direct evidence that they originate in an equivalent Fc region of the lower vertebrate proteins. Unlike the other lower vertebrate immunoglobulins so far characterized, the 9S sea lamprey immunoglobulin possesses a high content of α-helix (>45 per cent by reference to poly-L-lysine in the 100 per cent α-helix conformation), which may explain the marked dependence of subunit molecular weight on solvent composition observed in our initial studies of the lamprey immunoglobulin (Litman *et al.* 1970a). As mentioned, α-helix has not yet been demonstrated in any other immunoglobulin or immunoglobulin subunit and thus has raised doubts regarding the relationship of the 9S lamprey molecule to other immunoglobulins.

Fluorescence polarization has recently been adopted as a means for comparing subunit flexibility of higher and lower vertebrate immunoglobulins. Richter *et al.* (1972) and Zagyansky (1973) have attached 1-dimethylamino-naphthalene-5-sulphonyl (DNS) chloride to HMW carp, frog, tortoise and LMW (7S) frog and turtle immunoglobulins and measured rotational correlation times of the DNS conjugates.[8] Assuming that the DNS derivatization occurred at equivalent sites in the molecule, it could be concluded that 7·2S tortoise and 7S frog immunoglobulins were considerably more rigid than the 7S IgG molecules isolated from rats or humans. Similarly, mammalian IgM possessed less restricted flexibility than did carp, frog or tortoise HMW immunoglobulin, although the latter three were less rigid than the LMW frog and tortoise molecules.[9] The correlation of these findings with interchain non-covalent bonding patterns would be particularly useful in comparative analysis of lower vertebrate immunoglobulins.

Solvent perturbation difference spectroscopy has become a useful technique for examining topographic distribution of the aromatic amino acids tyrosine and tryptophan in polypeptides (Herskovits & Sorensen 1968). The method relies on the enhanced extinction coefficient of tyrosine and tryptophan in nondenaturing solvents (methanol, ethylene glycol, glycerol, sucrose, etc.) of varying geometric diameter. The accessibility of a perturbant for a given aromatic residue depends on the size of the perturbant and the polypeptide foldings in the immediate vicinity of the aromatic chormophore. We have examined the solvent perturbation difference spectrum of human IgM and bowfin HMW immunoglobulin and found them to be similar; burying of tryptophan and only marginal exposure of tyrosine to the solvent environment were the predominant characteristics of the spectra (Litman *et al.* 1971b). When African lungfish LMW immunoglobulin was compared to human or rabbit IgG, an entirely different result was obtained. Although the tryptophan content (residues/mole) of the lungfish LMW and mammalian immunoglobulins were equivalent, no exposure of tryptophan was detected in rabbit and human IgG, while 40 per cent of the tryptophan in the lungfish LMW molecule was exposed (Litman, unpublished). These findings suggest major differences in polypeptide chain folding between the dipnoid fish and mammalian immunoglobulins.

Several groups have utilized electron microscopy of negatively stained immunoglobulin preparations to study molecular dimensions and subunit arrangements of lower vertebrate immunoglobulins. Parkhouse *et al.* (1970) compared the HMW immunoglobulin of the clawed toad to mammalian IgM molecules and concluded that the Xenopus protein was most likely a hexamer as opposed to the mammalian IgM pentamer. Shelton and Smith (1970) isolated carp HMW antibody to dinitrophenol and sheep red blood cells (immune haemagglutinin) and found negatively stained preparations to be composed of four arms connected at a central core; they concluded that the molecule possessed a tetrameric configuration. Acton *et al.* (1971c) similarly analysed the HMW immunoglobulins isolated from immune paddlefish, gar and catfish serum and found them to be tetramers with a span of 300–400 Å across the arms and 95–100 Å in the central region of the molecule. These findings were in accord with the other physicochemical observations suggesting the molecule to be composed of four major subunits, each consisting of two heavy and two light chains. While limited resolution of the photomicrographs does not allow further interpretation of interchain relationships, electron microscopy has been invaluable in establishing the various polymer configurations of HMW immunoglobulins.

Immunoglobulin primary structure

Electrophoretic heterogeneity

Perhaps no issues in the field of comparative immunoglobulin structure are more deserving of attention than those relating to the relative heterogeneity of antibody. As the immunoglobulins are committed to recognition of diverse antigenic structures, it is apparent that a complex molecular polymorphism capable of fulfilling the antibody functional requirements be expressed and maintained. Marchalonis and Edelman (1966b) interpreted the diffuse banding of dogfish shark heavy and light chains in starch gel electrophoresis as an indication of molecular heterogeneity in the immunoglobulins of this lower vertebrate species. Similar conclusions were drawn from the banding patterns of paddlefish (Pollara *et al.* 1968), leopard shark (Suran & Papermaster 1967) and lemon shark (Clem & Small 1967) heavy or light chains in polyacrylamide gel electrophoresis in urea.

A recent study from our laboratory compared the distribution in isoelectric focusing of fully reduced and alkylated light chains derived from the immunoglobulins of nine species representing the major lines of vertebrate phylogenetic development (Merz *et al.*, 1975). The light chains exhibited profuse heterogeneity and remarkably similar banding patterns; three distinct electrophoretic fractions (pI 8·2, 8·5 and 8·9) were shared by each of the different light chain preparations. While these findings suggest similar primary structures for certain of the light chains, more definitive analyses such as peptide mapping and actual amino acid sequencing will be necessary to confirm the possible interspecies homologies.

Restrictions in the heterogeneity of specifically purified lower vertebrate antibody similar to those observed in mammals subjected to comparable immunization have been noted. Kubo *et al.* (1971) found the heavy and light chains of specifically purified chicken antibody to dinitrophenol to exhibit a more homogeneous electrophoretic distribution that the component chains of chicken immunoglobulin. Clem and Leslie observed a similar restriction in electrophoretic heterogeneity of the light chains from some purified preparations of nurse shark HMW (1971) and chicken IgM (1973) antibody to streptococcal A-variant carbohydrate. It would be of interest to correlate the restrictions in heterogeneity with the relative degree of specificity and average association constant exhibited by the purified antibody.

Amino acid and peptide composition

As mentioned above, analysis of amino acid composition has been useful to distinguish between the heavy chain classes of lower vertebrate immunoglobulins (Marchalonis & Edelman 1966a,b). While interspecies comparison of amino acid composition is not associated with the same level of confidence as amino acid sequencing for establishing evolutionary relationships, composition analysis has been employed successfully in determining the relatedness between members of several protein families (Marchalonis & Weltman 1971). Marchalonis (1972) compared the amino acid compositions of heavy chains derived from the 'IgM like' immunoglobulins of six lower vertebrate species to human immunoglobulin heavy chains of the μ-, γ- and α-classes. The interspecies differences in amino acid composition were then statistically compared to the relative differences in composition of cytochrome c and haemoglobin protein families which underwent rather conservative and moderate rates of evolution respectively. The immunoglobulin heavy chains of the μ-type evolved at a rate comparable to that of cytochrome c. The obvious extension of this approach to other heavy chain types will be of benefit in ascertaining the relationships of IMW and LMW immunoglobulins encountered in species at and above the phylogenetic level of the dipnoid fishes.

Although classic peptide composition analysis (peptide mapping) tends to overestimate the degree of relatedness and underestimate primary structure differences in heterogeneous protein populations, it has also aided in distinguishing heavy chain classes in lower vertebrate immunoglobulins. Marchalonis and Edelman (1965) and Clem and Small (1967) interpreted the similar peptide maps of heavy chains isolated from HMW and LMW dogfish shark and lemon shark immunoglobulins as indicating lack of heavy chain class divergence in Elasmobranch immunoglobulins. Acton *et al.* (1972a) interpreted the peptide map differences between HMW and LMW marine toad immunoglobulins as evidence for heavy chain class divergence at the level of the amphibians. Sanders *et al.* (1973) found chicken IMW immunoglobulin and human IgG heavy chains to share nine peptides with common mobilities; however, amino acid composition analysis of the peptides indicated significant differences in their primary structure. More extensive interspecies comparisons of peptide composition are not currently available.

Amino acid sequence

Although primary structure analysis is the most definitive means for establishing phylogenetic relationships of proteins, only limited amounts of sequence data are available for the immunoglobulins from species below the phylogenetic level of the mammals. This deficiency is related, in large part, to the comparable degree of amino acid heterogeneity found in the immunoglobulins of higher and lower vertebrates. The recent demonstration that lower vertebrate species respond to immunization with streptococcal vaccines by producing antibody of limited heterogeneity promises to expand our base of primary structure data for lower vertebrate immunoglobulins. Summarized in Table 10.2 are the sequences of lower vertebrate immunoglobulin heavy and light chains. Also included for reference are the sequences of mammalian immunoglobulin κ and λ light chains and heavy chain variable regions. In viewing the data, it should be remembered that:

(1) the lower vertebrate immunoglobulins are heterogeneous and only the predominant residue(s) at a given position are presented;
(2) the majority of currently available lower vertebrate heavy and light chain

sequences represent only unblocked residues; most heterogeneous lower vertebrate immunoglobulin populations contain a significant proportion of blocked sequences which may lack significant homology with comparable sequences in other species. Conclusions of possible homology based solely on unblocked sequences may thus be unfounded, and original sources should be consulted for details concerning the percentage of unblocked residues and composition of PCA blocked peptides;

(3) the majority of lower vertebrate immunoglobulin sequences encompass from 6–10 residues, resulting in analysis of only 4–5 per cent of a light chain and approximately 2 per cent of a heavy chain. Any conclusions regarding interspecies homology reached from such a limited portion of the molecule should be viewed cautiously.

Suran and Papermaster (1967a,b) and Pollara *et al.* (1968) determined the N-terminal amino acid sequence of both leopard shark and paddlefish immunoglobulin heavy and light chains. The sequences were found to be homologous to one another and to mouse and human κ-chains. From these studies the authors concluded that heavy and light chains shared a common genetic origin and that κ-chains evolved prior to λ-chains. Goodman *et al.* (1970) detected PCA blocked sequences in both the heavy and light chains of leopard shark immunoglobulin and have sequenced the peptides as well as the unblocked amino terminal residues of both chains (Klaus *et al.* 1971b). The single PCA blocked peptide isolated from the light chain and the three heavy chain PCA peptides demonstrated only slight homology to human heavy chain variable regions. The 40 per cent unblocked sequence of the heavy chains was homologous to human heavy chains but the degree of homology within V_H, V_κ and V_λ was about the same. The 25 per cent unblocked light chain sequence was equally related to the V_κ and V_λ but not to V_H.[10]

Litman *et al.* (1973e) sequenced the N-terminal 10 amino acids of the African lungfish and detected a homology to mammalian κ- and λ-light chains. Two deletions in the amino acid sequence at positions 2 and 3 were noted if reference were made to human κ-light chains. Inspection of N-terminal amino acid sequences of chicken, rabbit and pig light chains revealed similar ‘deletions’ as well as ‘additions’, and comparable findings have been detected at other positions in the amino acid sequence of human κ- and λ-light chains. It is tempting to speculate that they may reflect a genetic mechanism capable of introducing certain three-dimensional folding properties in a more effective manner than by the process of simply mutation.

More extensive sequence analyses have been performed on both the heavy and light chains of avian species. Kubo *et al.* (1970) sequenced the N-terminal 17 residues of chicken immunoglobulin light chains and concluded they were homologous to mammalian λ-light chains. Grant *et al.* (1971) confirmed these studies and extended the sequences to include almost one-third of the entire light chain. The authors also sequenced the light chains of turkey immunoglobulin and found them to differ from chicken light chains in only two of 74 positions. From these studies it was concluded that κ- and λ-light chains evolved 250 million years ago, prior to the separation of the avian and mammalian lines of evolution. It is difficult at present to extend the conclusions regarding κ- and λ-divergence any further back in evolutionary time, although the finding of serologically distinct light chain classes in the immunoglobulin of a reptile are suggestive of an earlier divergence (Saluk *et al.* 1970).[11]

The sequences of avian immunoglobulin heavy chains have indicated a close homology to mammalian heavy chains. Kubo *et al.* (1971) sequenced the heavy chains of chicken antibody specific for the DNP grouping and found the unblocked heavy chain sequences to be homologous to the V_{HIII} subgroup of mammalian heavy chains. Kehoe and Capra (1974) have simultaneously analysed the unblocked sequences of pooled heavy chains derived from the immunoglobulins of four other avian species, turkey, duck, goose and pigeon, and detected a close interspecies homology.[12] When these sequences were compared to those of unblocked heavy chains isolated from the immunoglobulins of phylogenetically diverse mammals (Capra *et al.* 1973), a definitive homology extending through eleven mammalian species and five avian species was realized. These data are most consistent with 'paucigene' as opposed to multigene theories of generation of immunoglobulin diversity in immunoglobulins.

No attempts have been made as yet to sequence the constant regions of heavy chains from the immunoglobulins of species phylogenetically distal to the Aves, although such studies would be invaluable in order to ascertain the phylogenetic relationships of IgG, IgA and IgM. Chuang *et al.* (1973) have introduced an alternative approach which relies on the estimation of degree of homology existing between the carboxy terminal sequences of mammalian immunoglobulin heavy chains. Assuming IgM to be the class of immunoglobulin appearing earliest in evolution, the authors concluded that IgA and IgG evolved independently from an ancestral μ-chain. The divergence of the α-chain was estimated as occurring approximately 200 million years ago, at about the time of avian evolution. More complete physicochemical characterization of the recently described IgA-like chicken immunoglobulin will be of use in substantiating the conclusions drawn from these studies.

Antibody active sites

Combining sites of antibody

As antibody activity is the principal physiologic function of the immunoglobulin molecule, it becomes essential that comparative physicochemical studies of lower and higher vertebrate immunoglobulins evaluate the nature, composition and location of the antigen-combining site. While antibody to any number of bacterial, viral, protein and carbohydrate antigens can be induced in lower vertebrates, studies of the antigen-combining site require well-defined antigenic determinants such as the substituted benzene derivatives. The dinitrophenol (DNP) hapten is one of the better characterized antigen systems and the combining site of mammalian antibody to DNP has been extensively characterized. A variety of techniques exist for quantitation of the DNP-anti DNP reaction (fluorescence quenching, equilibrium dialysis, precipitin analysis) and identification of active site contact residues (induced shifts in DNP spectra, affinity labelling), thus making the DNP-anti DNP system an obvious choice for analysis of combining site properties in lower vertebrate immunoglobulins.

Leslie and Clem (1970) provided the first comprehensive analysis of the lower vertebrate immune response to DNP substituted protein and amino acid homopolymer carriers. From their studies, they concluded that:

(1) several lower vertebrates were capable of manifesting an immune response to DNP as measured by capacity to neutralize DNP-coated bacteriophage,
(2) the phage neutralizing capacity of lower vertebrates was significantly less than that of rabbits immunized for comparable periods of time and
(3) the sera from several species contained significant amounts of 'natural' neutralizing activity that could interfere with evaluation of the immune response.

Voss *et al.* (1969) immunized nurse sharks with DNP substituted keyhole limpet haemocyanin (KLH) and found antibody activity to be associated with the HMW and LMW immunoglobulin fractions. Shark antibody to DNP induced a shift in the spectrum of ε-DNP-L-lysine similar to the shifts in the spectrum of DNP induced by mammalian antibody. The spectral shifts are thought to be related to the presence of tryptophan in the combining site regions of the antibody (Little & Eisen 1967). HMW and LMW antibody to DNP exhibited an average association constant (K_0) of 2×10^5 l/mole and 5 and 1 combining sites respectively for ε-DNP-L-lysine. The authors demonstrated the complications that a second, low affinity ($K_0 \sim 10^3$) antibody population would place on the estimation of valence in both the HMW and LMW preparations. Low affinity antibody populations previously have been shown to account for underestimation of the valence of rabbit IgM (Onoue *et al.* 1968). Clem and Small analysed the immune response of the giant grouper to DNP substituted carriers (1970). Grouper HMW immunoglobulin to DNP consisted of two binding populations exhibiting a valence of 4, with K_0 values of 8×10^4 M^{-1} and $2{\cdot}2 \times 10^6$ M^{-1} for the low and high affinity antibody respectively. The purified LMW immunoglobulin population also exhibited both high and low affinity binding site populations with K_0 values of $1{\cdot}2 \times 10^6$

-8×10^6 M^{-1} associated with the early immune high affinity binding populations (assuming a valence of 1 for the LMW antibody). In contrast to the increase in antibody K_0 during the course of immunization in mammalian, reptilian and avian species or the lack of change in K_0 during DNP immunization of another marine teleost, the gray snapper (Russell *et al.* 1970), the K_0 of grouper HMW and LMW antibody to DNP decreased during active immunization.[13] While this finding clearly distinguishes one aspect of the lower vertebrate immune response to haptens from comparable immune responses in higher vertebrates, the functional comparisons of antibody (e.g. active site K_0 values) are difficult to evaluate. It is highly probable that different immunoglobulin classes modulate active site characteristics (geometry, relative hydrophobicity, etc.) and limit the maximum association constant a given antibody can exhibit for a hapten. Therefore IgM-like proteins may only bind haptens at association constants of $\sim 10^4$–10^6, while immunoglobulins more closely resembling IgG may bind haptens at K_0 values of $\sim 10^6$–10^8. In fact, LMW reptilian (Litman *et al.* 1973a) and avian (Gallagher & Voss 1969) immunoglobulins exhibit K_0 values for dinitrophenol ligands well within the accepted range of K_0 values for mammalian antibody.

In an attempt to further explore the active site characteristics of lower vertebrate antibody to DNP derivatives, we analysed the induced shifts in the absorption spectrum of DNP and affinity labelling characteristics of turtle and duck antibody directed at 2′4′-DNP (Litman *et al.* (1973a). The molecular basis of induced spectral shifts has been mentioned above. Affinity labelling involves the binding of hapten analogues possessing at least one function capable of modifying (covalent derivatization) reactive amino acid(s). As the affinity-labelling reagent is recognized by the antibody as a hapten analogue, the chemical modification(s) are largely restricted to the immediate environment of the combining site. Once the affinity label is covalently bound in the active site, the following can be determined:

(1) the ratio of affinity label on heavy and light chains,
(2) the identity of the modified amino acid;
(3) the location of the modified residue in the primary structure (Singer & Doolittle 1966).

Table 10.3 summarizes our analyses of the induced shifts in the absorption spectrum of bound ε-DNP-L-lysine and the affinity-labelling characteristics of turtle and duck antibody to DNP. Both antibody species induced spectral shifts which could be interpreted as indications of the involvement of tryptophan in the active site of these antibodies. The significant differences in the spectra of ε-DNP-L-lysine in the presence of turtle, duck and rabbit antibody most likely reflect variations in the chemical microenvironment of the combining sites. Affinity labelling with a DNP analogue, m-nitrobenzene-

Table 10.3. Comparison of active sites directed at dinitrophenol (DNP) ligands

	Turtle LMW Ig	Duck LMW Ig	Rabbit IgG
Molecular weight	120,000	118,000	150,000
Induced shift in absorption spectra of ε-DNP-L-Lysine (difference maxima)	390, 468 nm	396, 474 nm	390 ± 2, 470 ± 3 nm$^{(1)}$
k_0, ε-DNP-L-Lysine pre MNBDF modification	$1{\cdot}7 \times 10^6$ M^{-1}	$3{\cdot}8 \times 10^5$ M^{-1}	$2\text{–}5 \times 10^6$ M^{-1}
k_0, ε-DNP-L-Lysine post MNBDF modification	$1{\cdot}7 \times 10^6$ M^{-1}	$3{\cdot}2 \times 10^5$ M^{-1}	—
Combining sites/molecule	$1{\cdot}7 \pm 0{\cdot}1$	$1{\cdot}5 \pm 0{\cdot}1$	$2{\cdot}0 \pm 0{\cdot}1$
Combining sites/molecule lost by MNBDF modification	0·5	0·2	0·5$^{(2)}$
Moles MNBDF incorporated per mole of antibody	0·4	0·3	0·6$^{(2)}$
Residue modified	tyrosine/ histidine (5:1)	tyrosine	tyrosine$^{(2)}$
Labelling ratio heavy/light chain	2·7:1	1·4:1	2:1$^{(2)}$

MNBDF is meta-nitrobenzenediazoniumfluoroborate. Turtle and duck LMW Ig (immunoglobulin) preparations contained 0·3 and 0·5 moles residual bound DNP/mole of antibody. (1) Little and Eisen (1967) (2) Good *et al.* (1967). Values for turtle LMW Ig, duck LMW Ig are from Litman *et al.* (1973a). Consult original manuscripts for details of MNBDF modifications.

diazoniumfluoroborate, modified tyrosine and histidine in turtle LMW immunoglobulin and tyrosine in duck LMW immunoglobulin; tyrosine has previously been shown to be the principal amino acid modified in the anti-DNP antibody from several mammalian species (Good *et al.* 1968). The ratio of heavy to light chain modification in turtle and duck antibody was in the accepted range (Good *et al.* 1967, 1968) for mammalian antibody to DNP. Although we have no information at present regarding the location of the affinity label within the primary structure of the turtle and duck antibody molecules, these preliminary studies suggest similar combining sites for reptilian, avian and mammalian antibody to dinitrophenol(s).[14]

Natural antibody

Another important aspect of antibody-combining sites pertains to the natural antibody demonstrated in the serum of both lower and higher vertebrates. Rudikoff *et al.* (1970) and Leslie and Clem (1970) detected antibody to the DNP grouping in the serum of non-immunized nurse sharks. This natural antibody could be functionally distinguished from immune antibody by the former's failure to bind to DNP-immunoadsorbents. Extensive analyses of the purified antibody have indicated its structural identity to nurse shark immunoglobulin (Clem *et al.* 1967) and have localized the binding activity to a pepsin derived Fab'_2 subunit. The purified natural antibody to DNP agglutinated several types of red blood cells and bound haptens other than DNP, while spectral shift studies with bis-α-ε-DNP-lysine suggested the participation of tryptophan in the active site (Voss *et al.* 1971). The more avid binding of bis-α-ε-DNP-lysine versus ε-DNP-lysine was felt to be due to relatively 'independent' combining sites for DNP in the individual Fab portions of the heavy and light chains; it is more likely, however, that the less polar α-ε-DNP-lysine permits a more avid association with the hydrophobic active site of the natural antibody. Based on certain primary structure considerations, we have suggested that immunoglobulins may exhibit generalized hydrophobic binding sites for a variety of ligands similar to the generalized binding sites Glazer (1970) postulated for several globulin proteins (Litman *et al.* 1970b). Natural antibody to DNP in sharks and other lower vertebrates may very well represent a phylogenetically early expression of such a phenomenon.

The sera of lower vertebrates also contain proteins which exhibit receptor sites for carbohydrates. The classification of these proteins and the nature of their reactions with carbohydrates are extremely important, as these molecules may represent a significant alternative recognition system to classical antibody. Springer and co-workers (Springer & Desai 1971, Bezkorovainy *et al.* 1971) isolated the 7S globulin with anti-human H(O) blood group specificity from the eel, a teleost fish. The purified protein possessed a molecular weight of 123,000 and was comprised of three non-covalently bonded subunits; each subunit in turn was comprised of four covalently bonded 10,000 molecular weight subunits. Five to eight moles of monosaccharide were bound per mole of protein and the agglutinin underwent precipitation upon binding monosaccharides in spite of fact that lattice formation with these carbohydrates was not possible. Circular dichroism in the far UV indicated significant conformational differences between the eel agglutinin and vertebrate immunoglobulin (Jirgensons *et al.* 1970). Normal nurse shark serum contains several structurally distinct proteins reactive with fructosans (Harisdangkul *et al.* (1972a). Unlike natural antibody to DNP, these proteins are not structurally related to nurse shark immunoglobulin. The reactive proteins have a molecular weight of ~280,500 and are comprised of four non-covalently linked subunits (Harisdangkul *el al.* 1972b). Baldo and Fletcher (1973) recently have described C-reactive protein-like precipitins in the plaice, a marine teleost. The proteins reacted with extracts of bacteria, fungi and worm and resembled mammalian C-reactive protein in electrophoretic mobility and behaviour in double diffusion reactions. Thus, the carbohydrate-binding proteins do not seem to resemble antibody but may instead be related to the acute phase proteins described in mammals. More complete physicochemical characterization will be necessary to substantiate this hypothesis.

Summary

The immunoglobulins from a sufficient number of phylogenetically critical species have been characterized, thereby permitting evaluation of the structural and functional evolution of this important class of macromolecule. Three major patterns of structural evolution can be discerned:

(1) species derived from the primitive Ostracoderms possess an inducible form of antibody, sharing a number of structural features with higher vertebrate immunoglobulin, yet differing in that they lack interchain disulphide bonding;
(2) species derived from the Placoderms (with the exception of those forms found along the evolutionary line of the Sarcopterygii) possess a single class of immunoglobulin resembling mammalian IgM; functional variability in these molecules may have been achieved through alterations in polymer composition (Hornick & Karush 1972);
(3) the Placoderm-derived vertebrates sharing common ancestors with the Sarcopterygii, and including representative amphibians, reptiles, avians and mammals, possess at least one class of immunoglobulin in addition to the IgM-like proteins.

The evolution of this second class of immunoglobulin was accompanied by variation in heavy chain size, presumably in the Fc region, and most likely associated with expansion of secondary biologic function. The variation was accomplished through mechanisms related to gene duplication and has been discussed at length (Marchalonis 1969, Zimmerman *et al.* 1971, Litman 1971a, Marchalonis & Cone 1973).

In the course of phylogenetic development, the immunoglobulins of Placoderm-derived vertebrates exhibited considerable variation in polymer composition, heavy chain length and intersubunit non-covalent bonding. However, other physicochemical properties such as intersubunit disulphide bonding, secondary structure, amino acid composition and electrophoretic heterogeneity were largely unchanged. The limited amounts of amino acid sequence data available for lower vertebrate immunoglobulin heavy and light chain variable regions indicate considerable degrees of interspecies homology.[15] The active sites of avian, reptilian and mammalian antibody to DNP are remarkably similar in their association constant for the DNP ligand, the participation of tryptophan in the active site and their affinity labelling characteristics. Although difficult to compare to other protein systems, it can be concluded that the evolution of immunoglobulins has been generally of a conservative nature.

The comprehensive physicochemical characterization of lower vertebrate immunoglobulin has provided us with valuable insights:

(1) a near complete evaluation in terms of general structural properties from a comparative standpoint of the evolution of this class of molecule;
(2) a view of alternate humoral immune recognition systems such as natural antibody and non-immunoglobulin, carbohydrate reactive proteins;
(3) an explanation of the mechanism involved in class and subclass antibody diversification;
(4) some perception of genetic mechanisms at work in encoding the variable regions of heavy and light chains.

More complete analyses of lower vertebrate immunoglobulin primary structure, particularly in the protein regions where hypervariability has been detected in mammalian immunoglobulin, will assist in evaluation of current theories regarding generation of antibody diversity (Hood & Talmage 1970).

Acknowledgments

I wish to thank Drs J. M. Kehoe and J. D. Capra for providing preprints of their work on the amino acid sequence of heavy chain variable regions and for many invaluable discussions. The assistance of Ronda Litman in preparation of the manuscript is most appreciated. Past support for our laboratory was provided by grants from The National Foundation March of Dimes, U.S. Public Health Service (AI-08677, NS-02024, HE-06314), University of Minnesota Graduate School and American Cancer Society to Dr R. A. Good or Dr G. W. Litman. Current support to the laboratory of Dr Litman is from NCI CA-08748, NCICA-17404 and the American Cancer Society BC-162.

References

Abel C.A., Spiegelberg H.L. & Grey H.M. (1968) The carbohydrate content of fragments and polypeptide chains of human γ-G-myeloma proteins of different heavy chain subclasses. *Biochemistry* **7,** 1271.

Acton R.T., Weinheimer P.F., Wolcott M., Evans E.E. & Bennett J.C. (1970) N-terminal sequences of immunoglobulin heavy and light chains from three species of lower vertebrates. *Nature* **228,** 991.

Acton R.T., Weinheimer P.F., Dupree H.K., Evans E.E. & Bennett J.C. (1971a) Phylogeny of immunoglobulins. Characterization of a 14S immunoglobulin from the gar, *Lepisosteus osseus. Biochemistry* **10,** 2028.

Acton R.T., Weinheimer P.F., Dupree H.K., Russel T.R., Wolcott M., Evans E.E., Schrohenloher R.E. & Bennett J.C. (1971b) Isolation and characterization of the immune macroglobulin from the paddlefish, *Polyodon spathula. J. Biol. Chem.* **246,** 6760.

ACTON R.T., WEINHEIMER P.F., HALL S.J., NIEDERMEIER W., SHELTON E. & BENNETT J.C. (1971c) Tetrameric immune macroglobulins in three orders of bony fishes. *Proc. Nat. Acad. Sci.* **68,** 107.

ACTON R.T., EVANS E.E., WEINHEIMER P.F., NIEDERMEIER W. & BENNETT J.C. (1972a) Purification and characterization of two classes of immunoglobulins from the marine toad, *Bufo marinus. Biochemistry* **11,** 2751.

ACTON R.T., NIEDERMEIER W., WEINHEIMER P.F., CLEM L.W., LESLIE G.A. & BENNETT J.C. (1972b) The carbohydrate composition of immunoglobulins from diverse species of vertebrates. *J. Immunol.* **109,** 371.

ACTON R.T., WEINHEIMER P.F., SHELTON E., NIEDERMEIER W. & BENNETT J.C. (1972c) Phylogeny of immunoglobulins-purification and physico-chemical characterization of the immune macroglobulin from the turtle, *Pseudemus seripta. Immunochemistry* **9,** 421.

ATWELL J.L., MARCHALONIS J.J. & EALEY E.H.M. (1973) Major immunoglobulin classes of the echidna, *Tachyglossus aculeatus. Immunology* **25,** 835.

BALDO B.A. & FLETCHER T.C. (1973) C-reactive protein—precipitins in plaice. *Nature* **246,** 145.

BEYCHOK S. (1968) Rotatory dispersion and circular dichroism. *Ann. Rev. Biochem.* **37,** 437.

BEZKOROVAINY A., SPRINGER G.F. & DESAI P.R. (1971) Physicochemical properties of the eel anti-human blood group H(O) antibody. *Biochemistry* **10,** 3761.

BIENENSTOCK J., PEREY D.Y.E., GAULDIE J. & UNDERDOWN B.J. (1973) Chicken γ-A: Physicochemical and immunochemical characteristics. *J. Immunol.* **110,** 524.

BRADSHAW C.M., CLEM L.W. & SIGEL M.M. (1971) Immunologic and immunochemical studies on the gar, *Lepisosteus platyrhincus. J. Immunol.* **106,** 1480.

CAPRA J.D., WASSERMAN R.L. & KEHOE J.M. (1973) Phylogenetically associated residues within the V_{HIII} subgroup of several mammalian species. Evidence for a 'paucigene' basis for antibody diversity. *J. Exp. Med.* **138,** 410.

CHARTRAND S.L., LITMAN G.W., LAPOINTE N., GOOD R.A. & FROMMEL D. (1971) The evolution of the immune response. XII. The immunoglobulins of the turtle. Molecular requirements for biological activity of the 5·7S immunoglobulin. *J. Immunol.* **107,** 1.

CHOI Y.S. & GOOD R.A. (1971) New immunoglobulin-like molecules in the serum of bursectomized-irradiated chickens. *Proc. Nat. Acad. Sci.* **68,** 2083.

CHUANG C., CAPRA J.D. & KEHOE J.M. (1973) Immunoglobulin evolution—Relationship between carboxyterminal region of a human α-chain and other immunoglobulin heavy chain constant regions. *Nature* **244,** 158.

CLEM L.W., DEBOUTAUD F. & SIGEL M.M. (1967) Phylogeny of immunoglobulin structure and function. II. Immunoglobulins of the nurse shark. *J. Immunol.* **99,** 1226.

CLEM L.W. & SMALL P.A. (1967) Phylogeny of immunoglobulin structure and function. I. Immunoglobulins of the lemon shark. *J. Exp. Med.* **125,** 893.

CLEM L.W. & SMALL P.A. (1970) Phylogeny of immunoglobulin structure and function. V. Valences and association constants of teleost antibodies to a haptenic determinant. *J. Exp. Med.* **132,** 385.

CLEM L.W. (1971) Phylogeny of immunoglobulin structure and function. IV. Immunoglobulins of the giant grouper, *Epinephelus itaira. J. Biol. Chem.* **246,** 9.

CLEM L.W. & LESLIE G.A. (1971) Production of 19S IgM antibodies with restricted heterogeneity from sharks. *Proc. Nat. Acad. Sci.* **68,** 139.

DAYHOFF M.O. (ed.) (1972–3) In *Atlas of Protein Sequence and Structure*, Vol 5, National Biomedical Research Foundation, Silver Spring, Md.

DIENER E. & MARCHALONIS J.J. (1970) Cellular and humoral aspects of the primary immune response of the toad, *Bufo marinus. Immunology* **18,** 279.

DREESMAN G.R. & BENEDICT A.A. (1965) Reductive dissociation of chicken γ-G immunoglobulins in neutral solvents without a dispersing agent. *Proc. Nat. Acad. Sci.* **54,** 822.

EDELMAN G.M. & GALL W.E. (1969) The antibody problem. *Ann. Rev. Biochem.* **38,** 415.

FROMMEL D., LITMAN G.W., CHARTRAND S., SEAL U.S. & GOOD R.A. (1971a) Significance of carbohydrate composition in immunoglobulin evolution. *Immunochemistry* **8,** 573.

FROMMEL D., LITMAN G.W., FINSTAD J. & GOOD R.A. (1971b) Evolution of the immune response. XI. Immunoglobulins of the horned shark: Purification, characterization and biological properties. *J. Immunol.* **106,** 1234.

GALLAGHER J.S. & VOSS E.W. (1969) Binding properties of purified chicken antibody. *Immunochemistry,* **6,** 573.

GLAZER A.N. (1970) On the prevalence of 'nonspecific' binding at the specific binding sites of globular proteins. *Proc. Nat. Acad. Sci.* **65,** 1057.

GOOD A.H., TRAYLOR P.S. & SINGER S.J. (1967) Affinity labeling of the active sites of rabbit anti 2,4-dinitrophenyl antibodies with m-nitrobenzene diazonium fluoroborate. *Biochemistry* **6,** 873.

GOOD A.H., OVARY Z. & SINGER S.J. (1968) Affinity labeling of the active sites of anti 2,4-dintrophenyl antibodies from different species. *Biochemistry* **7,** 1304.

GOOD R.A. & PAPERMASTER B.W. (1964) Ontogeny and phylogeny of adaptive immunity. *Advances in Immunology* **4,** 1.

GOODMAN J.W., KLAUS G.G., NITECKI D.E. & WANG A.-C. (1970) Pyrrolidonecarboxylic acid at the N-terminal positions of polypeptide chains from leopard shark immunoglobulins. *J. Immunol.* **104,** 260.

GRANT J.A., SANDERS B. & HOOD L. (1971) Partial amino acid sequences of chicken and turkey immunoglobulin light chains. Homology with mammalian λ chains. *Biochemistry* **10,** 3123.

GREENFIELD N. & FASMAN G.D. (1969) Computed circular dichroism spectra for the evaluation of protein conformation. *Biochemistry* **8,** 4108.

GREY H.M. (1969) Phylogeny of immunoglobulins. *Advances in Immunology* **10,** 51.

HADJI-AZIMI I. (1971) Studies on *Xenopus laevis* immunoglobulins. *Immunology* **21,** 463.

HALL S.J., EVANS E.E., DUPREE H.K., ACTON R.T., WEINHEIMER P.F. & BENNETT J.C. (1973) Characterization of a teleost immunoglobulin: the immune macroglobulin from the channel catfish, *Ictalurus punctatus. Comp. Biochem. Physiol.* **46,** 187.

HALPERN M.S. & KOSHLAND M.E. (1970) Novel subunit in secretory IgA. *Nature* **228,** 1276.

HARISDANGKUL V., KABAT E.A., MCDONOUGH R.J. & SIGEL M.M. (1972a) A protein in normal nurse shark serum which reacts specifically with fructosans. I. Purification and immunochemical characterization. *J. Immunol.* **108,** 1244.

HARISDANGKUL V., KABAT E.A., MCDONOUGH R.J. & SIGEL M.M. (1972b) A protein in normal nurse shark serum which reacts specifically with fructosans. II. Physicochemical studies. *J. Immunol.* **108,** 1259.

HERSKOVITS T.T. & SORENSEN M. (1968) Studies of the location of tyrosyl and tryptophyl residues in proteins. I. Solvent perturbation data of model compounds. *Biochemistry* **7,** 2523.

HOOD L., EICHMANN K., LACKLUND H., KRAUSE R.M. & OHMS J.J. (1970) Rabbit antibody light chains and gene evolution. *Nature* **228,** 1040.

HOOD L. & TALMAGE D.W. (1970) Mechanism of antibody diversity: germ line basis for variability. *Science,* **168,** 325.

HORNICK C.L. & KARUSH F. (1972) The role of multivalence. *Immunochemistry* **9,** 325.

JIRGENSONS B., SPRINGER F.G. & DESAI P.R. (1970) Comparative circular dichroism studies of individual eel and human antibodies. *Comp. Biochem. Physiol.* **34,** 721.

JOHNSTON W.J., ACTON R.T., WEINHEIMER P.F., NIEDERMEIER W., EVANS E.E., SHELTON E.

& BENNETT J.C. (1971) Isolation and physico-chemical characterization of the 'IgM-like' immunoglobulin from the sting ray, *Dasyatis americana*. *J. Immunol.* **107,** 870.

KEHOE J.M. & CAPRA J.D. (1974) Phylogenetic aspects of immunoglobulin variable region diversity. In *Contemporary Topics in Molecular Immunology*, volume 3. ed. Inman S.P. Plenum Press, New York.

KLAPPER D.G., CLEM L.W. & SMALL P.A. (1971) Proteolytic fragmentation of elasmobranch immunoglobulins. *Biochemistry* **10,** 645.

KLAUS G.G.B., HALPERN M.S., KOSHLAND M.E. & GOODMAN J.W. (1971a) A polypeptide chain from leopard shark 19S immunoglobulin analogous to mammalian J chain. *J. Immunol.* **107,** 1785.

KLAUS G.G.B., NITECKI D.E. & GOODMAN J.W. (1971b) Amino acid sequences of free and blocked N-termini of leopard shark immunoglobulins. *J. Immunol.* **107,** 1256.

KÖHLER H., SHIMIZU A., PAUL C., MOORE V. & PUTNAM F.W. (1970) Three variable-gene pools common to IgM, IgG and IgA immunoglobulins. *Nature* **227,** 1318.

KUBO R.T., ROSENBLUM I.Y. & BENEDICT A.A. (1970) The unblocked N-terminal sequence of chicken IgG λ-like light chains. *J. Immunol.* **105,** 534.

KUBO R.T., ROSENBLUM I.Y. & BENEDICT A.A. (1971) Amino terminal sequences of heavy and light chains of chicken anti-dinitrophenyl antibody. *J. Immunol.* **107,** 1781.

LEBACQ-VERHEYDEN A.M., VAERMAN J.P. & HEREMANS J.F. (1972) A possible homologue of mammalian IgA in chicken serum and secretions. *Immunology* **22,** 165.

LESLIE G.A. & CLEM L.W. (1969a) Phylogeny of immunoglobulin structure and function. III. Immunoglobulins of the chicken. *J. exp. Med.* **130,** 1337.

LESLIE G.A. & CLEM L.W. (1969b) Production of anti-hapten antibodies by several classes of lower vertebrates. *J. Immunol.* **103,** 613.

LESLIE G.A. & CLEM L.W. (1970) Reactivity of normal shark immunoglobulins with nitrophenol ligands. *J. Immunol.* **105,** 1547.

LESLIE G.A., CLEM L.W. & ROWE D. (1971) The molecular weight of human IgD heavy chains. *Immunochemistry* **8,** 565.

LESLIE G.A. & CLEM L.W. (1972) Phylogeny of immunoglobulin structure and function. VI. 17S, 7·5S and 5·7S anti-DNP of the turtle, *Pseudamys scripta*. *J. Immunol.* **108,** 1656.

LESLIE G.A. & CLEM L.W. (1973) Chicken antibodies to group A streptococcal carbohydrate. *J. Immunol.* **110,** 191.

LESLIE G.A. & MARTIN L.N. (1973) Studies on the secretory immunologic system of fowl. III. Serum and secretory IgA of the chicken. *J. Immunol.* **110,** 1.

LINTHICUM D.S. & HILDEMANN W.H. (1970) Immunologic responses of pacific hagfish. III. Serum antibodies to cellular antigens. *J. Immunol.* **105,** 912.

LITMAN G.W., FROMMEL D., FINSTAD J., HOWELL J., POLLARA B.W. & GOOD R.A. (1970a) The evolution of the immune response. VIII. Structural studies of the lamprey immunoglobulin. *J. Immunol.* **105,** 1278.

LITMAN G.W., GOOD R.A., FROMMEL D. & ROSENBERG A. (1970b) Biophysical studies of the immunoglobulins: The conformational significance of the intrachain disulfide linkages. *Proc. Nat. Acad. Sci.* **67,** 1085.

LITMAN G.W., FROMMEL D., CHARTRAND S., FINSTAD J. & GOOD R.A. (1971a) Significance of heavy chain mass and antigenic relationships in immunoglobulin evolution. *Immunochemistry* **8,** 345.

LITMAN G.W., FROMMEL D., FINSTAD J. & GOOD R.A. (1971b) Evolution of the immune response. IX. Immunoglobulins of the bowfin: Purification and characterization. *J. Immunol.* **106,** 747.

LITMAN G.W., FROMMEL D., FINSTAD J. & GOOD R.A. (1971c) Evolution of the immune response. X. Immunoglobulins of the bowfin: Subunit and multichain structure. *J. Immunol.* **107,** 881.

LITMAN G.W., FROMMEL D., ROSENBERG A. & GOOD R.A. (1971d) Circular dichroic analysis of immunoglobulins in phylogenetic perspective. *Biochim. Biophys. Acta* **36**, 647.

LITMAN G.W., WANG A.C., FUDENBERG H.H. & GOOD R.A. (1971e) N-terminal amino acid sequence of African lungfish immunoglobulin light chain. *Proc. Nat. Acad. Sci.* **68**, 2321.

LITMAN G.W., CHARTRAND S., FINSTAD C. & GOOD R.A. (1973a) Active sites of turtle and duck antibody to 2′4′ dinitrophenol. *Immunochemistry* **10**, 323.

LITMAN G.W., LITMAN R.S., GOOD R.A. & ROSENBERG A. (1973b) Molecular dissection of IgG: Conformational interrelationships of the subunits of human IgG. *Biochemistry* **12**, 2004.

LITTLE J.R. & EISEN H.N. (1967) Evidence for tryptophan in the active sites of antibodies to polynitrobenzenes. *Biochemistry* **6**, 3119.

MARCHALONIS J. & EDELMAN G.M. (1965) Phylogenetic origins of antibody structure. I. Multichain structure of immunoglobulins in the smooth dogfish (*Mustelus canis*). *J. exp. Med.* **122**, 601.

MARCHALONIS J. & EDELMAN G.M. (1966a) Phylogenetic origins of antibody structure. II. Immunoglobulins in the primary immune response of the bullfrog, *Rana catesbiana. J. exp. Med.* **124**, 901.

MARCHALONIS J. & EDELMAN G.M. (1966b) Polypeptide chains of immunoglobulins from the smooth dogfish (*Mustelus canis*). *Science* **154**, 1567.

MARCHALONIS J.J. & EDELMAN G.M. (1968) Phylogenetic origins of antibody structure. III. Antibodies in the primary immune response of the sea lamprey, *Petromyzon marinus. J. exp. Med.* **127**, 891.

MARCHALONIS J.J., EALEY E.H.M. & DIENER E. (1969) Immune response of the tuatara, *Sphenodon punctatum. Aust. J. Exp. Biol. Med. Sci.* **47**, 367.

MARCHALONIS J.J. (1969) Isolation and characterization of immunoglobulin-like proteins of the Australian lungfish (*Neoceratodus forsteri*). *Aust. J. Exp. Biol. Med. Sci.* **47**, 405.

MARCHALONIS J.J., ALLEN R.B. & SAARNI E.S. (1970) Immunoglobulin classes of the clawed toad, *Xenopus laevis. Comp. Biochem. Physiol.* **35**, 49.

MARCHALONIS J.J. & SCHONFELD S.A. (1970) Polypeptide chain structure of sting ray immunoglobulin. *Biochim. Biophys. Acta* **221**, 604.

MARCHALONIS J.J. (1971) Isolation and partial characterization of immunoglobulins of goldfish (*Carassius auratus*) and carp (*Cyprinus carpio*). *Immunology* **20**, 161.

MARCHALONIS J.J. & WELTMAN J.K. (1971) Relatedness among proteins: A new method of estimation and its application to immunoglobulins. *Comp. Biochem. Physiol.* **36**, 609.

MARCHALONIS J.J. (1972) Conservatism in the evolution of immunoglobulin. *Nature New Biology* **236**, 84.

MARCHALONIS J.J. & COHEN N. (1973) Isolation and partial characterization of immunoglobulin from a urodele amphibian. *Immunology* **24**, 395.

MARCHALONIS J.J. & CONE R.E. (1973) The phylogenetic emergence of vertebrate immunity. *Aust. J. Exp. Biol. Med. Sci.* **51**, 461.

MERZ D.C., FINSTAD C.L., LITMAN G.W. & GOOD R.A. (1975) Aspects of vertebrate immunoglobulin evolution. Constancy in light chain electrophoretic behavior. *Immunochemistry* **12**, 499.

NOVOTONY J., FRANEK F. & SORM F. (1970) Large scale isolation, characterization and classification of pig immunoglobulin κ-chains. *Eur. J. Biochem.* **14**, 309.

ONOUE K., GROSSBERG A.L., YAGI Y. & PRESSMAN D. (1968) Immunoglobulin M antibodies with ten combining sites. *Science* **162**, 574.

PARKHOUSE R.M.E., ASKONAS B.A. & DOURMASHKIN R.R. (1970) Electron microscopic studies of mouse immunoglobulin M; Structure and reconstitution following reduction. *Immunology* **18**, 575.

POLLARA B., SURAN A., FINSTAD J. & GOOD R.A. (1968) N-terminal amino acid sequences of immunoglobulin chains in *Polyodon spathula. Proc. Nat. Acad. Sci.* **59,** 1307.

POLLARA B., CHARTRAND S.L. & GOOD R.A. (1970a) An unusual immunoglobulin in *Polyodon spathula. Fed. Proc.* **29,** 772.

POLLARA B., LITMAN G.W., FINSTAD J., HOWELL J. & GOOD R.A. (1970b) The evolution of the immune response. VII. Antibody to human 'O' cells and properties of the immunoglobulin in lamprey. *J. Immunol.* **105,** 738.

PORTER R.R. (1959) The hydrolysis of rabbit γ-globulin and antibodies with crystalline papain. *Biochem. J.* **73,** 119.

PUTNAM F.W., FLORENT G., PAUL C., SHINODA T. & SHIMIZU A. (1973) Complete amino acid sequence of the mu heavy chain of a human IgM immunoglobulin. *Science* **182,** 287.

RICHTER R., NUHN P., AMBROSIUS H., ZAGYANSKY YU.A., TUMERMAN L.A. & NEZLIN R.S. (1972) Restricted flexibility of carp 15S immunoglobulin molecules as revealed by fluorescence polarization. *FEBS Letters* **27,** 184.

ROMER A.S. (1970) In *The Vertebrate Body*, fourth edition. W. B. Saunders, Philadelphia.

RUDIKOFF S., VOSS E. & SIGEL M.M. (1970) Biological and chemical properties of natural antibodies in the nurse shark. *J. Immunol.* **105,** 1344.

RUSSELL W.J., VOSS E.W. & SIGEL M.M. (1970) Some characteristics of anti-dinitrophenyl antibody of the gray snapper. *J. Immunol.* **105,** 262.

SALUK P.H., KRAUSS J. & CLEM L.W. (1970) The presence of two antigenically distinct light chains (κ and λ?) in alligator immunoglobulins. *Proc. Soc. Exp. Biol. Med.* **133,** 365.

SANDERS B.G., TRAVIS J.C. & WILEY K.L. (1973) Chicken low molecular weight immunoglobulin heavy chains: A comparison with the gamma chain of man. *Comp. Biochem. Physiol.* **45,** 189.

SHELTON E. & SMITH M. (1970) The ultrastructure of carp (*Cyprinus carpio*) immunoglobulin: A tetrameric macroglobulin. *J. Mol. Biol.* **54,** 615.

SINGER S.J. & DOOLITTLE R.F. (1966) Antibody active sites and immunoglobulin molecules. *Science* **153,** 13.

SPRINGER G.F. & DESAI P.R. (1971) Monosaccharides as specific precipitinogens of eel anti-human blood group H(O) antibody. *Biochemistry* **10,** 3749.

SURAN A.A. & PAPERMASTER B.W. (1967a) N-terminal sequences of heavy and light chains of leopard shark immunoglobulins: Evolutionary implications. *Proc. Nat. Acad. Sci.* **58,** 1619.

SURAN A.A., TARAIL M.H. & PAPERMASTER B.W. (1967b) Immunoglobulins of the leopard shark. I. Isolation and characterization of 17S and 7S immunoglobulins with precipitating activity. *J. Immunol.* **99,** 679.

THOENES G.H. & HILDEMANN W.H. (1970) Immunological responses of pacific hagfish. II. Serum antibody production to soluble antigen, p. 711. In *Developmental Aspects of Antibody Formation and Structure*, volume II, ed. Sterzl J. & Riha I. Czechoslovak Academy of Sciences, Prague.

VOSS E.W., RUSSELL W.J. & SIGEL M.M. (1969) Purification and binding properties of nurse shark antibody. *Biochemistry* **8,** 4866.

VOSS E.W., RUDIKOFF S. & SIGEL M.M. (1971) Comparative ligand binding by purified nurse shark antibodies and anti-2,4 dinitrophenyl antibodies from other species. *J. Immunol.* **107,** 12.

WANG A.C., PINK J.R.L., FUDENBERG H.H. & OHMS J. (1970) A variable region subclass of heavy chain common to immunoglobulins G, A and M and characterized by an unblocked amino terminal residue. *Proc. Nat. Acad. Sci.* **66,** 657.

Weinheimer P.F., Mestecky J. & Acton R.T. (1971) Species distribution of J chain. *J. Immunol.* **107,** 1211.

Wilde C.E. III & Koshland M.E. (1973) Molecular size and shape of J chain from polymeric immunoglobulins. *Biochemistry* **12,** 3218.

Zagyansky Yu.A. (1973) Phylogenesis of the general structure of immunoglobulins. Rigidity of 7S immunoglobulins and restricted flexibility of the 17S immunoglobulins of the tortoise, *Testudo horsfieldi. FEBS Letters* **35,** 309.

Zimmerman B., Shalatin N. & Grey H.M. (1971) Structural studies on the duck 5·7S and 7·8S immunoglobulins. *Biochemistry* **10,** 482.

Zimmerman B. & Grey H.M. (1972) Noncovalent interactions between immunoglobulin polypeptide chains. Stability to dissociation by denaturants. *Biochemistry* **11,** 78.

Footnotes to Chapter 10

1. Analysis of the 1,000,000 Molecular Weight hagfish immunoglobulin employing polyacrylamide gel electrophoresis in sodium dodecyl sulfate suggest that the immunoglobulin is comprised of only light chain-like (33,000 – 17,000 Molecular Weight) subunits. De Ioannes, A.E. and Hildemann, W.H. (1975) in *Immunologic Phylogeny*, Ed. Hildemann, W.H. and Benedict, A.A. *Adv. Exptl. Med. and Biol.* **64,** 151.

2. In addition see Sigel, M.M. *Ann. N.Y. Acad. Sci.* (1974) **234,** 183.

3. Recent studies suggest that in terms of heavy chain mass and carbohydrate composition, the LMW immunoglobulins of two amphibian species, the marine toad *Bufo marinus* and the clawed toad *Xenopus laevis* are more like the IMW immunoglobulins of dipnoid and avian species than mammalian IgG to which these proteins have been compared. Atwell, J.L. and Marchalonis, J.J. (1975) *J. Immunogen.* **1,** 367.

4. See Vaerman, J. P. *et al.* (1975) in *Immunologic Phylogeny*, Ed. Hildemann, W. H. and Benedict, A.A. *Adv. Exptl. Med. and Biol.* **64,** 185 for a discussion of the occurrence of IgA-like immunoglobulin in the secretions of avians and the lack of evidence for such molecules in the secretions of reptiles. IgM-like molecules may be the principal form of secretory immunoglobulin in amphibians and reptiles. Portis, J.L. and Coe, J.E. (1975) *Nature* **258,** 547.

5. Bullfrog (*Rana catesbiana*) LMW (IMW?, see footnote #3) immunoglobulin apparently lacks inter heavy-light chain disulfide bonding. Steiner, L.A. *et al.* (1975) in *Immunologic Phylogeny*, Ed. Hildemann, W.H. and Benedict, A.A. *Adv. Exptl. Med. and Biol.* **64,** 173.

6. The first 1/2 cystine residue of nurse shark (*Ginglymostoma cirratum*) heavy and light chains are in homologous positions to the first intra-chain disulfide 1/2 cystine residue in mammalian immunoglobulin heavy and light chains. Sledge *et al.* (1974) *J. Immunol.* **112,** 941.

7. The J chain from the catfish (*Ictalurus punctatus*) has been characterized and found to lack significant primary structure (peptide map) homology or antigenic cross reactivity with mammalian IgM. Mestecky, J. *et al.* (1975) *J. Immunol.* **115,** 993.

8. In addition see Zagyansky, Y.A. (1975) *Arch. Biochem. Biophys* **116,** 371.

9. A superior approach to analysis of segmental flexibility in which a dansyl hapten is immobilized in the antigen combining site of anti-dansyl antibody has been proposed. Differences in the time dependent emission anisotropy of dansyl-lysine in the active sites of horse and pig IgM and HMW nurse shark (*Ginglymostoma cirratum*) antibody were noted and it was concluded that the HMW shark immunoglobulin apparently possesses a lesser degree of segmental flexibility than mammalian IgM. Cathou, R.E. and Holowka, D.A. (1975) in *Immunologic Phylogeny*, Ed. Hildemann, W.H. and Benedict, A.A. *Adv. Exptl Med. and Biol.* **64,** 207.

10. The V (variable) region subgroup designations are those proposed by the Conference on Nomenclature for Animal Immunoglobulins, *Bulletin World Health Organization* (1969) **41,** 975.

11. The sequence of the 28 N terminal residues of nurse shark heavy and light chains (footnote 6) represents the most extensive sequence to date of an immunoglobulin from a species below the phylogenetic level of the avians,

12. See in addition Wasserman *et al.* (1974) *J. Immunol.* **113,** 954.

13. Nurse sharks (*Ginglymostoma cirratum*) immunized with DNP-lysine substituted Streptococcal vaccine do not show increases in association constants for DNP when followed for periods as long as two years. Clem, L.W. *et al.* (1975) in *Immunologic Phylogeny*, Ed. Hildemann, W.H. and Benedict, A.A. *Adv. Exptl. and Biol.* **64,** 231.

14. Combining site depth, another parameter of active site structure, has been estimated in rainbow trout (*Salmo gairdneri*) antibody to DNP using an electron paramagnetic resonance technique. The depth of the trout active site was 10–12 Å equivalent to the depth of mammalian antibody to DNP. Roubal, W.T. *et al.* (1974) *J. Immunol.* **113,** 309.

15. Idiotypic dissimilarities between different purified nurse shark antibodies to streptococcal carbohydrates have been noted and are suggestive of the presence of hypervariable segments in the heavy and light chain variable regions of immunoglobulins from this species (see footnote 13).

Chapter 11. Immunoglobulin Classes of Lower Vertebrates Distinct from IgM Immunoglobulin

John L. Atwell and John J. Marchalonis

Introduction

Comments on evolutionary generalizations

General properties of the amphibian antibody response

Physicochemical characterization of amphibian immunoglobulins
Immunoglobulins of the urodeles

Physicochemical characterization of amphibian immunoglobulins *continued*
Immunoglobulins of anurans

Comparison of reduced 7S immunoglobulins from various vertebrate classes

7S immunoglobulins in evolution

Introduction

The immune system manifests a gradual but increasing degree of complexity in the phylogenetic progression from the more primitive vertebrate classes to the more advanced ones (Good & Papermaster 1964). This statement holds true for types of immunocompetent cells, organization of the lymphoid system, and for the variety of immunoglobulin classes occurring within a species. It is the goal of this chapter to analyse the structural properties of immunoglobulins of lower vertebrates which are distinct from the primitive and ubiquitous IgM antibody class (see Litman Chapter 10). Low molecular weight immunoglobulins distinct from IgM clearly are present in amphibians, and these were once considered to be direct homologues of the IgG molecules which constitute the predominant immunoglobulin class of mammals (Marchalonis & Edelman 1966). Moreover, most workers glibly refer to the 7S antibodies of avian species as IgG, assuming a profound structural homology between these antibodies and the IgG molecules of mammals. Data pertinent to avian antibodies are considered in detail by Benedict (Chapter 13). In this chapter, we will examine certain physicochemical properties of '7S' immunoglobulins of amphibians, reptiles, birds and lower mammals and will develop the thesis that antibodies directly homologous to mammalian IgG do not occur below the phylogenetic level of prototherian mammals.

Comments on evolutionary generalizations

When considering the origins of immunoglobulin classes, we would emphasize that any attempts to gain an understanding of evolutionary processes from studies of living forms are predicated upon a major assumption; namely, that living organisms which are considered primitive (e.g. sharks) retain the biochemical characteristics of their ancestors. However, evolutionary events within a single vertebrate class might parallel events which occurred during the divergence of classes. Parallel evolutionary developments would be fostered by the existence of similar environmental selective pressures. Although the selective pressures which prompted the emergence of distinct immunoglobulin classes via tandem duplication of cistrons encoding heavy chain constant regions are not clearly understood (Spiegleberg 1974), these factors were operative upon all the tetrapod classes of vertebrates. In fact, immunoglobulins distinct from IgM in heavy chain type preceded the emergence of amphibians and exist in lungfish (Marchalonis 1969, Litman *et al.* 1971a). Therefore, all vertebrate classes were probably subjected to some pressures to increase their range of immunoglobulin types. This selection was directed towards generating new constant region functions, rather than tuning up the parameters of antigen binding.

The appearance of the amphibians was a significant event in the evolution of vertebrates because it gave vertebrates a toe hold on the terrestrial environment. Moreover, amphibians, particularly the anurans, demonstrate a more complex lymphoid system than do the fishes. This is exemplified by the extensive lymphomyeloid complex (Cooper *et al.* 1971) and the jugular bodies (Diener & Nossal 1966) which show similarities to lymph nodes of mammals. Similar structures are lacking in fishes. In terms of the present discussion, we would note that anuran amphibians possess multiple classes of immunoglobulins (Marchalonis & Edelman 1966, Hadji-Azimi 1971, Lykakis 1969, Acton *et al.* 1972, Geczy *et al.* 1973). The appearance of 7S non-IgM antibodies might have resulted from confrontation with the collection of new environmental pressures which amphibians faced in their transition from an aquatic to a terrestrial environment.

The most exact criterion for the determination of the evolutionary relationship among proteins is by statistical comparison of the nucleotide codons which determine their amino acid sequences (Fitch 1966). Unfortunately, the amino acid sequence data available for heavy chains of nonmammalian species are fragmentary and deal only with the amino terminus of the molecule (Acton *et al.* 1970, Pollara *et al.* 1968, Kubo *et al.* 1971, Klaus *et al.* 1971, Litman *et al.* 1971b). These data indicate that strong homologies exist among the variable region sequences of diverse vertebrate species, but they are irrelevant to an understanding of constant region inter-relationships. Other parameters have been applied. For example, studies have been performed to determine whether immunoglobulins of non-mammalian species cross-reacted antigenically with mammalian immunoglobulins. It was found that the μ-chain of chicken IgM was antigenically related to human μ-chain, but no such similarity was observed for chicken 7S immunoglobulin (Mehta *et al.* 1972). Other γ-chain properties of an adventitious nature were also investigated. Staphylococcal A protein, for example, binds to human γ-chains and to the IgG molecules of virtually all mammalian species; it does not bind to the putative IgG molecules of chickens or amphibians (Kronvall *et al.* 1970). In the present discussion, we will rely heavily upon physicochemical criteria such as mass and electrophoretic behaviour on polyacrylamide gels of polypeptide chains as indices of comparison. Although such an approach is less stringent than comparison of amino acid sequences, it provides an objective means of assessing similarities and differences among heavy chains of antibodies of various species. We will combine this type of analysis with comparisons of biological properties in an attempt to sort out the relationships among the 7S non-IgM antibodies of the tetrapod vertebrates.

General properties of the amphibian antibody response

Three distinct classes of amphibians; apoda, urodela, and anura presently exist (see Chapter 8). A good deal of information is available on humoral immunity in anurans (see Marchalonis 1971 for review). A few studies have been performed on antibodies of urodeles (Ching & Wedgwood 1967, Fougereau & Houdayer 1968, Fougereau *et al.* 1973, Marchalonis & Cohen 1973), but no data on antibodies of apodans occur in the literature. Early reports of antibody production in anurans suggested that these species were poor responders and perhaps were incapable of mounting an immune response (Goodner 1926, Bissett 1948). Subsequent work, however, showed that the responsiveness was temperature and dose dependent and that anurans could respond to a wide variety of antigens with a vigour comparable to that of higher vertebrates (Trnka & Franek 1960, Alcock 1965, Marchalonis & Edelman 1966, Uhr *et al.* 1962, Lykakis 1969, Manning & Turner 1972, Rosenquist & Hoffman 1972, Evans *et al.* 1966, Maniatis *et al.* 1969, Coe 1970).

The nature of the antibody response of amphibians appears to be particularly dependent on the nature of the antigen used to elicit the response. In the toad, *Bufo marinus*, *Salmonella adelaide* flagellar antigens elicited only the production of high molecular weight (19S) antibody (Diener & Nossal 1966, Diener & Marchalonis 1970). This antigen also failed to elicit an anamnestic secondary response. Other groups independently found comparable results in toads with similar antigens (Evans *et al.* 1966, Acton *et al.* 1972). The limited response is solely a reflection on the antigen used, since serum protein antigens (Alcock 1965, Manning & Turner 1972, Hadji-Azimi 1971), erythrocyte antigens (Atwell & Marchalonis 1975) and bacteriophage antigens (Marchalonis & Edelman 1966, Lin *et al.* 1971) are all able to elicit responses producing antibody of two different sizes and classes. This differential response which is strongly dependent upon the nature of the antigen is best illustrated in the study of responses to the dinitrophenol (DNP) hapten in the bullfrog, *Rana catesbeiana* (Rosenquist & Hoffman 1972). Dinitrophenylated keyhole limpet haemocyanin injected in Complete Freund's Adjuvant would induce anti-DNP antibodies predominantly of the low molecular weight class. Dinitrophenylated *Salmonella typhimurium*, on the other hand, induced antibody predominantly in the high molecular weight class. Antibody titres of bullfrogs injected with DNP-*S. typhimurium* remained high for more than twelve months, whereas the anti-DNP activity induced by DNP-KLH rose to a peak titre with a subsequent decrease to a level below detection. All bullfrogs were shown to contain a high natural antibody titre to DNP. DNP-KLH did not induce a significant high molecular weight antibody response above this high background level. These studies might reflect the phenomenon of thymus dependency of antibody responses to certain antigens in mammals. Proteins including haemocyanin and albumins are highly thymus-dependent in mice and cooperation between T and B lymphocytes is obligatory to the generation of optimal responses (see Chapter 2 for discussion of T/B cooperation). In such responses, antibodies appear transiently in the IgM immunoglobulins but IgG antibodies eventually predominate. The secondary response consists almost completely of IgG antibodies. In contrast, antigens such as *E. coli* lipopolysaccharide, *Salmonella* flagella, pneumococcal polysaccharides and polyvinylpyrrolidone are capable of inducing antibodies in athymic mice (Andersson & Blomgren 1971). Thymus-independent antigens usually induce only IgM antibodies. Anuran amphibians might prove valuable in studies of the mechanisms of T/B cooperation and induction of antibodies in the absence of a thymus. Turner and Manning (1974), for example, have recently found that antibody formation to human IgG and sheep erythrocytes (thymus-dependent antigens in mice) was completely eliminated by thymectomy of larval *Xenopus*.

The time course for antibody production in anurans is much slower than in mammals. The conversion of the antibody response from predominantly high molecular weight (19S) antibody to low molecular weight (7S) antibody appears to be generally slower and not as complete as it is in mammals. The time course for antibody class conversion for the same antigen can also be quite varied between different anuran species. In the bullfrog, *Rana catesbeiana*, 90 per cent of the antibody activity to the bacteriophage f_2 was found in the low molecular weight fraction 8 weeks after immunization (Marchalonis & Edelman 1966). In another species, *Bufo marinus*, the same antigen elicited a response in which the majority of the antibody activity persisted in the high molecular weight fraction 8 weeks after immunization (Lin *et al.* 1971). A second injection 4 weeks after the first gave an accelerated anamnestic response with a higher level of antibody activity appearing earlier than in the primary response. The conversion from 19S to 7S antibody, even in the secondary response, was not as complete as that seen by Marchalonis and Edelman (1966) in *Rana*. In *Bufo*, the 19S antibody was always the predominant class. The 7S antibody does not appear to have a negative feedback effect on IgM antibody production as does IgG antibody of mammals (Uhr & Möller 1968). We have found similar results in *Bufo marinus* using horse erythrocytes as antigen. Even after 8–10 weeks post-immunization, the majority of the antibody activity remained with the HMW Ig fraction (Atwell & Marchalonis 1975), Lykakis (1969) also made comparable observations in the clawed toad, *Xenopus laevis*, using bovine γ-globulin as antigen. We can conclude that the amphibian immune response possesses properties which characterize it as being intermediate in complexity between that of the primitive fishes and that of the more modern mammals. Precise control mechanisms regulating the amounts of high and low molecular weight antibody present at different times during the response appear not to be as highly developed in amphibia as they are in the mammals. The results of Marchalonis and Edelman (1966) on antibody conversion in the bullfrog suggest that we cannot rule out completely the possibility that the more advanced Ranid frogs may have developed a slightly more complex immune system, more similar to that of mammals, than their more 'primitive' amphibian relatives. Even in this case, however, the neutralization coefficient of the IgM antibody increased throughout the course of the immunization period. Therefore, no evidence for negative feedback by 7S antibody was observed. In general, the amphibian immune response cannot be said to be exactly similar to that of mammals, since IgM antibody production is not usually stimulated in mammals upon secondary challenge as has been found in the amphibians (Lin *et al.* 1971).

Physicochemical characterization of amphibian immunoglobulins

The previous section has shown that the number of studies on immunity in amphibia is large and these studies have extended over a considerable time period. However, only within the last 10 years has the development of the technology for the study of mammalian immunoglobulins enabled the physicochemical characterization of lower vertebrate immunoglobulin molecules.

Immunoglobulins of the urodeles

The information on urodele immunoglobulins is quite sparse, but the available information is pertinent to the interpretation of the pattern of immunoglobulin classes that are found in the anuran amphibians. Urodeles definitely make antibodies of the '19S' class, which has a polypeptide chain structure that is similar to the IgM of mammals (Marchalonis & Cohen 1972, Fougereau & Houdayer 1968). The heavy and light chains are present in proportion to their mass; thereby indicating an equal number of light and heavy chains per molecule. This observation corresponds to that found in the IgM immunoglobulins from other vertebrate classes (Fougereau *et al.* 1973). The class distinctive heavy chains possess a similar gel penetration to human μ-heavy chains when analysed by polyacrylamide gel electrophoresis in buffers containing the anionic detergent, sodium dodecylsulphate (SDS) (Fougereau *et al.* 1973, Marchalonis & Atwell 1973). We have previously discussed in detail the reliability of comparing two Ig heavy chains by this method (Atwell & Marchalonis 1975), and suggest that it is reasonable to conclude that two polypeptide chains are of similar molecular weight if they exhibit similar gel penetrations and possess a similar carbohydrate content. The relative mobility of glycoproteins on this gel is generally not indicative of their true molecular weight (Segrest *et al.* 1971) and independent estimates of molecular weight must be obtained. Two detailed studies using urodele species suggest that no immunoglobulin molecular smaller than a 19S IgM is present at all in the serum. Fougereau *et al.* (1973) showed that the axolotl, *Ambystoma mexicanum* displayed a complete absence of any protein, in the Sephadex G200 '7S' fraction of the serum γ-globulin fraction separated by starch block electrophoresis. In addition, no antibody activity was detected in this fraction. Marchalonis and Cohen (1973) found similar results in a study on immunized mud puppies, *Necturus maculosis.* In both cases there was a high molecular weight immunoglobulin present and this was characterized as an IgM immunoglobulin. The Necturus IgM is antigenically related to both *Bufo marinus* and *Xenopus laevis* IgM (Marchalonis & Cohen 1973). This was shown by a sensitive radioimmunoassay technique, which was able to show a greater cross-reaction to the more primitive anuran, *Xenopus*, than to the other.

Axolotls usually exist in an arrested larval form which can be artificially induced to metamorphose to an adult stage by adding thyroxin to their tank water. Fougereau and Houdayer (1968) report that they find only one antibody class formed in response to immunization with FH5 bacteriophage in either the larval or adult form. Earlier experiments by Ching and Wedgwood (1967) on the axoltl, *Siredon mexicanum*, showed that on primary challenge with the antigen ØX 174, only high molecular weight antibody was made in both the larval and adult forms. After secondary stimulation, however, they report that all the adult specimens and one larva possessed both slowly and rapidly sedimenting antibodies to ØX 174 when analysed by sucrose gradients. They also found that after intensive, multiple antigenic challenge, both slowly and rapidly sedimenting antibody could be detected in larvae one year later. Unfortunately, neither antibody containing fraction was isolated and characterized. It is therefore difficult to determine the structural relationship of these antibodies to the other known antibodies. Ching and Wedgwood's report of a second antibody class in the axolotl urodeles was not substantiated in either the extensive work of Fougereau *et al.* (1973) in axolotls or that of Marchalonis and Cohen (1973) in mud puppies, both of which were discussed above. No 7S immunoglobulin molecules were found in the serum by either group. All that can be concluded at present is that urodeles express at least one antibody class, and its structure is similar to polymeric IgM found in other vertebrate species.

If IgM antibody is the only major immunoglobulin class present in urodeles it raises some interesting speculations about the evolution of the different amphibian subgroups and the evolutionary appearance of the low molecular weight Ig present in anuran amphibians. These will be discussed at a later stage in this chapter.

Immunoglobulins of anurans

In order to establish that two different immunoglobulin classes are present in an animal it is necessary to show differences between their class-specific heavy chains, both antigenically and in terms of physicochemical criteria.

The first study on the structure of anuran immunoglobulins was that of Marchalonis and Edelman (1966) on the bullfrog, *Rana catesbeiana*. They found two anti-f_2 phage antibody fractions of different molecular weights, which were immunologically related but not identical. The light chains were antigenically identical and the heavy chains expressed disparate antigenic determinants. The 19S antibody fraction had a faster anodal mobility than the 7S antibody fraction. Reduction of the 19S immunoglobulin with mercaptoethanol in 8 M urea produced polypeptide chains whose mobilities on urea-formate starch gel electrophoresis were similar to mammalian μ- and light chains. Similarly, the light chains of the 7S immunoglobulin exhibited a characteristic light chain mobility, but the heavy chains had a mobility intermediate between that of the faster human γ-chains and the slower human μ-chains. Intact molecular weights were not determined but heavy chain molecular weights were estimated by high speed equilibrium ultracentrifugation. The heavy chain of the 19S immunoglobulin had a mass of around 72,000 daltons, which is typical of a μ-heavy chain. The heavy chain of the 7S immunoglobulin gave a value of 53,600, which suggested a similarity to mammalian γ chains. This paper established the presence of a new 7S immunoglobulin class in anura which is distinct from a 7S IgM. The molecular weight estimate supported its designation as an IgG, but the gel electrophoretic mobility of the heavy chain did not show an exact similarity to human γ-chains. Acid-urea gel electrophoresis separates proteins on the basis of both their size and charge. But if the mobility difference between this heavy chain and γ-chains is to be explained solely on charge differences, it is certainly not evident by differences in the amounts of charged amino acids in the heavy-chain amino acid compositions.

A molecular weight estimate of 53,000 has also been reported for the heavy chains of the 7S immunoglobulin of *Bufo marinus* (Acton *et al.* 1972) and *Xenopus laevis* (Marchalonis *et al.* 1970). The *Bufo* estimate was obtained by gel filtration and the *Xenopus* estimate was made by acid-urea gel electrophoresis, according to the method of Parish and Marchalonis (1969). The intact molecular weight of the Bufo 7S immunoglobulin was estimated from sedimentation studies to be 160,000 (Acton *et al.* 1972). Molecular weights of intact 7S immunoglobulins were not reported for *Xenopus*.

In 1971 Hadji-Azimi performed further experiments on *Xenopus* immunoglobulins. Separation of immune serum on a column of Sephadex G200 which had been calibrated for the elution position of human IgG, showed the low molecular weight peak of antibody activity symmetrically over the *Xenopus* protein peak and emerging slightly ahead of a position where intact human IgG would emerge. The molecular weight of the intact 7S Ig was not determined. Analysis of the polypeptide chains of both 19S and 7S immunoglobulin by polyacrylamide gel electrophoresis in SDS containing buffers under reducing conditions show a similarity of both light chains to one another and to mammalian light chains. The heavy chain from the 19S immunoglobulin has similar properties to those of the mammalian μ-chain. The heavy chain of the 7S Ig showed an intermediate mobility between μ- and γ-chains. The mobility difference between this amphibian heavy chain and mammalian γ-chains cannot be attributed to carbohydrate alone as the hexose content of the *Xenopus* chain was 2 per cent by weight. The heavy chain of *Bufo* 7S immunoglobulin has also been shown to have an intermediate mobility between μ- and γ-chains on acid-urea polyacrylamide gels (Diener & Marchalonis 1970).

Because of these anomalies between the published molecular weight values and electrophoretic behaviour of heavy chains of anuran 7S immunoglobulins, we decided to reinvestigate rigorously the properties of these molecules using the 7S immunoglobulins of *Bufo* and *Xenopus* for comparison. We found that the low molecular weight *Bufo* immunoglobulin eluted from Sephadex G200 significantly ahead of an ^{125}I-labelled human IgG marker, as shown in Fig. 11.1. This was similar to the results obtained by Hadji-Azimi (1971) for *Xenopus* 7S immunoglobulin. We estimated the molecular weight of the *Bufo* molecule by means of this calibrated column to be 168,000$\pm$4,000 (Atwell & Marchalonis 1975). This value is significantly higher than that of human IgG which has a molecular weight of approximately 150,000 (Edelman *et al*). 1968. We also found that the heavy chain had

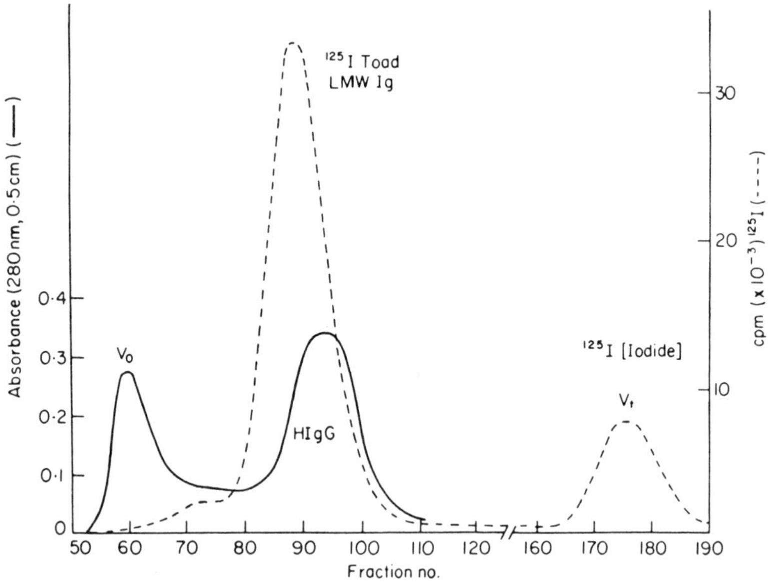

Fig. 11.1. Simultaneous gel filtration of toad (*Bufo marinus*) and human 7S immunoglobulins on Sephadex G200. Human IgG is detected by absorbance (——) and the peak at V_o, the void volume, is the absorbance of Blue Dextran. Toad 7S immunoglobulin was labelled with ^{125}I (iodide). Free ^{125}I (iodide) is found at the column volume, V_t.

an intermediate mobility between μ- and γ-standards when analysed by polyacrylamide gel electrophoresis both in the acid-urea system (Parish & Marchalonis 1969) and the SDS detergent system (Laemmli & Favre 1973). We estimated the molecular weight of the heavy chain of the 7S immunoglobulin using the acid-urea gel system to be 61,000$\pm$2,300. This significant difference in mass from γ-chains (50,000 daltons, Edelman *et al.* 1968) was supported by gel filtration studies. The toad heavy chain eluted significantly earlier than the human γ-chain marker from a Sephadex G200 column in 4 M urea, 1 M propionic acid. The light chains, on the other hand, co-eluted. The molecular weight estimate of the heavy chain from the standardized column of 61,500$\pm$2,500 was in extremely good agreement with that calculated from the polyacrylamide gels (Atwell & Marchalonis 1975). Since both techniques use an only partially shared set of molecular parameters as a basis for their separation, it would be hard to argue that the values obtained are the result of artefacts in the estimation. The heavy chain of *Bufo* 19S immunoglobulin had a molecular weight estimated on acid-urea gels of 67,400$\pm$2,300 which agrees reasonably well with other estimates of μ-type heavy chains (Atwell & Marchalonis 1975).

One other interesting point about the structure of anuran immunoglobulins is the report by Parkhouse *et al.* (1970) that *Xenopus laevis* IgM appears, under the electron microscope, to exist as a hexamer comprised of Y-shaped subunits. This observation contrasted with findings that mammalian IgM exists as a pentamer of such subunits. Unlike *Xenopus*, IgM from an ordinary frog, *Rana temporaria*, is pentameric in the electron microscope (Parkhouse, personal communication). There have been no intact molecular weight estimates of *Xenopus* IgM. The heavy chain of Xenopus IgM appears to have a molecular weight befitting a μ-type heavy chain ($71{,}500 \pm 2{,}800$) (Marchalonis *et al.* 1970) although Parkhouse suggests that it is a little smaller than that of the mouse (Parkhouse, personal communication). Hadji-Azimi (1971) by contrast reports a high molecular weight (76,000) for *Xenopus* μ-chain. It would be interesting to see whether the IgM hexameric structure is reflected in a higher intact molecular weight.

Comparison of reduced 7S Igs from various vertebrate classes

We were interested in comparing the results we had obtained in the marine toad with other anurans and also with low molecular weight 7S immunoglobulins in the higher vertebrate classes, the reptiles, birds and mammals. We chose gel electrophoresis under reducing conditions in a discontinuous buffer system, containing the detergent, SDS (Laemmli & Favre 1973). Small amounts of many different samples can be quickly and easily compared. All immunoglobulin heavy chains are glycoproteins, with each heavy chain class having different carbohydrate contents. The mobility of a carbohydrate containing protein relative to a non-carbohydrate containing protein of the same total molecular weight is retarded in the SDS system because the carbohydrate portion of the molecule does not bind the negatively charged detergent (Segrest *et al.* 1971). This lowers the charge density per unit mass on the molecule, relative to a non-carbohydrate containing molecule, thus lowering the mobility of the molecule in free solution. It follows that charge differences between molecules of the same size will be more apparent upon electrophoresis in gels of lower acrylamide concentration than in ones where the molecular sieving in a higher concentration gel becomes the major term affecting the separation. A detailed discussion of these effects can be found elsewhere (Atwell & Marchalonis 1975).

IgG heavy chains from several mammalian species all have identical gel penetrations to human γ-chains in the SDS gel system (Atwell & Marchalonis 1975). We have also shown that μ-chains from many vertebrate classes also have identical mobilities to human μ-chains (Marchalonis & Atwell 1973). These results supported our theoretical considerations and so we concluded that carbohydrate-containing heavy chains with the same carbohydrate content which run to similar positions on SDS gels could be considered to be of similar mass. We feel that such a technique is valid for preliminary comparisons. Exact comparisons, of course, require detailed information on the amino acid sequences of the proteins under consideration.

Studies using the SDS-polyacrylamide electrophoresis technique confirmed earlier work with immunoglobulins of a monotreme mammal, the echidna or spiny ant-eater, *Tachyglossus aculcatus* (Atwell *et al.* 1973). As depicted in Fig. 11.2, the major type of antibody in this primitive mammal

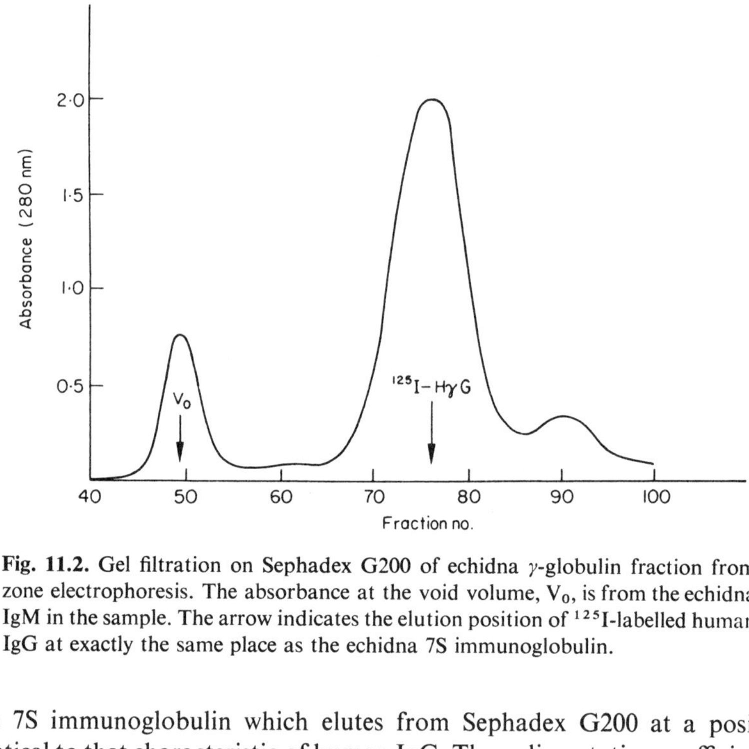

Fig. 11.2. Gel filtration on Sephadex G200 of echidna γ-globulin fraction from zone electrophoresis. The absorbance at the void volume, V_0, is from the echidna IgM in the sample. The arrow indicates the elution position of ^{125}I-labelled human IgG at exactly the same place as the echidna 7S immunoglobulin.

is a 7S immunoglobulin which elutes from Sephadex G200 at a position identical to that characteristic of human IgG. The sedimentation coefficient of this echidna antibody was 6·7S and its molecular weight was 150,000. The heavy chain of the echidna 6·7S immunoglobulin was found to be similar to the human γ-chain because these two chains expressed identical mobilities when analysed by polyacrylamide gel electrophoresis in SDS-containing buffers. This is shown in Fig. 11.3. Further evidence of similarity was suggested by two observations: first, application of a sensitive radioimmunoassay indicated a possible antigenic cross-reaction between IgG molecules of man and echidna (Marchalonis & Atwell 1973); in the second place, Kronvall *et al.* (1969) reported that a protein in echidna serum bound to staphylococcal A protein. This bacterial protein exhibits a binding affinity for the Fc portions of mammalian γ-chains. Further investigations using the SDS-polyacrylamide

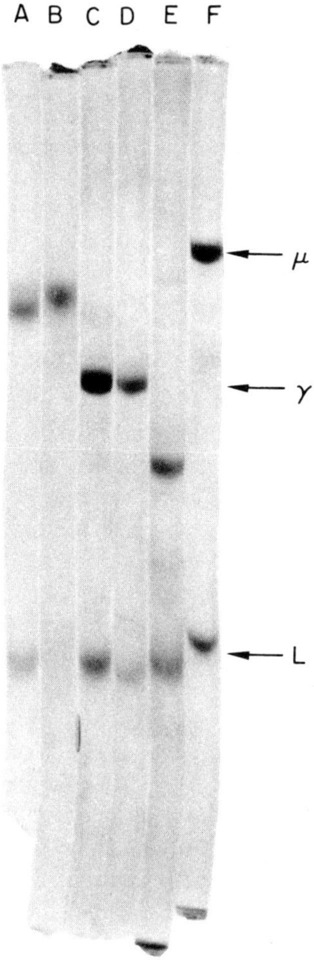

Fig. 11.3. Comparison of reduced low molecular weight immunoglobulins by electrophoresis in alkaline SDS gels. Direction of migration is downwards, the faster moving band in each case being the light chain, the other band the heavy chain. (A) Toad 7S immunoglobulin; (B) Chicken 7S immunoglobulin (IgY); (C) Echidna IgG; (D) Human IgG; (E) Lungfish IgN; (F) Human IgM. μ, γ and L indicate the position of migration of known μ, γ and light chains.

gel electrophoresis technique confirmed that the low molecular weight immunoglobulin of marsupials which was termed IgG in the absence of physiochemical characterization (Rowlands & Dudley 1968) did in fact possess heavy chains similar to γ-chains of eutherian mammals (Atwell & Marchalonis 1975). Our study involved immunoglobulins of the brush-tailed possum, *Trichosurus vulpecula.* Although these studies must be considered preliminary, we believe that it is reasonable to propose that γ-heavy chains are present in all three mammalian subclasses. Moreover, classes in addition to IgM and IgG occur in marsupials as witnessed by recent demonstrations of IgE-like (Lynch & Turner 1974) and IgA-like immunoglobulins (Bell *et al.* 1974) in the quokka, *Setonix brachyurus*, however direct demonstration of homology with the human classes has not been shown.

Since our studies suggested that IgG antibodies occur in all mammalian subclasses, but are lacking in amphibians, it was necessary to consider immunoglobulins of the non-mammalian vertebrates, reptiles and birds, which can trace their ancestry back to amphibians. Our discussion here will be brief because avian and reptilian antibodies are considered in detail elsewhere in this volume (Chapters 12 and 13). Molecular weight values considerably higher than those of mammalian γ-chain were reported for heavy chains of 7S immunoglobulins of avian species; the chicken (Leslie & Clem 1969), the duck (Zimmerman *et al.* 1971) and reptilian species, the turtle (Leslie & Clem 1972, Benedict & Pollard 1971). The reported molecular weight values ranging from 65,000 to 67,000 were close to the molecular weight of the heavy chain of the 7S immunoglobulin marine toad (Atwell & Marchalonis 1975). Using the chicken 7S immunoglobulin for comparison, we determined that its heavy chain gave an identical SDS gel mobility to heavy chains from both *Bufo* and *Xenopus* 7S immunoglobulins. This mobility was intermediate between that of human μ- and γ-chains. This is shown in Fig. 11.3. The marine toad and the chicken have total carbohydrate contents of about 5 per cent (Acton *et al.* 1972, Leslie & Clem 1969). *Xenopus* 7S immunoglobulin has a hexose content of about 2 per cent (Hadji-Azimi 1971) and by comparison with other immunoglobulin carbohydrate distributions, the total carbohydrate content is probably of the same order. The similarity in size and carbohydrate content of these molecules is completely mirrored in their similar gel mobilities. Geczy *et al.* (1973) find that the low molecular weight Ig from *Rana catesbeiana*, the species upon which the earlier work of Marchalonis and Edelman was performed (1966), has a heavy chain which also has an intermediate mobility between μ- and γ-chains on SDS gels. By this criterion, it appears to be comparable to other amphibian, reptilian and avian low molecular weight immunoglobulins.

Such similarities would suggest that there may be a relatively close relationship between these molecules and quite a dissimilarity from mammalian IgG.

7S immunoglobulins in evolution

A critical reappraisal of the physicochemical properties of the 7S immunoglobulin from anuran amphibians shows that it differs markedly from the 7S IgG immunoglobulin which is present in all mammals. The parameters with which we classify lower vertebrate immunoglobulins indicate a greater resemblance to the 7S immunoglobulin than has been found in both birds and reptiles.

It is pertinent to consider whether this immunoglobulin in the three vertebrate classes represents an immunoglobulin class which is completely distinct from any major immunoglobulin class present in mammals. The 64,000–68,000 molecular weight heavy chain present in this immunoglobulin is somewhat similar in properties to the mammalian IgG heavy chain. Differing molecular weights have been reported for mammalian and heavy chains. Cebra and Small (1967) estimated the rabbit α-chain molecular weight at 64,000. Other values such as 55,000 for a mouse IgA myeloma protein (Seki *et al.* 1968) and 56,300 and 52,000 for α-chains from human IgA_1 and IgA_2 Ig classes (Dorrington & Rockey 1970) have also been reported. Such variations in molecular weight consequently make it difficult for comparisons to be made. Naturally, it is unwise to confer homology solely by similar molecular weights of heavy chains. It is therefore interesting to note that serum IgA in animals apart from humans exists predominantly in a dimeric form (Wang & Fudenberg 1974). The 7S Ig under discussion from amphibia, aves and reptilia have molecular weights in non-dissociating conditions characteristic of a monomer. The fact that there exists in chickens both an IgA-like immunoglobulin and a 7S Ig (IgY) (Lebacq-Verheyden *et al.* 1972, Bienenstock *et al.* 1973), is perhaps the most compelling evidence to date as to their unrelatedness. Moreover, the IgA molecules of the chicken are comprised of light chains and α-chains which are not linked via disulphide bonds (Vaerman *et al.* 1974). This situation is similar to that found in IgA molecules of the IgA_2 Am+ type in man (Grey *et al.* 1968) and murine molecules bearing the Balb/c allotype (Warner & Marchalonis 1972).

It was considered above that urodeles probably lack 7S immunoglobulins. What does this mean in terms of the relatedness of the 7S Ig in anurans to the similar protein present in reptiles and birds? All amphibian subclasses are presumed to have arisen from a common set of ancestral species (Romer 1966). Likewise, if we are to accept the homology of the amphibian 7S Ig with that of reptiles and birds, it would be natural to expect that the genetic event giving rise to this new class of Ig heavy chain would have occurred in the common ancestors of all three vertebrate subclasses. This would imply that the progenitors of the urodeles should have also received this gene. The phenotypic absence of the gene product in the species of urodeles studied does not necessarily mean that the gene is absent. It is possible that its expression is suppressed. If this gene never was present in urodeles, it implies that the anuran 7S immunoglobulin is the product of a gene which arose by a separate set of genetic events than that generating the similar sized product of reptiles and birds. This possibility cannot be discounted at the moment.

One other piece of biological evidence supports our contention of the dissimilarity of lower vertebrate 7S Igs from mammalian IgG. Protein A from the staphylococcal cell wall will react with a certain portion of the Fc portion of γ-chains from human IgG resulting in precipitation (Kronvall *et al.* 1970). Other mammalian sera or immunoglobulins either show a similar precipitation reaction or inhibit the precipitation of protein A and human IgG. This property was not shared by any lower vertebrate sera apart from mammals. This reaction, which appears to be a specific γ-chain marker supports our hypothesis for the restriction of γ-heavy chains to mammals.

Fig. 11.4 illustrates schematically the possible domain structure of the

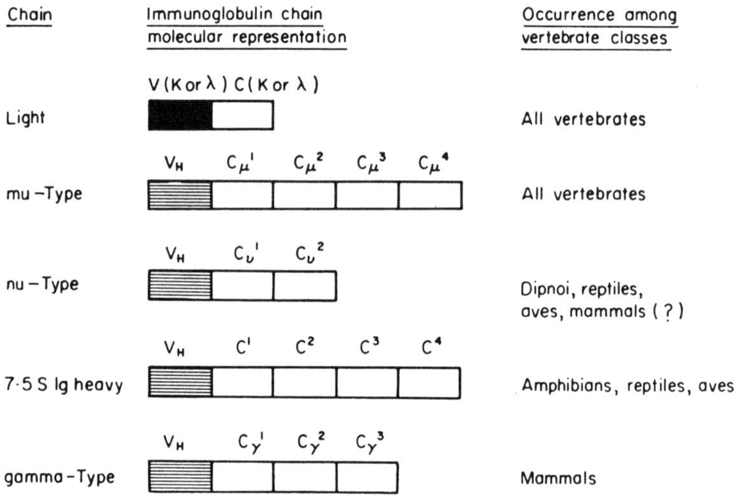

Fig. 11.4. Molecular representation of different immunoglobulin chains. The length of each chain is proportional to its carbohydrate free molecular weight. Each chain is divided into domain regions, each of approximately 11,000 daltons, the variable region domain indicated by the dark or hatched area denoted V and the constant region domains by the clear areas denoted C.

amphibian 7S Ig heavy chain compared to other vertebrate immunoglobulin chains. α-Chains were omitted as the variation in molecular weights could result in a heavy chain of four or five domains. The calculations are based on the proposal by Hill *et al.* (1966) that the primordial gene ancestral to all immunoglobulins probably coded for a polypeptide chain of approximately 110 amino acids to about 11,000 daltons in size. All genes coding for immunoglobulin variable regions would have arisen by successive tandem gene duplications and deletions. The nature of the internal sequence homologies within μ-chains (Putnam *et al.* 1973), γ-chains (Edelman & Gall 1969) and light chains (Hilschmann & Craig 1965) support such a theory. Assuming that lower vertebrate immunoglobulins have this same periodic structure, the number of domains per heavy chain were calculated from the carbohydrate-free molecular weight (Marchalonis 1970, Zimmerman *et al.* 1971). The amphibian 7S immunoglobulin heavy chain contains enough protein for there to be five domains, similar in fact to μ-chains and of course the heavy chain from the 7S immunoglobulin in reptiles and birds. This similarity to μ-heavy chains is suggestive of a possible close relationship between these chains early in evolution. Their distinction came about when sufficient mutations were accumulated to produce a product antigenically different from μ-chains, binding different proportions of carbohydrate and performing different biological functions.

Although the molecular properties described here and in Chapters 10, 12 and 13 allow us to make a reasonable guess at the domain structures of immunoglobulins of lower vertebrates, they do not enable us to give familiar mammalian names to the immunoglobulins. The assignment of an immunoglobulin to a definite class requires knowledge of antigenic and functional properties which ultimately derived from amino acid sequence of the molecules. We propose to consider the 7S immunoglobulins of amphibians, reptiles and birds to be directly homologous and term them IgRAA where RAA symbolizes reptiles, aves and amphibians. Amphibians, thus, possess IgM and IgRAA immunoglobulins; reptiles, IgM, IgN and IgRAA; and birds, IgM, IgN, IgRAA and IgA. The relative amounts of the various classes would differ from species to species. In the duck, for example, IgN is the major class of serum immunoglobulin (Grey 1967), whereas this class is not readily detectable in the serum of chickens. IgRAA (IgY in the terminology of Leslie & Clem 1969) is the predominant antibody type in the latter. Minor immunoglobulin classes such as IgE and IgD are difficult to identify conclusively even in mammalian species such as the mouse. Homocytotropic antibody has been observed in chickens (Faith & Clem 1973) and marsupials (Lynch & Turner 1974); therefore immunoglobulins functionally homologous to IgE occur in birds and lower mammals. Antigenic and structural evidence are required to confirm the identification.

The emergence of non-IgM 7S immunoglobulins in amphibians, reptiles and birds most likely represents a burst of duplication of the cistron encoding the ancestral μ-chain which was independent of that which generated the gamma chain of mammals. Therefore, the amphibian 7S immunoglobulin might be considered an evolutionary parallel of human IgG rather than a direct homologue. Of course the heavy chain amphibian molecule and human γ-chain are homologous in a more general sense because they both derive from a primitive gene specifying μ-like heavy chain. This general similarity is reflected in amino acid compositions (Atwell & Marchalonis 1975) and in homologous properties of the variable region (Litman, Chapter 10). A lack of direct homology between 7S immunoglobulins of non-mammalian species and mammals raises another major issue. There is a tendency at present to presume that 7S immunoglobulins of chickens, for example, are subject to the same sorts of regulatory influences operative in the generation of murine IgG antibodies. Insufficient data are presently available to warrant such comparisons.

The selective pressures which brought about the emergence of distinct immunoglobulin classes remain obscure. One can argue that a need exists to diversify the range of effector functions conditioned by constant regions of the heavy chain (Spiegleberg 1974). Tandem duplication of genes encoding both variable and constant regions of immunoglobulins appears to be an integral part of immunoglobulin evolution (Gally & Edelman 1972). Immunoglobulin genes of man and mouse are organized into three unlinked translocons; namely, that specifying κ-light chains, that specifying λ-light chains and that specifying heavy chains. A series of genes determining the structures of both variable and constant sequences occur in each cluster. The heavy chain translocon consists of an array of V-region genes (at least three distinct families) probably associated with a constant region array comprised of genes specifying the various heavy chains and their subclasses. The order of arrangement has been represented as follows: V_{HI}-V_{HII}-V_{HIII}—$C_{\mu1}$-C-$_{\mu2}$ $C_{\gamma3}$-$C_{\gamma2}$-$C_{\gamma1}$-$C_{\gamma4}$-$C_{\alpha1}$-$C_{\alpha2}$-C_{δ}-C_{ε}. The arrangement of γ-chain sub-classes has been determined by linkage studies (Natvig & Kunkel 1973). If we accept the proposal that tandem duplication is an essential part of immunoglobulin evolution and carry the argument to the level of domains or internal homology units (Fig. 11.4) it is clear that the immune system can generate great diversity to be acted upon by selection. Certain obvious advantages would be presented by a 7S molecule rather than a 19S immunoglobulin. The 7S molecule would not be restricted to intravascular spaces, but might diffuse into extravascular spaces. IgG can do this, whereas polymerized IgM cannot. Further modifications can occur within the family of 7S immunoglobulins if a domain becomes modified to impart a new function such as binding to surface receptors on lymphocytes, macrophages or mast cells. In man, for example, monocytes have receptors for the Fc regions of IgG1 and IgG2 but do not bind IgG3, IgG4 or IgM (Spiegleberg 1974). These differences in cytophilic binding might bring about major differences in antigen processing which could sway the balance between immunity or tolerance. The proliferation of subclasses in man and mouse might also entail the emergence of selectively neutral genes which are not removed (Kimura & Ohta 1971). In contrast some immunoglobulin genes would be strongly selected because of a major function which has not changed throughout evolutionary time. The role of IgM 7S units as lymphocyte surface receptors for antigen (Marchalonis 1974, Warner 1974) serves as an example of this situation.

Since duplication of heavy chain genes often entails deletion or addition of domains, the possibility arises that the immunoglobulin generating system might produce other molecules in addition to readily recognizable immunoglobulins. β_2-microglobulin have been found associated with the surfaces of lymphocytes and other cells represent such a product of duplication of the gene segment encoding the third constant region of immunoglobulin gamma chain (Cunningham *et al.* 1973). The natural course of immunoglobulin evolution, then, would most likely be to generate subclasses and free domains unless selective pressures removed the newly created genes. This tendency to generate subclasses (which might be raised to class status as mutational differences accumulate) is illustrated by the reported presence of two distinct 16S IgM immunoglobulins in the goldfish (Trump 1970) and four antigenically distinct IgM immunoglobulins in certain sharks (Gitlin *et al.* 1973). The paucity of subclasses in the rabbit and the echidna might reflect the situation where the selective pressures for suppression of subclasses are acting strongly to promote rigorous suppression.

Acknowledgments

This work was supported in part by grants from the Australian Research Grants Council and the United States Public Health Service (AI 12565-01). This is publication No. 2109 from the Walter and Eliza Hall Institute of Medical Research.

References

ACTON R.T., WEINHEIMER P.F., WOLCOTT M., EVANS E.F. & BENNETT J.C. (1970) N-terminal sequences of immunoglobulin heavy and light chains from three species of lower vertebrates. *Nature (Lond)* **228,** 991.

ACTON R.T., EVANS E.E., WEINHEIMER P.F., NIEDERMEIER W. & BENNETT J.C. (1972) Purification and characterization of two classes of immunoglobulins from the marine toad, *Bufo marinus, Biochemistry* **11,** 2751.

ALCOCK D.M. (1965) Antibody production in the common frog, *Rana temporaria. J. Path. Bact.* **90,** 31.

ANDERSSON B. & BLOMGREN H. (1971) Evidence for thymus-independent humoral antibody production in mice against polyvinylpyrollidone and *E. coli* lipopolysaccharide. *Cellular Immunol.* **2,** 411.

ATWELL J.L., MARCHALONIS J.J. & EALEY E.H.M. (1973) Major immunoglobulin classes of the echidna *Tachyglossus aculeatus. Immunology* **23,** 835.

ATWELL J.L. & MARCHALONIS J.J. (1975) Phylogenetic emergence of immunoglobulin classes distinct from IgM. *J. Immunogenetics* **1,** 391.

BELL R.G., STEPHENS C.J. & TURNER K.J. (1974) Marsupial Immunoglobulins resembling eutherian IgA in the serum and secretions of *Setonix brachyurus* (quokka). *J. Immunol.* **113,** 371.

BENEDICT A.A. & POLLARD L.W. (1972) Three classes of immunoglobulins found in the sea turtle, *Chelonia mydas. Folia Microbiol.* **17,** 75.

BISSET K.A. (1948) The effect of temperature upon antibody production in cold-blooded vertebrates. *J. Path. Bact.* **60,** 87.

BIENENSTOCK J., PEREY D.Y.E., GAULDIE J. & UNDERDOWN B.J. (1973) Chicken γA: Physicochemical and immunochemical characteristics. *J. Immunol.* **110,** 524.

Cebra J.J. & Small P.A. Jr (1967) Polypeptide chain structure of rabbit immunoglobulins. III. Secretory IgA from colostrum. *Biochemistry* **6,** 503.

Ching Y.C. & Wedgwood R.J. (1967) Immunologic responses in the axolotl, *Siredon mexicanum. J. Immunol.* **99,** 191.

Coe J.E. (1970) Specificity of antibody produced in the bullfrog (*Rana catesbeiana*). *J. Immunol.* **104,** 1166.

Cooper E.L., Brown B.A. & Baculi B.S. (1971) New observations on lymph gland (LMI) and thymus activity in larval bullfrogs, *Rana catesbeiana*. In *Advances in Exp. Med. and Biol.* (Morphological and Functional aspects of Immunity, ed. Lindahl-Keissling K., Alm G. & Hanna M.G. Jr) **12,** 1.

Cunningham B.A., Wang J.L., Berggard I. & Peterson P.A. (1973) The Complete Amino Acid Sequence of B_2-microglobulin. *Biochemistry* **12,** 4811.

Diener E. & Marchalonis J.J. (1970) Cellular and humoral aspects of the primary immune response of the toad, *Bufo marinus, Immunology* **18,** 279.

Diener E. & Nossal G.J.V. (1966) Phylogenetic studies on the immune response. I. Localization of antigens and immune response in the toad, *Bufo marinus. Immunology* **10,** 535.

Dorrington, K.J. & Rockey, J.H. (1970) Differences in the molecular size of the heavy chains from γA_1 and γA_2 globulins. *Biochimica et Biophysica acta*, **200,** 584.

Edelman G.M. & Gall W.E. (1969) The Antibody Problem. *Ann. Rev. Biochem.* **38,** 415.

Edelman G.M., Gall W.E., Waxdall M.J. & Konigsberg W.H. (1968) The covalent structure of human γG globulin. I. Isolation of the whole molecule, the polypeptide chains and the tryptic fragments. *Biochemistry* **7,** 1950.

Evans E.E., Kent S.P., Bryant R.E. & Moyer M. (1966) Antibody formation and immunological memory in the marine toad. In *Phylogeny of Immunity*, ed. Smith R.T., Miescher P.A. & Good R.A. University of Florida Press, Gainesville.

Faith R.E. & Clem I.W. (1973) Passive cutaneous anaphylaxis in the chicken. Biological fractionation of the mediating antibody population. *Immunology* **25,** 151.

Fitch W.M. (1966) An improved method of testing for evolutionary homology. *J. Mol. Biol.* **16,** 9.

Fougereau M. & Houdayer M. (1968) Immunoglobulines et réponse immunitaire chez l'axolotl (*Ambystoma mexicanum*) *Ann. Inst. Pasteur* **115,** 968.

Fougereau M., Houdayer M. & Dorson M. (1973) Réponse immunitaire et structure multicaténaire des immunoglobulines d'un téléostéen: la truite arc-en-ciel (*Salmo gairdoneri*) et d'un amphibien urodèle: l'axolotl (*Ambystoma mexicanum*), p. 121. In *The Phylogenetic and Ontogenetic Study of the Immune Response and its Contribution to the Immunological Theory*, ed. Liacopoulas P. & Panijel J. INSERM, Paris.

Gally J.A. & Edelman G.M. (1972) The genetic control of immunoglobulin synthesis. *Ann. Rev. Genetics* **6,** 1.

Geczy C.L., Green P.C. & Steiner L.A. (1973) Immunoglobulins of the developing amphibian, *Rana catesbeiana, J. Immunol.* **111,** 1261.

Gitlin D., Perricelli & Gitlin J.D. (1973) Multiple immunoglobulin classes among sharks and their evolution. *Comp. Biochem. Physiol.* (*B*) **44,** 225.

Good R.A. & Papermaster B.W. (1964) Ontogeny and phylogeny of adaptive immunity. *Advan. Immunol.* **4,** 1.

Goodner K. (1926) Studies in anaphylaxis. IV. Allergic manifestations in frogs. *J. Immunol.* **11,** 335.

Grey H.M. (1967) Duck immunoglobulins. I. Structural studies on a 5·7S and 7·8S γ-globulin. *J. Immunol.* **98,** 811.

Grey H.M., Abel C.A., Yount W.J. & Kunkel H.G. (1968) A subclass of human γA-globulins (γA2) which lacks disulphide bonds linking heavy and light chains. *J. Expt. Med.* **128,** 1223.

HADJI-AZIMI I. (1971) Studies on *Xenopus larvis* immunoglobulins. *Immunology* **21,** 463.

HILL R.E., DELANEY R., FELLOWS R.E. JR & LEBOVITZ H.E. (1966) The evolutionary origins of immunoglobulins. *Proc. Natl. Acad. Sci.* (*Wash.*) **56,** 1762.

HILSCHMANN N. & CRAIG L.C. (1965) Amino acid sequence studies with Bence-Jones proteins. *Proc. Natl. Acad. Sci.* (*Wash*). **53,** 1403.

KIMURA M. & OHTA T. (1971) Protein polymorphism as a phase of molecular evolution. *Nature* (*Lond.*) **229,** 467.

KLAUS G.G.B., NITECKI D.E. & GOODMAN J.W. (1971) Amino acid sequences of free and blocked N-termini of leopard shark immunoglobulins. *J. Immunol.* **107,** 1250.

KRONVALL G., SEAL U.S., FINSTAD J. & WILLIAMS R.C. JR (1970) Phylogenetic insight into evolution of mammalian F_c fragment of γG globulin using staphylococcal protein A. *J. Immunol.* **104,** 140.

KUBO R.T., ROSENBLUM L.Y. & BENEDICT A.A. (1971) Amino terminal sequences of heavy and light chains of chicken anti-dinitrophenyl antibody. *J. Immunol.* **107,** 1781.

LAEMMLI U.K. & FAVRE M. (1973) Maturation of the head of bacterophage T4. I. DNA packaging events. *J. Mol. Biol.* **80,** 575.

LEBACQ-VERHEYDEN A.M., VAERMAN J.P. & HEREMANS J.F. (1972) A possible homology of mammalian IgA in chicken serum and secretions. *Immunology* **22,** 165.

LESLIE G.A. & CLEM L.W. (1969) Phylogeny of immunoglobulin structure and function. III. Immunoglobulins of the chicken. *J. Exptl. Med.* **130,** 1337.

LESLIE G.A. & CLEM L.W. (1972) Phylogeny of immunoglobulin structure and function. IV. 17S, 7·5S and 5·7S anti-DNP of the turtle, *Pseudamys scripta. J. Immunol.* **108,** 1656.

LIN H.H., CAYWOOD B.E. & ROWLANDS D.T. JR (1971) Primary and secondary immune responses of the marine toad (*Bufo marinus*) to bacteriophage f2. *Immunology* **20,** 373.

LITMAN G.W., FROMMEL D., CHARTRAND S.L., FINSTAD J. & GOOD R.A. (1971a) Significance of heavy chain mass and antigenic relationships in immunoglobulin evolution. *Immunochemistry* **8,** 345.

LITMAN G.W., WANG A.C., FUDENBERG H.H. & GOOD R.A. (1971b) N-terminal amino-acid sequence of African lungfish immunoglobulin light chains. *Proc. Natl. Acad. Sci.* (*Wash*). **68,** 2321.

LYKAKIS J.J. (1969) The production of two molecular classes of antibody in the toad, *Xenopus laevis,* homologous with mammalian γM (19S) and γG (7S) immunoglobulins. *Immunology* **16,** 91.

LYNCH N.R. & TURNER K.J. (1974) Immediate hypersensitivity of the marsupial, *Setonix brachyurus* (quokka). Characterization of the homocytotrophic antibody. *Aust. J. Biol. Exptl. Med. Sci.* **52,** 755.

MANIATIS G.M., STEINER L.A. & INGRAM V.M. (1969) Tadpole antibodies against frog hemoglobin and their effect on development. *Science* **165,** 67.

MANNING M.J. & TURNER R.J. (1972) Some responses of the clawed toad, *Xenopus laevis* to soluble antigens administered in adjuvant.

MARCHALONIS J.J. (1969) Isolation and characterization of immunoglobulin-like proteins of the Australian lungfish (*Neoceratodus forsteri*). *Aust. J. Expt. Biol. Med. Sci.* **47,** 405.

MARCHALONIS J.J. (1970) Phylogenetic origins of antibody structure. *Transplant. Proc.* **2,** 318.

MARCHALONIS J.J. (1971) Immunoglobulins and antibody production in amphibians. *Am. Zool.* **11,** 171.

MARCHALONIS J.J. (1974) Lymphocyte receptors for antigen. *J. Med.* **5,** 329.

MARCHALONIS J.J. & ATWELL J.L. (1973) Phylogenetic emergence of distinct immunoglobulin classes, p. 153. In *The Phylogenetic and Ontogenetic Study of the Immune Response and its contribution to the Immunological Theory*, ed. Liacopoulos T. & Panijel J. INSERM, Paris.

MARCHALONIS J.J. & COHEN N. (1973) Isolation and partial characterization of immunoglobulin from a urodele amphibian (*Necturus maculosis*). *Immunology* **24,** 395.

MARCHALONIS J.J. & EDELMAN G.M. (1966) Phylogenetic origins of antibody structure. II. Immunoglobulins in the primary immune response of the bullfrog, *Rana catesbeiana. J. Exptl. Med.* **124,** 901.

MEHTA P.D., REICHLIN M. & TOMASI T.B. JR (1972) Comparative studies of vertebrate immunoglobulins. *J. Immunol.* **109,** 1272.

NATVIG J.B. & KUNKEL H.G. (1973) Human immunoglobulins: classes, subclasses, genetic variants and idiotypes. *Advan. Immunol.* **16,** 1.

PARISH C.R. & MARCHALONIS J.J. (1970) A simple and rapid acrylamide gel method for estimating the molecular weights. *Analy. Biochem.* **34,** 436.

PARKHOUSE R.M.E., ASKONAS B.A. & DOURMASHKIN R.R. (1970) Electron microscopic studies of mouse immunoglobulin M; structure and reconstitution following reduction. *Immunology*, **18,** 575.

POLLARA B., SURAN A., FINSTAD J. & GOOD R.A. (1968) N-terminal amino acid sequences of immunoglobulin chains in *Polyodon spathula. Proc. Nat. Acad. Sci.* (*Wash.*) **59,** 1307.

PUTNAM F.W., FLORENT G., PAUL C., SHINODA T. & SHIMIZU A. (1973) Complete amino acid sequence of the mu heavy chain of human IgM immunoglobulin. *Science* **182,** 287.

ROMER A.S. (1966) *Vertebrate Paleontology*, University of Chicago Press, Chicago.

ROSENQUIST G.L. & HOFFMAN R.Z. (1972) The production of anti-DNP antibody in the bullfrog, *Rana catesbeiana. J. Immunol.* **108,** 1499.

ROWLANDS D.T. JR & DUDLEY M.A. (1968) The isolation of the immunoglobulins of the adult opossum (*Didelphys virginiana*). *J. Immunol.* **100,** 736.

SEGREST J.P., JACKSON R.L., ANDREWS E.P. & MARCHESI V.T. (1971) Human erythrocyte membrane glycoprotein: a re-evaluation of the molecular weight as determined by SDS polyacrylamide gel electrophoresis. *Biochem. Biophys. Res. Comm.* **44,** 390.

SEKI T., APPELLA E. & ITANO H.A. (1968) Chain models of 6·6S and 3·9S mouse myeloma γA immunoglobulin molecules. *Proc. Natl. Acad. Sci.* (*Wash.*) **61,** 1071.

SPIEGLEBERG H.L. (1974) Biological activities of immunoglobulins of different classes and subclasses. *Adv. Immunol.* **19,** 259.

TRNKA Z. & FRANEK F. (1960) Studies on the formation and characteristics of antibodies in frogs. *Folia Microbiol.* **5,** 374.

TRUMP G.N. (1970) Goldfish immunoglobulins and antibodies to bovine serum albumin. *J. Immunol.* **104,** 1267.

TURNER R.J. & MANNING M.J. (1974) The thymic dependence of amphibian antibody responses. *Europ. J. Immunol.* **4,** 343.

UHR J.W., FINKLESTEIN M.S. & FRANKLIN E.C. (1962) Antibody response to bacteriophage ØX 174 in non mammalian vertebrates. *Proc. Soc. Exp. Biol. Med.* **111,** 13.

UHR J.W. & MÖLLER G. (1968) Regulatory effect of antibody on the immune response. *Advan. Immunol.* **8,** 81.

VAERMAN J.P., LEBACQ-VERHEYDEN A.M. & HEREMANS J.F. (1974) Absence of disulphide bridges between heavy and light chains from IgA from chicken bile. *Immunol. Comm.* **3,** 239.

WANG A.C. & FUDENBERG H.H. (1974) IgA and evolution of immunoglobulins. *J. Immunogenetics*, **1,** 3.

WARNER N.L. (1974) Membrane immunoglobulin and antigen receptors on B and T lymphocytes. *Advan. Immunol.* **19,** 67.

WARNER N.L. & MARCHALONIS J.J. (1972) Structural differences in mouse IgA myeloma proteins of different allotypes. *J. Immunol.* **109,** 657.

ZIMMERMAN, B., SHALATIN N. & GREY H.M. (1971) Structural studies on the duck 5·7S and 7·8S immunoglobulins. *Biochemistry* **10,** 482.

Chapter 12. Immunoglobulins and Antibody Production in Reptiles

H. Ambrosius

Introduction

Antibody production: a survey of the reptilian orders
Rhynchocephalia
Crocodilia
Lacertilia
Serpentes
Chelonia

Immunoglobulins
Rhynchocephalia
Crocodilia
Lacertilia
Serpentes
Chelonia

General problems in antibody production and the biological properties of reptilian antibodies
Antigen elimination

General problems in antibody production and the biological properties of reptilian antibodies *continued*
Material transfer of antibody into eggs and the ontogeny of antibody production
Immunological memory
Morphology and kinetics of appearance of antibody-producing cells
Valence and affinity of reptilian antibodies
Antigen binding sites of reptilian antibodies
Maturation of the immune response

Factors influencing antibody production in reptiles
Influence of the antigen type
Influence of the temperature
Influence of adjuvants
Influence of seasonal factors

Introduction

Reptiles were among the first non-mammalian species to be used as experimental animals during the classical period of research in immunology. In 1897 Widal and Siccard reported the production of antitoxins and agglutinins in the pond turtle *Cistudio lutaria*. In addition, the grand old man in immunity research, Elias Metschnikoff (1902) studied the immune response of *Alligator mississipiensis* and found tetanus and cholera antitoxins.

Since that time, especially in the last ten years, many publications have appeared. The emergent results vary from one another according to the taxonomic group of reptiles under investigation. Therefore, it would appear necessary to pay attention to species-specific characteristics (Cohen 1971) and to the evolutionary branches of the class.

Antibody production: a survey on the reptilian orders

Rhynchocephalia

In the tuatara, *Sphenodon punctatum*, Marchalonis *et al.* (1969) and Diener (1970) observed the formation of antibodies following the injection of *Salmonella adelaide* flagellin. The titre maximum appeared 2 to 3 months after the immunization and for 6 months following immunization the antibody activity could only be found in the high molecular weight fraction (18S).

Crocodilia

Alligator mississippiensis has been studied by Metschnikoff (1902), Lerch *et al.* (1967) and Saluk *et al.* (1970) and the species *Caiman sclerops* by Evans *et al.* (1965). Antibodies have been found to be produced against bacterial as well as soluble protein antigens. As Lerch *et al.* (1967) pointed out, the alligators contained antibodies against haemocyanin in the blood serum from the second to the sixth week following the primary antigen contact. These antibodies belong to two kinds of immunoglobulins which differ in electrophoretic mobility and molecular weight.

Lacertilia

Lizards have been investigated by several authors (Table 12.1). The most

Table 12.1. Lizard antibodies

Species	Antigen	Author
Zonurus giganteus	Tetanus and diphtheria anatoxine	Grasset 1931
Z. giganteus	Salmonella, Meningococcus	Grasset *et al.* 1935
Lacerta viridis	Bac. proteus, Bac. septicaemia ranarum	Buch 1940
L. muralis	Salmonella, Arizona	Dimow 1966
Tiliqua scincoides	Bact. antigens	Willis 1932
T. rugosa	Salmonella, BSA, rat erythrocytes	Wetherall *et al.* 1972
Dipsosaurus dorsalis *Sauromalus obesus* *Phrynosoma solare* *Iguana iguana*	Salmonella typhosa	Evans *et al.* 1965
Ophisaurus apodus	serum proteins, BGG	Ambrosius 1970 Ambrosius *et al.* 1969 Hemmerling 1971 Hemmerling *et al.* 1971
Calotes versicolor	Sheep erythrocytes	Kanakambika *et al.* 1972

extensive studies are those by Ambrosius *et al.* (1969), Hemmerling and Ambrosius (1971), and Wetherall and Turner (1972). 19S and 7S antibodies of different immunoglobulin classes were found.

Serpentes

Antibody production in snakes has been studied by Grasset *et al.* (1935), Svet-Moldavski (1954), Timourian *et al.* (1961), Frair (1963), Evans (1965), Dimow and Slawtschew (1967), and Salanitro and Minton (1973). Antibodies could be found following immunization with viruses, bacterial antigens, heterologous erythrocytes, protein antigens, and after infection with parasitic nematodes. Salanitro and Minton (1973) found 19S and 7S antibodies.

Table 12.2. Turtle and tortoise antibodies

Species	Antigen	Author
Chrysemys picta	Erythrocytes	Noguchi 1902
C. picta	Haemocyanin, BSA	Grey 1963, 1966
Chrysemys elegans	BSA, HSA, RGG, EA	Coe 1972
C. elegans	Bact. salmonicida	Gee 1941
Clemmys caspica	Leptospiren	v. d. Hoeden 1966
Cistudio lutaria	Typhus toxine	Widal *et al.* 1897
Emys orbicularis	BGG	Lykakis 1968
E. meleagris	Erythrocytes	Noguchi 1902
Terrapene carolina	Salmonella	Evans *et al.* 1965
Pseudemys scripta	Serum proteins	Frair 1963
P. seripta	Salmonella	Acton *et al.* 1972
P. seripta	DNP-BGG	Leslie *et al.* 1972
Testudo angulata	Bacterial antigens	Grasset *et al.* 1931, 1935
T. ibera	Brucella	Maung 1963
T. hermanni	Protein antigens	Ambrosius 1965, 1966, 1967, 1970, 1972 Ambrosius *et al.* 1965, 1969, 1972
T. hermanni	DNP-proteins	Frenzel *et al.* 1971 Ambrosius *et al.* 1972
Agrionemys horsfieldii	Sheep erythrocytes	Rothe *et al.* 1968 Kassin *et al.* 1969
A. horsfieldii	DNP-BGG	Richter *et al.* 1972
A. horsfieldii	DNP-proteins	Ambrosius *et al.* 1972
Chelydra tricarinata	Bact. salmonicida	Gee *et al.* 1941
C. serpentina	Serum proteins	Frair 1963
C. serpentina	HRBC, Brucella	Chartrand *et al.* 1971
C. serpentina	DNP-Brucella	Litman *et al.* 1973
Chelonia mydas	BSA, DNP-BGG	Benedict *et al.* 1972

Chelonia

The groups of reptiles most studied in antibody production are the turtles and tortoises (Table 12.2). These animals synthesize IgM-similar high molecular weight antibodies and 7S and/or 5·7S antibodies. These low molecular weight antibodies seem to be similar to the comparable antibodies found in birds.

Immunoglobulins

Different species amongst the diverse orders of reptilia possess different immunoglobulins and therefore each will be considered separately in the sections that follow.

Rhynchocephalia

The blood serum of the tuatara, *Sphenodon punctatum*, contains two types of immunoglobulins (Marchalonis *et al.* 1969). The 18S immunoglobulin resembles the IgM in polypeptide chain structure. It is a pentameric molecule, the subunits consisting of two light chains and two heavy chains. In acrylamide gel electrophoretic comparison the migration of the chains is identical to that of the L-chains and μ-chains of human IgM.

The 7S immunoglobulin is antigenically related to the 18S Ig, having the same type of light chains. The heavy chains of the 7S Ig, however, differ from those of the 18S Ig, indicating a distinct immunoglobulin class. The migration of the heavy chain of the 7S Ig in acrylamide gel electrophoresis is similar to the human γ-chain. Although the immunization period lasted for more than 8 months, antibody activity was only found in the 18S Ig (Marchalonis *et al.* 1969).

Crocodilia

Clem and Leslie (1969) and Saluk *et al.* (1970, 1973) have detected two kinds of immunoglobulins in the alligator. The high molecular weight 19S Ig has a mol. wt. of 900,000 and is a pentameric molecule (Saluk *et al.* 1973). By means of sedimentation equilibrium analysis, Saluk *et al.* (1973) found the data which is cited in Table 12.3.

Table 12.3. Immunoglobulins of alligator (Saluk *et al.* 1973)

	Molecular weight				Probable
	H-chain	L-chain	Subunit	Total	isotype
High mol. wt. Ig	70,000	20,000	175,000	900,000	IgM
Low mol. wt. Ig	56,000	20,000	—	160,000	?

In both types of alligator immunoglobulin, two kinds of light chains have been found (Saluk *et al.* 1970). These differ in antigenicity but show identical electrophoretic mobility. Because both types of L-chains could be found in all individual sera tested, they are probably under the control of independently segregating genes, perhaps comparable to χ and λ in mammals.

Lacertilia

Since Hemmerling's investigation of the Scheltopusik, *Ophisaurus apodus* (Ambrosius *et al.* 1969), it has been believed that lizards can produce at least two types of immunoglobulins which are sensitive to 2-mercapto-ethanol. This has subsequently been confirmed by Wetherall (1969), Ambrosius (1970), Hemmerling (1971), Hemmerling and Ambrosius (1971), and Wetherall and Turner (1972). Both the high and low molecular weight antibodies are to be found in early and late immune sera, but the quantities of the low molecular weight antibodies increases with time after immunization.

In recent works from our Laboratory Dietlind Hädge and H. Fiebig (unpublished) studied the structure of the immunoglobulins of *Ophisaurus*. They isolated three types of immunoglobulins with antibody activity. In contrast to earlier investigations they detected the high molecular weight Ig in the β-2 region. In the α-2 region a protein can be found with unspecific binding activity to some proteins and which is present in blood serum in a high quantity. This is not an immunoglobulin.

The 7S fraction of antiserum contains two types of immunoglobulin which are antigenically different and also differ from one another in their electrophoretic mobility (Fig. 12.1). Following immunization with serum proteins, BGG, DNP-BGG, and DNP-*Brucella*, the most antibody activity is to be found in the Ig with β-1 mobility. This corresponds to the 7S antibody described earlier. The second low molecular weight Ig with β-2 mobility is present in the antiserum in much lower concentration. As acrylamide-electrophoresis in SDS shows, the molecular weight of the heavy chain of the β-1

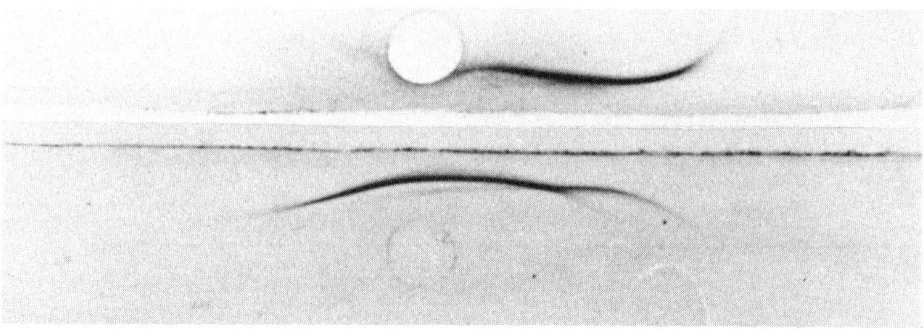

Fig. 12.1. Immunoelectrophoresis of purified antibodies of the lizard, *Ophisaurus apodus*, developed by rabbit-anti-Ophisaurus whole serum. Upper part IgM antibodies, lower part low molecular weight antibodies. Anode on the left side. Courtesy Dr Fiebig.

Ig is somewhat lower, that of the β-2 Ig somewhat higher than the mol. wt. of the γ-chain (Fig. 12.2). A summary of the data is given in Table 12.4.

The structural data as well as the binding data (see p. 316) for the immunoglobulin of lizards suggest that lizards possess a high molecular weight pentameric similar to IgM. The 7·3S Ig with β-2 mobility may correspond to the IgY of birds (Leslie & Clem 1969). The 6·8S Ig, which in electrophoresis migrates as a β-1 protein, seems to be an isotype unique to this reptilian group.

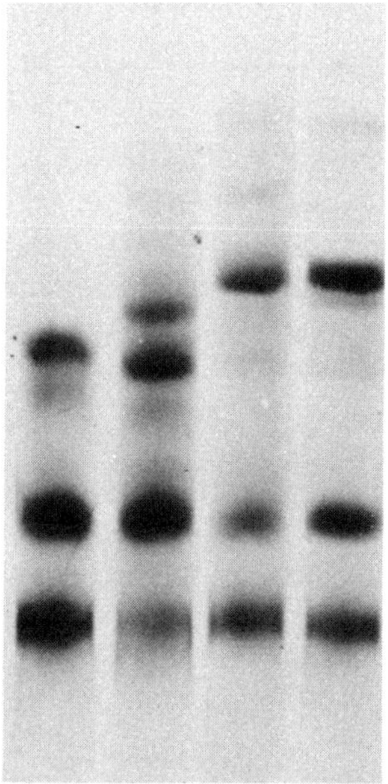

Fig. 12.2. SDS-acrylamide electrophoresis of reduced immunoglobulins. From left to right: (1) rabbit IgG; (2) Ophisaurus 7·3S and 6·8S antibodies; (3) Ophisaurus IgM; (4) human IgM. In the upper part the H-chains, in the lower part the L-chain, on the bottom myoglobin as marker. Courtesy Dr Fiebig.

Serpentes

At this time we have only the report of Salanitro and Minton (1973) that colubrid snakes produce 7S antibody to BSA and 19S antibody to KLH.

Chelonia

Since the first investigation by Grey (1963) in *Chrysemys picta* and Maung (1963) in *Testudo ibera*, numerous investigations have been carried out into the structure of the immunoglobulins of turtles (Lykakis 1968, Grey 1969,

Table 12.4. Immunoglobulins of lizards

Species	S-value	Molecular weight H-chain	L-chain	Total	Carbohydrate content (%) Hexose	Hexosamine
Ophisaurus*	17·7	70,000	23,000	~900,000	5·3	2·7
Tiliqua†	19·1	77,000	22,400	953,000	6·7	—
Ophisaurus*	6·8	48,000	23,000	142,000	1·1	0·9
Tiliqua†	6·8	51,000	22,400	158,000	1·8	—
Ophisaurus*	7·3	63,000	23,000	~170,000		

* Fiebig and Hädge (unpublished data).
† Wetherall (1969).

Chartrand *et al.* 1971, Frommel *et al.* 1971, Acton *et al.* 1972, Benedict & Pollard 1972, Coe, 1972, Leslie & Clem 1972) and of tortoises (Ambrosius 1966, 1967, 1968, 1970, Ambrosius *et al.* 1969, 1972, Rothe & Ambrosius 1968). Thus this group of reptiles supplies the most exact information about the immunoglobulin structure and the sequence of the appearance of the isotypes in the course of immunization.

Because the differences between the various species are not very marked and our investigation with *T. hermanni* lasted more than 7 years, we will first give a description of the dynamics of the production of the different isotypes in that species following immunization. The tortoises (*T. hermanni* GMELIN) were kept at an average temperature of 25°C and immunized with 70 mg pig serum proteins. The immunization schedule is given in Table 12.5. In all cases

Table 12.5. Immunization schedule of *Testudo hermanni*

Immunization in days after the immunization 1	2	3	4	5	6	7	8	9	10	11	12
221	0										
431	210	0									
537		106	0								
710			173	0							
717				17	0						
734					17	0					
752						18	0				
769							17	0			
795								26	0		
815									20	0	
1696										881	0

the same animals were used throughout the investigation (Ambrosius *et al.* 1969, 1972).

The separation of the various antisera with Sephadex G 200 chromatography and the demonstration of antibody activity by passive haemagglutination showed a high molecular weight (HMW) antibody to be synthesized initially following the first immunization. Some months later this was followed by a low molecular weight (LMW) antibody (Fig. 12.3). The two antibodies were sensitive to treatment with 2-mercapto-ethanol (ME). After the second immunization the two antibody types usually appeared at about the same time, followed nearly one week later by another LMW antibody, which was stable under ME treatment (Fig. 12.4). Production of the latter increased

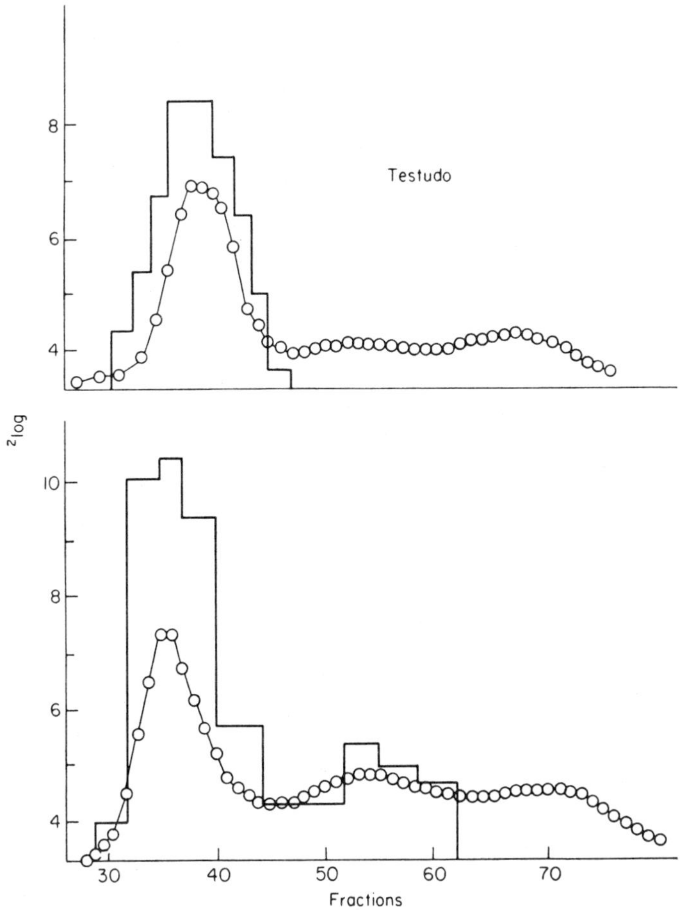

Fig. 12.3. Gel filtration of an early (27th and 36th days) and a late (99th and 124th days) primary antiserum of the tortoise, *Testudo hermanni*. Antibody activity determined by passive haemagglutination.

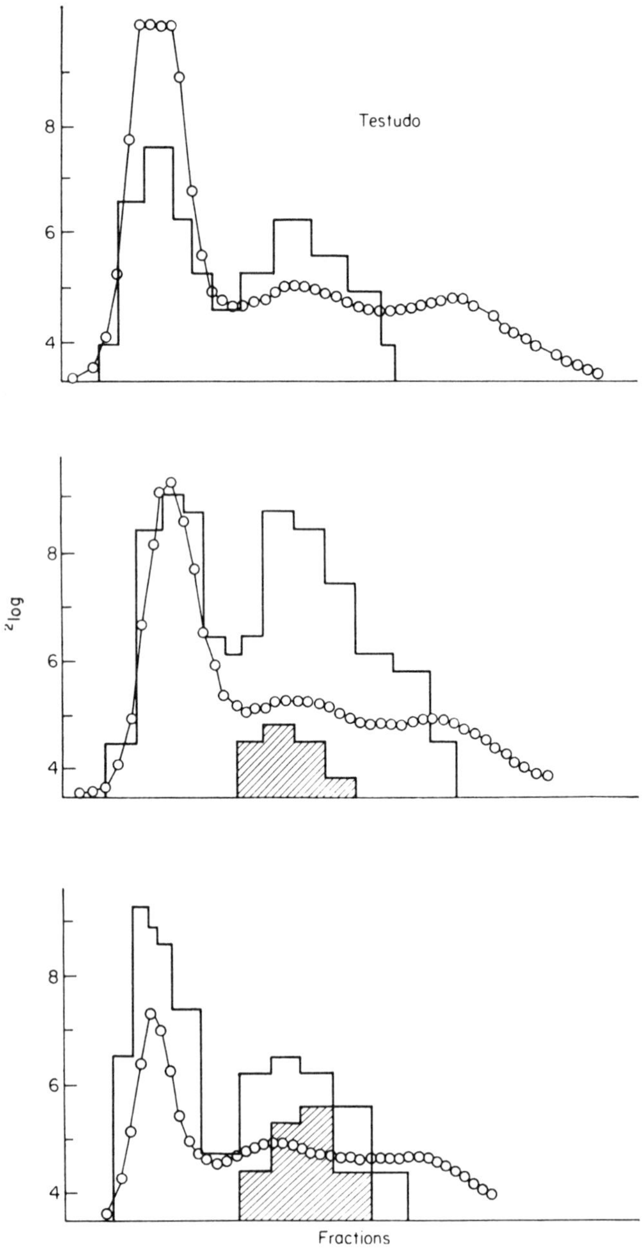

Fig. 12.4. Gel filtration of antisera (10th, 17th, 51st days) following the second immunization, the ME-resistant antibody is shown by cross-hatched area.

with each additional immunization proportionally to the decrease of the HMW antibody and, at the same time, a further, extremely LMW, ME-sensitive, antibody appeared from about the fourth immunization onwards (Fig. 12.5). Collection of fractions from the third peak of chromatographic separation, and their rechromatography with Sephadex G 200, confirmed the presence of this fourth antibody type. Repeatedly immunizing the tortoises at short-time intervals, resulted in a marked increase in the LMW, ME-stable,

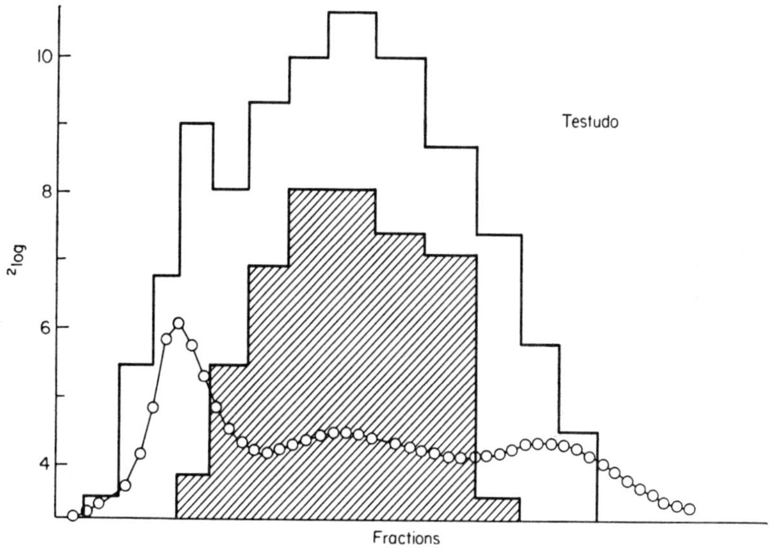

Fig. 12.5. Gel filtration of an early serum (10th day) after the eighth immunization. Note the proportion of the ME-sensitive antibodies in the third peak.

antibody (Fig. 12.6). During a resting period of 2·5 years, however, the titre of the latter decreased much more than that of the other immunoglobulins (Fig. 12.7). Following an additional (twelfth) immunization immediately after this period, the distribution of the immunoglobulins closely corresponded to that found after the fourth immunization. Thus in the tortoise we find a sequence of HMW and LMW antibodies following the diverse immunizations comparable to the IgM–IgG sequence in mammals, but the whole reactivity of the reptile is slower than that of the mammal. A summary of data for the different antibody types of *Testudo* is given in Table 12.6.

Data comparable to the above have been obtained by several other authors. Thus, after immunization in *Chrysemys picta*, Grey (1963, 1969) and Coe (1972) first found an HMW antibody, followed later on by LMW antibodies. The early antibodies could be inactivated by ME treatment, but the late antibodies were stable. Both HMW and LMW antibodies have also

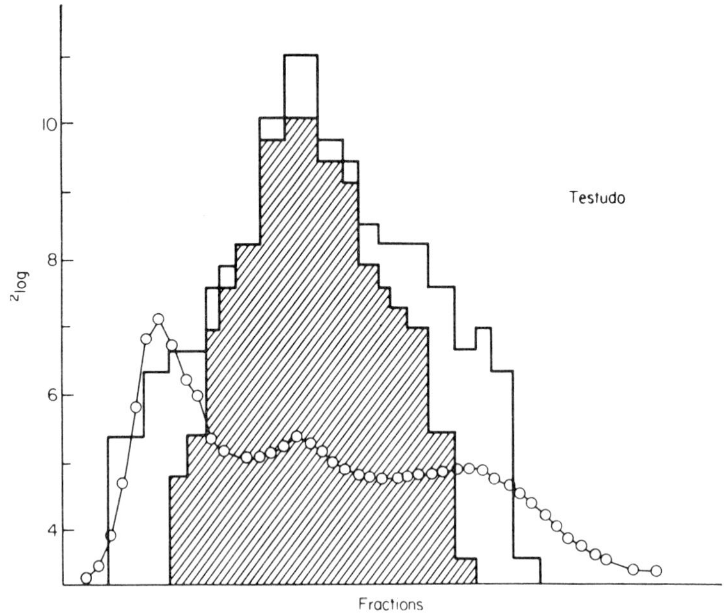

Fig. 12.6. Gel filtration of an early hyperimmunserum (11th day, 11th immunization).

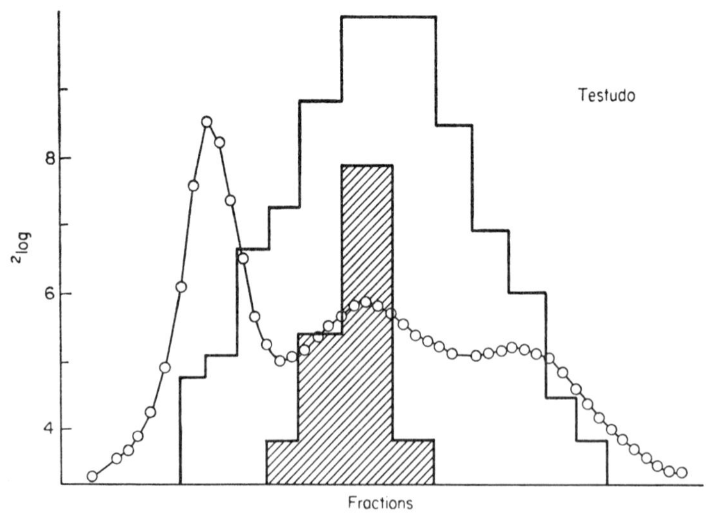

Fig. 12.7. Gel filtration of an extremely late antiserum (860th day) after the 11th immunization.

Table 12.6. Antibody types of *Testudo hermanni*

	$Early_1$	$Early_2$	$Late_1$	$Late_2$
Molecular type	High mol. wt.	Low mol. wt.	Low mol. wt.	Extremely low mol. wt.
ME-stability	Sensitive	Sensitive	Resistant	Sensitive
Electroph. mobility	β_2	γ	γ	β_1
S_c 20°C value	19	7	7	5·7

been found in *Emys orbicularis* by Lykakis (1968), in *Chelydra serpentina* by Chartrand *et al.* (1971), in *Chelonia mydas* by Benedict and Pollard (1972), and in *Pseudemys scripta* by Leslie and Clem (1972). The extremely LMW antibody could also be detected in *Chelydra serpentina*, *Chelonia mydas*, and *Pseudemys scripta* (Chartrand *et al.* 1973, Benedict & Polland 1972, Leslie & Clem 1972). The differences in the dynamics of the appearance of the immunoglobulins may in part depend on the different immunization schedules, and partly reflect species-specific characters.

An extensive analysis of the immunoglobulin structure of turtles and tortoises has been done by Chartrand *et al.* (1971), Acton *et al.* (1972), Leslie and Clem (1972), and in our group by Eva-Maria Andreas, H. Fiebig and Dietlind Hädge (unpublished). In antigenic comparison we found that the two 7S antibodies, one of them ME-sensitive, the other ME-resistant, belong to the same isotype. They differ in only very few antigenic determinants and may represent different subclasses.

The extremely LMW antibody (5·7S) is antigenically similar to the 7S antibody, in that it has the same heavy chain but lacks one or two domains in the Fc portion (Ambrosius *et al.* 1972).

The structural data on the immunoglobulins of turtles and tortoises available at this time are summarized in Tables 12.7 and 12.8.

Table 12.7. High molecular weight immunoglobulins of tortoises and turtles

Species	S-value	Molecular weight H-chain	L-chain	Total	Carbohydrate content (%) Hexose	Hexosamine
*Testudo**	19	70,000	23,000	~900,000	2·8	1·3
Pseudemys†	17·7	67,000	22,500	~850,000	4·3	2·2
Pseudemys‡	17	70,000	22,500	850,000	2·5	—
Chelydra§	18·8	70,000	23,500	~900,000	—	—

* Andreas, Fiebig and Hädge (unpublished data)
† Acton *et al.* (1972).
‡ Leslie and Clem (1972).
§ Chartrand *et al.* (1971).

Table 12.8. Low molecular weight immunoglobulins of tortoises and turtles

Species	S-value	Molecular weight H-chain	L-chain	Total	Carbohydrate content (%) Hexose	Hexosamine
*Testudo**	7	63,000	23,000	183,000	1·5	0·7
Pseudemys†	7·5	67,500	22,500	180,000	2·1	—
*Testudo**	5·7	35,000	23,000	120,000	—	—
Pseudemys†	5·7	35,000	22,500	120,000	0·35	—
Chelydra‡	5·7	38,000	22,500	120,000	0·63	0·05

* Andreas, Fiebig and Hädge (unpublished data).
† Leslie and Clem (1972).
‡ Chartrand *et al.* (1971).

As can be seen in the Tables and in Fig. 12.8, the HMW immunoglobulin is similar to the IgM of mammals. But the 7S immunoglobulin differs remarkably from the IgG (Fig. 12.8), in that it seems to be comparable to the IgY of birds (Leslie & Clem 1969, Zimmerman *et al.* 1971). The 5·7S immunoglobulin with the shortened heavy chain resembles the 5·7S antibody of the duck (Zimmerman *et al.* 1971). At this time it is not possible to decide whether other extremely LMW immunoglobulins in teleosts, dipnoi, and mammals (Marchalonis 1970, Richter *et al.* 1972, Thomas *et al.* 1972) are

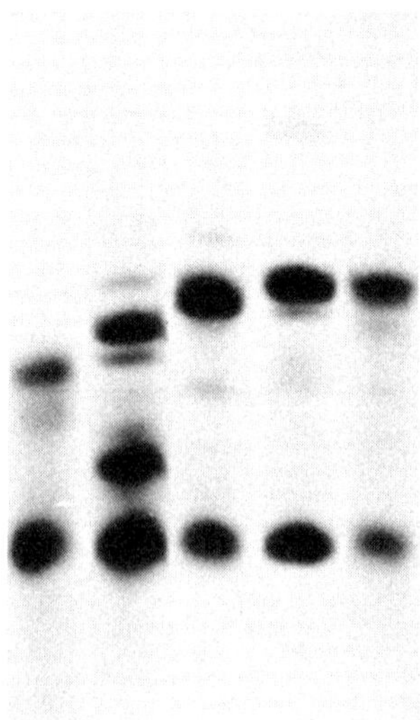

Fig. 12.8. SDS-acrylamide electrophoresis of reduced immunoglobulins. From left to right: (1) bovine IgG; (2) 7S and 5·7S antibodies of tortoise; (3) tortoise IgM; (4) carp IgM; (5) human IgM. In the upper part the H-chains, in the lower part the L-chains. Courtesy Dr Andreas.

directly similar to this type of immunoglobulin. Here, as in many other cases, extensive studies in antigenic comparison are needed to clarify the situation.

General problems in antibody production and the biological properties of reptilian antibodies

Antigen elimination

In reptiles the elimination of antigens, solely in the first part of the immune response, is comparable to the processes which can be shown experimentally to exist in mammals. Thus, in *Testudo hermanni* following immunization with ^{131}I-bovine γ-globulin, we found the typical phases of distribution in body fluids; normal elimination followed by immune elimination (Fig. 12.9).

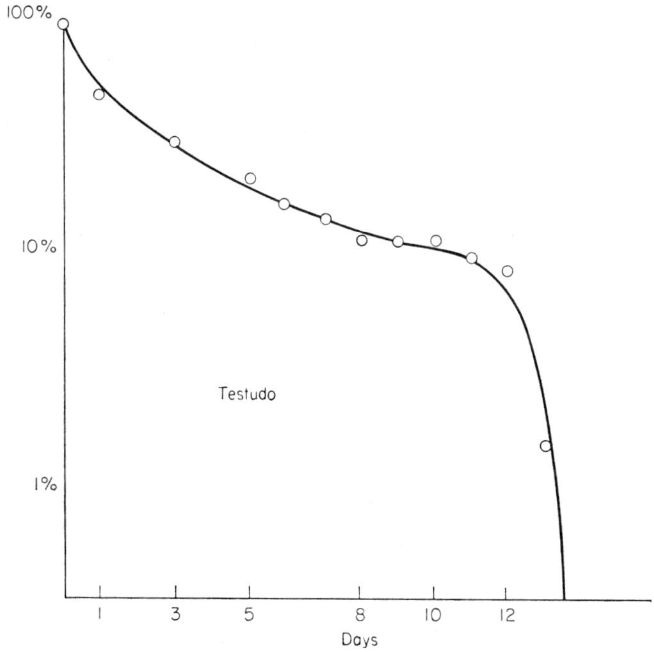

Fig. 12.9. Elimination of radioactive-labelled protein antigen in the tortoise, *Testudo hermanni.*

However, traces of the antigen could be found in the animals for a long time. This preservation of the antigen in the body is very curious but has been noted by several authors. Widal and Sicard (1897) noted that in the blood of the turtle, *Cistudio lutaria*, bacterial antigen and agglutinins occur together. This conservation of antigen has also been found in *Testudo graeca* by Blanc *et al.* (1960), in *T. ibera* by Maung (1963), in *Emys orbicularis* by Combiesco *et al.*

(1963), and in *Lacerta muralis* and *Vipera ammodytes* by Dimow (1968) and Dimow and Slawtschew (1967). We cannot speculate about the exact distribution of the antigen in the tissues since no information is available. However, the capacity of reptilian antibodies to form soluble antigen-antibody complexes in the region of equivalence (Hemmerling 1971) might influence the distribution of antigen.

Maternal transfer of antibody into eggs and the ontogeny of antibody production

The only information we have regarding the transfer of antibodies into eggs is based upon investigation of turtles (Grasset *et al.* 1931, Maung 1963, Chartrand *et al.* 1971, Leslie & Clem 1972). In all species examined, an antibody transfer has been found. As Chartrand *et al.* (1971) and Leslie and Clem (1972) pointed out, there are striking differences between the diverse immunoglobulin classes. Only the extremely LMW 5·7S antibody can cross the intervening barriers and get into the yolk of the egg. There are interesting connections here with the capacity for complement binding as discussed by Chartrand *et al.* (1971). We know from studies with IgG from man, rabbit, and mouse that the segment of the γ-chain associated with complement binding activity was assigned to the C_H2 region. Enzymatically-derived polypeptides composed of the C_H3 region only were inactive. Moreover, Kehoe and Fougereau (1969) isolated a peptide of 60 amino acids, derived from the C_H2 region of a mouse IgG_{2a} myeloma, that possessed almost all of the complement binding activity of that molecule. Because turtle 5·7S immunoglobulin interacts with amphibian or reptilian complement, it must be suggested that the site for complement attachment lies on the C-terminal C_H region of the molecule. In mammals, passage of immunoglobulins across fetal membranes is a highly selective process directly related to the Fc molecular fraction. The fact that only the 5·7S turtle immunoglobulin can be found in the eggs indicates a specific transfer in reptiles comparable to IgG transfer to the fetus in some mammals. These data also suggest that the site involved in cellular interaction may be located on the C_H2 region, as is the complement binding site.

The only information we have regarding the ontogeny of antibody production in reptiles is that provided by Sidky and Auerbach (1968) and Kanakambika and Muthukkaruppan (1972). In the turtle, *Chelydra serpentina*, the ability to produce antibodies is not only lacking at the time of hatching, but it takes more than 3 months of post-hatching development to reach a level of immunological reactivity comparable to that of adults (Sidky & Auerbach 1968). The authors point out that in nature these young turtles probably enter their first hibernation before they reach full immune competence.

The picture presented by the lizard *Calotes versicolor* is very different (Kanakambika & Muthukkaruppan 1972). In this species, following immunization with sheep erythrocytes, the hatchlings produce nearly as many haemolytic plaque-forming cells as the adult animals. Thus different reptiles show great differences in the time of maturation of their immune systems.

Immunological memory

One of the most controversial problems in the literature is whether reptiles are able to show a typical secondary response. Some authors could not find a typical immunological memory, especially when using bacterial antigens (Maung 1963, Grey 1963, Marchalonis *et al.* 1969, see also Acton *et al.* 1972). In other cases, mostly using protein antigens, a typical secondary response has been observed (Ambrosius 1966, 1967, 1968, Ambrosius & Lehmann 1965, Ambrosius *et al.* 1972, Lerch *et al.* 1967, Acton *et al.* 1972, Benedict *et al.* 1972, Wetherall & Turner, 1972, Wright & Shapiro 1973). A characteristic example from our studies of the tortoise, *Testudo hermanni*, may illustrate the capacity of reptiles to show an immunological memory. The animals, kept at 25°C, were immunized with 50 mg pig serum proteins per kg body weight; 170 days later they received the second injection and on day 380 the third antigen injection. As can be seen in Fig. 12.10 the titre in the passive haemagglutination following the second and the third antigen contacts was much higher than in the primary response, and these high titres lasted for a long time.

An example of the influence of the antigen type on the immunological memory is the work with the desert iguana, *Dipsosaurus dorsalis*. Previous studies with the antigen *Salmonella typhosa* have failed to demonstrate a

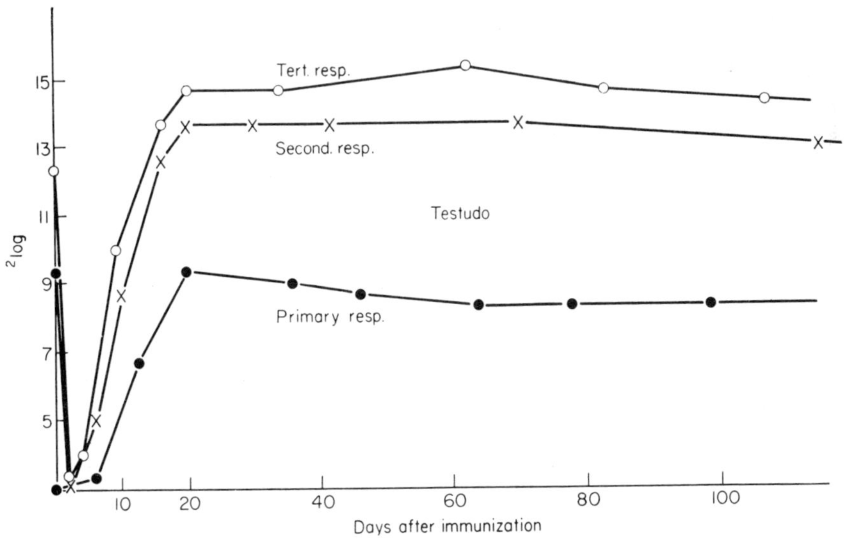

Fig. 12.10. Antibody titres (pass. haemagglutination) in *Testudo hermanni* following the first, second, and third immunization.

secondary response (Evans 1963, Evans *et al.* 1965). However, Wright and Schapiro (1973) obtained in the same species an enhanced secondary response with haemocyanin, characterized by the rapid appearance of antibody, a three- to four-fold increase in titre over that of the primary response, and the persistence of antibodies for long periods of time.

Summarizing, the controversial data in the literature about the appearance of a typical secondary response centre around two factors: the state of the antigen and the period between the first and the second antigen contact. Only with protein antigens which induce a true primary response can we induce a characteristic secondary response too. The second antigen contact should come after a period long enough to allow for the maturation processes in the immune system to be completed, which means at least several weeks.

Morphology and kinetics of appearance of antibody-producing cells

Few investigations have been carried out to determine the cellular basis of antibody production (Rothe & Ambrosius 1968, Kassin & Pevnitskii 1969, Kanakambika & Muthukkaruppan 1972) or the ultrastructure of antibody synthesizing cells (Ambrosius & Hoheisel 1969, 1973). The dynamics of haemolytic plaque-forming cells in tortoises (Rothe & Ambrosius 1968) and in lizards (Kanakambika & Muthukkaruppan 1972) are very similar to those of mammals. Fig. 12.11 shows the results of an experiment with the tortoise,

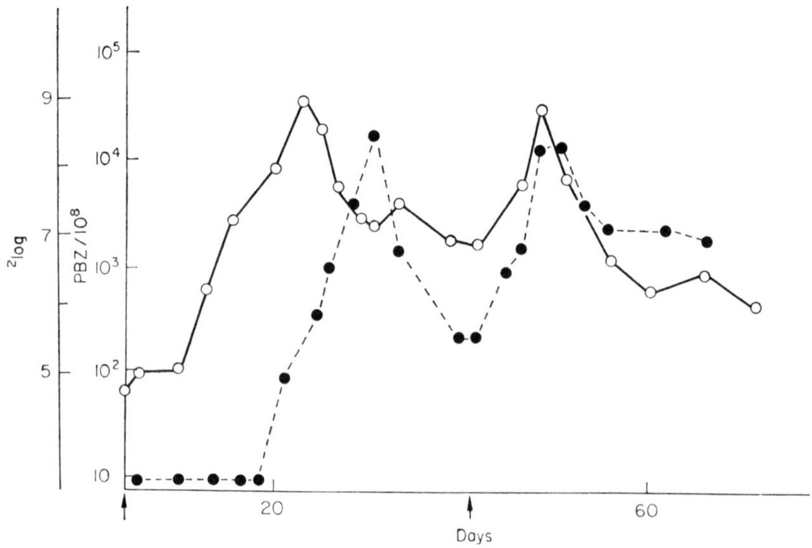

Fig. 12.11. Number of PFC (○——○) of spleen cells and haemolysin titre (●——●) following immunization of the tortoise, *Agrionemys horsfieldii*, with sheep erythrocytes. Data of Rothe and Ambrosius (1968). Arrows represent the date of immunization.

Agrionemys horsfieldi. The animals were immunized with $1{\cdot}6 \times 10^9$ sheep red blood cells. The number of plaque-forming cells (PFC) in the spleen peaked at three weeks following the immunization, the maximum titre of haemolysing antibodies in the blood serum nearly 8 days later. In the primary response, the course of the haemolysins followed the course of PFC with a time lapse of nearly one week. This interval is much longer than the one or two days usual in mammals. However, in the secondary response the two curves were almost identical. It is interesting that none of the rosette-forming or agglutinating cells were PFC.

Most of the PFC have been found in the spleen, a considerable number in the blood, but almost none in the thymus, bone marrow, cloacal complex, lung, liver or kidneys (Kanakambika & Muthukkaruppan 1972, Rothe & Ambrosius 1968). That agrees with the observation of Kanakambika and Muthukkaruppan (1972) that lizards cannot produce antibodies against sheep red blood cells if they have been splenectomized from 7 days to 2 hours before testing. Thus the spleen must be considered the main antibody-producing organ in reptiles.

PFC from the spleen or blood of the tortoise *Agrionemys horsfieldi* have been investigated by electron microscopy (Ambrosius & Hoheisel 1969, 1973). In the spleen very immature and mature plasmocytic cells were found in nearly equal proportions. The mature plasma cells possessed short elements of endoplasmic reticulum dilated in irregular sacs (Fig. 12.12). They may represent a primitive type of protein secreting and/or storing cells. In the majority of the antibody-producing cells signs of phagocytosis and pinocytosis were seen. The spectrum of the PFC in the blood stretched from activated lymphocytes to plasma cells, some of them with a peculiar arrangement of short RER cisternae (Figs. 12.12, 12.13, 12.14). All of the PFC contained numerous free ribosomes and polysomes in their cytoplasm and showed phagocytic activity.

Valence and affinity of reptilian antibodies

The nature of the binding properties of antibodies required the induction of anti-hapten antibodies. These could be induced with DNP-conjugates and also dimethylnaphthalinsulfonyl-(Dansyl)-conjugates (Frenzel & Ambrosius 1971, Fiebig 1972, 1973, Ambrosius, Frenzel & Fiebig 1972, Benedict & Pollard 1972, Litman *et al.* 1973).

The binding properties of HMW anti-DNP antibodies of the tortoise, *Agrionemys horsfieldi*, and the lizard, *Ophisaurus apodus*, have been investigated (Fiebig 1972, 1973, Ambrosius *et al.* 1972, Fiebig *et al.* 1974). With DNP-PLL, DNP-HSA, and DNP-BGG the antibodies induced have been mostly LMW. A measurably higher IgM response could be elicited by immunization with DNP-haemocyanin or DNP-Brucella.

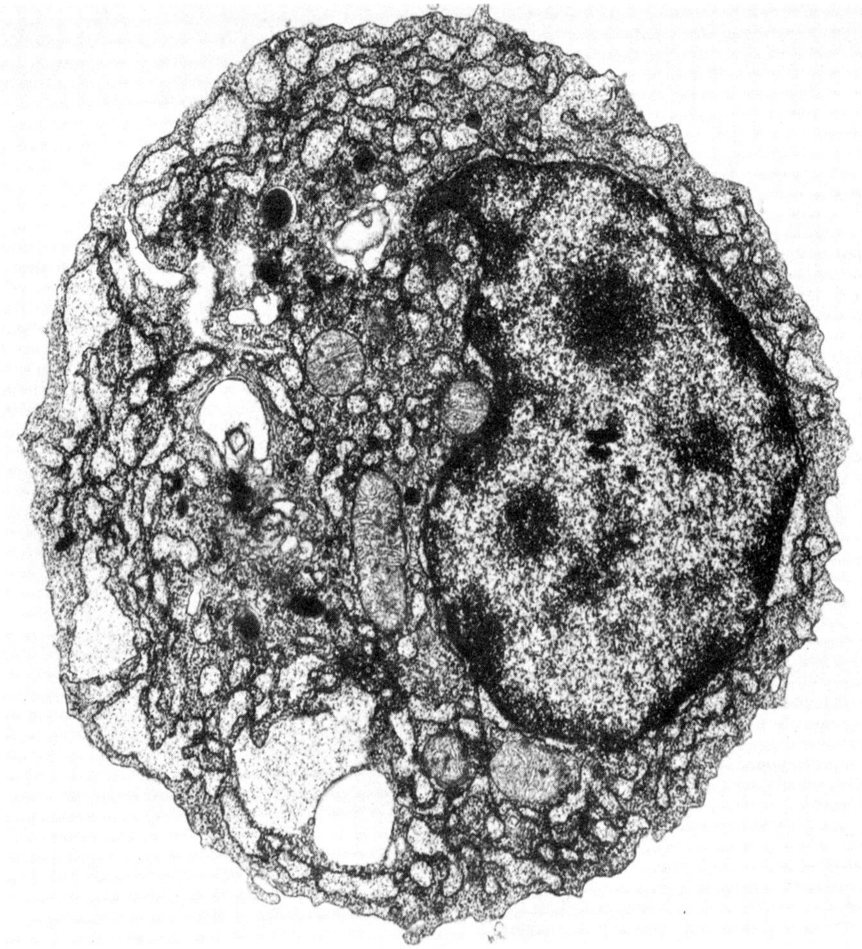

Fig. 12.12. Mature plasma cell from the spleen of the tortoise, *Agrionemys*, as plaque-forming cell, × 16,000.

The results with specific purified IgM anti-DNP antibodies in equilibrium dialysis with ε-DNP-lysine give data which can be calculated to give five binding sites per molecule (Fig. 12.15). In HMW anti-DNP antibodies of *Ophisaurus* only four to five binding sites could be found (Ambrosius *et al.* 1972). Studies using various vertebrate species, e.g. sharks (Voss *et al.* 1969), bony fishes (Russell *et al.* 1970, Fiebig 1972, 1973, Ambrosius & Fiebig 1972, Fiebig & Ambrosius 1975), birds (Fiebig, unpublished), and mammals (Frank & Humphrey 1968, Lindqvist & Bauer 1966, Onoue *et al.* 1965, Voss & Eisen 1968, Mukkur 1972), suggest that the 7S subunit of HMW antibodies

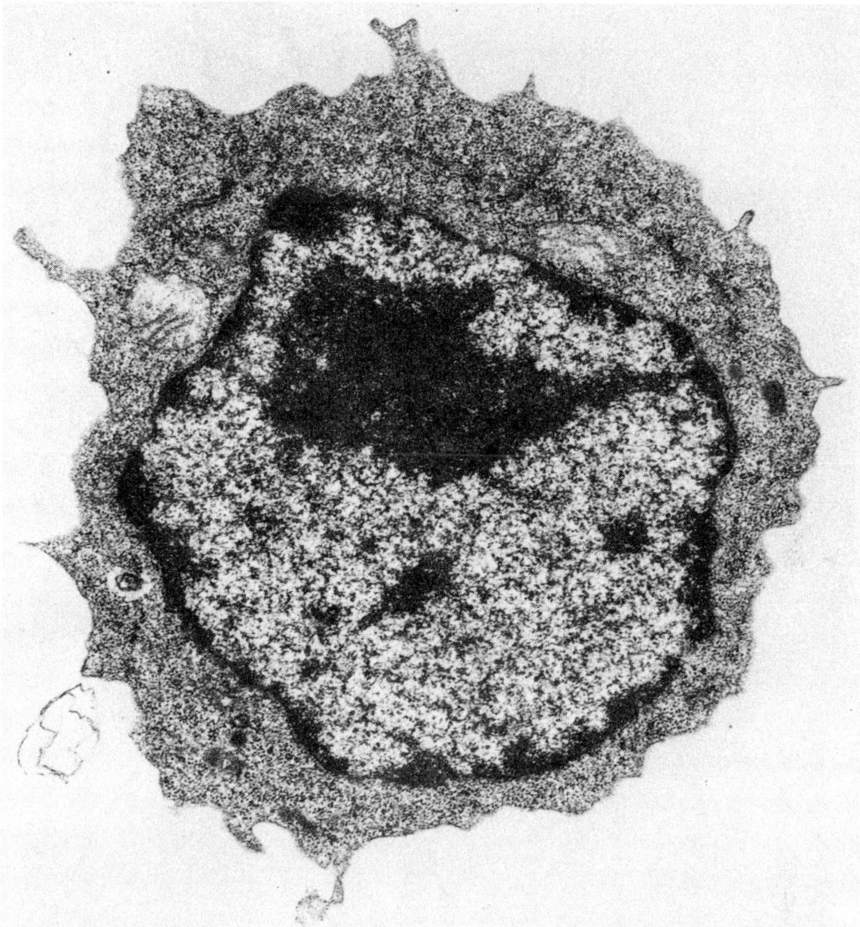

Fig. 12.13. Lymphoid plaque-forming cell from the blood of the tortoise, *Agrionemys*, ×20,000.

is functionally monovalent. Contrary to these data, other studies establish the presence of ten binding sites, five of them with high, five of them with low affinity (Clem & Small 1970, Voss & Sigel 1972, Kishimoto & Onoue 1971, Oriol *et al.* 1971). The mostly low affinity of the antibodies is probably the reason for the measurement of only a part of the binding sites. The average association constant of *Agrionemys* IgM anti-DNP antibodies is K_0 10^4 to $K_0 = 1 \times 10^5$ M^{-1} depending on the antigen used (Fiebig 1972, 1973, Ambrosius *et al.* 1972). The IgM antibodies of *Ophisaurus* have identical values.

Bivalence has been demonstrated in tortoise 7S and lizard 7·3S antibodies

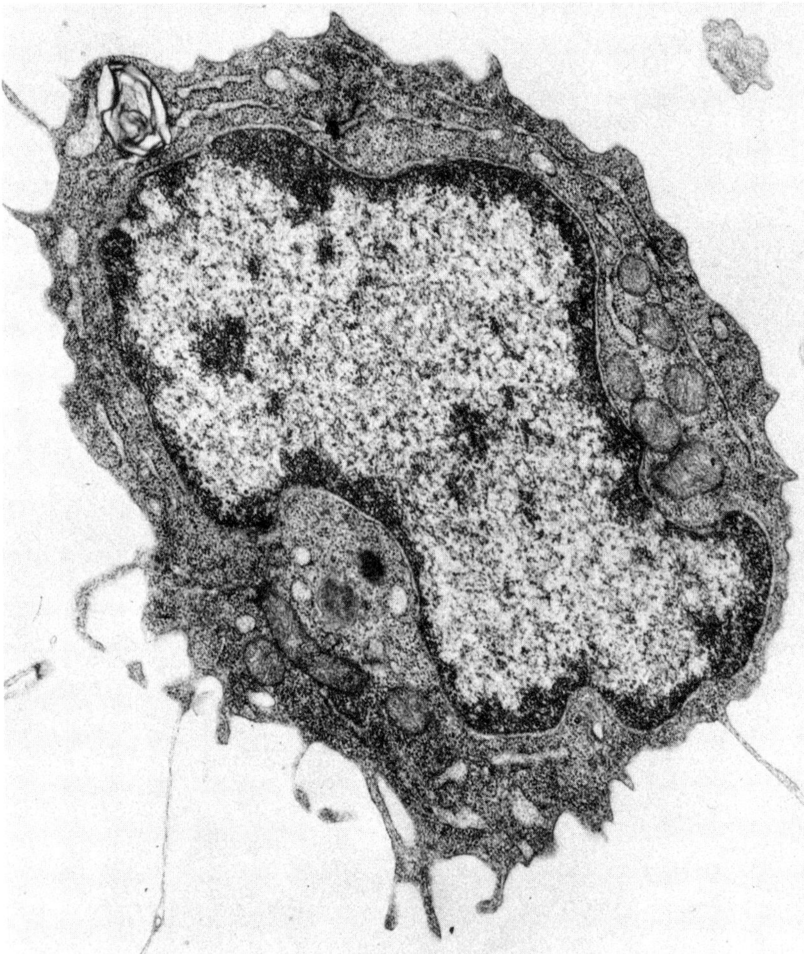

Fig. 12.14. Most frequent type of plaque-forming cell from the blood of the tortoise, *Agrionemys*, corresponding to plasmoblast or immature plasma cell, ×20,000.

(mol. wt. of H-chain 63,000–64,000). These antibodies show a low heterogeneity with regard to the binding properties. The average association constant for ε-DNP lysine is relatively low, for *Ophisaurus* $K_0 = 1 \times 10^4\ M^{-1}$, for *Agrionemys* K_0 10^4–10^5 M^{-1} (Fiebig 1972, 1973, Ambrosius *et al.* 1972, Fiebig *et al.* 1974).

The 6·8S is the dominant LMW antibody of *Ophisaurus* (H-chain mol. wt. 48,000) and is well characterized. Its most striking property is its bad precipitability (Hemmerling 1970) but the formation of soluble antigen-antibody

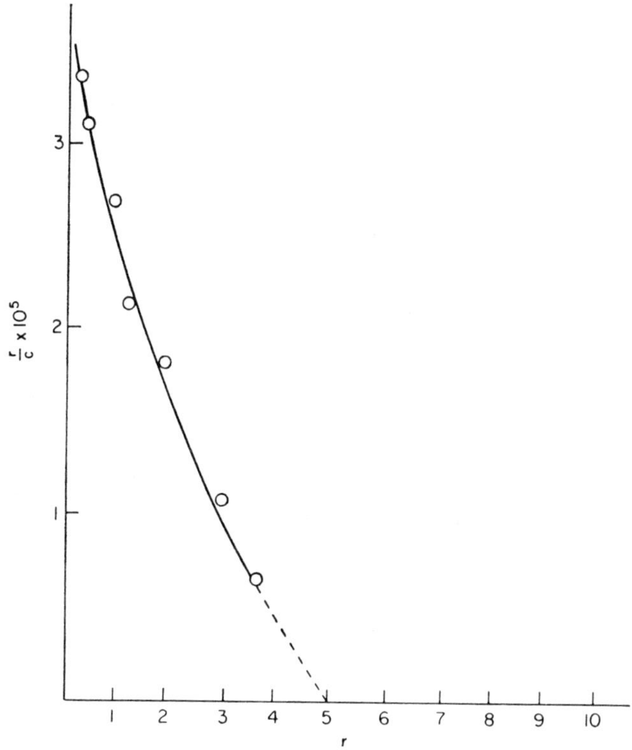

Fig. 12.15. Valence of IgM antibodies of *Agrionemys*. Equilibrium dialysis of purified anti-DNP antibodies with the hapten ε-DNP-lysine. The extrapolated valence is 5. The intrinsic average association constant $K_0 = 5{\cdot}2 \times 10^4\ \text{M}^{-1}$. Courtesy Dr Fiebig.

complexes has been demonstrated (Hemmerling 1971). A similar behaviour in several mammalian antibodies has been described (Klinman *et al.* 1964, Christian 1970). Mammalian IgG antibodies have been shown to possess two identical binding sites (Klinman *et al.* 1964) but the molecule is functionally monovalent, which may be due to the flexibility of the Fab fraction or the position of the binding sites. On the other hand, in *Ophisaurus* no data can be found to suggest that the antibody is more than monovalent (Fig. 12.16). But because the strength of the binding is relatively low, $K_0 = 3{\cdot}5 \times 10^4\ \text{M}^{-1}$, the existence of a second binding site with still lower affinity, which cannot be detected with the usual techniques, cannot be excluded.

In tortoises, the 5·7S antibody shows bivalence and a strong binding site heterogeneity (Fig. 12.17). The association constants normally fall in the range between 10^5 and $10^6\ \text{M}^{-1}$, but in some cases values of nearly $10^8 \times \text{M}^{-1}$ have been obtained. Since the population of the high affinity binding sites in no case exceeds the valence 1 an intramolecular asymmetry in the binding

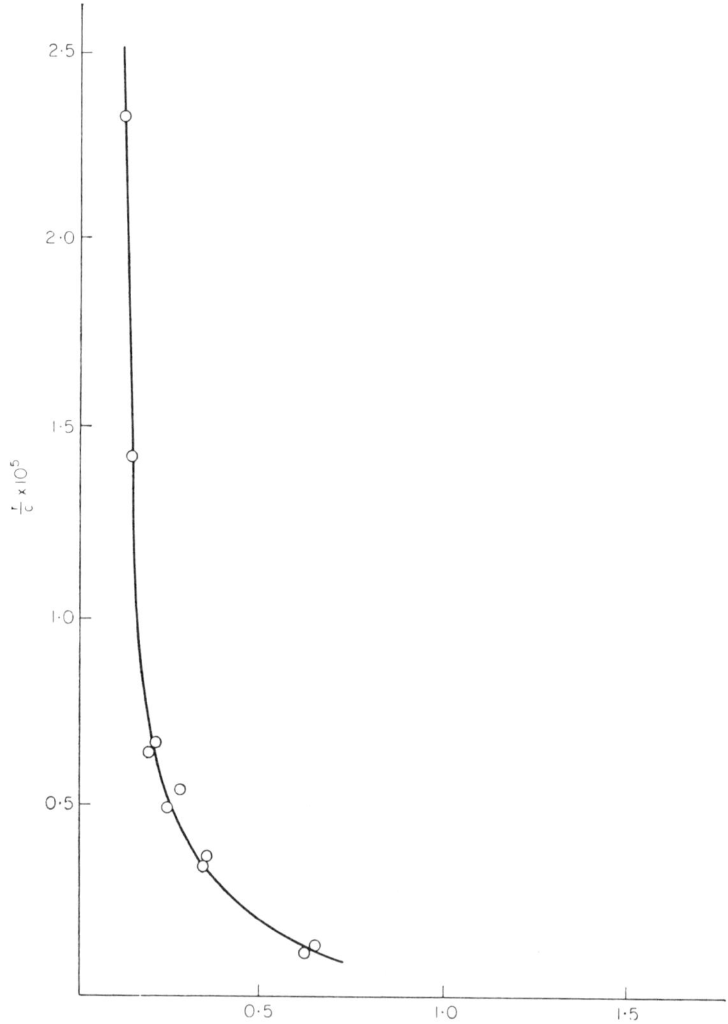

Fig. 12.16. Binding data of the 6·8S *Ophisaurus* anti-DNP antibody to the hapten ε-DNP-lysine, determined by equilibrium dialysis. The observed valence is 1. The intrinsic average association constant $K_0 = 3{\cdot}8 \times 10^4$ M^{-1}. Courtesy Dr Fiebig.

affinity cannot be excluded. Litman *et al.* (1973) found a valence of 1·7 for the 5·7S anti-DNP antibody of *Chelydra*, with an average association constant $K_0 = 1{\cdot}7 \times 10^6$ M^{-1}, but no allusions to similar affinity differences in the binding sites.

Antigen binding sites of reptilian antibodies

The antigen binding sites of reptilian antibodies were only investigated in the

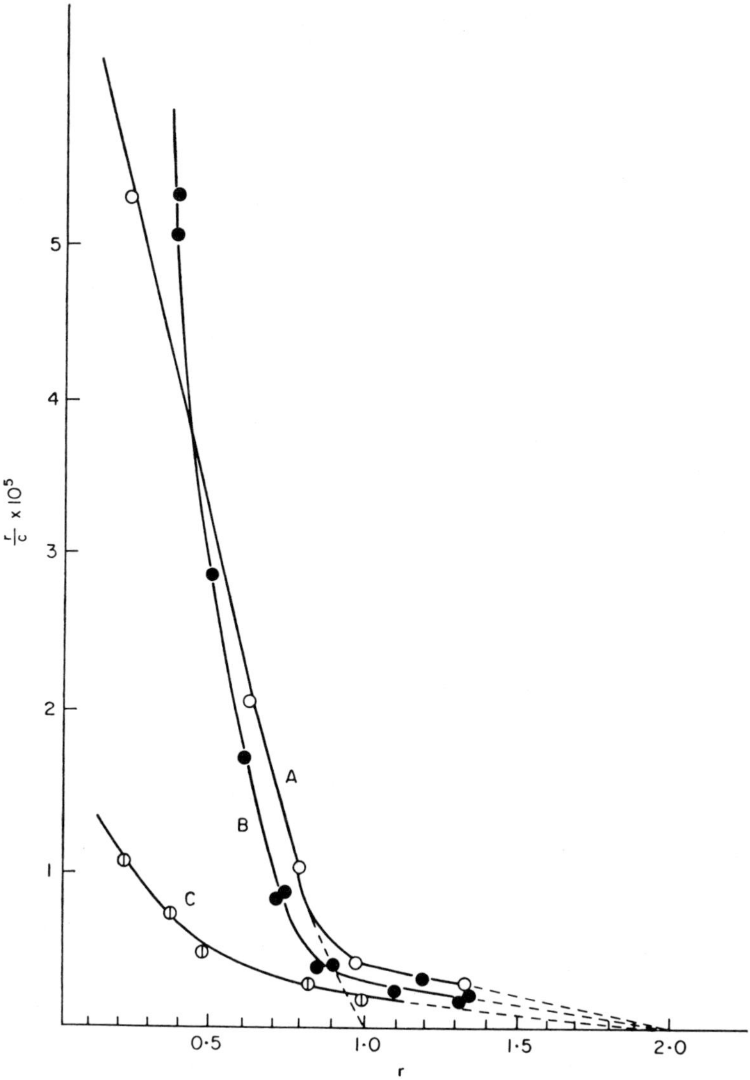

Fig. 12.17. Binding data of low molecular weight *Agrionemys* anti-DNP antibodies.

5·7S antibody: ● = $K_0 = 4{\cdot}8 \times 10^5$ M^{-1}, ○ = $K_0 = 3{\cdot}1 \times 10^5$ M^{-1}, 7S antibody: ⦶ = $K_0 = 1{\cdot}2 \times 10^5$ M^{-1}. Courtesy Dr Fiebig.

DNP system. These investigations are made feasible because DNP antibodies show a decrease in the fluorescence of tryptophan residues upon binding of the DNP hapten (Eisen 1964). This phenomenon of fluorescence quenching has been observed with anti-DNP antibodies of different vertebrate classes; in sharks (Voss *et al.* 1969), and in mammals (Eisen 1964). The interaction of tryptophan at the antibody binding site can be detected by absorption difference spectra (Fig. 12.18). They show the shift of the spectrum of ε-DNP lysine

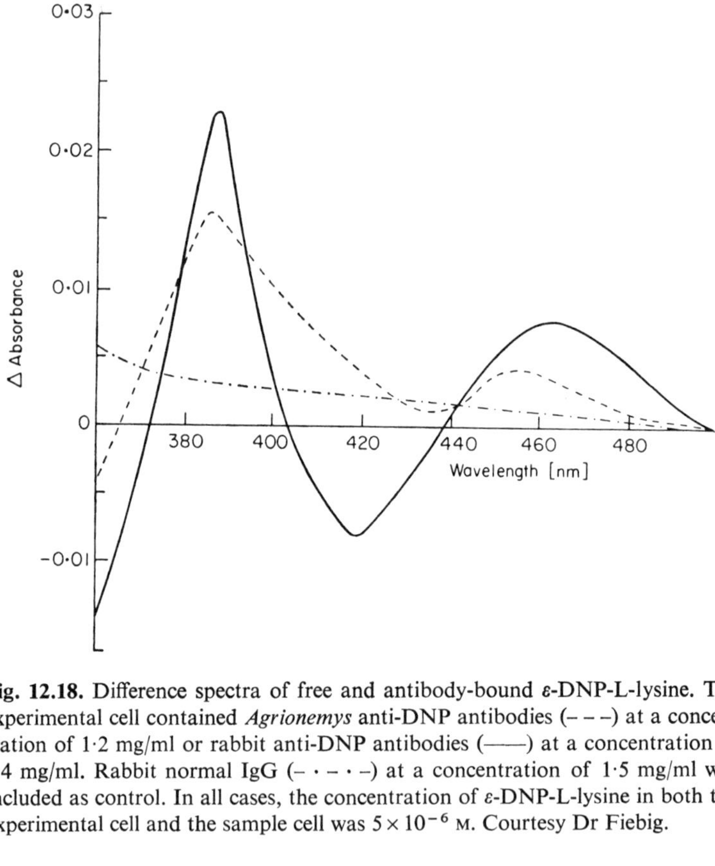

Fig. 12.18. Difference spectra of free and antibody-bound ε-DNP-L-lysine. The experimental cell contained *Agrionemys* anti-DNP antibodies (– – –) at a concentration of 1·2 mg/ml or rabbit anti-DNP antibodies (——) at a concentration of 1·4 mg/ml. Rabbit normal IgG (– · – · –) at a concentration of 1·5 mg/ml was included as control. In all cases, the concentration of ε-DNP-L-lysine in both the experimental cell and the sample cell was 5×10^{-6} M. Courtesy Dr Fiebig.

into the visible range following the specific binding. This interaction can be interpreted in the participation of hydrophobic binding strength and the complexes of the charge transfer in the antibody-hapten binding strength (Eisen & Siskind 1964).

In *Agrionemys* 5·7S antibodies, Fiebig (unpublished) found very similar difference spectra to those obtained by Litman *et al.* (1973) in 5·7S antibodies of *Chelydra* (Fig. 12.18). The similarity of the spectra with comparable spectra of antibodies from sharks (Voss *et al.* 1969), birds (Litman *et al.* 1973) and various mammals (Little & Eisen 1967) does at least speak for a similarity in the structure of the binding sites of anti-DNP antibodies from species of different phylogenetic evolutionary orders.

By affinity labelling experiments with metanitrobenzene diazonium fluoroborate in the 5·7S antibody of *Chelydra,* Litman *et al.* (1973) demonstrated the participation of tyrosine and histidine in the active site of the antibody.

The tryptophane fluorescence quenching can be used for analysis of the binding conditions. For comparison, the quenching value at maximum saturation of the binding sites in the excess of hapten, Q_{max}, is suitable. For IgM anti-DNP antibodies of the *Ophisaurus* against DNP, Q_{max} with 42 per cent was detected, the comparable antibodies of *Agrionemys* with 38 per cent. The maximum fluorescence quenching in the LMW antibodies of *Agrionemys* increase in the course of the immune response. That change is coupled with the increase in affinity (Fiebig 1972, 1973). In high affinity antibodies Q_{max} amounts to 60 per cent. This value lies in the same range, as described for anti-DNP antibodies of birds and mammals (Gallagher & Voss 1968, Eisen 1964, Eisen & Siskind 1964).

Late anti-DNP antibodies of *Agrionemys* differentiate DNP derivatives with different carbon chains better than do early antibodies (Fig. 12.19). That phenomenon can be interpreted as increase in specificity of the antibodies in the maturation of the immune response for the lysine residue of the hapten coupled to the protein carrier.

Comparable to high affinity rabbit anti-DNP antibodies (Little & Eisen 1969) *Agrionemys* antibodies also bind 2,4,6-trinitrophenol derivatives. By measurement of the temperature dependence of the binding constant: $H^0 = 6{\cdot}9$ kcal/mol and $S^0 = 1{\cdot}8$ Cl/mol were calculated. These values are in the same range as those of comparable mammalian antibodies (Eisen & Siskind 1964).

Maturation of the immune response

The maturation of the immune response, the ability to increase the affinity of the antibodies in the course of immunization, is a very important capacity. Its first appearance in the evolution represents a remarkable qualitative step.

The IgM anti-DNP antibodies of *Agrionemys* and *Ophisaurus* show almost no maturation in affinity. Only in the earliest phase could a slight increase of affinity be found; but then affinity of the IgM antibodies remains constant for a long time (Tables 12.9 and 12.10). In the secondary response the affinity has not changed in comparison to the primary response. An increase in affinity was not detected in the 7·3S and 6·8S antibodies of *Ophisaurus* during the course of secondary immunization. The LMW antibodies of *Agrionemys,* in contrast, showed a typical maturation in affinity. The affinity increased

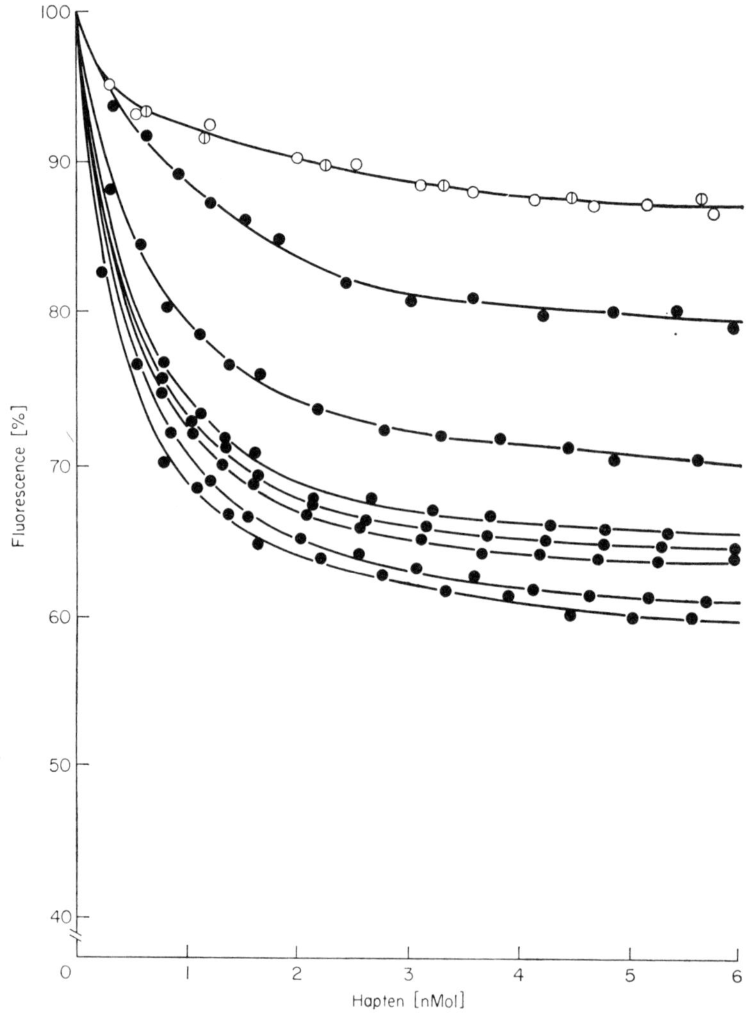

Fig. 12.19. Fluorescence quenching of the low molecular weight *Agrionemys* anti-DNP antibodies by various DNP haptens. To early antibodies (primary response, day 45) 2·4-dinitro-aniline (⦶) and ε-DNP-lysine (○) were added. To the late antibodies (secondary response, day 41) different DNP derivatives (●) were added; from top to bottom: dinitrophenol, dinitroaniline, α-DNP-glycine, β-DNP-alanine, γ-DNP-amino-butyric acid, ε-DNP-lysine, and ε-DNP-aminocaproic acid. Courtesy Dr Fiebig.

Table 12.9. Affinity of *Ophisaurus* anti-DNP antibodies (data from Fiebig 1972)

	High mol. wt. antibodies		Low mol. wt. antibodies	
	Primary resp. Day 21	Secondary resp. Day 14	Primary resp. Day 21	Secondary resp. Day 14
K_0 ($\times 10^4$ M^{-1})	0·6	0·6	3·2	3·8
Heter. index	0·80	0·80	0·56	0·56
Ab. conc. (μg/ml)	88	116	55	82

Table 12.10. Affinity of *Agrionemys* anti-DNP antibodies (data from Fiebig 1972)

	High mol. wt. antibodies			Low mol. wt. antibodies		
	Primary resp.		Secondary resp.	Primary resp.		Secondary resp.
	Day 45	Day 162	Day 41	Day 45	Day 162	Day 41
K_0 ($\times 10^5$ M^{-1})	0·6	~0·5	0·8	2·0	10	600
Heter. index	0·85	—	0·90	0·53	0·50	0·40
Ab. conc. (μg/ml)	25	10	40	30	20	380

five-fold in the primary response and 300-fold in the secondary response. In this case the binding strength attained values comparable to those of mammalian anti-DNP antibodies (Tables 12.9 and 12.10).

The increasing difference between the affinity of IgM and LMW antibodies in the tortoise (Fiebig 1972, 1973, Ambrosius *et al.* 1972, Ambrosius & Fiebig 1972, Ambrosius 1973) (Fig. 12.20) is remarkable. It means that the animal produces, at the same time, antibodies of different isotypes against the same hapten, but with quite different affinities or antigen binding sites. The strong differences of the association constants of IgM and of LMW antibodies seem to suggest, not only a different regulation of IgM and of LMW antibody response, but also a very early separation of cell clones for the production of the different antibody isotypes.

Factors influencing antibody production in reptiles

Influence of the antigen type

In reptiles, as in other vertebrates, the type of the antigen determines the dynamics of the immune response. Typical examples of the influence of the antigen on the kinetics of the response, the immunological memory and the

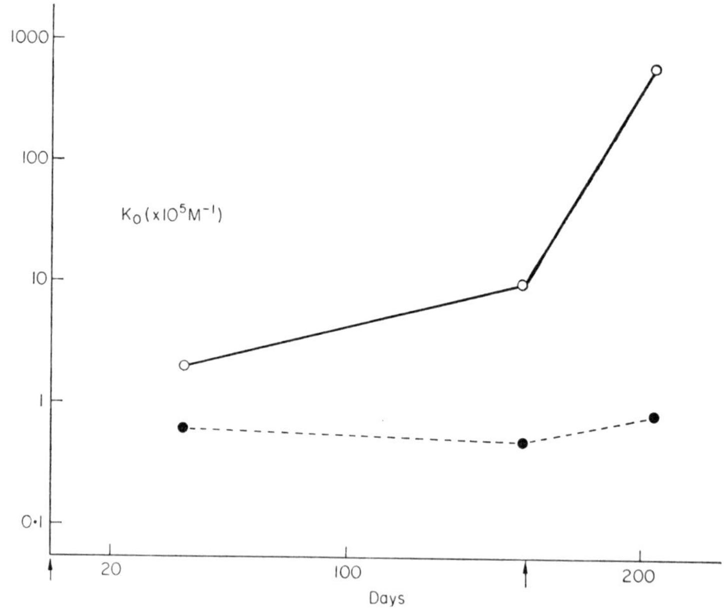

Fig. 12.20. Affinity of anti-DNP antibodies of the tortoise, *Agrionemys horsfieldii*, in the course of the immune response. Arrows represent the date of immunization.
○——○ = low molecular weight antibodies.
● - - - - ● = IgM antibodies

isotype of the antibodies produced, were given by Wetherall (1969) and Wetherall and Turner (1972). Contrary to sheep erythrocytes, which only induce a poor antibody response, the response to *Salmonella* and to BSA were vigorous, but more striking was the difference in the isotype elicited by the various antigens. Only IgM antibodies were produced by the lizard in response to immunization with *Salmonella*. The antibody found in the animals 240 days after the immunization was entirely macroglobulin. Both 19S and 7S antibodies were elicited during the response to rat erythrocytes; even 240 days later both 19S and 7S antibodies were present in appreciable quantities. In the vigorous reaction of the lizard to BSA both 19S and 7S antibodies were produced. However, the macroglobulin response was transitory and 65 days post immunization only 7S antibodies were evident.

That modified protein antigens elicit a different immune reaction has been observed by Frenzel and Ambrosius (1971) and Ambrosius *et al.* (1972). Tortoises, *Testudo* or *Agrionemys*, following the immunization with normal protein antigens, such as BGG or serum proteins, retained a high level of antibodies after the titre maximum for a very long time. The quantity of the antibodies detectable by passive haemagglutination 6 months later is therefore almost constant in most cases. Quite another situation can be seen following the immunization with dinitrophenylated proteins. Here, after reaching the maximum titre, the antibodies disappeared relatively fast. This may depend on the relatively uniform antigenic determinants in the modified antigen in contrast to the heterogeneous determinants in the normal protein.

In the lizard, *Ophisaurus apodus*, the situation where the isotype of the LMW antibodies dominated those produced depends on the particular protein antigen used. Thus, pig serum proteins induced the production of precipitating and, moreover, of non-precipitating antibodies (Hemmerling 1971). Using bovine IgG, only non-precipitating antibodies were elicited. Because we know that the 7·3S antibody of *Ophisaurus* (H-chain mol. wt. 63,000) is a precipitating antibody but the 6·8S antibody (H-chain mol. wt. 48,000) is a non-precipitating one (Fiebig & Hädge, unpublished) it is reasonable to assume that in this case the particular antigen influenced the antibody isotype which was produced.

The affinity of reptilian antibodies will also be affected by the antigen type. For instance, in tortoises the particulate carrier of DNP conjugates markedly influenced the isotype and the affinity of the antibodies (Fiebig 1972). The tortoise, *Agrionemys horsfieldi*, has been immunized with DNP_{22}-PLL, DNP_{21}-HSA, DNP_{42}-BGG or DNP-*Brucella abortus*. A strong macroglobulin response has been elicited by the immunization with DNP-Brucella. Even following the second antigen contact, measurable amounts of IgM antibodies were found. The affinity of the IgM antibodies did not change distinctly, so in the primary response the average association constant was $K_0 = 1 \times 10^4\ M^{-1}$, in the secondary response $K_0 = 5 \times 10^4\ M^{-1}$.

The three soluble antigens only induced the production of LMW antibodies, but there were striking differences between the LMW antibodies elicited by the diverse antigens including DNP-*Brucella*. The poorest response was obtained following immunization with DNP-PLL, in which only the binding strength of the antibodies could be measured in the secondary response; this was low, $K_0 = 1 \times 10^4\ M^{-1}$. The other two soluble antigens elicited a good antibody reaction and showed a typical anamnestic response. So the quantity of the antibodies in the secondary response was three to eight times higher than in the primary reaction. The affinity of the antibodies produced remained almost the same in the course of the immune response. The average association constants showed values between $5 \times 10^4\ M^{-1}$ in the primary and $9 \times 10^4\ M^{-1}$ in the secondary response. Contrary to this, the LMW antibody response following immunization by DNP-*Brucella* was not strong but the affinity increased very remarkably in the course of the response. So, in the primary reaction the association constant was $1{\cdot}6 \times 10^4\ M^{-1}$, and in the secondary response it increased to $33 \times 10^4\ M^{-1}$. In this case the LMW antibodies were mostly from the 5·7S type.

In the same investigation (Fiebig 1972) in the tortoise, several DNP conjugates were found to influence the heterogeneity of the produced antibodies. DNP-PLL elicited an antibody population with restricted heterogeneity; the heterogeneity index 'a' was 0·9, which shows the population was nearly homogeneous. Conversely, DNP-HSA and DNP-*Brucella* induced antibody populations with normal heterogeneity, the index lying between 0·3 and 0·6.

Influence of the temperature

It has long been known that the immune response in poikilothermic vertebrates is temperature dependent. Since another chapter in this book deals with that problem (Chapter 9) only few references will be given here. Metschnikoff initially observed in 1902 that crocodiles synthesize antibodies in a range of 32–37°C but do not at 20°C. A number of similar results have been subsequently published for other reptilian species (Buch 1940, Svet-Moldavsky 1954, Blanc *et al.* 1960, Evans *et al.* 1959, 1965, Evans 1963, Maung 1963, Ambrosius & Lehmann 1965, Vorobjeva 1965, Wetherall & Turner 1972). Nevertheless, at this time the experiments in reptiles have not clarified the question whether the temperature mainly influences the production or the secretion of the antibodies or affects primarily the induction period of the immune response. Since some reptilian species can live in a broad range of temperature suitable experiments in that order of vertebrates are promising.

Influence of adjuvants

In contrast to Grey (1963) who, studying the antibody production in the turtle, *Chrysemys picta*, found almost no differences between the experimental groups immunized with or without adjuvants, in some cases in the tortoise, *Testudo hermanni*, we observed distinct differences (Ambrosius & Lehmann 1964, 1965, Ambrosius 1966, 1967). Following immunization with pig serum proteins in the primary response, those animals given antigen adsorbed to aluminium hydroxide produced antibodies faster and achieved titres two tubes higher than did those animals which did not receive adjuvant. With incomplete Freund's adjuvant the titre increased by two further tubes.

These titre differences were maintained for some months. However, in the secondary response the differences between the animal groups were not distinct. Thus, the adjuvants seem to influence mainly the period of cell proliferation in the beginning of the primary response.

Adjuvants not only influence the quantity of antibodies produced but also the isotype mostly synthesized. In the primary response of tortoise, *Testudo hermanni*, incomplete Freund's adjuvant raised the antibody titre in contrast to animals immunized without adjuvant (Ambrosius 1967). In the secondary response, however, we obtained differences in the antibody isotypes produced in the two groups of animals. In the animals without adjuvant the 2-mercapto-ethanol sensitive antibodies dominated, whereas in the other group 2-mercapto-ethanol resistant antibodies were prevalent.

In the lizard, *Tiliqua rugosa*, Wetherall (1969) found a strong effect of complete Freund's adjuvant (CFA) on immunization with sheep erythrocytes or BSA. For example, doses of 1 mg or less of BSA injected i.p. without CFA did not produce a measurable response by 40 days. When the BSA was emulsified with CFA, however, following the immunization, measurable responses could be obtained with even 10 μg doses.

Influence of seasonal factors

Contrary to the fact that nearly all physiological factors are affected by seasonal factors, we have very poor information about the influence on the immune response. Some authors observed that 'winter animals' were poorer responders than 'summer animals' in spite of the same temperature conditions in the experiments (Sirotinin 1959, Maung 1963, Sidky & Auerbach 1968, Cohen 1971). In 1965 we extensively studied the influence of the season on the antibody response of the tortoise, *Testudo hermanni* (Ambrosius 1966). Groups of animals, kept at 25°C, were immunized with serum proteins at different times of the year. The antibody titre was determined by passive haemagglutination. As can be seen in Fig. 12.21, there were striking differences in the elected animal groups. The immunological reactivity of the

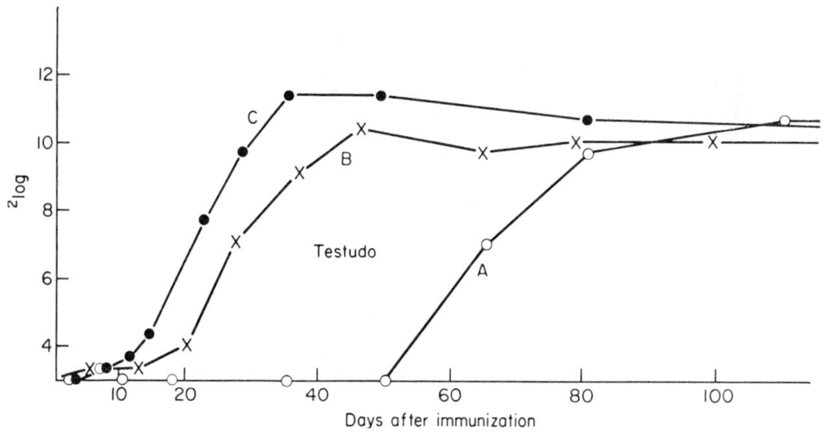

Fig. 12.21. Different immune responses of the tortoise, *Testudo hermanni*, after immunization at different dates.

A = 2 October.
B = 21 November.
C = 21 April.

tortoises in a few weeks in the autumn were poor, but some weeks later the animals showed an immune response not very distinct from the reaction of the other groups. The poor reactivity probably depends on the preparation of the hibernation. That particular physiological situation had changed a few weeks later. Presumably this seasonal factor mainly affects the phases in the beginning of the immune response but the antibody titre that will be reached later on is as high as in animals immunized in the other seasons of the year.

If tortoises in the seasonal phase of poor responsiveness were immunized with protein antigen in incomplete Freund's adjuvant, the particular physiological state was overcome and a normal immune response without prolongation of the initial phase of the response results. This example shows clearly the significance to take into consideration the influence of seasonal factors on immunological experiments. That may be true, not only in reptiles, but also in other vertebrate species.

References

ACTON R.T., NIEDERMEIER W., WEINHEIMER P.F., CLEM I.W., LESLIE G.A. & BENNETT J.C. (1972) The carbohydrate composition of immunoglobulins from diverse species of vertebrates. *J. Immunol.* **109,** 371.

ACTON R.T., WEINHEIMER P.F., SHELTON E., NIEDERMEIER W. & BENNETT J.C. (1972) Phylogeny of immunoglobulins—purification and physico-chemical characterization of the immune macroglobulin from the turtle, *Pseudemus seripta. Immunochemistry* **9,** 421.

AMBROSIUS H. (1965) Zu einigen Problemen der vergleichenden Immunbiologie. *Verh. d. D. Zool. Ges. Jena 1965* 492.

AMBROSIUS H. (1965) The choice of experimental animals for the production of antisera. *Fed. of Europ. Biochemical Soc. Vienna 1965.*

AMBROSIUS H. (1966) Beiträge zur Immunbiologie poikilothermer Wirbeltiere. IV. Weitere immunologische und immunchemische Untersuchungen an Schildkröten. *Z. Immun. forsch.* **130,** 41.

AMBROSIUS H. (1966) Untersuchungen zur Phylogenie der Immunglobuline. *Verh. d. D. Zool. Ges. Göttingen 1966* 279.

AMBROSIUS H. (1967) Untersuchungen über die Immunglobuline niederer Wirbeltiere. *Allergie und Asthma* **13,** 111.

AMBROSIUS H. (1968) Die Entwicklung immunologischer Reaktionen in der Phylogenese. *Wiss. Z. d. Friedr.-Schiller-Univ. Jena, Math.-Nat. Reihe* **17,** 104.

AMBROSIUS H. (1970) Some aspects of the phylogeny of immunity. *Ann. Immunol.* **II,** 177.

AMBROSIUS H. & FIEBIG H. (1972) Evolution of antibody affinity. Colloque INSERM: Phylogenic and ontogenic study of the immune response. *Paris 1972* 135.

AMBROSIUS H. & FRENZEL E.-M. (1972) Anti-DNP antibodies in carp and tortoises. *Immunochemistry* **9,** 65.

AMBROSIUS H., FRENZEL E.-M. & FIEBIG H. (1972) Untersuchungen zur Struktur und Affinität der Antikörper von Schildkröten. *Annales Immunologiae Hungaricae* **XVI,** 15.

AMBROSIUS H., HEMMERLING J., RICHTER R. & SCHIMKE R. (1969) Immunoglobulins and the dynamics of antibody formation in poikilothermic vertebrates (Pisces, Urodela, Reptilia) *Proc. of a Symp. held in Prague June, 1969* 727.

AMBROSIUS H. & HOHEISEL G. (1969) Electron-microscopic study of antibody-producing (plaque-forming) spleen cells of the tortoise *Agrionemys horsfieldi* Gray. *Experientia* **25,** 1177.

AMBROSIUS H. & HOHEISEL G. (1973) Ultrastructure of antibody-producing cells of reptiles. I. Spleen cells of the tortoise (*Agrionemys horsfieldi* Grey). *Acta biol. med. germ.* **31,** 733.

AMBROSIUS H. & HOHEISEL G. (1973) Ultrastructure of antibody-producing cells of reptiles. II. Blood cells of the tortoise (*Agrionemys horsfieldi* Gray). *Acta biol. med. germ.* **31,** 741.

AMBROSIUS H. & LEHMANN R. (1964) Poikilotherme Wirbeltiere als Versuchstiere beim Studium des Wirkungsmechanismus immunologischer Adjuvantien. *Acta biol. med. german.* **12,** 615.

AMBROSIUS H. & LEHMANN R. (1965) Beiträge zur Immunbiologie poikilothermer Wirbeltiere. II. Immunologische Untersuchungen an Schildkröten (*Testudo hermanni* Gmelin) *Z. Immun. forsch.* **128,** 81.

AUERBACH R. (1970) In vitro studies of immune capacity of amphibians and reptiles. *Transplantation Proceedings* **II,** 307.

BENEDICT A.A. & POLLARD L.W. (1972) Three classes of immunoglobulins found in the sea turtle, *Chelonia mydas. Folia Microbiol.* **17,** 75.

BLANC G., DELAGE B. & ASCIONE L. (1960) Comportement des salmonelles inoculées par voie sanguine a *Testudo graeca. Bull. Soc. Path. Exot.* **53,** 131.

BLANC G., DELAGE B. & ASCIONE L. (1960) Comportement des salmonelles inoculées parvoie sanguine a *Testudo graeca. Bull. Soc. Path. Exot.* **53,** 774.

BUCH P.L. (1940) Humoral immunity from the viewpoint of comparative pathology. III. On the formation of agglutinins in cold-blooded animals (russ). *Med. Sh.* **10,** 1153.

CHARTRAND S.I., LITMAN G.W., LAPOINTE N., GOOD R.A. & FROMMEL D. (1971) The evolution of the immune response. XII. The immunoglobulins of the turtle. Molecular requirements for biologic activity of 5·7S immunoglobulin. *J. Immunol.* **107,** 1.

CLEM L.W. & LESLIE G.A. (1969) Phylogeny of immunoglobulin structure and function, p. 62. In *Developmental Immunology*, ed. Adinolfi M. Spastics Intern. Med. Publ., London.

CLEM L.W. & SMALL P.A. (1970) Phylogeny of immunoglobulin structure and function. V. Valencies and association constants of teleost antibodies to a haptenic determinant. *J. exp. Med.* **132,** 385.

CHRISTIAN C.L. (1970) Character of non-precipitating antibodies. *Immunology* **18,** 457.

COE J.E. (1972) Immune response in the turtle (*Chrysemys picta*). *Immunology* **23,** 45.

COHEN N. (1971) Reptiles as models for the study of immunity and its phylogenesis. *J. Am. Vet. Med. Assoc.* **159,** 1662.

COMBIESCO D., STURDZA N. & NICOLESCO M. (1963) Neue Untersuchungen über die Infektionsquellen bei Leptospirose. Erstmalige Isolierung der serologischen Typen L. bataviae und L. saxkoebing in Rumänien (franz.) *Arch. Rumain. Path. exp. Microbiol.* **22,** 5.

DIENER E. (1970) Evolutionary aspects of immunity and lymphoid organs in vertebrates. *Transplantation Proceedings* **II,** 309.

DIMOW I. (1968) Versuche zur künstlichen Infektion von Eidechsen (*Lacerta muralis*) mit Salmonella- und Arizonabakterien. *Zentralbl. f. Vet. medizin Reihe B*, **13,** 587.

DIMOW I. & SLAWTSCHEW R. (1967) Versuche der Experimentalinfizierung von Schlangen Vipera ammodytes mit Salmonella- und Arizonabakterien. *Path. Microbiol.* **30,** 495.

DOWNS C.M. (1928) Anaphylaxis VII. Active anaphylaxis in turtles. *J. Immunol.* **15,** 77.

EISEN H.N. (1964) Determination of antibody affinity for hapten by means of fluorescence quenching. *Methods Med. Res.* **10,** 115.

EISEN H.N. & SISKIND G.W. (1964) Variations in affinities of antibodies during the immune response. *Biochemistry* **3,** 996.

EVANS E.E. (1963) Antibody response in Amphibia and Reptilia. *Fed. Proc.* **22,** 1132.

EVANS E.E. (1963) Comparative immunology. Antibody response in *Dipsosaurus dorsalis* at different temperatures. *Proc. Soc. Exp. Biol. and Med.* **112,** 531.

EVANS E.E. & COWLES R.B. (1959) Effect of temperature on antibody synthesis in the reptile, *Dipsosaurus dorsalis. Proc. Soc. Exp. Biol. and Med.* **101,** 482.

EVANS E.E., KENT S.P., ATTLEBERGER M.H., SEIBERT CH., BRYANT R.E., BOOTH B. (1965) Antibody synthesis in poikilothermic vertebrates. *Ann. N.Y. Acad. Sci.* **126,** 629.

FALCOFF E. & FAUCONNIER B. (1965) In vitro production of an interferon-like inhibitor of viral multiplication by a poikilothermic animal cell, the tortoise (*Testudo greca*). *Proc. Soc. Exp. Biol. Med.* **118,** 609.

FIEBIG H. (1972) Vergleichende Untersuchung der Affinität von Anti-Hapten-Antikörpern von Vertretern verschiedener Wirbeltierklassen. Dissertation, Karl-Marx-Universität, Leipzig.

FIEBIG H. (1973) Die Entwicklung der Antikörperaffinität in der Phylogenese. *Allergie u. Immunologie* **19,** 248.

FIEBIG H. & AMBROSIUS H. (1975) Bindungseigenschaften von IgM-Anti-DNP-Antikörpern des Karpfens. *Acta biol. med. germ.* **34,** 1681.

FIEBIG H., HÄDGE D. & FRENZEL E.-M. (1974) Unpublished data.

FRAIR W. (1963) Blood group studies with turtles. *Science* **140,** 1412.

FRANK M.M. & HUMPHREY J.H. (1968) The subunits in rabbit anti-forssman IgM antibody. *J. exp. Med.* **127,** 967.

FRENZEL E.-M. & AMBROSIUS H. (1971) Anti-Hapten-Antikörper bei niederen Wirbeltieren. *Acta biol. med. germ.* **26,** 165.

FROMMEL D., LITMAN G.W., CHARTRAND S.L., SEAL U.S. & GOOD R.A. (1971) Carbohydrate composition in the evolution of the immunoglobulins. *Immunochemistry* **8,** 573.

GALLAGHER I.S. & VOSS E.W. (1969) Binding properties of purified chicken antibodies. *Immunochemistry* **6,** 573.

GEE L.L. & SMITH W.W. (1941) Defences against trout furunculosis. *J. Bact.* **41,** 266.

GRASSET E. & ZOUTENDYK A. (1931) Immunological studies in reptiles and their relation to aspects of immunity in higher animals. *Publ. South African Inst. Med. Res.* **4,** 377.

GRASSET E., ZOUTENDYK A. & SCHAAFSMA A. (1935) Sur la production d'agglutinines antibactériennes chez les reptiles. *C. r. Soc. Biol.* **119,** 67.

GREY H.M. (1963) Phylogeny of the immune response. Studies on some physical chemical and serologic characteristics of antibody produced in the turtle. *J. Immunol.* **91,** 819.

GREY H.M. (1966) Structure and kinetics of formation of antibody in the turtle. p. 227. In *Phylogeny of Immunity*, eds Smith R.T., Miescher P.A. & Good R.A., Gainesville.

GREY H.M. (1969) Phylogeny of immunoglobulins. *Adv. in immunology* **10,** 51.

HEMMERLING J. (1970) Untersuchungen über die Antikörperbildung und die Immunglobuline von Eidechsen am Beispiel von Ophisaurus apodus (PALLAS). Dissertation, Sekt. Biowissenschaften, Karl-Marx-Universität, Leipzig.

HEMMERLING J. (1971) Properties of soluble antigen-antibody complexes in lower vertebrates, p. 44. In *Antigen-antibody reactions*, eds Ambrosius H., Malberg K. & Schäffner H. Jena.

HEMMERLING J. & AMBROSIUS H. (1971) Beiträge zur Immunbiologie poikilothermer Wirbeltiere. VII. Immunglobuline und Antikörperbildung beim Scheltopusik, Ophisaurus apodus (Reptilia, Lacertilia, Anguidae). *Acta biol. med. germ.* **27,** 783.

HOEDEN VAN DER J. (1966) Leptospiral antibodies in cold-blooded animals. *Ann. Soc. belge Méd. trop.* **46,** 171.

KANAKAMBIKA P. & MUTHUKKARUPPAN VR. (1972) Immunological competence in the newly hatched lizard, *Calotes versicolor. Proc. Soc. Exp. Biol. Med.* **140,** 21.

KANAKAMBIKA P. & MUTHUKKARUPPAN VR. (1972) The immune response to sheep erythrocytes in the lizard, *Calotes versicolor. J. Immunol.* **109,** 415.

KANAKAMBIKA P. & MUTHUKKARUPPAN VR. (1972) Effect of splenectomy on the immune response in the lizard, *Calotes versicolor. Experientia* **28,** 1225.

KASSIN L.F. & PEVNITSKII L.A. (1969) Detection of antibody-forming cells in turtle spleen with a modified method of local hemolysis in gel. *Byul. Eksp. Biol. Med.* **67,** 70.

KISHIMOTO T. & ONOUE K. (1971) Properties of combining sites of rabbit IgM antibodies. *J. Immunol.* **106,** 341.

KLINMAN N.R., ROCKEY J.H., KARUSH F. (1964) Valence and affinity of equine nonprecipitating antibody to a haptenic group. *Science* **146,** 401.

LERCH E.G., HUGGINS S.E. & BARTEL A.H. (1967) Comparative immunology. Active immunization of young alligators with hemocyanin. *Proc. Soc. Exp. Biol. Med.* **124,** 448.

LESLIE G.A. & CLEM L.W. (1969) Phylogeny of immunoglobulin structure and function. III. Immunoglobulins of the chicken. *J. Exp. Med.* **130,** 1337.

LESLIE G.A. & CLEM W. (1972) Phylogeny of immunoglobulin structure and function. VI. 17S, 7·5S and 5·7S anti-DNP of the turtle, *Pseudamys scripta. J. Immunol.* **108,** 1656.

LINDQVIST K. & BAUER D.C. (1966) Precipitin activity of rabbit macroglobulin antibody. *Immunochemistry* **3,** 373.

LITMAN G.W., CHARTRAND S.L., FINSTAD C.L. & GOOD R.A. (1973) Active sites of turtle and duck low molecular weight antibody to 2′4′dinitrophenol. *Immunochemistry* **10,** 323.

LITTLE J.R. & EISEN H.N. (1967) Evidence for tryptophane in the active sites of antibodies to polynitrobenzenes. *Biochemistry* **6,** 3119.

LITTLE J.R. & EISEN H.N. (1968) Physical and chemical differences between rabbit antibodies to the 2,4-dinitrophenyl and 2,4,6-trinitrophenyl groups. *Biochemistry* **7,** 711.

LYKAKIS J.J. (1968) Immunglobulin production in the European pond tortoise, *Emys orbicularis,* immunized with serum protein antigens. *Immunology* **14,** 799.

MARCHALONIS J.J. (1970) Phylogenetic origins of antibody structure. *Transplantation Proceedings* **II,** 318.

MARCHALONIS J.J., EALEY E.H.M. & DIENER E. (1969) Immune response of the tuatara, *Sphenodon punctatum. Aust. J. exp. Biol. med. Sci.* **47,** 367.

MAUNG H.T. (1963) Immunity in the tortoise, *Testudo ibera. J. Pathol. Bacteriol.* **85,** 51.

METCHNIKOFF E. (1902) Immunität bei Infektionskrankheiten. Jena.

MUKKUR T.K.S. (1972) Valence and association constant of bovine colostral immunoglobuline antibody. *Immunochemistry* **9,** 1049.

NOGUCHI H. (1902) A study of immunization haemolysins, agglutinins, precipitine, and coaguline in cold-blooded animals. *Univ. of Penna. Med. Bull.* **15,** 301.

ONOUE K., YAGI Y., GROSSBERG A. & PRESSMAN D. (1965) Number of binding sites of rabbit macroglobuline antibody and its subunits. *Immunochemistry* **2,** 401.

ORIOL R., BINAGHI R. & COLTORTI E. (1971) Valence and association constant of rat macroglobulin antibody. *J. Immunol.* **104,** 932.

POLLARA B., FINSTAD J.P. & GOOD R.A. (1966) The phylogenetic development of immunoglobulins, p. 88. In *Phylogeny of Immunity*, eds Smith R.T., Miescher P.A. & Good R.A. Gainesville.

RICHTER R., FIEBIG H. & AMBROSIUS H. (1972) Evolution der Immunglobuline. *Wiss. Zschr. Friedrich-Schiller-Univ., Jena, Math.-Nat. R.* **21,** 803.

ROTHE F. & AMBROSIUS H. (1968) Beiträge zur Immunbiologie poikilothermer Wirbeltiere.

V. Die Proliferation Antikörper bildender Zellen bei Schildkröten. *Acta. biol. med. germ.* **21,** 525.

Russel W.J., Voss E.W. & Sigel M.M. (1970) Some characteristics of anti-dinitrophenyl-antibody of the gray snapper. *J. Immunol.* **105,** 6165.

Salanitro, S.K. & Minton, S.A. (1973) Immune response of snakes. COPEIA, 1973, 504.

Saluk P.H., Krauss J. & Clem L.W. (1970) The presence of two antigenically distinct light chains (κ and λ?) in alligator immunoglobulins. *Proc. Soc. Exp. Biol. Med.* **133,** 365.

Saluk P.H., Krauss J. & Clem L.W. (1973) Unpublished data.

Sidky Y.A. & Auerbach R. (1968) Tissue culture analysis of immunological capacity of snapping turtles. *J. Exp. Zool.* **167,** 187.

Sirotinin N.N. (1962) A comparative physiological study of the mechanism of antibody formation. *Proc. Symp. Mechanisms of Antibody Formation*, Prague, 113.

Svet-Moldawski G.J. (1954) Serologische Reaktivität bei wechselwarmen Wirbeltieren. Die Bildung virusneutralisierender Antikörper bei Reptilien unter verschiedener Körpertemperatur (russ.). *Bjull. eksperim. Biol. i. med.* **38,** 54.

Thomas W.R., Turner K.J., Eadie M.E. & Yadav M. (1972) The immune response of the quokka (*Setonix brachyurus*). The production of a low molecular weight antibody. *Immunology* **22,** 401.

Timourian H., Dobson C. & Sprent J.F.A. (1961) Precipitating antibodies in the carpet snake against parasitic nematodes. *Nature*, **192,** 996.

Vorobjeva M.S. (1965) Experimental study of humoral immunity in reptiles infected with tick-borne encephalitis virus. *Vop. Virusol* **10,** 36.

Voss E.W. Jr & Eisen H.N. (1972) Anti-hapten chicken antibodies of the 7S class. *J. Immunol.* **109,** 944.

Voss E.W. & Sigel M.M. (1972) Valences and temporal change in affinity of purified 7S and 18S nurse shark anti-2,4 dinitrophenyl antibodies. *J. Immunol.* **109,** 665.

Wetherall J.D. (1969) Immunoglobulins of the lizard, *Tiliqua rugosa.* Doctoral thesis, University of Adelaide.

Wetherall J.D. & Turner K.J. (1972) Immune response of the lizard, *Tiliqua rugosa. Aust. J. exp. Biol. med. Sci.* **50,** 79.

Widal & Sicard (1897) Influence de l'organisme sur les proriétés acquises par les humeurs du fait de l'infection. (L'agglutination chez quelques animaux a sang froid.) *C. r. Soc. Biol.* **49,** 1047.

Willis R.A. (1932) A bacillary disease of the blue-tongued lizard (*Tiliqua scincoides*). *Med. J. Austral.* **1,** 149.

Wright R.K. & Schapiro H.C. (1973) Primary and secondary immune response of the desert iguana, *Dipsosaurus dorsalis. Herpetologica* **29,** 275.

Zimmermann B., Shalatin N. & Grey H.M. (1971) Structural studies on the duck 5·7S and 7·8S immunoglobulins. *Biochemistry* **10,** 482.

Chapter 13. Immunoglobulins and Antibody Production in Avian Species

Albert A. Benedict and Karen Yamaga

Introduction

Immunoglobulins: 7S immunoglobulins
Galliformes
  Structure
  Biological properties
Anseriformes
  Structure
  Biological properties
Other birds
  Structure
  Biological properties

17S immunoglobulins
Galliformes
  Structure
  Biological properties
Anseriformes

IgA-like immunoglobulins: Galliformes

5·7S immunoglobulins: Anseriformes
  Structure
  Biological properties

Antibody production to soluble antigens

Conclusions

Introduction

Both birds and mammals evolved from reptiles, and both became homeothermic and highly successful organisms, but the two groups evolved entirely separately. It is pertinent to know the extent to which the structural and biological properties of the immunoglobulins have been conserved in these distinct evolutionary branches. Some structural differences have developed, most notable of which is that the molecular weight of the H chain of the major 7S immunoglobulin of the chicken is higher than the molecular weight of the mammalian γ-chain. Nevertheless, the chief biological functions associated with mammalian immunoglobulins are also associated with avian immunoglobulins. Furthermore, multiple classes of immunoglobulins have also been clearly demonstrated in birds. Whether or not birds have evolved multiple classes and subclasses of immunoglobulins as diverse as mammalian immunoglobulins should prove to be important information on the phylogeny of immunoglobulins.

Similarities and differences between mammalian immunoglobulins and avian immunoglobulins however may only reflect inadequate coverage of the various orders of Aves. Of about 8600 living species of Class Aves (estimate of the total number of birds, past and present, is approximately 154,000 species) (Brodkorb 1971) only the duck (*Anas platyrhynchos*) and members of the order Galliformes, in particular the domestic fowl (*Gallus domesticus*), have been studied in detail with respect to the immune response and to the structure and function of the immunoglobulins. Therefore, 'avian immunology' in reality refers to 'chicken and duck immunology', and the general characteristics of 'avian immunology' cannot be defined until members of other orders have been studied.

This review has as its aim an integrated, but not an exhaustive, review of each avian immunoglobulin and some characteristics of the immune response in birds. The cellular aspects of the immune response are covered elsewhere.

Immunoglobulins: 7S immunoglobulins

Galliformes

STRUCTURE

Introduction

The low molecular weight chicken antibody has characteristics that resemble those of mammalian IgG; these include: (1) a sedimentation coefficient of about 7S; (2) elution from DEAE-cellulose in low ionic strength buffers; and (3) synthesis in increased amounts following earlier synthesis of high molecular weight antibody (Benedict *et al.* 1963a). However, the molecular weight of the chicken 7S immunoglobulin heavy (H) chains exceeds the mammalian γ-chain by about 10,000. Therefore, the avian low molecular weight immunoglobulin will be referred to as 7S Ig. With the recognition of class-specific amino acid residues from sequence studies such as those reported on human γ- (Edelman *et al.* 1969) and μ-chains (Putman *et al.* 1973), it will be possible to determine whether the 7S and 19S immunoglobulin molecules of other mammals and lower vertebrates should be designated 'IgG' and 'IgM', respectively.

In the purification of chicken, pheasant, and quail immunoglobulins attention should be given to the high lipid content of hen serum, the tendency of 7S Ig to aggregate during fractionation, the polymerization of 7S Ig in high concentrations of salt, and the precipitation of 7S Ig during dialysis against low ionic strength buffers which are commonly used for chromatographic separation of serum proteins (Benedict 1967a).

Electrokinetic Properties

In immunoelectrophoresis 7S Ig forms the usual cathodal migrating arc. In starch block electrophoresis γ_1- and γ_2-peaks are resolved (Benedict *et al.* 1963d). Different values have been obtained for the isoelectric point of 7S Ig. By moving boundary electrophoresis, the pI was 5·0 (Tenenhouse & Deutsch 1966). Using isoelectric focusing, Gallagher and Voss (1970) reported a pI value of 6·6 for the monomeric form of chicken 7S Ig and 5·6 for the polymerized protein. In an isoelectric focusing pH gradient of 5–8, three major peaks for normal 7S Ig were obtained with approximate pI values of 5·5, 5·8 and 6·3, respectively (Wakeland & Benedict, unpublished data). Discrepancies in pI values may result from varying amounts of aggregated 7S Ig since a lower value was obtained with a polymerized protein.

Molecular Weights

At infinite dilution, the $S_{20,w}$ of 7S Ig in 0·015 M phosphate (pH 7·0) containing 0·15 M NaCl was 7·3 (Hersh & Benedict, unpublished data). Recent sedimentation equilibrium studies gave a molecular weight of about 170,000 for chicken (Hersh *et al.* 1969, Leslie & Clem 1969a, Gallagher & Voss 1970) and for pheasant (*Phasianus colchicus*) and quail (*Coturnix coturix*) 7S Ig (Hersh *et al.* 1969). The molecular weights of the chicken H- and L-chains determined by high speed sedimentation equilibrium were 60,800 $\pm$ 1400 and 23,700 $\pm$ 800, respectively (Kubo 1970), and by gel filtration these weights were 67,500 and 22,000, respectively (Leslie & Clem 1969a). By gel filtration molecular weights of the H- and L-chains of the Numigall (a hybrid of a domestic cock and a guinea hen) were 68,000 and 20,000, respectively (Oriol *et al.* 1972). Based on an average carbohydrate content of about 5·5 per cent associated with an H-chain (Acton *et al.* 1972, Howell *et al.* 1973) the recalculated molecular weight (using 61,000) is about 58,000. This is the same value obtained for a sugar-free duck 7S Ig H-chain (Zimmerman *et al.* 1971). Therefore, the chicken and duck H-chains probably consist of five domains, each about 11,000–12,000 in molecular weight. The structure of chicken 7S Ig is consistent with the four-chain model (Porter 1962) involving one pair of L- and one pair of H-chains held together by interchain disulphide bonds (Dreesman & Benedict 1965a, Gold *et al.* 1966).

L-Chains

Little can be said about structural similarities and differences between chicken and mammalian 7S Ig L-chains based on amino acid composition (Kubo 1970, Hood *et al.* 1967). On the other hand, the major N-terminal sequences of chicken and turkey (*Meleagris gallopavo*) L-chains had a marked homology with the N-terminal sequences of human λ-chains (Kubo *et al.* 1970, 1971, Grant *et al.* 1971). Assuming a deletion of the first two N-terminal residues and a deletion at position 9, pooled normal L-chains and anti-DNP L-chains were predominantly *unblocked* λ-chains with alanine as the major terminal residue. Turkey L-chains differed from the corresponding peptides in chicken L-chains in only two of a total of 74 residues. Also in the C-regions both chicken and turkey L-chains were more closely related to human λ- than to κ-chains (Grant *et al.* 1971). Gaps, or insertions, were shared by the avian and human λ-chains at positions 9, 111, 203 and 204. Perhaps highly significant in the evolution of the V-region was the finding that a highly conserved pentapeptide (Arg-Phe-Ser-Gly-Ser) sequence extending from positions 68–72 was present in L-chains from chicken, duck, turkey, the nurse shark and nine mammals (Stanton *et al.* 1974). This same conserved sequence also was present in κ-chains.

The *blocked* N-terminal λ-chain, which is the predominant λ-chain in humans, has not been detected in chicken L-chains. The avian N-terminal V-region is relatively homogeneous in contrast to mammalian counterparts in which there are major subsets of Vλ- and Vκ-regions. To date, we have detected only one antigenic type of chicken L-chain. In accord with this apparent homogeneity, chicken L-chains from anti-DNP 7S Ig often show restricted heterogeneity in alkaline urea starch gel (Kubo *et al.* 1971).

Kubo *et al.* (1971) reported that about 90 per cent of pheasant L-chains had a blocked N-terminal residue, and that only 5–10 per cent alanine was recovered as the N-terminal residue. Chicken and pheasant L-chains show close antigenic identity (Leslie & Benedict 1970b) which suggests that the pheasant L-chain is the blocked λ-type.

Grant *et al.* (1971) speculate that 'λ and κ genes must have diverged prior to the divergence of avian and mammalian lines (about 250 million years ago)' because it is likely that the ancestor to sharks and mammals must have had κ-genes as the shark L-chains show homology with human κ-chains, and because the ancestor to birds and mammals must have had λ-genes.

H-chains

There is no information on the location of the additional domain of about 100 amino acids in the H-chain. Tryptic peptide maps of chicken H-chains and those of human γ- (Travis & Sanders 1973) and peptic peptide maps of chicken H-chains and rabbit γ-chains (Benedict *et al.* 1972) revealed little homology between the chicken and the mammalian H-chains. Radioautographs of peptic digests of radiolabelled chicken H-chains had two large spots near the origin which were not seen in the rabbit γ-chains (Benedict *et al.* 1972). Peptides in the same region were identified as carbohydrate-peptides (Travis & Sanders 1973). The percentage composition of the amino acids residues were similar for chicken H- and human γ-chains, except for three more cysteines in the chicken H chains which was to be expected for a longer chain (Travis & Sanders 1973).

Normal pooled H-chains and anti-DNP H-chains had alanine as the free N-terminal residue (Kubo *et al.* 1971). Based on 20 N-terminal residues anti-DNP H-chains resembled the mammalian V_HIII subgroup (Kubo *et al.* 1971). This is the major subgroup in other animal species (Kehoe & Capra 1972), but it accounts only for 15–25 per cent of the H-chains in normal human sera (Wang *et al.* 1971).

Binding Site

Chicken anti-DNP 7S Ig has two binding sites as indicated by the extrapolation of curves in Scatchard plots. Valences less than two often have been seen, but this might be due to the presence of low-affinity antibody (Gallagher & Voss 1969, Voss & Eisen 1972, Benedict *et al.* 1972, Yamaga 1975).

Intramuscular injection of DNP-BGG in Freund's Complete Adjuvant (FCA), produced anti-DNP which specifically purified had K_0 values about 10^6 M^{-1} (Gallagher & Voss 1969). Repeated intravenous injections of DNP-BGG also yielded antibody with moderate binding constants (10^6–$10^7 M^{-1}$) as determined by using 7S globulin fractions according to the method of Werblin and Siskind (1972b) (Yamaga 1975). Under optimal conditions of antigen dosage and timing anti-DNP antibodies with K_0 values as high as those obtained in rabbits ($> 10^0$ M^{-1}) can be produced in chickens (Yamaga 1974).

Tryptophan fluorescence of chicken anti-DNP was quenched when ε-DNP-L-lysine was bound in the active site (Voss & Eisen 1972). The ligand undergoes the same kind of spectral shift as it does with anti-DNP antibodies from a variety of animals (Little & Eisen 1967). The binding of a variety of nitrobenzyl compounds by chicken anti-DNP antibody was about the same order of relative binding as with rabbit anti-DNP antibody (Gallagher & Voss 1969).

Employing the paired-labelled method of Roholt & Pressman (1968), the hapten binding sites of chicken anti-DNP antibody appeared to contain an iodinatable residue since binding activity was decreased by iodination of the antibody, and the presence of the hapten during iodination protected the site (Benedict *et al.* 1972). Peptides were isolated from peptic digests of the paired-iodinated antibody which appeared to have come from the binding site. Identification of peptides from the site by iodination indicated the presence of a tyrosine or histidine in the site (Pressman *et al.* 1970).

Homogeneity

A number of anti-DNP 7S Ig antibodies obtained from individual chickens injected with antigen in FCA seem to have limited heterogeneity as judged from autoradiographs of peptic digests (Benedict *et al.* 1972), acrylamide gel electrophoresis (Kubo, unpublished data) and isoelectric focusing (Benedict

& Yamaga, unpublished data). Repeated attempts to detect 7S Ig H-chain subclasses have been unsuccessful, although antigenic and electrophoretic heterogeneity have been reported (Barabas & Barabas 1969, Wilkinson & French 1969). According to the following criteria, the 7S Ig appears to be relatively homogeneous: (1) the L-chains are predominantly λ; (2) the H-chains are predominantly a single subgroup (V_HIII); (3) the absence of proven H-chain subclasses; and (4) restricted heterogeneity of anti-DNP H- and L-chains in starch gel electrophoresis.

Carbohydrate composition

The hexose content is higher in chicken 7S Ig than in human IgG (Tenenhouse & Deutsch 1966, Dreesman 1966). Recent quantitative carbohydrate analyses by a radiochromatographic method (Howell *et al.* 1973) and by gas chromatography (Acton *et al.* 1972) revealed a total carbohydrate of 5·5–6·0 per cent for chicken 7S Ig (molecular weight of 170,000) (Table 13.1). This value is about twice that of human IgG (Acton *et al.* 1972). Frommel *et al.* (1971) obtained a somewhat lower value (4·1 per cent) which is a reflection of lower total hexose and hexosamine concentrations. The hexosamine : hexose ratio varied from 0·5 (Acton *et al.* 1972) to 0·86 (Howell *et al.* 1973). The carbohydrate contents of chicken anti-DNP antibody and of normal chicken 7S Ig were 5·5 per cent and 6·0 per cent, respectively (Howell *et al.* 1973); thus, the methods used to isolate the Ig might account for the differences.

Acton *et al.* (1972) reported the carbohydrate composition of the immunoglobulins and their chains from species representing the major classes of vertebrates. They found some carbohydrate associated with L-chains from various species, and relatively large amounts were isolated from chicken (2·5 per cent) and pheasant (> 1·08 per cent) L-chains; and from L-chains of a lower species, the catfish (2·49 per cent). Nevertheless, most of the carbohydrate was associated with the H-chain. Based on a molecular weight of 67,500 the carbohydrate composition of chicken H-chains was 6·18 per cent (Acton *et al.* 1972). The antigenically related pheasant H-chain contained 3·61 per cent, which is more closely aligned with the human γ-chain (3·09 per cent).

The mannose:galactose ratio was greater than one in the 7S immunoglobulins of humans (3·1) and of birds (chicken 5·2; pheasant 3·6; duck 2·4). Below Aves this ratio was of the order of one. Whether carbohydrate composition of the immunoglobulins will serve as a marker in the phylogenetic relationship of these proteins will have to await further studies. Information on the structure of the glycopeptides might serve as a more useful phylogenetic tool. In this connection, there was as little homology of the amino acid sequences of the carbohydrate peptides between human γ- and chicken 7S Ig H-chains as between human γ- and μ-chains (Travis & Sanders 1973).

Table 13.1. Carbohydrate composition of chicken and duck immunoglobulins

Immunoglobulin	Mannose (%)		Galactose (%)	Glucosamine (%)	Fucose (%)	Sialic acid (%)	Total (%)	Reference
Chicken 7S		2·0*		1·25	0·45	0·4	4·1	Frommel *et al.* (1971)
	2·77		0·61	1·7	0·19	0·23	5·5	Acton *et al.* (1972)
	2·9		0·3	2·8			6·0	Howell *et al.* (1973)
	2·8†		0·2†	2·5†			5·5†	Howell *et al.* (1973)
Chicken 17S	2·18		1·41	2·21	0·17	0·63	6·6	Acton *et al.* (1972)
Duck 5·7S		0·28*		0·28	0·12	0·09	0·77	Zimmerman *et al.* (1971)
Duck 7S	1·92		1·54	2·2	0·74		6·4	Acton *et al.* (1972)
		3·11*		1·6	0·42	0·26	5·4	Zimmerman *et al.* (1971)
Duck 17S	2·06		1·91	1·20	0	0·18	5·4	Acton *et al.* (1972)

* Calculated as hexoses.

† All preparations were normal immunoglobulins except these, which were anti-DNP antibody.

Enzymatic Digestion

Chicken 7S Ig hydrolysed with papain and reducing agent was split to 3·5S fragments (Michaelides *et al.* 1964, Dreesman & Benedict 1965b). Unlike mammalian IgG, approximately 30–50 per cent of the products were dialysable peptides. The Fab and Fc fragments were electrophoretically slow and fast, respectively. Pheasant and quail 7S Ig were hydrolysed by papain in a similar manner (Leslie & Benedict 1970a). The molecular weights of chicken Fab and Fc were 55,700 and 56,900, respectively (Kubo 1970). The sum of these weights $[(2 \times 55{,}700)+(56{,}900) = 168{,}300]$ is in excellent agreement with the mass of the undigested molecule. The Fc is easily purified as a precipitate by dialysis against 1·5 M NaCl (Kubo & Benedict 1969a). The conditions for crystallization of Fc were unlike those used for crystallization of mammalian Fc (Kubo & Benedict 1969a). Crystals shaped as hexagonal prisms terminated by hexagonal pyramids form at 37°C, but they were not stable at low temperatures.

In the absence of reducing agents, the yields of various fragments of chicken 7S Ig from pepsin digestion were dependent upon the digestion time, pH, and the type of preparation (Kubo 1970, Leslie & Benedict 1970a). Unlike rabbit and human IgG, which are converted to 5S $F(ab')_2$ fragments by digestion at pH 4·5, chicken pseudoglobulins (water-soluble) were converted mostly to Fab′ (3·5S). The Fab′ and papain-produced Fab showed a line of complete identity in immunodiffusion. Digestion of the pseudoglobulins at a higher pH (5·0) produced a mixture of 7S, 5·4S and 3·4S fragments (Tenenhouse & Deutsch 1966, Leslie & Benedict 1970a). Digestion of euglobulins (water-insoluble) at pH 4·5 yielded mostly Fab′. Under these conditions the major product of pepsin cleavage is Fab′ fragments. Digestion of purified anti-DNP 7S Ig with pepsin in the presence of ligand followed by extensive dialysis to remove the hapten yielded mostly 4·8S $(Fab')_2$ (Voss & Eisen 1972). Apparently the hapten inhibited cleavage of the molecules to predominantly Fab′ fragments. Even though pheasant 7S Ig is antigenically and structurally related to chicken Ig, digestion of pheasant Ig with pepsin at pH 4·5 resulted in mainly $F(ab')_2$ and a small amount of Fab′ (Leslie & Benedict 1970a). Behaving in an intermediate manner between chicken and pheasant, pepsin digestion of Japanese quail 7S Ig produced a mixture of 5·4S and 3·2S fragments.

Reductive Dissociation

Unlike mammalian IgG chicken 7S Ig reduced with 2-mercaptoethanol (ME) and alkylated, released some L chains at neutral or slightly alkaline solutions in the absence of dissociating agents, such as weak acids, urea, or detergents (Dreesman & Benedict 1965a). Sulphhydryl reducing agents have been used to distinguish IgM from IgG antibodies; however, this criterion should be used cautiously with chicken antibodies. Even with 0·1 M ME the 7S Ig antibodies lose some agglutinating and precipitating capacities with antigen (Benedict *et al.* 1963b, d, Rosenquist & Gilden 1963).

Kubo (1970) studied reductive dissociation of chicken 7S Ig in more detail. As shown in Table 13.2, about 1·3 disulphide bonds per molecule were

Table 13.2. The number of disulphide bonds broken per molecule of chicken 7S Ig reduced with mercaptoethanol (ME), and the release of the L-chains (Kubo 1970)

ME* (M)	Solvent	S–S bonds broken per molecule of 7S Ig reduced†	Relative percentage of Sephadex fraction‡ Aggregate	7S Ig	L-chain (pH 8·2)	L-chain (pH 2·4)
0	0·2 M tris, pH 8·0	0·2	6·7	93·3	0	0
0·005	0·2 M tris, pH 8·0	0·6				
0·01	0·2 M tris, pH 8·0	1·3	6·3	93·7	0	4·3
0·03	0·2 M tris, pH 8·0	3·0				
0·05	0·2 M tris, pH 8·0	3·5	6·2	92·3	1·5	10·9
0·1	0·2 M tris, pH 8·0	4·8	12·9	81·3	5·8	12·1
0·2	0·2 M tris, pH 8·0	6·6	30·8	55·2	14·0	12·9
0·2	5 M guanidine	13·6				
0·5	5 M guanidine	13·6				

* Samples of unreduced 7S Ig were treated with the indicated concentration of ME and then analysed for the —SH groups released by the method of Ellman (1959).

† Numbers expressed were averaged from duplicate determinations at two different protein concentrations.

‡ Calculated from peaks eluted from Sephadex G-200 equilibrated with either borate buffer, pH 8·2 or 1 M propionic acid, pH 2.4.

reduced with 0·01 M ME, but no dissociation of L-chains was detected by gel filtration at pH 8·2 of the reduced protein. Gel filtration in propionic acid (pH 2·4) yielded 4·3 per cent L-chains. Reduction with 0·05–0·2 M ME resulted in the reduction of 3–4 and 6–7 disulphide bonds per molecule, respectively, with the release of L-chains at pH 8·2. Dissociation of L-chains in neutral buffer may be explained as resulting from some conformational change due to reduction which is unfavourable for the association of the H- and L-chains. Alternatively, the non-covalent bonds of chicken 7S Ig may be weaker than those which occur in the Ig of mammalian species. Also, λ-chains may dissociate easier than κ-chains (Cohen & Gordon 1965). Kubo (1960) also found that L-chains were released at pH 2·4 from human IgG reduced with 0·01 M ME while rabbit IgG was converted to half molecules (Palmer & Nisonoff

1964) when treated in the same manner. Similar to mouse (Williamson & Askonas 1968), human and guinea pig IgG, the L–H disulphide bonds in the majority of the chicken molecules were more susceptible to reduction than the H–H bonds. Reduction of pheasant and quail 7S Ig in the absence of a dispersing agent also resulted in dissociation of L-chains (Leslie & Benedict 1969).

Aggregation

Chicken 7S Ig has a sedimentation coefficient of 10–14S in 1·5 M NaCl (high salt) (Hersh & Benedict 1966). These values are higher than expected from the density and viscosity of the 1·5 M NacCl solutions used. The curve of the sedimentation coefficient *versus* concentration of the 7S Ig in high salt showed a pronounced positive curvature at low protein concentrations (Hersh & Benedict 1966). Such a curve is associated with polymerization reactions of some proteins in which re-equilibrium between species occurs rapidly (Nichol *et al.* 1964). The polymers had an average molecular weight of 560,000, suggesting an aggregate of 3–4 molecules depending on the geometry of the aggregates. Aggregation in high salt has been observed by others (Van Orden & Treffers 1968, Kubo & Benedict 1969b, Gallagher & Voss 1970). Dimers of anti-DNP antibody with molecular weights of 347,000 and 390,000 were reported as the major species formed in 2·0 M NaCl and 3·0 M NaCl, respectively (Gallagher & Voss 1970). The 7S Ig of all the gallinaceous birds studied by Kubo and Benedict (1969b) (chicken, pheasant, quail, turkey) and by Benedict (unpublished data) (guinea fowl, jungle fowl, currassow) aggregated in 1·5 M NaCl; whereas rabbit, porcine, bovine, sheep and human IgG did not (Kubo & Benedict 1969b). Turkey 7S Ig showed a more limited tendency to aggregate in high salt than the Ig of some of the other gallinaceous birds. That aggregation in high salt is a property of the gallinaceous 7S Ig is borne out by preliminary studies in our laboratory that the 7S Ig of the following non-gallinaceous birds do not seem to aggregate in 1·5 M NaCl; namely, cassowary, dove, duck, emu, goose, pigeon, rhea. The possible relationship of salt-aggregation to the precipitin reactions will be discussed below.

Antigenic relationships

Chickens, pheasants and Japanese quail were found to be closely related to each other by means of common antigenic determinants on the H-chains, L-chains, and Fab and Fc fragments (Leslie & Benedict 1970b). Chicken and pheasant 7S Ig were more closely related antigenically than quail was to either of these. The L-chains of the chicken and pheasant were antigenically identical. As shown in Fig. 13.1, with rabbit anti-chicken 7S Ig there was

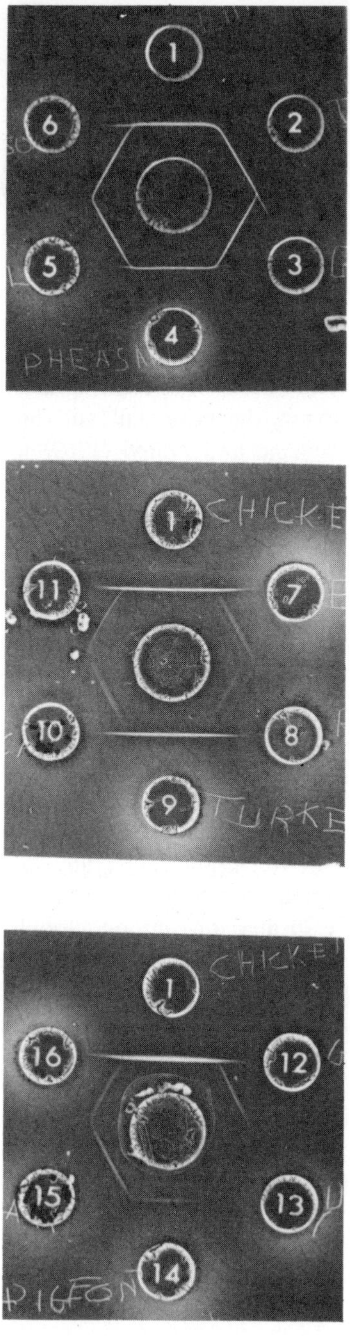

Fig. 13.1. Double-diffusion in agar gel of the cross-reactivity of various avian sera with a rabbit anti-chicken 7S Ig antiserum (centre wells). Avian sera: (1) chicken (*Gallus domesticus*); (2) jungle fowl (*Gallus gallus*); (3) guinea fowl (*Numida meleagris*); (4) pheasant (*Phasianus colchicus*); (5) quail (*Coturnix coturix*); (6) curassow (*Crax rubra*); (7) emu (*Dromiceius n. hollandiae*); (8) rhea (*Rhea americana*); (9) turkey (*Meleagris gallopavo*); (10) pelican (*Pelecanus erythrorhynches*); (11) duck (*Anas platyrhynchos*); (12) goose (*Anser anser*); (13) dove (*Streptopelia risoria*); (14) pigeon (*Columba livia*); (15) cassowary (*Casuarius unappendiculatus*); (16) emu (*Dromiceius n. hollandiae*). (Benedict & Kubo, unpublished data).

strong cross-reactivity with other gallinaceous birds (jungle fowl, guinea fowl, curassow, turkey) and weak cross-reactivity with non-gallinaceous birds (duck, dove, emu, goose, pelican, pigeon, rhea) (Benedict & Kubo, unpublished data). The sera of three closely-related large ratites (cassowary, emu, rhea) (Sibley & Ahlquist 1972) formed two precipitin bands (Fig. 13.1); in immunoelectrophoresis they both migrated in the γ-globulin region. With rabbit anti-duck 7S Ig antiserum, antigenic determinants were found on the chicken 7S Ig which were not present on the duck 5·7S molecule (Zimmerman *et al.* 1971). The locations of these cross-reacting determinants are not known.

Cross-reactivity between the Numigall and human IgG was reported (Oriol *et al.* 1972). Skameme and Ivanyi (1969) found common antigenic determinants on the chicken 7S Ig and 17S Ig H-chains which are hidden in the 7S Ig molecule but apparently accessible on the macroglobulin molecule.

Allotypes

For thousands of years birds have been subjected to selective breeding practices which have generated countless genetic variations. Birds may be valuable for elucidating the genetic and chemical basis for immunoglobulin polymorphisms. Unfortunately, these kinds of analyses have been limited. Using alloantisera raised against antibody-coated bacteria, Skalba (1964) detected several allotypic specificities in chicken serum proteins. Four were associated with γ-globulins while eight were found in the β-globulin fraction (perhaps transferrin) (Skalba 1966). McDermid *et al.* (1969) noted that some apparently normal chicken sera formed precipitins with other chicken sera, but whether these alloantigens were located on immunoglobulins was not established. Schierman and McBride (1968) detected allotypes presumably present on the 7S Ig, and David *et al.* (1961) reported several specificities. The alloantisera against two specificities reacted with intact 7S Ig as well as yolk immunoglobulin but not with preparations treated with ME or enzymes (David 1972).

Before meaningful genetic studies on immunoglobulins can be performed, it is necessary to establish that the allotypes actually are located on Ig molecules. The structural location and the distribution of the allotypic determinants among the classes of immunoglobulins need to be determined.

BIOLOGICAL PROPERTIES

Precipitin reaction

Chicken 7S Ig differs in a number of respects from typical mammalian antisera, most notable of which is that the maximum precipitation of immune complexes occurs in 1·5 M NaCl (high salt) (Wolfe 1942, Wolfe & Dilks 1946, Goodman *et al.* 1951, Benedict *et al.* 1963c). Pheasant and owl anti-

BSA antisera also behave in this manner (Goodman & Wolfe 1952), but pigeon antisera do not (Guttman, personal communication in Kubo *et al.* 1973). Whether this salt dependence for immune precipitation of antibody occurs in other non-gallinaceous birds, in addition to the owl and pigeon, remains to be determined.

The high salt dependence has resulted in a substantial literature since it was first observed by Hektoen (1918). Kabat & Mayer (1961) state that '. . . it is not at all clear how the antibody content of chicken antisera can be reliably determined'. Indeed this would seem to be the case if the precipitin reaction was the sole method of assay. Antigen-binding techniques used with chicken antibody, such as equilibrium dialysis (Gallagher & Voss 1970), the Farr (Farr 1958) method (Dreesman *et al.* 1965), radioelectrocomplexing (Simons & Benedict 1974), and fluorescence quenching (Voss & Eisen 1972) do not require high salt for optimal binding. At high concentrations of salt the average intrinsic constant and the valence of chicken anti-DNP 7S Ig was the same as measured at physiological conditions (Gallagher & Voss 1970, Voss & Eisen 1972). Therefore, the salt dependence probably relates to secondary effects on the antibodies. Several groups have explained the high salt effect on the basis of co-precipitation of normal serum components, particularly macroglobulins (Gengozian & Wolfe 1957, Makinodan *et al.* 1960, Orlans *et al.* 1961, Orlans *et al.* 1964, Van Orden & Treffers 1968), Co-precipitation of normal serum factors probably does not explain the high salt effect (Kubo 1967). The effect of salt on chicken anti-BSA 7S Ig fractions (macroglobulin-free) was the same as on whole antiserum. Furthermore, specifically purified anti-BSA (Vasan & Benedict, unpublished data) and specifically purified anti-DNP antibody (Gallagher & Voss 1970) required high salt for optimal precipitation with antigen.

As described above, the 7S Ig aggregates in high salt (Hersh & Benedict 1966, Kubo & Benedict 1969b), and it was proposed that because of aggregation the 7S Ig antibody precipitated better in high salt. Based on this observation, and the finding that Fab and $F(ab')_2$ do not precipitate in high salt but Fc does, Kubo (1970) proposed a model which is depicted by Kubo *et al.* (1973). According to this model non-precipitating 7S Ig formed trimers in high salt by aggregation of the Fc portions of the molecules, thus allowing accommodation of the binding sites for cross-linking with antigen. This theory and the one proposed by Gallagher & Voss (1969, 1970) are not mutually exclusive. They proposed that high salt induced a conformational change which allowed for polar orientation of the active sites and thus lattice formation. This hypothesis was based on their observations that increased immune precipitation of chicken anti-DNP antibody also occurred in physiological salt concentrations at pH 5·0. At this pH, which is below the pI, the antibody did not aggregate, and the intrinsic association constant was the same as that obtained at pH 7·0. Therefore, it was suggested that low pH in low ionic strength solution induced a conformation reorientation in the absence of aggregation similar to that induced by high salt. Based on ultracentrifugation and fluorescence depolarization studies, unfolding of the 7S Ig at pH 5·0 was indicated (Gallagher & Voss, personal communication). It will be interesting to know whether high salt induces similar changes. In extreme antibody excess, the molar ratio of Ab/Ag in precipitates formed in low pH and in high salt were 11·8 and 5·9, respectively (Gallagher & Voss 1970). The ratio at low pH is similar to that expected of bivalent rabbit anti-DNP antibody in extreme antibody excess. This indicates that the mechanisms of increased precipitation at pH 5·0 and in high salt might be different. Recently, Voss and Eisen (1972) noted in immunodiffusion plates enhanced precipitation of anti-DNP $F(ab')_2$ with antigen in high salt even though Kubo (1970) found that pepsin-produced chicken and pheasant $F(ab')_2$ did not aggregate in high salt. This is in accord with the interpretation given by Voss & Eisen (1972), namely, the portion of the molecule responsible for high salt precipitation is not localized in the Fc domains. Indeed, 'monogamous' binding of bivalent antibody with multivalent ligands (Hornick & Karush 1969) might occur in low salt, whereas cross-linking occurs in high salt (Voss & Eisen 1972). Nevertheless, the fact that aggregation takes place in high salt must be considered in any explanation. Also to be considered in this connection is that anti-BSA antisera obtained following a single injection of BSA (primary response) contained a 7S non-haemagglutinating (passive haemagglutination) antibody which precipitated with antigen chiefly in high salt. However, hyperimmune sera contained a 7S haemagglutinating antibody which precipitated well in low salt with antigen (Benedict *et al.* 1963c, Orlans 1967).

In addition to the precipitin reaction, the haemagglutination titres of chicken anti-BSA antisera, particularly primary antisera, could be greatly increased by the use of high salt in a test in which formalized tanned BSA-sensitized sheep erythrocytes were used (Pinckard & Benedict, unpublished data). Therefore, lattice formation was enhanced by high salt for this reaction as well as in the precipitin reaction.

Complement fixation

It has been generally accepted that chicken antibodies do not fix guinea-pig complement (C). This deficiency lies in the inability of chicken antibody to activate guinea-pig C1 (Benson *et al.* 1961, Rose & Orlans 1962), but the addition of chicken C1 to chicken antibody–antigen complexes can activate the other guinea-pig components (Benson *et al.* 1961). The following observations suggested that this was possible. Bushnell and Hudson (1927) and Rice (1947) reported that unheated chicken anti-pullorum sera fixed guinea-pig C with homologous antigen. Heated chicken anti-sheep red blood cell antibody also failed to lyse sheep cells with guinea-pig C, whereas lysis occurred with chicken C (Rose & Orlans 1962, Benson *et al.* 1961). Thus a direct complement fixation (DCF) test was proposed by addition of fresh unheated chicken serum to heated chicken antiserum, antigen, and guinea-pig C (Brumfield & Pomeroy 1959). This test was refined by using purified chicken C1, guinea-pig serum, free of C1, and RBC sensitized with chicken haemolysin (Stolfi *et al.* 1971).

Most CF tests with avian sera have been done with antisera to infectious agents, particularly to ornithosis (psittacosis). When tested with particulate antigens, chicken, duck, goose, turkey and pheasant anti-ornithosis sera did not fix guinea-pig C while antisera from psittacine birds and some pigeons did (Rice 1961). For this reason the indirect complement fixation (ICF) reaction was devised for detection of non-complement fixing antibodies (Rice 1947, 1948, Karrer *et al.* 1950). As indicated by the ICF and DCF reactions, pigeon sera contain both CF and non-complement fixing antibodies (Piraino 1966).

The nature of the antigen apparently has some influence on the fixation of guinea-pig C by *turkey* antibody. A soluble antigen extracted from a Chlamydial agent (Meningopneumonitis) with a detergent (Benedict & O'Brien 1956) was capable of fixing guinea-pig C with turkey antibody as efficiently as with rabbit antibody (Benedict & McFarland 1956, 1958); yet particulate antigens failed to do so. Dreesman *et al.* (1967) proposed that the ICF (measured with particulate antigen) and the DCF (measured with soluble antigen) detected different turkey anti-ornithosis antibodies. The role of the antigen (soluble *versus* particulate) in permitting activation of guinea-pig C by turkey anti-ornithosis antisera is not known. It is tempting to speculate that the sites on the 7S Ig involved in guinea-pig C1 activation were masked, but they may be made available by proper conformational change induced by antigen. Alternatively, the soluble antigen might be detecting 7S antibodies having the ability to fix guinea-pig C but with different specificities than those antibodies directed to the particulate antigen. Whatever the case, the soluble antigen did not fix guinea-pig C with *chicken* anti-ornithosis antibody (Benedict & McFarland 1958); therefore, the abilities of turkey and chicken antibodies to fix guinea-pig C differ. Based on this knowledge of the ornithosis system, admittedly limited, birds can be listed in decreasing order of their ability to fix guinea-pig C as follows: psittacine (fixes with particulate antigen), pigeon (fixes with particulate but also contains non-CF antibody), turkey (fixes with soluble antigen only), chicken (does not fix with particulate or soluble antigen). Further work on this interesting subject is warranted.

Immediate-type hypersensitivity

Although systemic anaphylaxis had been known for quite some time to occur in birds (Gahringer 1926) only in recent years have the conditions for sensitization been studied. Celada and Ramos (1961) found the sensitivity to passive cutaneous anaphylaxis (PCA) low in chickens. The reason was that reactions are readily induced in young chicks (Kubo & Benedict 1968, Conway *et al.* 1968) and in adult pathogen-free chickens (Ettinger & Hirata 1971) but they are not induced in conventionally raised adult birds. Histologically the reaction is typical of PCA and not of an Arthus type (Ettinger *et al.* 1970). Following intradermal injection of antibody a short latent period of 3–4 hours before intravenous injection of antigen is required for maximal reactions (Kubo & Benedict 1968). Nevertheless, chicken antisera with very high concentrations of anti-BSA precipitins will give weak reactions after a latent period of 3 days (Luoma 1974). As determined by the precipitin reaction, 0·28 μg of chicken anti-BSA N gave minimal reactions in 3-week-old chicks. Optimal reactions were obtained with an antigen dosage of 0·06 mg of BSA/g of body weight (Kubo & Benedict 1968).

There are several possibilities to explain the refractory state of adult chickens to PCA. Ettinger & Hirata (1971, 1973) proposed that 'as chickens grow older in conventional environments their skin receptor sites for homocytotropic antibodies are pre-empted by antibodies of various specificities'. To substantiate this hypothesis they rendered 7-day-old chicks PCA-negative by replacing their blood with blood from conventional adult chickens 24 hours before testing. Also adult germ-free chickens lost their ability for PCA after they were held in a conventional environment for a period as short as 1 month. However, there is presumptive evidence that all of the skin receptor sites of adult birds are not occupied by homocytotropic antibodies of various specificities (Faith & Glem 1973). A second possibility which in part might explain this phenomenon is the existence of a factor in the blood of young birds that 'facilitates' PCA (Ettinger & Hirata 1973). The fact that young chickens are more sensitive to histamine than adult birds (Faith & Clem 1973) must be considered too. In addition to the above, the difference between PCA in young and adult chickens might be due to: (1) blood C levels (the role of C in chicken PCA reactions has not been studied); (2) the susceptibility of the mast cells to release vasoactive substances as a result of the antigen–antibody reaction; and (3) the distribution of mast cells. In this regard, mast cells in adult chickens are associated mainly with the connective tissues of the digestive system (Carlson & Hacking 1972).

The immunoglobulin responsible for PCA has all of the immunologic and structural characteristics of the major 7S Ig found in chicken serum (Faith & Clem 1973). Nevertheless, it is homocytotropic because it does not sensitize mice (Celada & Ramos 1961), guinea-pigs (Ovary 1960), and ducks (Faith & Clem 1973) to PCA, but it does sensitize the skin of a closely-related species, the quail (Faith & Clem 1973). Some of the properties of the antibody responsible for PCA resemble those of the mammalian IgG-type of homocytotropic antibodies, and other properties are characteristic of mammalian IgE. Similar to the IgG-type antibody, the antibody responsible for PCA was reported to be resistant to treatment with ME and to be 'not particularly labile to heating' (Faith & Clem 1973). Also characteristic of the IgG-type, the chicken antibody migrated electrophoretically as a γ_1-globulin, and the optimal period for fixation to skin was short (Kubo & Benedict 1968). On the other hand, similar to mammalian IgE, chicken anti-BSA antisera had the following characteristics in respect to PCA (Luoma 1974): (1) considerable activity to induce PCA was lost when antisera were heated at 63°C for 30 minutes; (2) activity was completely abolished when antisera were treated with 0·1 M ME for one hour, alkylated with iodoacetamide and dialysed against buffer [Faith & Clem (1973) treated their antisera with ME in a similar manner, but apparently did not alkylate]: and (3) some sera contained antibodies which fixed to chicken skin for 3 days. Although failure to detect anaphylactic antibody in the egg yolk (Faith & Clem 1973) is characteristic of IgE antibody, Luoma (1974) prepared a saline extract of egg yolk which contained anti-BSA 7S Ig precipitins and which produced strong PCA. Whether the chicken has IgE and/or a subpopulation of an IgG-type of homocytotropic antibody is not known, but such information would be of considerable significance for problems concerned with the evolution of multiple classes of immunoglobulins.

Chickens also elicit macroscopically-typical Arthus reactions (Luoma & Benedict 1974). In direct or reversed passive Arthus (RPA) reactions cutaneous haemorrhage and moderate oedema appear in 3–4 hours in highly sensitized animals. Although adult chickens do not respond to direct cutaneous anaphylaxis, they do elicit direct Arthus reactions. Surprisingly, as in PCA, RPA reactions were induced more easily in young chicks than in older birds. The maximal response occurred in 3- to 4-week-old chicks. The refractory state of adult birds to RPA reactions and not to direct reactions is puzzling.

The severity of RPA reactions was related to the concentration of high salt precipitins (Luoma & Benedict 1974). For minimal reactions about 0·12 mg of chicken AbN were required. A similar amount of rabbit antibody also induced minimal reactions in chicks. This amount is considerably higher than that which is necessary to elicit minimal reactions in some other animals (Fischel & Kabat 1947, Benacerraf & Kabat 1950, Ovary & Bier 1952), but similar to the mouse which also has low sensitivity to RPA reactions particularly to rabbit antibody (Benedict & Tips 1954). Chicken antiserum heated to 63°C for 30 minutes failed to induce RPA reactions in chickens.

Chicken antibody cannot effectively elicit RPA in the guinea pig. Whereas 0·300 mg of rabbit anti-BSA N gave a strong reaction in guinea pigs, this amount of chicken antibody elicited only a doubtful reaction. Since chicken antibody does not activate guinea-pig C1, it is not surprising that chicken antibody did not initiate a C-dependent allergic response in guinea pigs.

Egg yolk immunoglobulins

Antibodies produced in response to a variety of antigens pass through the yolk of the egg to the developing chick (Jukes *et al.* 1934, Brandly *et al.* 1946, Buxton 1952). The 7S Ig found in the yolk is immunochemically and physicochemically identical to the major 7S Ig found in the serum (Faith & Clem 1973). The 17S Ig is not transferred through the egg. Orlans & Rose (1972) reported an IgA-like Ig in the yolk, and two antigenically distinct H-chain subtypes were found in yolk (Wilkinson & French 1969). These have not been characterized further. Most likely there is selective transfer of immunoglobulin to the yolk (Patterson *et al.* 1962, Malkinson 1965) which might be comparable to the selective placental transfer of immunoglobulins in mammals (Brambell 1958, Gitlin *et al.* 1964).

Anseriformes

STRUCTURE

Grey (1963) reported a 7S antibody in ducks which was somewhat heavier than mammalian 7S antibody. Later, ducks were shown to have high molecular weight (17S) and 5·7S immunoglobulins (Unanue & Dixon 1965, Grey 1967a,b). For the purposes of this review the duck immunoglobulins with a $S_{20,w}$ value of 7·8S (Grey 1967a) will be referred to as '7S Ig'.

In several respects (Grey 1967a,b, Zimmerman *et al.* 1971) duck 7S Ig resembles the chicken 7S Ig: (1) the molecular weight is 178,000; (2) the H- and L-chains have molecular weights of 62,000–66,000 and 23,000, respectively; therefore the H-chains have a molecular weight which can be accounted for by a structure with five domains; (3) the amino acid composition of the H-chain differed significantly from the amino acid composition of human γ-chain; (4) the total carbohydrate content is higher than the carbohydrate content of mammalian IgG; values of 5·0 per cent (Zimmerman *et al.* 1971) and 6·4 per cent (Acton *et al.* 1972) have been obtained; (5) the hexose content is 3·1 per cent; (6) the H-chain has a greater number of cysteines than human γ-chains—however, the percentage per protein is about the same as human γ-chain; (7) papain-produced Fc has a greater anodal migration than Fab; and (8) rabbit anti-duck 7S Ig detects antigenic determinants on chicken 7S Ig not present on the duck 5·7S Ig, and rabbit anti-chicken γ-globulin antiserum reacts better with chicken 7S Ig than with duck 5·7S protein.

Except for the following, little else is known about the structure of the 7S Ig. Only three N-terminal amino acid residues of the L-chain have been reported (Hood *et al.* 1970) and they are the same as the N-terminal residues of chicken L-chains (Kubo *et al.* 1970); namely, Ala-Leu-Thr. The kinetics of dissociation of pre-formed BSA-anti BSA complexes is altered by reduction in that there was about a 75 per cent increase in half-dissociation time (Grey 1967b).

The goose also has 17S, 7S, and 5·7S immunoglobulins (Benedict &

Pollard, unpublished data). In response to DNP-BGG, all three immunoglobulins had anti-DNP antibody.

BIOLOGICAL PROPERTIES

Duck anti-ornithosis antisera failed to fix guinea-pig C in the presence of homologous antigens (Rice 1947, Rice 1961, Karrer *et al.* 1950); but the 7S Ig antibody was capable of fixing duck C (Grey 1967b). The 7S Ig also was capable of sensitizing the duck skin for PCA reactions (Grey 1967b), but whether it can act as a heterocytotropic antibody is not known.

Other birds

STRUCTURE

Unfortunately, there are no data on the structure of the immunoglobulins of other birds. As indicated before, the 7S Igs of several non-gallinaceous birds do not seem to undergo salt-induced aggregation. Pigeon (*Columba livia*) anti-BSA antibodies resembling 7S and 17S immunoglobulins were demonstrated by radioimmunoelectrophoresis (Guttman *et al.* 1971).

BIOLOGICAL PROPERTIES

Pigeon anti-BSA homocytotropic skin sensitizing antibodies were reported to resemble mammalian IgE because (1) the latent period for PCA in pigeons was maximal at 72 hours; (2) reactions could be detected up to 14 days after transfer; (3) skin sensitizing ability was destroyed by heating at 56°C for 4 hours; and (4) PCA could not be transferred to chickens, guinea-pigs or hamsters (Guttman *et al.* 1971). Unlike the gallinaceous birds, the precipitin reaction with pigeon 7S antibody does not appear to be dependent on salt concentrations (Guttman, personal communication in Kubo *et al.* 1973).

A number of different species of birds, particularly seashore birds, have antibodies which fix guinea-pig complement with the ornithosis agent (Pollard 1947, Pollard *et al.* 1947) and others (herons and egrets) had anti-ornithosis antibodies detected by the ICF (Moore *et al.* 1959). A systematic study is needed on the ability of antisera from a number of different species to fix guinea-pig C.

17S immunoglobulins

Galliformes

STRUCTURE

Introduction

In addition to the classical 7S γ-globulin antibodies the synthesis of high molecular weight chicken antibodies (17S Ig) in response to soluble antigens was realized (Benedict *et al.* 1962) at about the same time as IgM antibody synthesis was found to be a general occurrence to protein antigens in mammals (Bauer & Stavitsky 1961, Benedict *et al.* 1962). The properties of chicken 17S Ig are similar to those of mammalian IgM; in fact, antisera to human μ-chain cross-reacts strongly with chicken 17S Ig (Mehta *et al.* 1972).

'Purified' preparations of chicken 17S Ig often are contaminated with aggregated 7S Ig. To reduce this contamination, large amounts of 7S Ig and α_2-macroglobulin can be removed from a serum by precipitation with 9 per cent Na_2SO_4 which leaves most of the 17S Ig in the supernatant fluid (Benedict 1967a). Following gel filtration of the IgM-rich fractions through Sephadex G-200, further purification can involve the passing of the 17S fraction through an anti-7S Ig Fc immunoadsorbent column.

In starch block electrophoresis 17S anti-BSA passive haemagglutinins migrate as γ_2- and γ_1-globulins (Benedict *et al.* 1963d). The isoelectric point has not been determined.

Molecular weights

In the ultracentrifuge the chicken 17S Ig sediments as two peaks which at infinite dilution extrapolate to 16·7 and 28·5, respectively (Benedict 1967b). As determined by sedimentation equilibrium the molecular weight was 880,000–890,000 (Hersh & Benedict, unpublished data, Leslie & Clem 1969). The molecular weights of the H- and L-chains as determined by high speed equilibrium were $62{,}600 \pm 2{,}000$ and $23{,}900 \pm 600$, respectively (Hersh & Benedict, unpublished data); and by gel filtration the weights of H- and L-chains were about 70,000 and 22,000, respectively (Leslie & Clem 1969). As viewed by electron microscopy the 17S Ig had a pentameric structure (Feinstein & Munn 1969).

Carbohydrate Composition

The total carbohydrate and hexoses of the chicken 17S Ig were determined by Acton *et al.* (1972) to be 6·6 per cent and 3·5 per cent, respectively, and by Frommel *et al.* (1971) to be 7·2 per cent and 3·2 per cent, respectively. The total carbohydrate for pheasant was 6·1 per cent (Acton *et al.* 1972). These values were similar to those of the 17S Ig of other species studied. After subtraction of the weight due to carbohydrate the molecular weight of the heavy chain is about 59,000; this is about the same molecular weight as the human μ-chain. The mannose/galactose ratio of chicken 17S (3·0) was similar to human IgM but higher than species below Aves. Pheasant 17S Ig had a mannose/galactose ratio of 1·1.

Reductive dissociation

Reduction with low concentrations of reducing agent produced subunits with a molecular weight of 180,000. On the basis of a pentameric structure a molecular weight of 900,000 would be expected. Reduction with 0·02 M ME produced subunits with a lower molecular weight (166,000) (Hersh & Benedict, unpublished data), and caused the dissociation of L-chains (Benedict 1967b). Thus, similar to chicken 7S Ig, reduced chicken 17S partially dissociates in neutral buffer without a dispersing agent. The L-chains were released in reduced preparations which were either alkylated with iodacetamide or not alkylated. Treatment with 0·005–0·02 M ME converted the 17S and 28S molecules to species with sedimentation coefficients between 6S and 7S. Reduction with higher concentrations of ME produced subunits with sedimentation coefficients less than six. Reduction with 0·1 M ME produced 5·84S subunits, and followed by removal of the ME by dialysis, the sedimentation coefficient increased to 6·61; whereas, treatment with 0·1 ME followed by alkylation and dialysis produced 6·95S subunits. The peculiar behaviour of the chicken 17S Ig following reduction is not understood. It is unlikely that the release of J-chains would account for the decrease of the sedimentation coefficient and molecular weight. In this connection, the J-chain has been identified with chicken 17S Ig and it cross-reacts with human J-chain (Kobayashi *et al.* 1973). A fast-moving band in disc gel electrophoresis resembles a J-chain released from pheasant 17S Ig (Weinheimer *et al.* 1971).

Binding Site

Sufficient amounts of chicken 17S anti-DNP antibodies for equilibrium dialysis studies can be obtained by repeated intravenous injections of antigen (Yamaga 1975). With specifically-purified preparations of anti-DNP, valences of less than 10 were obtained. This may be due to the presence of varying amounts of high and low affinity binding sites. The affinity constants were of the order of 10^6 M^{-1}.

BIOLOGICAL PROPERTIES

The chicken 17S anti-BSA antibody precipitates optimally in 0·15 M NaCl (low salt) and the course of the precipitin reaction (Kubo 1967) is similar to that of the rabbit IgM precipitin reaction (Lindqvist & Bauer 1966). Whether the 17S Ig fixes C, and can induce immediate-type allergic responses remains to be determined.

Anseriformes

The duck 17S Ig has a total carbohydrate content of 5·34 per cent, similar to the chicken 17S Ig (Acton *et al.* 1972). No other data have been reported.

IgA-like immunoglobulins: Galliformes

Definitive proof that the chicken possesses an immunoglobulin homologous to mammalian IgA must await amino acid sequence homology and antigenic cross-reactivity of the H-chains (Vaerman & Heremans 1968). In 1972, however, Lebacq-Verheyden *et al.* (1972a), Orlans & Rose (1972) and Bienenstock *et al.* (1972) published persuasive evidences that such an immunoglobulin exists.

Historically, many investigators suggested that local immunity could be established in the respiratory tract of chickens and several postulated the existence of an IgA-like Ig in birds. Prior to 1972, few attempts were made to identify the immunoglobulins found in secretions. For example, Hitchner & Johnson (1948) demonstrated that intranasal vaccination with attenuated Newcastle Disease Virus rendered chickens less susceptible to respiratory infection when challenged with virulent virus. Parenteral vaccination had little effect. Similarly, vaccination by the aerosol route was more effective than by other routes (Beard & Easterday 1967, Heuschele & Easterday 1970a). Immunofluorescence studies showed the presence of antibody-producing cells in the lamina propria of the intestine (Jankovak & Mitrovic 1967) or in tracheal sections (Heuschele & Easterday 1970b). No attempt was made to identify the antibody. There have been occasional reports that chicken serum may contain at least three electrophoretically distinct antibodies. Dreesman *et al.* (1965) reported a β-migrating protein with anti-azobenzoate binding activity in addition to the anti-azobenzoate 7S and 17S antibodies. Patterson *et al.* (1965) also reported that anti-ferritin antisera displayed three bands by immunoelectrophoresis, one of which had a β-mobility. Initial attempts to find an Ig distinct from the 7S or 17S Ig in secretions from the respiratory and gastrointestinal tracts of chickens were unsuccessful (Leslie *et al.* 1971).

At present, the following data indicate that the chicken possesses a mammalian IgA homologue. First, the IgA-like Ig is the major immunoglobulin in bile and in high concentrations in other secretions (saliva; intestinal, bronchial, oviduct washes), whereas it represents a minor immunoglobulin relative to the 7S Ig in sera and in crude yolk extracts (Lebacq-Verheyden *et al.* 1972a,b, Orlans & Rose 1972, Bienenstock *et al.* 1972, 1973a,b, Leslie & Martin 1973). Immunohistological studies showed that the relative predominance of immunoglobulins in the spleen is in the order of 7S, 17S and IgA-like Igs while in the lamina propria the order is IgA-like, 17S and 7S Igs (Lebacq-Verheyden *et al.* 1972b, Bienenstock *et al.* 1973b). The fact that numerous tissues associated with the secretory system contain cells with the IgA-like Ig and that organ cultures of tissues synthesized this immunoglobulin (Bienenstock *et al.* 1973b) indicates that it may be produced locally both in the respiratory and gastrointestinal tracts.

Structurally, the IgA-like Ig contains L-chain determinants but is distinct from the 7S and 17S Igs based on cross-adsorption studies. Antibody activity has been detected against ferritin (Lebacq-Verheyden *et al.* 1972a), DNP-BSA (Bienenstock *et al.* 1972), and against streptococcal vaccine (Leslie & Martin 1973). Finally, human secretory component selectively bound the IgA-like Ig isolated from serum (Bienenstock *et al.* 1972, 1973a). Approximately 10–17 per cent of the human secretory component was associated with the heavy fraction (12–19S region) of normal chicken sera. Only trace amounts were observed with chicken 17S Ig. The IgA-like Ig was found in the void volume after filtration through Sephadex G-200 of intestinal or bile globulins (Bienenstock *et al.* 1972, 1973a, Leslie & Martin 1973). Intestinal IgA-like Ig sedimented at 11·9 to 16·2S (Bienenstock *et al.* 1973a). Bile IgA-like Ig has an estimated molecular weight of 350,000–360,000 by polyacrylamide gel electrophoresis (Leslie & Martin 1973). Serum contained predominantly polymeric but also monomeric forms. Treatment with low concentrations of reducing agent did not dissociate the molecule (Bienenstock *et al.* 1973a); at higher concentrations, subunits similar in size to those obtained from the reduction of 17S Ig were formed (Leslie & Martin 1973).

5·7S immunoglobulins: Anseriformes

STRUCTURE

The duck 5·7S Ig has a molecular weight of 118,000 and it is composed of two H-chains and two L-chains with molecular weights of 35,000 and 23,000, respectively (Zimmerman *et al.* 1971). Kubo *et al.* (1973) point out that the 5·7S Ig H-chain fits the formula V_1C_2. A phylogenetic formula, V_1C_n ($n = 1, 2 \ldots$) describes the evolution of an immunoglobulin polypeptide chain.

Phenylalanine was the C-terminal residue of the H-chain, and no other amino acid was released after prolonged digestion with carboxypeptidase (Zimmerman *et al.* 1971). The amino acid composition of the H-chain was similar to the duck 7S H-chain, but differed significantly from human γ-chain. There were 5·2 and 1·7 carboxymethyl cysteines per chain following partial reduction of the H- and L-chains, respectively. These values were considered to be somewhat higher than those obtained from mammalian IgG chains. The H-chains contained 11·2 carboxymethyl cysteines after complete reduction and alkylation. The carbohydrate content was low (0·6 per cent), and it was associated with the Fd fragment and L-chain. Mild reduction lowered the molecular weight to 58,000 and resulted in the formation of 'half molecules' in the absence of dissociating agents. Grey (1967b) presented evidence that the 5·7S Ig was neither a breakdown product nor a precursor of the 7S Ig. It is antigenically deficient in respect to the 7S Ig and unique class determinants have not been demonstrated.

BIOLOGICAL PROPERTIES

Reduction with 0·1 M ME for 1 hour followed by alkylation decreased the antigen-binding capacity considerably, and abolished the haemagglutinating capacity (Grey 1967b). The 7S Ig was unaffected by reduction in these respects.

The 5·7S antibody failed to fix duck complement and to elicit a PCA reaction in the duck. No other information has been reported.

Table 13.3 summarizes some of the properties of chicken and duck immunoglobulins.

Antibody production to soluble antigens

Introduction

In chickens, the range of immune responsiveness to a variety of antigens is not unlike that found in mammals. Antibodies are synthesized to proteins, polypeptides, polysaccharides, hapten conjugates and a wide variety of cellular and viral antigens. The role of the thymus and bursa of Fabricius in the chicken immune response and the development of lymphoid tissues are covered in Chapter 16. Some characteristics of the immune response to soluble antigens will be reviewed briefly here.

Interpreting some of the data concerned with antibody production may be misleading because different methods of measuring antibody have been used. Tests based on secondary (precipitation, agglutination, CF) and tertiary (*in vivo*) immune reactions often fail to measure considerable amounts of antibody detectable by primary interactions between antigen and antibody (Farr & Minden 1970). Because of the greater avidity of 17S antibodies, reactions such as haemagglutination and viral neutralization may exaggerate the 17S response (Greenbury *et al.* 1963, Benedict 1965, Hornick & Karush 1969). The use of ME sensitivity to distinguish between chicken 17S and 7S antibody should be used cautiously because some chicken 7S Igs are sensitive to 0·1 M ME. Thus, ME sensitivity is not a definitive criterion for 17S antibody (Benedict *et al.* 1963b). Even when reactions based on primary interactions are utilized, such as the Farr (1958) method, 17S haemagglutinating antibody may not be detected (Benedict 1965).

Proteins and Synthetic Polypeptides

Ewing & Strauss (1903) and Hektoen (1918) found that chickens produce large amounts of antibody to mammalian serum proteins. Later it was shown that chickens differ from mammals and some other birds (see below) in that relatively high levels of antibody can be obtained within a week following a single intravenous injection of soluble protein (BSA) in saline (Wolfe 1942, Wolfe & Dilks 1946, 1948). Generally, it has been accepted that this vigorous response might be due, in part, to the phylogenetic differences between the mammalian antigens and fowls. However, not all birds respond to BSA with vigorous antibody production. Turkeys (Wolfe & Dilks 1949, Dreesman *et al.* 1967), pigeons (Wolfe & Dilks 1949, Guttman *et al.* 1971), guinea fowl (Wolfe & Dilks 1949), Japanese quail (Leslie & Benedict 1969) and Adelie penguins (*Pygoscelis adeliae*) (Allison & Feeney 1968) respond very poorly to BSA. Even after several injections in FCA some turkeys failed to synthesize anti-BSA precipitating antibody (Dreesman *et al.* 1967). In view of these findings, birds in general cannot be considered as vigorous responders, at least to BSA. Perhaps the intensive breeding which produced different genetic backgrounds was responsible for the evolution of high and low responders to some antigens.

The doses used to elicit antibody by the intravenous route in chickens generally have been high (40 mg/kg body weight). Increased precipitating antibody was not obtained when a series of daily smaller doses were injected (Blazkovec & Wolfe 1965). In fact, induction of adult tolerance to proteins in birds was difficult and required massive doses (up to 5 g/kg body weight) of antigen (Mueller & Wolfe 1961, Ivanyi *et al.* 1966). Even at these doses some birds still produced antibody.

The presence of anti-BSA 17S antibody was reported in chickens (Benedict *et al.* 1962). Generally, both 17S and 7S antibodies were detected early in the response and often 17S antibody appeared slightly before the 7S antibody. After repeated injections of BSA, mainly 7S antibody was formed (Benedict 1967a). As in other animals, the relative concentrations of 17S and 7S antibodies appear to depend, in part, on the dose of antigen (Valentova *et al.* 1966).

More precipitating antibody was synthesized in the secondary response when the interval between the first and second intravenous injections was lengthened (3 weeks to 36 weeks) (Blazkovek & Wolfe 1965). Animals injected with very small doses (0.1 μg) of human serum albumin (HSA) may not elicit detectable antibody initially, but can prime for a secondary response (Valentova *et al.* 1967).

Outbred and inbred chickens respond to a single injection of 2 mg of the linear random copolymer L-glu^{60}L-ala^{30}L-tyr^{10} (GAT) in FCA by synthesis of both 17S and 7S antibodies (Benedict *et al.*, unpublished data). Intravenous injection of this antigen stimulates the synthesis of chiefly 17S antibodies. One highly inbred line of chickens was found to contain non-responders.

Grey (1967b) reported that 8 days following immunization of ducks with

Table 13.3. Some properties of chicken and duck immunoglobulins

Property	Chicken 7S	Chicken 17S	Duck 5·7S	Duck 7S	Duck 17S	Reference
Molecular weight ($\times 10^{-3}$)						
Ig	170	890	118	178		Hersh *et al.* (1969), Leslie & Clem (1969b), Kubo (1970), Grey (1967a), Zimmerman *et al.* (1971)
H-chain	60·5	62·6	35	62		
L-chain	23·7	23·9	23	23		
Fab	55·7		48			
Fc	56·9					
Concentration in 'normal' serum (mg/ml)	2·7 (young) 5·3 5·9 7·5 (>1 yr old)	0·7				Cooper *et al.* (1969), Leslie & Clem (1970), Van Meter *et al.* (1969), Tam (1975)
Reduction at neutral pH in the absence of a dissociating agent	Release of free L-chains	Release of free L-chains	'Half-molecules'			Dreesman & Benedict (1965a), Benedict (1967b), Zimmerman *et al.* (1971)
Lability of disulphide bonds to mild reduction	H-L > H-H	Probably H-L > H-H	Probably H-H > H-L			Kubo (1970), Zimmerman *et al.* (1971)
Enzymatic hydrolysis						
Papain	Fab; Fc		Fab	Fab; Fc		Dreesman & Benedict (1965b), Kubo (1970), Grey (1967a), Zimmerman *et al.* (1971)
Pepsin	Fab′ (major); some $F(ab')_2$; and pFc					
Trypsin	tFab; tFc; $tF(ab')_2$					
Aggregation in 1·5 M NaCl (high salt)	Yes ($S_{20,w}$ = 14S)					Hersh & Benedict (1965)

Immune precipitation in high salt	Enhanced	Decreased				Wolfe (1942), Kubo (1967)
L-chain N-terminal amino acid sequence*	Mostly unblocked λ† (anti-DNP)			(Ala-Leu-Thr)		Kubo *et al.* (1971), Hood *et al.* (1970)
H-chain N-terminal amino acid sequence (anti-DNP)	Resembles V_HIII‡					Kubo *et al.* (1971)
Total carbohydrate (%)	5·5	6·6	0·6	6·4	5·4	Acton *et al.* (1972), Zimmerman *et al.* (1971)
Metabolic half-life (days)	3·0 (neonatal) 1·5 (adults) 4·3 (adults) 4·1 (adults)	1·7 (adults)	~3			Patterson *et al.* (1962), Wostmann & Olson (1964), Leslie & Clem (1970), Grey (1967b)
Complement fixation	Guinea-pig C (−) Chicken C (+)		Duck C (−)	Guinea-pig C (−) Duck C (+)		Bushnell & Hudson (1927), Rice (1947), Grey (1967b)
Antibody in passive cutaneous anaphylaxis	Homocytotropic; sensitizes young birds optimally		No homocytotropic reactions induced	Homocytotropic (Heterocytotropic?)		Celada & Ramos (1961), Kubo & Benedict (1968), Conway *et al.* (1968), Grey (1967b)
Antibody in reverse passive Arthus reaction	Sensitizes young birds optimally. Guinea-pig poorly sensitized			Guinea-pigs sensitized with duck antiserum		Luoma & Benedict (1974), Ward & Cochrane (1965)

* Amino acid position:

	1	2	3	4	5	6	7	8	9	10	11	12	13	14	15	16	17	18	19	20	21	22	23
†	[ ]	-[ ]	-Ala	-Leu	-Thr	-Gln	-[ ]	-Pro	-Ala	-Ser	-Val	-Ser	-Ala	-Gln	-Leu	-Gly	-Glu	-Thr	-Val	-Ser	-Leu	-Thr	-Cys-
‡	Ala	-Val	-Thr	-Leu	-Asp	-Glu	-Ser	-Gly	-Gly	-Gly	-Leu	-Gln	-Thr	-Pro	-Gly	-Gly	-	-Leu	-	-Leu	-Val	-Cys-	

BSA in Freund's incomplete adjuvant (FIA) slightly more antibody activity was in the 7S Ig than in the 5·7S Ig fractions. 'No clear-cut production' of 17S Ig was demonstrated. Similar responses occurred in ducks immunized with rabbit glomerular basement membrane (Unanue & Dixon 1965). In the goose we have observed that early in immunization anti-BSA and anti-DNP 7S Ig antibodies are in slightly higher concentrations than the 5·7S antibodies, and that a continued synthesis of both of these antibodies occurred for several months. The 17S Ig antibody was not detected in some antisera by radio-immunoelectrophoresis. This type of temporal sequence of antibody synthesis is not limited to these animals. In a more thorough study, 17S anti-DNP and anti-BSA antibodies rarely have been detected in large sea turtles (*Chelonia mydas*) (100–350 lbs) early in the primary response, yet synthesis of both 7S and 5·7S antibodies persisted in varying ratios for a period of 5 years following a single injection of antigen (Benedict & Pollard 1972). In fact, 2-month-old sea turtles (~30 g) synthesize only 7S anti-DNP and anti-BSA antibodies following a single injection of antigen, and their levels of 5·7S protein are very low at this age but increase with age. It would appear from these data that the 7S Ig resembles the 17S in other animals in regards to early synthesis in the immune response and perhaps in regards to ontogenetic development. It would be interesting to determine whether this occurs in other animals in which the 5·7S protein is found (Marchalonis 1969, Clem 1971).

Polysaccharides

Similar to men and mice, chickens (Medlin *et al.* 1973) are capable of responding to soluble pneumococcal polysaccharide. The antibody titres as detected by passive haemagglutination and by the haemolytic plaque technique were low. As in other animals, the response was strongly dose-dependent with high doses being partially tolerogenic.

Haptens

Early reports indicated that intravenous injections of hapten-protein conjugates in chickens resulted in poor anti-hapten production similar to that expected in mammals. Multiple intravenous injections of *p*-azobenzoate-bovine γ-globulin resulted in low titres of passive haemagglutinating antibody (Gold & Benedict 1962, Riha 1965). Little or no haemagglutinating or precipitating anti-DNP antibody could be elicited by intravenous or intramuscular injection of DNP–BGG without FCA (Orlans *et al.* 1968). More recently, moderate anti-DNP responses have been obtained (Leslie & Clem 1969b, Yamaga 1975). Factors which may have influenced the amount of anti-DNP antibody detected are (1) limited coupling ratios of DNP to protein resulting in a poor anti-DNP response (Ashley & Ovary 1965); (2) the genetic background of the animals (Balcarova *et al.* 1973); and (3) the sensitivity of the assay. Both 17S and 7S anti-DNP antibodies were synthesized after a single intravenous injection, but the primary response was fleeting (Yamaga 1975). In radio-immunoelectrophoresis, binding was most intense by 6 days but very weak by 20 days. At very low doses (0·02 mg) some birds failed to respond with detectable antibody, but they were primed for a secondary response. The secondary response was characterized by prompt appearance of both 17S and 7S antibodies and persistence of 17S binding for 2 months or more. The amounts and affinity constants of antibody synthesized to various doses of DNP-BGG are discussed below (see *Maturation of antibody affinity*).

As observed with other animal sera, some chicken pre-immune sera bound DNP proteins weakly. In radio-immunoelectrophoresis, the binding proteins were identified as 7S Ig, 17S Ig, and α_2-macroglobulin. The α_2-macroglobulin had low binding because it was not removed by a DNP-lysyl immunoadsorbent column.

Effect of Adjuvants

Striking changes develop in chickens injected with FCA and to a lesser extent in birds given Freund's incomplete adjuvant (FIA). Immunization of birds with HSA in FCA or FIA resulted in a biphasic anti-HSA response (White 1970, Steinberg *et al.* 1970, French *et al.* 1970, Aitken 1973). As measured by the Farr (1958) technique, the amount of antibody in the first phase was similar to that obtained after a single intravenous injection of protein in aqueous solution. The response reached a peak at 8–12 days and decreased to a low level by 18 days. Later, a prolonged second rise of antibody occurred which peaked between 6–9 weeks. This second phase was most pronounced in birds injected with FCA; moderate in those given FIA; and not detected without adjuvant. Limited studies showed that antibodies from birds given either FCA or FIA increased in avidity.

Associated with FCA was the development of a massive granuloma at the site of the injection (White 1970, French *et al.* 1970). It is thought that most of the antibody produced in the second phase was synthesized locally since intense plasma cell infiltration developed in the granuloma and anti-HSA could be extracted from the granuloma in high yields when compared with other tissues. In the first phase most of the antibody synthesis occurred in the red pulp of the spleen. Thus, it is possible that cells were primed in the spleen and then migrated to the granuloma where they underwent a secondary response. In addition, it is conceivable, although no attempt was made to determine the class of antibody synthesized, that the initial phase might be due to 17S antibody followed by a progressive increase in the 7S antibody. These effects may depend in part on thymus-derived (T) cells since neonatal thymectomy and whole body X-irradiation decreased the size of the granuloma and the antibody response in the second phase (White 1970).

Even injection of FCA without antigen resulted in increased levels of 'non-specific' 7S Ig, as determined by radial immunodiffusion (Tam & Benedict 1975). These immunoglobulins were not directed to *Mycobacterium*. Chickens immunized with either FIA in saline, or BSA incorporated in FIA, or *Mycobacterium* in saline did not synthesize such demonstrable increases in 7S Ig. Changes in the relative amounts of other serum proteins also occurred in birds immunized with FCA. By cellulose acetate electrophoresis there was a sharp decrease in albumin with an increase in α-, β-, and γ-proteins. These have been identified as inflammatory proteins, perhaps similar to the C-reactive proteins found in mammals (Tillet & Francis 1930) and reported in chickens (Patterson & Mora 1964). The inflammatory serum proteins were purified and the α- and γ-proteins had sedimentation coefficients of about 5S; the β-protein sedimented at about 7S (Tam & Benedict 1975).

Maturation of Antibody Affinity

The mechanism involved in the synthesis of high affinity antibody has been explained as a selection process (Siskind & Benacerraf 1969, Werblin *et al.* 1973). The selective pressure is exerted, in part, by a limiting antigen concentration. When antigen concentration is low, cells with high binding receptors are thought to capture antigen preferentially, proliferate and secrete high affinity antibody; cells with receptors of low affinity persist but they are not preferentially stimulated. Furthermore, the cells responsible for the secondary response reflect the population of cells present immediately before boosting (Steiner & Eisen 1967, Paul *et al.* 1967, Siskind & Benacerraf 1969, Feldbush & Gowans 1971). If an animal is boosted after the selection process has occurred, an immediate burst of synthesis of high affinity antibody would be expected. Also, recent studies (Gershon & Paul 1971, Elfenbein *et al.* 1973) have indicated that the T cell may be involved in the maturation process. The role of FCA in the affinity maturation process could be evaluated in the chicken because the chicken responds to intravenous injections of DNP-BGG by synthesizing anti-DNP antibody in sufficient quantities to study by equilibrium dialysis. Thus, comparisons were made between intravenous immunization in aqueous solution versus intramuscular injection in FCA (Yamaga 1975).

Groups of birds were injected intravenously with various priming doses of antigen (0·02–20 mg). Birds in each group were boosted with 2 mg of DNP-BGG intravenously at various times later (1–8 weeks) and bled 1 week after the second injection. Affinities and amounts of antibody in the 7S globulin fractions were determined by equilibrium dialysis as described by Werblin & Siskind (1972b). Regardless of the priming dose or the time interval between injections no maturation in antibody affinity was observed; the $-\Delta F$ did not exceed 9·2. Moreover, the Sips' plots generated from these preparations were linear indicating that the selection process had not developed. However, there was a marked difference in the amount of antibody produced. The lowest yields of antibody were from those birds injected with either a very low (0·02 mg) or a very high (20 mg) priming dose for all time intervals when compared with those birds given intermediate doses (0·2 or 2 mg). Although these animals were apparently partially tolerant, the affinities of the antibody were the same. These results differed from those obtained by Theis & Siskind (1968) but agreed with those obtained later (Werblin & Siskind 1972a, Heller & Siskind 1973). Although protocols differed among these studies, the contrasting results might be reconciled by assuming that cells are rendered tolerant in a random manner and that the loss of some high affinity cells becomes conspicuous when they cannot be preferentially stimulated during the maturation process.

Birds also had been given multiple widely-spaced intravenous injections of 2 mg over a 1–2 year period. Preparations were obtained 16 weeks after four injections or 1 week after five or six injections. The antibody of highest affinity ($-\Delta F = 9{\cdot}16$) was not much greater than the affinity of antibody from chickens given only two intravenous injections. In contrast, when chickens were injected with a single dose of antigen in FCA the antibody affinity increased dramatically in a manner similar to that observed in rabbits (Werblin & Siskind 1973). For example, a chicken immunized with a single intramuscular injection of 2 mg DNP-BGG in FCA yielded antibody with a $-\Delta F$ of 9·6; 4 months later, the $-\Delta F$ of the antibody rose to 10.4. The curves were non-linear indicating that there was a selection for high affinity antibodies. Dose dependency appeared to be similar to that found in rabbits. Antibody affinity could be affected by FCA in at least two ways: (1) it establishes an antigen depot allowing for the slow release of antigen causing continual stimulation (Siskind & Benacerraf 1969); (2) *Mycobacterium* activates T cells which promote maturation (Gershon & Paul 1971, Elfenbein *et al.* 1973). In order to delineate the relative importance of these two factors, birds were injected with antigen in FIA. Preliminary work suggests that maturation is more limited but still apparent when compared with birds given FCA. Thus, although the evidence is indirect and incomplete, the following sequence of events may occur. Injection of FCA results in the formation of a granuloma which may contain T cells. The T cells may produce 'allogeneic factor' which augments the proliferation or differentiation of B cells (Elfenbein *et al.* 1973). This allows the antigen present as a depot to select high affinity cells more efficiently.

The effect of FCA in chickens can be summarized as follows: (1) induces a biphasic antibody response (moderate with FIA); (2) forms a granuloma which may be the site of local antibody synthesis (macroscopically not visible with FIA); (3) induces the appearance of inflammatory proteins; (4) non-specifically stimulates 7S Ig synthesis (5) augments the maturation of antibody affinity (moderate with FIA; minimal in aqueous solutions); (6) elicits delayed-type hypersensitivity (wattle reactions) (White 1970).

Conclusions

Vaerman and Heremans (1968) have suggested several criteria for establishing immunoglobulin homologies. These criteria were restated and ably used by Kubo *et al.* (1973) to evaluate the relationships between the immunoglobulins of lower vertebrates. In decreasing order of importance these criteria are: (1) amino acid sequences and antigenic cross-reactivity; (2) relatively specific properties of an immunoglobulin, such as those associated with human IgA and IgE; and (3) phenomena not necessarily unique to any single immunoglobulin, such as carbohydrate or amino acid composition, electrophoretic mobility, molecular weight, and complement fixation. It is clear that most of the data presented here on the biological and physical properties of avian immunoglobulins are chiefly third-order criteria.

Nevertheless, functionally, the immune responses (both humoral and cellular) of birds—at least some gallinaceous species—resemble the mammalian responses. Unlike many lower vertebrates (Kubo *et al.* 1973), but similar to mammals, birds are brisk antibody responders to a variety of antigens. In contrast to the sluggish responses seen in some amphibians, reptiles and fishes, antibodies are synthesized in birds in relatively high concentrations in short periods of time. Similarly, the affinity constants of chicken anti-DNP antibodies increase with time and approach the high values found in some mammals. In many lower vertebrates anti-DNP antibodies have relatively lower binding constants: and 'maturity' of affinity is a rather slow process. Parenthetically, in lower vertebrates the cellular immune response might be a more effective protective mechanism against microbial agents than the humoral antibody response.

Structurally, avian and mammalian immunoglobulins have unique antigenic determinants responsible for class distinctions, whereas in some lower vertebrates the low molecular weight immunoglobulins are 'classes' by virtue of their apparent antigenic deficiencies with respect to the high molecular weight immunoglobulins. Perhaps a greater degree of structural diversity will be found in birds than in lower animals.

Relationships between vertebrate classes may be puzzling, however, if only third-order criteria are available. The following examples serve to illustrate this point. Chickens and ducks have in common with some reptiles and amphibians a major 7S immunoglobulin which exceeds human IgG in molecular weight by an additional H-chain domain. Ducks share with turtles, the giant grouper (*Epinephelus itaira*) (Clem 1971) and the Australian lungfish (*Neoceratodus forsteri*) (Marchalonis 1969) an immunoglobulin

(5·7S) with an H-chain which seems to have one domain less than the mammalian γ-chain. The ratios of mannose:galactose of the chicken and duck 7S Ig are closer to the ratios for human IgG than to the ratios for certain amphibia and fishes (Acton *et al.* 1972). We agree that immunoglobulin homologies will be more firmly established with the completion of the amino acid sequence analyses and precise antigenic analyses of the H-chains.

Of particular importance in relation to the phylogeny of avian immunoglobulins is the need to study representatives of orders other than Galliformes (Pono, personal communication).

Acknowledgments

Some of the studies reported here were supported by the United States Public Health Service Grant AI-05660.

References

Acton R.T., Niedermeier W., Weinheimer P.F., Clem L.W., Leslie G.A. & Bennett J.C. (1972) The carbohydrate composition of immunoglobulins from diverse species of vertebrates. *J. Immunol.* **109,** 371.

Aitken I.D. (1973) The serological response of the chicken to a protein antigen in multiple emulsion oil adjuvant. *Immunology* **25,** 957.

Allison R.G. & Feeney R.E. (1968) Penguin blood serum proteins. *Arch. Biochem. Biophys.* **124,** 548.

Ashley H. & Ovary Z. (1965) Effect of bovine gamma globulin on subsequent immunization with dinitrophenylated bovine gamma globulin. *Proc. Soc. Exp. Biol. Med.* **119,** 311.

Balcarova J., Hala K. & Hraba T. (1973) Differences in antibody formation to the dinitrophenol group in inbred lines of chickens. *Folia Biol.* (*Praha*) **19,** 19.

Barabas A.Z. & Barabas H. (1969) Preparation of specific anti-chicken immunoglobulin sera. *Clin. Exp. Immunol.* **4,** 603.

Bauer D.C. & Stavitsky A.B. (1961) On the different molecular forms of antibody synthesized by rabbits during the early response to a single injection of protein and cellular antigens. *Proc. Nat. Acad. Sci. U.S.A.* **47,** 1667.

Beard C.W. & Easterday B.C. (1967) The influence of the route of administration of Newcastle Disease Virus on host response. I. Serological and virus isolation studies. *J. Infect. Dis.* **117,** 55.

Benacerraf B. & Kabat E.A. (1950) A quantitative study of the Arthus phenomenon induced passively in the guinea pig. *J. Immunol.* **64,** 1.

Benedict A.A. (1965) Sensitivity of passive hemagglutination for assay of 7S and 19S antibodies in primary rabbit anti-bovine serum albumin sera. *Nature* **206,** 1368.

Benedict A.A. (1967a) Production and purification of chicken immunoglobulins, vol. 1, p. 229. In *Methods in Immunology and Immunochemistry*, ed. Williams C.A. & Chase M.W. Academic Press, New York and London.

Benedict A.A. (1967b) Studies on chicken γM immunoglobulin. VII. *International Congress of Biochemistry, Tokyo* 979.

BENEDICT A.A. & MCFARLAND C. (1956) Direct complement-fixation test for diagnosis of ornithosis in turkeys. *Proc. Soc. Exp. Biol. Med.* **92,** 768.

BENEDICT A.A. & MCFARLAND C. (1958) Newer methods for detection of avian ornithosis. *Ann. N.Y. Acad. Sci.* **70,** 501.

BENEDICT A.A. & O'BRIEN E. (1956) Antigenic studies on the psittacosis-lymphogranuloma venereum group of viruses. II. Characterization of complement-fixing antigens extracted with sodium lauryl sulfate. *J. Immunol.* **76,** 293.

BENEDICT A.A. & POLLARD L.W. (1972) Three classes of immunoglobulins found in the sea turtle, *Chelonia mydas. Folia Microbiol.* **17,** 75.

BENEDICT A.A. & TIPS R.L. (1954) Actively and passively induced Arthus reactions in the mouse. *Proc. Soc. Exp. Biol. Med.* **87,** 618.

BENEDICT A.A., BROWN R.J. & AYENGAR R. (1962) Physical properties of antibody to bovine serum albumin as demonstrated by hemagglutination. *J. Exp. Med.* **115,** 195.

BENEDICT A.A., BROWN R.J. & HERSH R.T. (1963a) The temporal synthesis and some chromatographic and ultracentrifugal characteristics of chicken antibodies. *J. Immunol.* **90,** 399.

BENEDICT A.A., BROWN R.J. & HERSH R. (1963b) Inactivation of high and low molecular weight chicken antibodies by mercaptoethanol. *Proc. Soc. Exp. Biol. Med.* **113,** 136.

BENEDICT A.A., HERSH R.T. & LARSON C. (1963c) The temporal synthesis of chicken antibodies: The effect of salt on the precipitin reaction. *J. Immunol.* **91,** 795.

BENEDICT A.A., LARSON C. & NIK-KHAH H. (1963d) Synthesis of chicken antibodies of high and low molecular weight. *Science* **139,** 1302.

BENEDICT A.A, ROHOLT O.A., YAMAGA K. & PRESSMAN D. (1972) Peptides from the site of chicken anti-DNP antibodies. *Immunol. Communications* **1,** 279.

BENSON H.N., BRUMFIELD H.P. & POMEROY B.S. (1961) Requirement of avian C1 for fixation of guinea pig complement by avian antibody-antigen complexes. *J. Immunol.* **87,** 616.

BIENENSTOCK J., PEREY D.Y.E., GAULDIE J. & UNDERDOWN B.J. (1972) Chicken immunoglobulin resembling γA. *J. Immunol.* **109,** 403.

BIENENSTOCK J., PEREY D.Y.E., GAULDIE J. & UNDERDOWN B.J. (1973a) Chicken γA: Physico-chemical and immunochemical characteristics. *J. Immunol.* **110,** 524.

BIENENSTOCK J., GAULDIE J. & PEREY D.Y.E. (1973b) Synthesis of IgG, IgA, and IgM by chicken tissues: Immunofluorescent and ^{14}C-amino acid incorporation studies. *J. Immunol.* **111,** 1112.

BLAZKOVEC A.A. & WOLFE H.R. (1965) Factors affecting the primary and secondary responses to bovine serum albumin in chickens. *Int. Arch. Allergy* **26,** 80.

BRAMBELL F.W.R. (1958) The passive immunity of the young mammal. *Biol. Rev.* **33,** 488.

BRANDLY C.A., MOSES H.E. & JUNGHERR E.L. (1946) Transmission of antiviral activity via the egg and the role of congenital passive immunity to Newcastle Disease in chickens. *Poultry Sci.* **25,** 3971.

BRODKORB P. (1971) Origin and evolution of birds, vol. 1, p. 19. In *Avian Biology*, ed. Farner D.S. & King J.R. Academic Press, New York and London.

BRUMFIELD H.P. & POMEROY B.S. (1959) Test based on normal serum component implementing fixation of complement by turkey antiserum. *Proc. Soc. Exp. Biol. Med.* **102,** 278.

BUSHNELL L.D. & HUDSON C.B. (1927) Complement fixation and agglutination tests for *Salmonella pullorum* infection. *J. Infect. Dis.* **41,** 388.

BUXTON A. (1952) On the transference of bacterial antibodies from the hen to the chick. *J. Gen. Microbiol.* **7,** 268.

CARLSON H.C. & HACKING M.A. (1972) Distribution of mast cells in chicken, turkey, pheasant, and quail, and their differentiation from basophils. *Avian Diseases* **16,** 574.

CELADA F. & RAMOS A. (1961) Passive cutaneous anaphylaxis in mice and chickens. *Proc. Soc. Exp. Biol. Med.* **108,** 129.

CLEM L.W. (1971) Phylogeny of immunoglobulin structure and function. IV. Immunoglobulins of the giant grouper, *Epinephelus itaira. J. Biol. Chem.* **246,** 9.

COHEN S. & GORDON S. (1965) Dissociation of κ- and λ-chains from reduced human immunoglobulins. *Biochem. J.* **97,** 460.

CONWAY A.M., VAN ALTEN P.J. & HIRATA A.A. (1968) Passive cutaneous anaphylactic-like reactions in young chicks. *Proc. Soc. Exp. Biol. Med.* **129,** 694.

DAVID C.S. (1972) Characterization of chicken b-locus (IgG) allotypes. *Genetics* **71,** 649.

DAVID C.S., KAEBERLE M.L. & NORDSKOG A.W. (1969) Genetic control of immunoglobulin allotypes in the fowl. *Biochem. Gen.* **3,** 197.

DREESMAN G.R. (1966) Chicken antibodies: Classes of immunoglobulins and enzymatic and reductive dissociation of IgG. Ph.D. Thesis, University of Hawaii, Honolulu.

DREESMAN G.R. & BENEDICT A.A. (1965a) Reductive dissociation of chicken γG-immunoglobulin in neutral solvents without a dispersing agent. *Proc. Nat. Acad. Sci. U.S.A.* **54,** 822.

DREESMAN G.R. & BENEDICT A.A. (1965b) Properties of papain-digested chicken 7S γ-globulin. *J. Immunol.* **95,** 855.

DREESMAN G.R., BENEDICT A.A. & MOORE R.W. (1967) Characteristics of direct and indirect complement-fixing antibodies obtained from turkeys infected with ornithosis agent. *J. Immunol.* **98,** 1167.

DREESMAN G.R., LARSON C., PINCKARD R.N., GROYON R.M. & BENEDICT A.A. (1965) Antibody activity in different chicken globulins. *Proc. Soc. Exp. Biol. Med.* **118,** 292.

EDELMAN G.M., CUNNINGHAM B.A., GALL W.E., GOTTLIEB P.D., RUTISHAUSER U. & WAXDAL M.J. (1969) The covalent structure of an entire γG immunoglobulin molecule. *Proc. Nat. Acad. Sci. U.S.A.* **63,** 78.

ELFENBEIN G.J., GREEN I. & PAUL W.E. (1973) The allogeneic effect: Increased affinity of serum antibody produced during a secondary response. *Eur. J. Immunol.* **3,** 640.

ETTINGER A.C. & HIRATA A.A. (1971) PCA reactions in adult specific pathogen-free chickens. *J. Immunol.* **107,** 278.

ETTINGER A.C. & HIRATA A.A. (1973) Effect of blood replacement on passive cutaneous anaphylactic reaction in chickens. *Proc. Soc. Exp. Biol. Med.* **144,** 229.

ETTINGER A.C., HIRATA A.A. & VAN ALTEN P.J. (1970) Differential susceptibilities of young and adult chickens to passive cutaneous anaphylactic reaction. *Immunology* **19,** 257.

EWING J. & STRAUS I. (1903) Precipitins and their medico-legal use. *Med. News* **83,** 871.

FAITH R.E. & CLEM L.W. (1973) Passive cutaneous anaphylaxis in the chicken: Biological fractionation of the mediating antibody population. *Immunology*, **25,** 151.

FARR R.S. (1958) A quantitative immunochemical measure of the primary interaction between I*BSA and antibody. *J. Infec. Dis.* **103,** 239.

FARR R.S. & MINDEN P. (1970) Antigen-antibody reactions, p. 332, In *Biology of the Immune Response*, ed. Abramoff P. & LaVia M.F. McGraw-Hill.

FEINSTEIN A. & MUNN E.A. (1969) Conformation of the free and antigen bound IgM antibody molecules. *Nature* **224,** 1307.

FELDBUSH T.L. & GOWANS J.L. (1971) Antigen modulation of the immune response. *J. Exp. Med.* **134,** 1453.

FISCHEL E.E. & KABAT E.A. (1947) A quantitative study of the Arthus phenomenon induced passively in the rabbit. *J. Immunol.* **55,** 337.

FRENCH V.I., STARK J.M. & WHITE R.G. (1970) The influence of adjuvants on the immunological response of the chicken. II. Effects of Freund's complete adjuvant on later antibody production after a single injection of immunogen. *Immunology* **18,** 645.

FROMMEL D., LITMAN G.W., CHARTRAND S.L., SEAL U.S. & GOOD R.A. (1971) Carbohydrate composition in the evolution of the immunoglobulins. *Immunochemistry* **8,** 573.

GAHRINGER J.E. (1926) Sensitization of pigeons to foreign protein. *J. Immunol.* **12,** 477.

GALLAGHER J.S. & VOSS E.W. JR (1969) Binding properties of purified chicken antibody. *Immunochemistry* **6,** 573.

GALLAGHER J.S. & VOSS E.W. JR (1970) Immune precipitation of purified chicken antibody at low pH. *Immunochemistry* **7,** 771.

GENGOZIAN N. & WOLFE H.R. (1957) Precipitin production in chickens. XV. The effect of aging of the antisera on precipitate formation. *J. Immunol.* **78,** 401.

GERSHON R.K. & PAUL W.E. (1971) Effect of thymus-derived lymphocytes on amount and affinity of anti-hapten antibody. *J. Immunol.* **106,** 872.

GITLIN D., KUMATE J., URRUSTI J. & MORALES C. (1964) Selection and directional transfer of $7S\gamma_2$-globulin across the human placenta. *Nature (Lond.)* **203,** 86.

GOLD E.F. & BENEDICT A.A. (1962) Formation of antibody to haptens. I. Primary and and secondary responses to *p*-amino benzoic acid and bovine γ-globulin in chickens rabbits. *J. Immunol.* **89,** 234.

GOLD E.F., CORDES S., LOPEZ M.A., KNIGHT K.L. & HAUROWITZ F. (1966) Studies on chicken γ-globulins and hapten-specific chicken antibodies. *Immunochemistry* **3,** 433.

GOODMAN M. & WOLFE H.R. (1952) Precipitin production in chickens. VIII. A comparison of the effect of salt concentration on precipitate formation of pheasant, owl, and chicken antisera. *J. Immunol.* **69,** 423.

GOODMAN M., WOLFE H.R. & NORTON S.R (1951) Precipitin production in chickens. VI. The effect of varying concentrations of NaCl on precipitate formation. *J. Immunol.* **66,** 225.

GRANT J.A., SANDERS B. & HOOD L. (1971) Partial amino acid sequences of chicken and turkey immunoglobulin light chains. Homology with mammalian λ chains. *Biochemistry* **10,** 3123.

GREENBURY C.L., MOORE D.H. & NUNN L.A.C. (1963) Reaction of 7S and 19S components of immune rabbit antisera with human group A and AB red cells. *Immunology* **6,** 421.

GREY H.M. (1963) Production of mercaptoethanol sensitive, slowly sedimenting antibody in the duck. *Proc. Soc. Exp. Biol. Med.* **113,** 963.

GREY H.M. (1967a) Duck immunoglobulins. I. Structural studies on a 5·7S and 7·8S γ-globulin. *J. Immunol.* **98,** 811.

GREY H.M. (1967b) Duck immunoglobulins. II. Biologic and immunochemical studies. *J. Immunol.* **98,** 820.

GUTTMAN R.M., TEBO T., EDWARDS J., BARBORIAK J.J. & FINK J.N. (1971) The immune response of the pigeon (*Columbia livia*). *J. Immunol.* **106,** 392.

HEKTOEN L. (1918) The production of precipitins by the fowl. *J. Infect. Dis.* **22,** 561.

HELLER K.S. & SISKIND G.W. (1973) Effect of tolerance and of antibody mediated immune suppression on the avidity of the cellular and humoral immune response. *Cellular Immunology* **6,** 59.

HERSH R.T. & BENEDICT A.A. (1966) Aggregation of chicken γG immunoglobulin in 1·5 M sodium chloride solution. *Biochim. Biophys. Acta* **115,** 242.

HERSH R.T., KUBO R.T., LESLIE G.A. & BENEDICT A.A. (1969) Molecular weights of chicken, pheasant and quail IgG immunoglobulins. *Immunochemistry* **6,** 762.

HEUSCHELE W.P. & EASTERDAY B.C. (1970a) Local immunity and persistence of virus in the tracheas of chickens following infection with Newcastle Disease Virus. I. Organ culture studies. *J. Infect. Dis.* **121,** 486.

HEUSCHELE W.P. & EASTERDAY B.C. (1970b) Local immunity and persistence of virus in the tracheas of chickens following infection with Newcastle Disease Virus. II. Immunofluorescent and histopathologic studies. *J. Infect. Dis.* **121,** 497.

HITCHNER S.B. & JOHNSON E.P. (1948) A virus of low virulence for immunizing fowls against Newcastle disease (*avian pneumoencephalitis*). *Vet. Med.* **43,** 525.

HOOD L., GRANT J.A. & SOX H.C. JR (1970) On the structure of normal light chains from mammals and birds: Evolutionary and genetic implications, vol. 1, p. 283. In *Developmental Aspects of Antibody Formation and Structure*, ed. Sterzl J. & Riha I. Academia Publishing House, Czechoslovak Academy of Sciences, Prague.

HOOD L., GRAY W.R., SANDERS B.G. & DREYER W.J. (1967) Light chain evolution. *Cold Spring Harbor Symp. Quant. Biol.* **32,** 133.

HORNICK C.L. & KARUSH F. (1969). *Topics in Basic Immunology*, p. 29, ed. Sela M. & Prynes M. Academic Press, New York and London.

HOWELL H.M., CONRAD H.E. & VOSS E.W. JR (1973) Hexose and hexosamine content of purified chicken anti-2,4-dinitrophenyl antibody by radiochromatographic analysis. *Immunochemistry* **10,** 761.

IVANYI J., VALENTOVA V. & CERNY J. (1966) The dose of antigen required for the suppression of the IgM and IgG antibody response in chickens. I. The kinetics and characterization of serum antibodies. *Folia Biol. (Praha)* **12,** 157.

JANKOVAK B.D. & MITROVIC K. (1967) Antibody-producing cells in the chicken as observed by fluorescent antibody technique. *Folia Biol. (Praha)* **13,** 406.

JUKES T.H., FRASER D.T. & ORR M.D. (1934) The transmission of diphtheria antitoxin from hen to egg. *J. Immunol.* **26,** 353.

KABAT E.A. & MAYER M.M. (1961) *Experimental Immunochemistry.* 2nd ed., Chas. C. Thomas, Springfield, Illinois.

KARRER H., MEYER K.F. & EDDIE B. (1950) The complement fixation inhibition test and its application to the diagnosis of ornithosis in chickens and in ducks. I. Principles and techniques of the test. *J. Infect. Dis.* **87,** 13.

KEHOE J.M. & CAPRA J.D. (1972) Sequence relationships among the variable regions of immunoglobulin heavy chains from various mammalian species. *Proc. Nat. Acad. Sci. U.S.A.* **69,** 2052.

KOBAYASHI K., VAERMAN J., BAZIN H., LEBACQ-VERHEYDEN A. & HEREMANS J.F. (1973) Identification of J-chain in polymeric immunoglobulins from a variety of species by cross-reaction with rabbit antisera to human J-chain. *J. Immunol.* **111,** 1590.

KUBO R.T. (1967) Chicken antibodies: Precipitin reaction of the bovine serum albumin chicken anti-bovine serum albumin system. M.S. Thesis, University of Hawaii, Honolulu.

KUBO R.T. (1970) Structural studies on chicken IgG immunoglobulin. Ph.D. Thesis, University of Hawaii, Honolulu.

KUBO R.T. & BENEDICT A.A. (1968) Passive cutaneous anaphylaxis in chickens. *Proc. Soc. Exp. Biol. Med.* **129,** 256.

KUBO R.T. & BENEDICT A.A. (1969a) Unusual conditions for crystallization of the Fc fragment of chicken IgG. *J. Immunol.* **102,** 1523.

KUBO R.T. & BENEDICT A.A. (1969b) Comparison of various avian and mammalian IgG Immunoglobulins for salt-induced aggregation. *J. Immunol.* **103,** 1022.

KUBO R.T., ROSENBLUM I.Y. & BENEDICT A.A. (1970) The unblocked N-terminal sequence of chicken IgG γ-like light chains. *J. Immunol.* **105,** 534.

KUBO R.T., ROSENBLUM I.Y. & BENEDICT A.A. (1971) Amino Terminal sequences of heavy and light chains of chicken anti-dinitrophenyl antibody. *J. Immunol.* **107,** 1781.

KUBO R.T., ZIMMERMAN B. & GREY H.M. (1973) Phylogeny of immunoglobulins, vol. 1, p. 417. In *The Antigens*, ed. Sela M. Academic Press, New York and London.

LEBACQ-VERHEYDEN A.M., VAERMAN J.-P. & HEREMANS J.F. (1972a) A possible homologue of mammalian IgA in chicken serum and secretions. *Immunology* **22,** 165.

LEBACQ-VERHEYDEN A.M., VAERMAN J.-P. & HEREMANS J.F. (1972b) Immunohistologic distribution of the chicken immunoglobulin. *J. Immunol.* **109,** 652.

LESLIE G.A. & BENEDICT A.A. (1969) Structural and antigenic relationships between avian immunoglobulins. I. The immune responses of pheasants and quail and reductive dissociation of their immunoglobulins. *J. Immunol.* **103,** 1356.

LESLIE G.A. & BENEDICT A.A. (1970a) Structural and antigenic relationships between avian immunoglobulins. II. Properties of papain- and pepsin-digested chicken, pheasant and quail IgG-immunoglobulins. *J. Immunol.* **104,** 810.

LESLIE G.A. & BENEDICT A.A. (1970b) Structural and antigenic relationships between avian immunoglobulins. III. Antigenic relationships of the immunoglobulins of the chicken, pheasant, and Japanese quail. *J. Immunol.* **105,** 1215.

LESLIE G.A. & CLEM L.W. (1969a) Phylogeny of immunoglobulin structure and function. III. Immunoglobulins of the chicken. *J. Exp. Med.* **130,** 1337.

LESLIE G.A. & CLEM L.W. (1969b) Production of anti-hapten antibodies by several classes of lower vertebrates. *J. Immunol.* **103,** 613.

LESLIE G.A. & CLEM L.W. (1970) Chicken immunoglobulins: Biological half-lives and normal adult serum concentrations of IgM and IgY. *Proc. Soc. Exp. Biol. Med.* **134,** 195.

LESLIE G.A. & MARTIN L.N. (1973) Studies on the secretory immunologic system of fowl. III. Serum and secretory IgA of the chicken. *J. Immunol.* **110,** 1.

LESLIE G.A., WILSON H.R. & CLEM L.W. (1971) Studies on the secretory immunologic system of fowl. I. Presence of immunoglobulins in chicken secretions. *J. Immunol.* **106,** 1441.

LINDQVIST K. & BAUER D.C. (1966) Precipitin activity of rabbit macroglobulin antibody. *Immunochemistry* **3,** 373.

LITTLE J.R. & EISEN H.N. (1967) Evidence for tryptophan in the active sites of antibodies to polynitrobenzenes. *Biochemistry* **6,** 3119.

LUOMA B. (1974) Arthus reactions in chickens. M.S. Thesis, University of Hawaii, Honolulu.

LUOMA B. & BENEDICT A.A. (1974) Arthus reactions in chickens. *Immunology* (submitted for publication).

MAKINODAN T., GENGOZIAN N. & CANNING R.E. (1960) Demonstration of a normal serum macroglobulin coprecipitating with the bovine serum albumin (BSA)—chicken anti-BSA precipitate. *J. Immunol.* **85,** 439.

MALKINSON M. (1965) The transmission of passive immunity to *Escherichia coli* from mother to young in the domestic fowl. *Immunology* **9,** 311.

MARCHALONIS J.J. (1969) Isolation and characterization of immunoglobulin-like proteins of the Australian lungfish (*Neoceratodus forsteri*). *Austral. J. Exp. Biol. Med. Sci.* **47,** 405.

MCDERMID E.M., PETROVSKY E. & YAMAZAKI H. (1969) Iso-antigens of serum proteins of the chicken. *Immunology* **17,** 413.

MEDLIN J., FEIGLOVA E. & NOUZA K. (1973) The development of the immune response to type III pneumococcal polysaccharide in chickens. *Folia Biol.* (*Praha*) **19,** 107.

MEHTA P.D., REICHLIN M. & TOMASI T.B. JR (1972) Comparative studies of vertebrate immunoglobulins. *J. Immunol.* **109,** 1272.

MICHAELIDES M.C., SHERMAN R. & HELMREICH E. (1964) The interaction of muscle phosphorylase with soluble antibody fragments. *J. Biol. Chem.* **239,** 4171.

MOORE R.W., WATKINS J.R. & DIXON J.R. (1959) Experimental ornithosis in herons and egrets. *Amer. J. Vet. Res.* **20,** 884.

MUELLER A.P. & WOLFE H.R. (1961) Precipitin production following massive injection of BSA in adult chickens. *Int. Arch. Allergy* **19,** 321.

NICHOL L.W., BETHUNE J.L., KEGELES G. & HESS E.L. (1964). *The Proteins*, vol. 2, p. 305, ed. Neurath H. Academic Press, New York and London.

ORIOL R., ROCHAS S., BARBIER Y., MOUTON D., STIFFEL C. & BIOZZI G. (1972) Studies on the immune response of the Numigall, a hybrid of domestic cock and guinea hen. *Eur. J. Immunol.* **2,** 308.

ORLANS E. (1967) Fowl antibody. VIII. A comparison of natural, primary and secondary antibodies to erythrocytes in hen sera; their transmission to yolk and chick. *Immunology* **12,** 27.

ORLANS E., RICHARDS C.B. & ROSE M.E. (1964) The composition of soluble complexes formed in antigen excess by fowl antibody to bovine γ-globulin. *Immunochemistry* **1,** 317.

ORLANS E. & ROSE M.E. (1972) An IgA-like immunoglobulin in the fowl. *Immunochemistry* **9,** 833.

ORLANS E., ROSE M.E. & MARRACK J.R. (1961) Fowl antibody. I. Some physical and immunochemical properties. *Immunology* **4,** 262.

ORLANS E., SAUNDERS B.J. & ROSE M.E. (1968) Fowl antibody. IX. The different responses to the hapten and carrier moieties of 2,4-dinitrophenyl-bovine γ-globulin. *Immunology* **14,** 53.

OVARY Z. (1960) Reverse passive cutaneous anaphylaxis in the guinea pig with horse, sheep and hen antibodies. *Immunology* **3,** 19.

OVARY Z. & BIER O.G. (1952) Quantitative study of Arthus reaction and of cutaneous anaphylaxis induced passively in the rat. *Proc. Soc. Exp. Biol. Med.* **81,** 584.

PALMER J.L. & NISONOFF A. (1964) Dissociation of rabbit γ-globulin into half molecules after reduction of one labile disulfide bond. *Biochemistry* **3,** 863.

PATTERSON L.T. & MORA E.C. (1964) Occurrence of a substance analogous to C-reactive protein in the blood of the domestic fowl. *Texas Reports Biol. Med.* **22,** 716.

PATTERSON R., SUSZKO I.M. & PRUZANSKY J.J. (1965) Some antigenic characterization and immunologic reactions of horse spleen ferritin. *Proc. Soc. Exp. Biol. Med.* **118,** 307.

PATTERSON R., YOUNGNER J.S., WEIGLE W.O. & DIXON F.J. (1962) Antibody production and transfer to egg yolk in chickens. *J. Immunol.* **89,** 272.

PAUL W.E., SISKIND G.W., BENACERRAF B. & OVARY Z. (1967) Secondary responses in haptenic systems: Cell population selection by antigen. *J. Immunol.* **99,** 760.

PIRAINO F.F. (1966) The occurrence of psittacosis virus complement-fixing (CF) non-complement-fixing (NCF) and neutralizing (N) antibodies in domestic pigeons. *J. Immunol.* **95,** 1107.

POLLARD M. (1947) Ornithosis in sea-shore birds. *Proc. Soc. Exp. Biol. Med.* **64,** 200.

POLLARD M., CAPLOVITZ C.D. & SWAUSCH C.D. (1947) The identification of an ornithosis virus from the willet. *Texas Reports Biol. Med.* **5,** 337.

PORTER R.R. (1962) The structure of gamma-globulin and antibodies, p. 177. In *Symposium on Basic Problems in Neoplastic Disease*, ed. Gelhorn A. & Hirschberg E. Columbia Univ. Press, New York.

PRESSMAN D., ROHOLT O.A. & GROSSBERG A.L. (1970) Chemical and structural differences between antibodies capable of binding a particular hapten group: Evidence for limited heterogeneity. *Ann. N.Y. Acad. Sci.* **169,** 65.

PUTNAM F.W., PAUL G.F.D., SHINODA T. & SHIMIZU A. (1973) Complete amino acid sequence of the mu heavy chain of a human IgM immunoglobulin. *Science* **182,** 287.

RICE C.E. (1947) A typical behavior of certain avian antisera for complement-fixation tests. *Canad. J. Comp. Med.* **11,** 236.

RICE C.E. (1948) Inhibitory effects of certain avian and mammalian antisera in specific complement-fixation systems. *J. Immunol.* **59,** 365.

RICE C.E. (1961) The use of complement-fixation tests in the study and diagnosis of viral diseases in man and animals—a review. *Canad. J. of Comp. Med.* **25,** 74.

RIHA I. (1965) The formation of specific 7S and macroglobulin type antibodies in chickens, p. 253. In *Molecular and Cellular Basis of Antibody Formation*, ed. Sterzl J. Academia Publishing House, Czechoslovak Academy of Sciences, Prague.

ROHOLT O.A. & PRESSMAN D. (1968) Structural differences between antibodies produced against the same hapten by individual rabbits. *Immunochemistry* **5,** 265.

ROSE M.E. & ORLANS E. (1962) Fowl antibody. IV. The estimation of haemolytic fowl complement. *Immunology* **5,** 642.

ROSENQUIST G.L. & GILDEN R.V. (1963) Chicken antibodies to bovine serum albumin. Molecular size and sensitivity to 2-mercaptoethanol. *Biochim. Biophys. Acta* **78,** 543.

SCHIERMAN L.W. & MCBRIDE R.A. (1968) Segregation of genes controlling allotypes in two inbred lines of fowl. *Genetics* (abstract) **60,** 222.

SIBLEY C.G. & AHLQUIST J.E. (1972) A comparative study of the egg white proteins on non-passerine birds. *Peabody Museum of Natural History, Yale Univ., Bulletin* **39,** 44.

SIMONS M.J. & BENEDICT A.A. (1974) Radioelectrocomplexing: A general radioimmunoassay procedure for the detection of primary binding of antigen and antibody. In *Contemporary Topics in Molecular Immunology*, Vol. 3, p. 205, Plenum Press.

SISKIND G.W. & BENACERRAF B. (1969) Cell selection by antigen in the immune response. *Adv. Immunol.* **10,** 1.

SKALBA D. (1964) Allotypes of hen serum proteins. *Nature* **204,** 894.

SKALBA D. (1966) Allotypic specificity in gamma- and beta-globulins of hen serum. *Bulletin De L'academie Polonaise Ses Sciences* **XIV,** 159.

SKAMENE E. & IVANYI J. (1969) Common antigenic specificity on the H-chains of chicken IgM and IgG. *Immunochemistry* **6,** 733.

STANTON T., SLEDGE C., CAPRA J.D., WOODS R., CLEM W. & HOOD L. (1974) A sequence restriction in the variable region of immunoglobulin light chains from sharks, birds, and mammals. *J. Immunol.* **112,** 633.

STEINBERG S.V., MUNRO J.A., FLEMING W.A., FRENCH V.I., STARK J.M. & WHITE R.G. (1970) The influence of adjuvants on the immunological response of the chicken. I. Effects on primary and secondary responses of various adjuvants in the primary stimulus. *Immunology* **18,** 635.

STEINER L.A. & EISEN H.N. (1967) The relative affinity of antibodies synthesized in the secondary response. *J. Exp. Med.* **126,** 1185.

STOLFI R.L., FUGMANN R.A., JENSEN J.J. & SIGEL M.M. (1971) A C1-fixation method for the measurement of chicken anti-viral antibody. *Immunology* **20,** 299.

TAM L.Q. & BENEDICT A.A. (1975) Elevated 7S immunoglobulin and acute phase proteins in adjuvant-injected chickens. *Proc. Soc. Exp. Biol. Med.* **150,** 340.

TENENHOUSE H.S. & DEUTSCH H.F. (1966) Some physical-chemical properties of chicken γ-globulins and their pepsin and papain digestion products. *Immunochemistry* **3,** 11.

THEIS G.A. & SISKIND G.W. (1968) Selection of cell populations in induction of tolerance: Affinity of antibody formed in partially tolerant rabbits. *J. Immunol.* **100,** 138.

TILLET W.S. & FRANCIS T. JR (1930) Serological reaction in pneumonia with a nonprotein fraction of pneumococcus. *J. Exp. Med.* **52,** 561.

TRAVIS J.C. & SANDERS B.G. (1973) Structural comparisons between chicken low molecular weight immunoglobulin heavy chains and human γ chains. *Biochem. Gen.* **8,** 391.

UNANUE E.R. & DIXON F.J. (1965) Experimental glomerulonephritis. V. Studies on the interaction of nephrotoxic antibodies with tissues of the rat. *J. Exp. Med.* **121,** 697.

VAERMAN J.-P. & HEREMANS J.F. (1968) The immunoglobulins of the dog. I. Identification of canine immunoglobulins homologous to human IgA and IgM. *Immunochemistry* **5,** 425.

VALENTOVA V., CERNY J. & IVANYI J. (1966) The characterization of the immunological memory of the IgM type of response in chickens. *Folia Biol. (Praha)* **12,** 207.

VALENTOVA V., CERNY J. & IVANYI J. (1967) Immunological memory of IgM and IgG type antibodies. I. Requirements of antigen dose for induction and of time interval for development of memory. *Folia Biol. (Praha)* **13,** 100.

VAN ORDEN D.E. & TREFFERS H.P. (1968) The effect of salt-induced aggregation on the gel filtration of chicken 7S antibodies. *J. Immunol.* **100,** 659.

VOSS E.W., JR & EISEN H.N. (1972) Anti-hapten chicken antibodies of the 7S class. *J. Immunol.* **109,** 944.

WANG A.C., FUDENBERG H.H. & PINK J.R.C. (1971) Heavy chain variable regions in normal and pathological immunoglobulins. *Proc. Nat. Acad. Sci. U.S.A.* **68,** 1143.

WARD P.A. & COCHRANE C.G. (1965) Bound complement and immunologic injury of blood vessels. *J. Exp. Med.* **121,** 215.

WEINHEIMER P.F., MESTECKY J. & ACTON R.T. (1971) Species distribution of J chain. *J. Immunol.* **107,** 1211.

WERBLIN T.R. & SISKIND G.W. (1972a) Effect of tolerance and immunity on antibody affinity. *Transplant. Rev.* **8,** 104.

WERBLIN T.R. & SISKIND G.W. (1972b) Distribution of antibody affinities: Techniques of measurement. *Immunochemistry* **9,** 987.

WERBLIN T.R., KIM Y.T., QUAGLIATA F. & SISKIND G.W. (1973) Studies on the control of antibody synthesis. III. Changes in heterogeneity of antibody affinity during the course of the immune response. *Immunology* **24,** 477.

WHITE R.G. (1970) Adjuvant stimulation of antibody synthesis, p. 91. In *Immunopathology 6th International Symposium*, ed. Miescher P.A. Grune & Stratton, New York and London.

WILKINSON P.C. & FRENCH V.I. (1969) Antigenic heterogeneity of chicken 7S immunoglobulin. *Immunochemistry* **6,** 498.

WILLIAMSON A.R. & ASKONAS B.A. (1968) Differential reduction of interchain disulfide bonds of mouse immunoglobulin G. *Biochem. J.* **107,** 823.

WOLFE H.R. (1942) Precipitin production in chickens. I. Interfacial titers as affected by quantity of antigen injected and aging of antisera. *J. Immunol.* **44,** 135.

WOLFE H.R. & DILKS E. (1946) Precipitin production in chickens. II. Studies of the *in vitro* rise of the interfacial titers and the formation of precipitins. *J. Immunol.* **52,** 331.

WOLFE H.R. & DILKS E. (1948) Precipitin production in chickens. III. The variation in the antibody response as correlated with the age of the animal. *J. Immunol.* **58,** 245.

WOLFE H.R. & DILKS E. (1949) Precipitin production in chickens. IV. A comparison of the antibody response of eight avian species. *J. Immunol.* **61,** 251.

WOSTMANN B.S. & OLSON G.B. (1969) Persistence of primary antibody formation caused by the absence of antigen of microbial origin in the germ-free chicken. *Immunology* **17,** 199.

YAMAGA K. & BENEDICT, A.A. (1975) Class, amounts and affinities of anti-dinitrophenyl antibodies in chickens. I. Production of 7S and 17S antibodies of equal affinity by intravenous injection of antigen. *J. Immunol.* **115,** 750.

ZIMMERMAN B., SHALATIN N. & GREY H.M. (1971) Structural studies on the duck 5·7S and 7·8S immunoglobulins. *Biochemistry* **10,** 482.

Addendum to Chapter 13

Notable advances have been made in avian immunogenetics during the past two years—particularly in those areas dealing with (1) the role of the major histocompatibility complex (MHC) in the control of immunologic reactions, and (2) allotypes. In addition to the control of transplantation antigens, the mammalian MHC has been viewed as a source of genes for the control of immune responsiveness, the synthesis of molecules involved in antigen recognition, lymphocyte interactions, and serum complement levels. With the MHC of man (HL-A) and of the mouse (H-2) serving as guides, it is most appropriate that the chicken MHC is also under closer scrutiny. The *B* blood group locus in the chicken [Briles, W.E., McGibbon, W.H. & Irwin, M.R. (1950) On multiple alleles affecting cellular antigen in the chicken. *Genetics*, **35,** 633] represents the avian counterpart of the mammalian MHC. It has been associated with allograft rejection [Schierman, L.W. & Nordskog, A.W. 1961) Relationship of blood type to histocompatibility in chickens. *Science* **134,** 1008] and the graft-versus-host reaction [Jaffe,W.P. & McDermid, E.M. (1962) Blood groups and splenomegaly in chicken embryos. *Science*, **137,** 984]. Recently, immune responsiveness to synthetic polypeptide antigens [Günther, E., Balcarová, J., Hála, K., Rüde, E. & Hraba, T. (1974) Evidence for an association between immune responsiveness of chicken to (T,G)-A—L and the major histocompatibility system. *Eur. J. Immunol.* **4,** 538; Benedict, A.A., Pollard, L.W., Morrow, P.R., Abplanalp, H.A. Maurer, P.H. & Briles, W.E. (1975) Genetic control of immune responses in chickens. I. Responses to a terpolymer of poly($glu^{60}ala^{30}tyr^{10}$) associated with the major histocompatibility complex. *Immunogenetics* **2,** 313] and to tuberculin [Karakoz, J., Krejčí, J., Hála, K., Blaszcyk, B., Hraba, T. and Pekárek, J. (1974) Genetic determination of tuberculin hypersensitivity in chicken inbred lines. *Eur. J. Immunol.* **4,** 545] were shown to be controlled by genes associated with the *B* locus. The MHC-linked Ir gene(s) controlling the response to poly($glu^{60}ala^{30}tyr^{10}$) involves recognition of the response to the carrier moiety [Benedict, A.A. & Pollard, L.W. (1975) Genetic control of immune responses in chickens. *In* Immunologic phylogeny, *Adv. in Exp. Med. & Biol.*, **64,** 421, W.H. Hildemann and A.A. Benedict, editors, Plenum Press, N.Y. and London]. In addition, the mixed leukocyte reaction [Miggiano, V., Birgen, I. & Pink, J.R.L. (1974) The mixed leukocyte reaction in chickens. Evidence for control by the major histocompatibility complex. *Eur. J. Immunol.* **4,** 397] and serum hemolytic complement levels [Chanh, T.C., Benedict, A.A. & Abplanalp, H.A. (1976) Association of serum hemolytic complement levels with the major histocompatibility complex in chickens, submitted to *J. Exp. Med.*] are controlled by genes associated with the *B* locus. Finding these MHC associations in a non-mammal strengthens the importance of the relationship between closely-linked genes controlling histocompatibility, immune responsiveness and complement activity. It is unlikely that these immunological functions are linked in species as different as chickens, mice and men by chance. As yet, none of these immunologic reactions can be assigned to any particular region within the *B* locus (complex?) as has been done with H-2. It will be important to determine whether there are a number of linked loci, as in H-2, or whether the immunologic functions are controlled by a less-evolved complex. In their review of the chicken MHC, Pazderka *et al.* [Pazderka, F. Longenecker, B.M., Law, G.R.J. & Ruth, R.F. (1975) The major histocompatibility complex of the chicken. *Immunogenetics*, **2,** 101] pointed out that the chicken 'is emniently suited' for a species-wide evaluation of the linkage between the MHC-associated functions because of the 'many differently selected populations large and stable enough to permit prolonged and repetitive sampling'. For these reasons the chicken also is suited for revealing the evolutionary genetic mechanisms affecting immunoglobulin structural genes as recent studies on allotypes indicate.

Recently, chicken allotypes were found on 17S Ig [Pink, J.R.L. (1974) An allotypic marker on chicken immunoglobulin M. *Eur. J. Immunol.* **4,** 679], on 7S Ig [Ivanyi, J. (1975) Polymorphism of chicken serum allotypes. *J. Immunogenetics* **2,** 69; Wakeland, E.K. & Benedict, A.A. (1975) Structural and genetic analysis of four chicken 7S immunoglobulin allotypes. *Immunogenetics* **2,** 531], and on a lipoprotein [Ivanyi, J. (1975) Polymorphism of chicken serum allotypes. *J. Immunogenetics* **2,** 69]. Genetic analysis of F_2 progeny of highly inbred chicken lines has demonstrated that both the 17S Ig [Pink, J.R.L. (1974) An allotypic marker on chicken immunoglobulin M. *Eur. J. Immunol.* **4,** 679] and 7S Ig [Wakeland, E.K. & Benedict, A.A. (1975) Structural and genetic analysis of four chicken 7S immunoglobulin allotypes. *Immunogenetics* **2,** 531] allotypes segregate as codominant alleles at autosomal loci. The loci controlling 7S Ig and 17S allotypes are closely linked [Pink, J.R.L. & Ivanyi, J. (1975) Linkage between genes coding for allotypic markers on chicken IgG and IgM. *Eur. J. Immunol.* **6,** 506]. At least two regions of the 7S Ig H chain contain genetic variations. Specificities are found in the Fd region, and in a region sensitive to papain digestion [Wakeland, E.K. & Benedict, A.A. (1975) The genetics of chicken 7S immunoglobulin allotypes. *In* Immunologic phylogeny, *Adv. in Exp. Med. & Biol.*, **64,** 431, W.H. Hildemann and A.A. Benedict, editors, Plenum Press, N.Y. and London], and both specificities are present on 95% of the serum 7S Ig of homozygous birds. These data strongly suggest that the 7S Ig H chain constant region is the product of a single locus and that chicken 7S Ig subclasses are either not present or are extremely low concentrations. Further, these allotypes are distributed among the serum 7S Ig molecules in a manner consistent with allelic exclusion [Wakeland, E.K., unpublished data].

The 7S Ig allotypic specificities probably represent stable, neutral mutations in the structure of the chicken 7S Ig H chains. In support of this, specificities in both the Fd and papain-sensitive regions have been detected in some, but not all, fowl, pheasant, and turkey sera [Foppoli, J. & Wakeland, E.K., Benedict, A.A., unpublished data]. We have made a preliminary survey of production line chickens for 7S Ig allotypes and extensive phenotypic diversity was found. Also, specificities in the Fd region do not appear to form stable, genetic associations with the other H chains specificities. Perhaps the phenotypic diversity reflects extensive genotypic diversity which has been generated by repeated intragenic recombination within the 7S Ig H chain structural genes. Thus, genetic analysis of the distribution within production line chickens of structurally well-defined allotypic specificities, may reveal the nature of some of the evolutionary mechanisms operating on Ig structural genes.

Chapter 14. Immunity in Prototherian and Metatherian Mammals

David T. Rowlands, Jr.

Introduction

Monotremata
Anatomy of the lymphoid system
Immune responses
Immunoglobulins
Summary

Marsupials
Anatomy of lymphoid tissues
Immune responses in marsupials
Immunoglobulins and complement
Cellular immunity
Response to infection
Summary

Introduction

Monotremes and marsupials have attracted relatively little interest in the immunological community despite their critical phylogenetic location being at a transition from poikilothermic vertebrates to eutherian mammals and sharing a common ancestor, *Therapsidae*, with eutherian mammals (Diener *et al.* 1967). It may be that the relatively small numbers of extant species of monotremes and the relative geographical isolation of both *Monotremata* and *Marsupalia*, out of the easy reach of many of the world's immunologists, accounts for this apparent lack of interest.

In the course of this presentation the available information concerning the characterization of lymphoid tissues, immunoglobulins, and immune responses in adult monotremes and marsupials will be summarized. Additional material will be provided in a later chapter concerning the role of the embryos of one species of marsupial (*Didelphis virginiana*) in studies of the ontogeny of immunity.

Monotremata

Anatomy of the lymphoid system

According to Diener (1970) both extant monotremes, the echidna (*Tachyglossus aculeatus*) and the Australian platypus (*Ornithorhynchus paradoxus*), have thymic, lymph node, and splenic lymphocytes. However, only the echidna seems to have received significant attention as an immunologic model (Diener & Ealey 1965, Diener *et al.* 1967, Diener, Ealey & Legge 1967, Diener 1970).

The anatomy and function of the lymph nodules of the echidna have been most extensively studied and display unique characteristics. These nodules lie within lymphatic channels (Fig. 14.1) and are connected to surrounding tissue through blood vessels. Because of their position in lymphatics, the nodules are seen to be unlike lymph nodes of eutherian mammals in that they have no clearly structured peripheral lymphatic sinuses but are, instead, bathed in the lymph of large lymphatic channels. In this way the lymphocytes of the echidna have ample opportunity to encounter foreign materials transported in the animals' lymph. Similarly, the internal structure of these lymphoid nodules is more nearly like the lymph glands of amphibia (Diener & Nossal 1966) than like the complex sinusoid populated lymph nodes of higher vertebrates. As in *Eutheria*, the lymphatic nodules of the echidna are heavily laced with reticulum fibres about which may be found abundant macrophages. Following antigenic stimulation, these phagocytic cells may take on the features of tingible-body macrophages with abundant foreign materials being housed in their cytoplasms. The arrangement of cells in the lymph nodules of the echidna is such that the outer one-third of each nodule is made up of closely packed lymphocytes; contrasting sharply with the more loosely organized, germinal centre-like appearance of the central portions of the nodules (Fig. 14.1). The principal nourishment for the lymphatic nodules of the echidna comes through vascular channels, which can be identified within the closely packed mass of lymphocytes as venules having cuboidal endothelium; a characteristic of the post-capillary venules of eutherian mammals. The central, loosely organized portions of the lymphoid nodules of echidna have no sinusoids and so are unlike the lymph node medulla seen in higher vertebrates. Instead, the central parts of lymphoid nodules in echidna are structurally more like germinal centres in being heavily populated with large poorly defined cells.

Diener and his associates (1967b) have examined the cellular responses in these lymphoid nodules following stimulation of the intact animals with antigens by using both radio-labelled antigens and incorporation of tritiated thymidine into lymphocytes. With these techniques, they were able to show that the centrally located portion of the tissues in the lymphatic nodules of echidna undergo a striking cellular proliferation (Fig. 14.2) within hours after the animals are immunized with the bacteria *Salmonella adelaide*. Of particular interest was the fact that the site of localization of antigens in the lymphatic tissues of the echidna usually differed markedly from the site of lymphoid cellular proliferation in these tissues. Bacterial antigens were typically located within the peripheral parts of the lymphatic nodules soon after injection of echidna with *S. adelaide*.

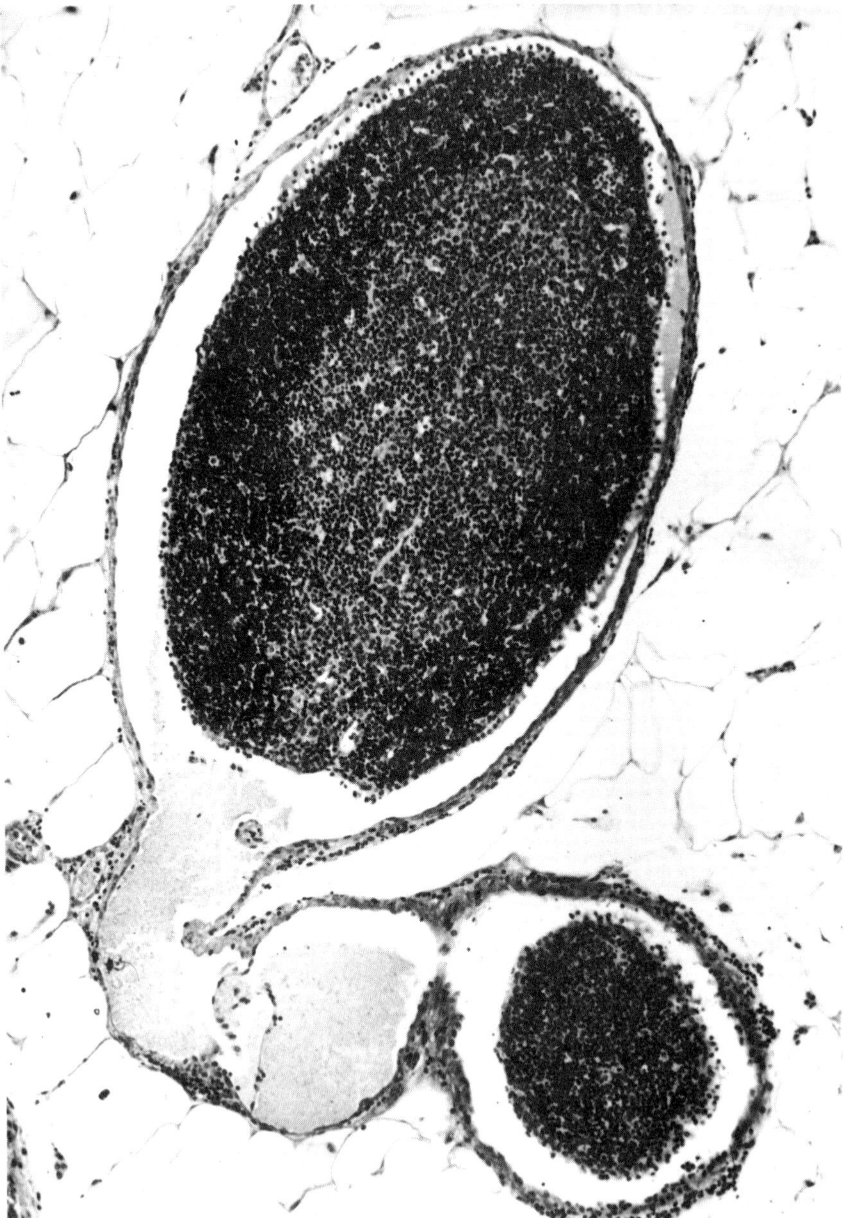

Fig. 14.1. Lymph nodules of echidna: The 'circular sinus' is defined by the nodule and the wall of the lymphatic vessel. The outer portions of nodules are made up of densely packed lymphocytes and their centres consist of more loosely organized cells. Hematoxylin and eosin ×140. Photograph provided by Dr E. Diener.

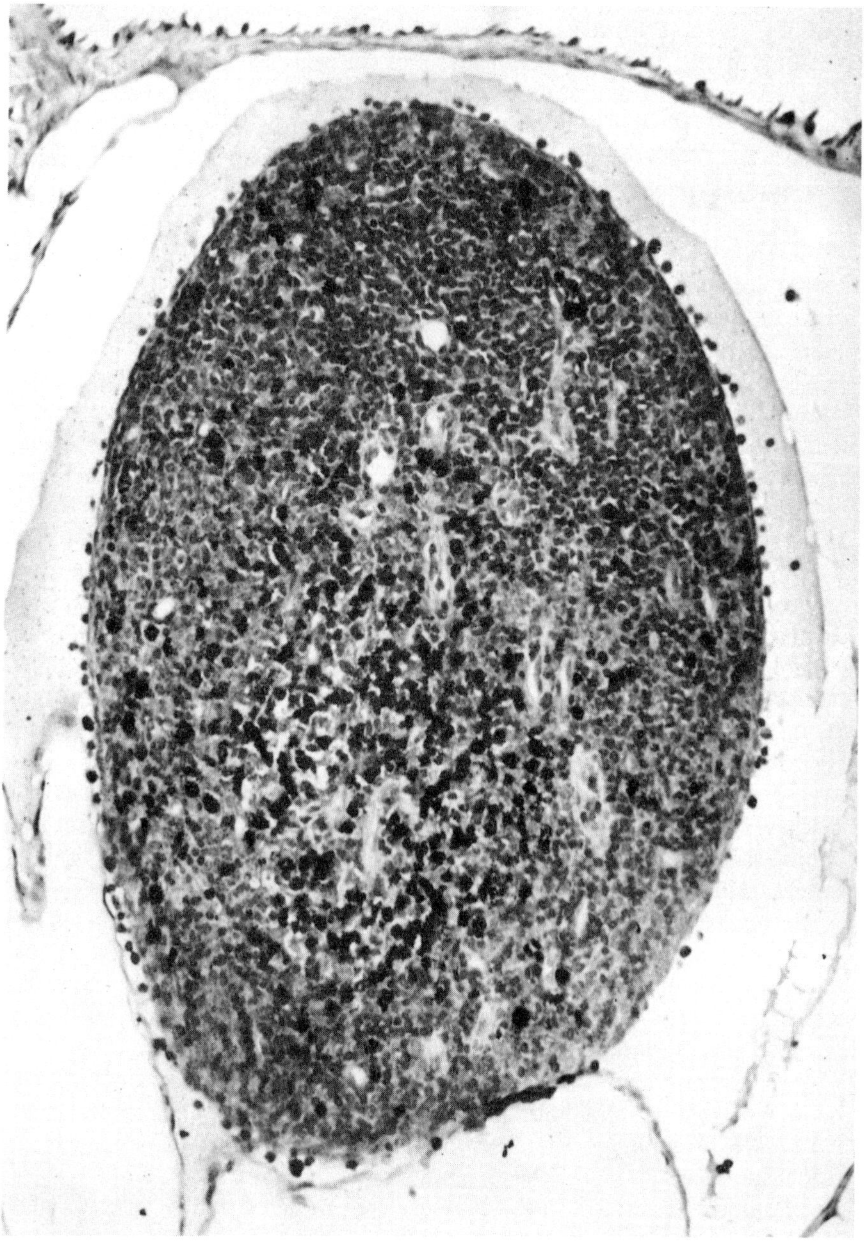

Fig. 14.2. Lymph nodule of the echidna, 3 hours after injection of 3H-thymidine. Autoradiograph exposed for 90 days. Note the single germinal centre as indicated by 3H-thymidine labelled cells ×200. Photograph provided by Dr E. Diener.

Less commonly, and most often in mesenteric lymph nodules, antigens localized to the central parts of the nodules rather than to the peripheral portions of the nodules. Localization of antigens to germinal centre-like areas was quite unlike that observed in similar studies of lymph nodes of rats (Nossal *et al.* 1964). However, the echidna shares, with rats and amphibia (Diener & Nossal 1966), the capacity to trap antigens within those macrophages which appear in close relationship to the reticulum fibre skeleton of the lymphoid structures.

Although Diener and his associates (Diener *et al.* 1967) did not identify a structure equivalent to the bursa of Fabricius, others have felt that such a structure may exist in the echidna. Schofield and Cahill (1969a,b) identified lymphoid elements within the gastrointestinal tract of the echidna. They suggested that the relationship of these lymphoid tissues to the gastrointestinal epithelium make these structures likely candidates as equivalents of the bursa of Fabricius. Proof of this assertion will, of course, require further experimentation.

Immune responses

Studies of the immune response, similarly, seem limited to a few experiments carried out in the echidna. Diener *et al.* (1967a) immunized the echidna by either intravenous or subcutaneous injections of a bacterium, *S. adelaide*. The resulting immune response, as detected by measurement of antibodies (anti-H) in the serum of these animals was characterized by great variability in antibody titres. But, in general, antibody activity was identified during the second post-immunization week. The peak of the immune response was reached slowly in the 5 animals studied; in 3 animals within 7 weeks, but in 2 animals not until 12–13 weeks had elapsed after immunization. The titres of serum antibodies fell after 13 weeks in all 5 animals.

Secondary immune responses can only be demonstrated with difficulty in the echidna as evidenced by the fact that only one of five animals given a second injection of antigen in the footpad displayed serum antibody levels which were significantly higher than those seen in the primary responses. However, the results of secondary immunization were improved when the antigen was given subcutaneously along the route of jugular drainage to the main masses of lymphoid nodules. Three of five animals studied in this manner showed a significant increase in serum antibodies after the second injection of antigen.

Antibodies obtained from echidna were evaluated with respect to their sensitivity to reduction with 2-mercaptoethanol (2-ME) (Diener *et al.* 1967a). Results of these studies were similar to what would be anticipated from similar experiments in higher vertebrates in that 2-ME resistant antibodies were prominent late in the primary responses and throughout the secondary responses in animals immunized in their footpads. Antibodies which were resistant to reduction were present, but less prominent, when the animals were immunized subcutaneously.

Immunoglobulins

Three protein peaks were identified when serum from echidna was passed over Sephadex G-200. As would be true in eutherian mammals, the first peak of echidna serum to come off the column after the void volume contained mostly 2-ME sensitive antibodies; the second peak contained mostly 2-ME resistant antibodies; while the third peak had no detectable antibody activity. Elution of antibodies from DEAE-cellulose ion exchange columns (pH 8·0, 0·05 M) produced single peaks of protein coincident with single peaks of antibody activity. The immunoglobulins harvested in this way had a sedimentation rate of 6·4S. The larger antibody was 17·2S. As one might expect, antiserum prepared in rabbits against these two immunoglobulins could be used to detect two distinct immunoglobulins with immunoelectrophoresis when the antiserum was reacted against whole serum of the adult echidna.

Atwell *et al.* (1973) carried the physical chemical characterization of the immunoglobulins of the echidna through a more detailed analysis, verifying that there are two distinct classes of immunoglobulins in the echidna serum. It was found that each of the immunoglobulins are made up of light and heavy polypeptide chains comparable in molecular size to those found in other vertebrates. The immunoglobulins having the greater molecular weight comprised 6–10 per cent of the total serum immunoglobulins of the echidna and contained 6·4 per cent hexose. These immunoglobulins (IgM) appeared to be pentamers and had molecular weights of $950,000 \pm 57,000$. Their heavy chains (μ) were $69,000 \pm 1700$ and the light chains, which are shared with the echidna IgG, were $22,550 \pm 500$. The IgG immunoglobulin molecules of echidna had molecular weights of $150,000 \pm 9000$ with the λ-chains being $49,000 \pm 1200$. The hexose content of these molecules was 1·5 per cent.

Summary

It can be readily seen that studies of both the immune system and the immune response of prototherians are limited, being essentially restricted to the echidna. The immunoglobulins found in echidna are like those of amphibia and eutherian mammals in being represented by more than one distinct class of immunoglobulin, as determined by the primary structures of their heavy chains. Studies of the immune response of echidna appear to be limited to a relatively small number of animals exposed to a single antigen (*S. adelaide*). However, the response to this antigen is more like that of lower vertebrates than like that of eutherian mammals in having both a relatively long latent period and a very slow rise to peak serum antibody titres. Portions of the antibodies were found to be resistant to 2-ME, and secondary immune responses were evident in only a portion of the animals studied. Echidna seem well equipped with appreciable masses of lymphocytes organized in thymus and spleen, and in curious appearing lymphatic nodules housed in lymphatic channels. These latter masses have been studied extensively and appear to be readily capable of taking up antigen. The lymphoid nodules are structurally primitive, appearing like the jugular nodules of amphibia except that they have germinal centre-like areas placed centrally in each of the lymphatic nodules.

Marsupials

As one might anticipate, since there are many more extant marsupials than monotremes and since marsupials are more generally available throughout several portions of the world, marsupials have received more attention from immunologists than have monotremes. However, despite these advantages our information concerning immunity in marsupials is fragmentary compared to what is available for eutherian mammals.

Anatomy of lymphoid tissues

Among marsupials, the North American opossum (*Didelphis virginiana*) seems to have attracted most immunologic interest; an especially fortuitous state since this species is among the most ancient of marsupials (Young 1962, Walker 1964). Opossums have a complex lymphoid system with thymus, lymph nodes, splenic white pulp and gastrointestinal lymphocytes making up the bulk of the lymphoid tissues in the adult. The thymus appears as a single, sail-shaped mass in the superior mediastinum. Distinct cortical and medullary components can be readily recognized within the thymus. The cortex of the thymus consists of masses of closely packed small and medium lymphocytes and the medulla is made up of a mixture of epithelial cells and scattered lymphocytes.

Although North American opossums seem to have only a single thymus, other marsupials have a second thymus (Yadav & Papadimitrou 1969). These have been designated as deep and superficial thymuses. However, the structures of the deep and superficial thymus glands appear identical to each other.

In other respects representative Australian marsupials are like the North American opossum and eutherian mammals with regard to the structures of their lymphatic tissues (Yadav 1973). Lymph nodes of adult opossums are not unlike those of most eutherian mammals in having distinct cortical and medullary components; with abundant lymphocytes and germinal centres in the cortex and sinusoids and mature plasma cells in the medulla. Lymph nodes are most heavily concentrated in the upper portion of the opossum's body. Similarly, the spleen has aggregates of lymphocytes surrounding intrasplenic vessels and these lymphoid masses also contain germinal centres. The functional relationships of the lymphocytic components within the opossum, both in terms of development (e.g. central versus peripheral lymphoid tissues) and in their relationship to antigen (e.g. uptake of particulate antigens by macrophages in the lymph nodes) seem likely to be as in eutherian mammals. However, as will be noted below, a number of studies have been designed to test the responsiveness of adult opossums to various classes of antigens; experiments which raise interesting questions as to the overall development of immune responsiveness in these animals.

Immune responses in marsupials

The immunologic responsiveness of adult opossums has been extensively evaluated with regard to a variety of antigens. Included among these are bacterial antigens, viral antigens, sheep red blood cells, and soluble antigens (e.g. serum proteins and haemocyanin). When adult opossums were given single injections of bacteriophage (Rowlands 1970) either emulsified in Freund's complete adjuvant or uniformily suspended in saline, there was a latent period, of about 7 days before antibodies could be detected as measured by bacteriophage neutralization using the agar overlay technique (Adams 1959, Rowlands 1967). There then followed a long phase of increase of antibodies within the serum of the opossums. The peak of this response was not reached before 14 days post-immunization and often not until 21 days after immunization. Although the peak levels of serum antibodies reached may be greater with antigens emulsified in adjuvant than in those immunized with antigens in saline, the differences are not very great. When a second immunization with the antigen used for primary immunization was carried out 35 days after the first injection of antigen (Rowlands 1970), the levels of serum antibodies reached were appreciably higher than was evident after primary antigenic stimulation. In addition, unlike what is seen in eutherian mammals treated in a similar fashion, there was an increase of IgM antibodies in the secondary as compared to the primary immune response (Fig. 14.3).

Extensive studies employing a variety of antigens, comparable to what has been used in eutherian mammals, have not been done in opossums. But, in preliminary studies, we have found that opossums can respond to haptens placed on several different protein carriers, to small proteins such as RNAase and lysosyme, as well as to bacterial viruses. We have not been able to demonstrate immune responses of opossums to the hapten dansyl chloride placed on several different protein carriers or to the small protein, sperm whale myoglobin.

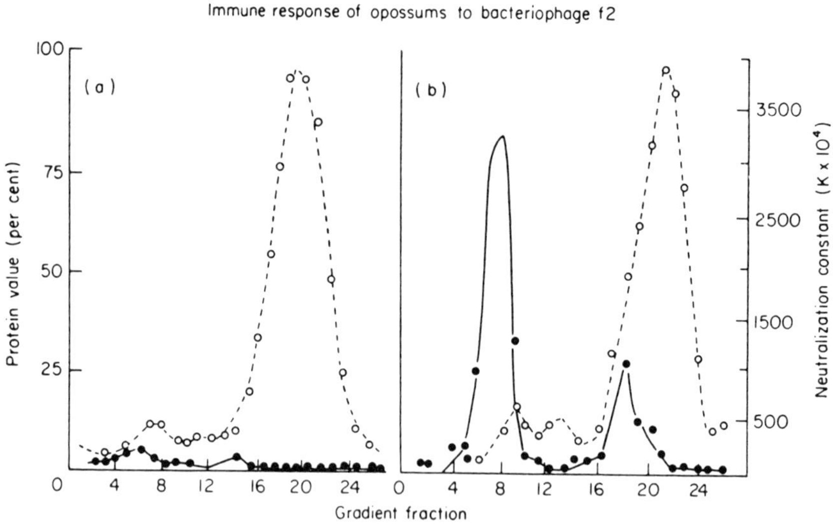

Fig. 14.3. Antibody response in adult opossums as studied by sucrose gradient centrifugation. (a) 7-day primary and (b) 7-day secondary responses. ●——● Antibody activity; ○- - - - -○ protein. There is an increase in both heavy and light antibody activity in the secondary as compared to the primary immune response. (Adapted from Fig. 3 of Rowlands 1970.)

Burrell and his students have carried out additional studies of the immune responses of adult opossums to a variety of antigens (Taylor 1968, Marx *et al.* 1971). They also reached the conclusion that humoral immunity is not so highly developed in opossums as in eutherian mammals. These investigators evaluated the immune responses of opossums to both particulate antigens (*Salmonella typhosa*, *Brucella abortus*, and sheep erythrocytes) and soluble antigens (bovine serum albumin, aggregated bovine serum albumin, alum precipitated diphtheria toxoid, and haemocyanin). Serum antibodies to each of the particulate antigens were recognized by the second week with peaks in serum antibody activity being identified at 3 weeks or later. Antibodies to the soluble antigens were only detectable with the sensitive passive haemagglutination technique. The responses usually did not appear until after the second post-immunization week, were not found in all immunized animals, and often could not be demonstrated after only a single injection of antigen.

Having reached a conclusion similar to ours, that the immune response of the opossum was not so vigorous as that of the rabbit, these investigators (Taylor 1968, Taylor & Burrell 1968, Marx 1970, Marx *et al.* 1971), examined the immune system of the opossum in greater detail. When the abilities of opossums were compared with rabbits with regard to their capacity to clear bacteria from blood, it was found that rabbits were more effective than opossums in removing bacteria in the first 2 minutes after injection of bacteria but that these two species of animals were equally effective in clearing bacteria after 60 minutes. Since further studies showed that opossums produced fewer plaques than rabbits using the Jerne technique to measure the immune response to sheep erythrocytes, it was concluded that the defect in immune response of the opossum lies in the efferent rather than in the afferent portions of the immune system.

Yadav (1973) has recently suggested that the defects in immune responses described in the North American opossum do not exist in other, phylogenetically more advanced marsupials. This investigator examined the immune responses of three species of Western Australian marsupials (*Setonix brachyurus*, *Macropus eugenii*, and *Trichosurus vulpecula*) to sheep erythrocytes, the flagella of *S. adelaide*, and the bacteriophage ØX 174. In each case the immune responses seemed more prompt than those in the North American opossum with antibodies at 7 days being equal to or in excess of the levels measured in serum taken 21 days after immunization. Second injections of the antigens 42 days after primary immunization showed variable results in *S. brachyurus* with increased antibody titres being found when *S. adelaide* or bacteriophage ØX 174 were used as antigens. But, evidence of an anamnestic response to sheep erythrocytes could not be demonstrated in these animals.

Immunoglobulins and complement

Two laboratories (Rowlands & Dudley 1968, Taylor & Burrell 1968) have independently arrived at similar conclusions regarding the fundamental nature of the immunoglobulins in opossums. Both groups identified large (19S) and small (7S) immunoglobulins and a third investigator (Genco & Liebert 1970) has identified a subclass of the smaller immunoglobulin.

Our studies showed that in addition to the similarities in size between these immunoglobulins and the IgM and IgG classes of immunoglobulins of other species of animals, the hexose content of these immunoglobulins (8–10 per cent for heavy and 2–3 per cent for light immunoglobulins) were comparable to those found in higher vertebrates. Although rigorous proof that immunoglobulins of opossums represent two distinct classes of immunoglobulins have not been provided, our unreported studies using starch gel analyses of reduced immunoglobulins suggest that this is the case. In this connection, it is of interest to point out that, in contrast to the case in 62 other mammalian species, only the opossum showed an inability of the Fc fragment of its IgG to react with the protein A fraction of staphylococci (Kornvall *et al.* 1970).

Antibody populations appearing to correspond to IgM and IgG classes of immunoglobulins of eutherian mammals were found in other species of marsupials and a secondary immune response appeared to be associated with increased IgG antibody activity (Yadav 1973). As in North American opossums (Rowlands & Dudley 1968, Rowlands 1970) and in other species of animals (Adler 1956, Rosenquist & Campbell 1966, Monoz 1967, Wagner & Freeman 1970), IgG antibodies were found to be only partially resistant to reduction with 2-mercaptoethanol (2-ME). Similarly, Yadav (1973) found a portion of the IgM antibodies in the marsupials studied by him to resist reduction with 2-ME. This investigator and his associates have also gathered evidence that certain immunoglobulins identified by him may be of a size which is appreciably smaller than that of IgG (Thomas *et al.* 1972, Yadav 1973); an observation similar to that made in other animal species (Rosen *et al.* 1967, Krough 1970, Kuwahara *et al.* 1966).

Complement has received less attention in marsupials than have the immunoglobulins. Wirtz and Westfall (1967) surveyed the conditions for opossum serum complement activation and found the total complement activity to be somewhat less in opossum than in guinea-pig serum but C1 was found to be increased. Dr P. Burkholder (unpublished observations) carried out a preliminary study of the opossum serum complement system and confirmed the observation that it was not unlike that of other vertebrates.

Cellular immunity

Cellular immunity in the opossum has been most extensively evaluated by Taylor (1968) working in Burrell's laboratory. He studied skin reactivity to tuberculin, the production of MIF, skin reactivity to a hapten, DNCB, and concluded that, while intact, cellular immunity appeared relatively late after sensitization in opossums and was much less striking than cellular immunity as seen in guinea-pigs. Taylor (1968) also demonstrated that cellular immunity could be transferred from a sensitized to a control opossum with cells from a peritoneal exudate or with cells from the spleens of sensitized animals but that the skin reactivity in such passively sensitized animals was also far less dramatic than that evident in other species of animals treated in similar manner.

Cellular immunity has also been demonstrated in both skin allograft rejection (Taylor 1968, LaPlante *et al.* 1969) and in allergic encephalomyelitis (Taylor 1968) in adult opossums. Rejection of primary skin grafts occurred in $14 \pm 4{\cdot}75$ days and second set skin graft rejection was accelerated ($6{\cdot}5 \pm 0{\cdot}9$ days). The encephalomyelitis observed in the experimental setting in the opossum was characterized by perivascular aggregates of lymphocytes, typical of the morphology of cellular immunity.

We (Fox, Wilson, Rowlands) have been able to confirm the observations that tuberculin sensitivity can be induced in adult opossums and that skin allografts are rejected as in other higher vertebrates. In addition, we have shown that the lymphocytes from sensitized adults respond to tuberculin in tissue culture as do lymphocytes from other laboratory mammals. However, we have been unable to demonstrate a mixed lymphocyte interaction in these animals. In order to optimize the chances of producing a positive response, we tested lymphocytes obtained from animals found in the same section of this country with each other as well as with cells from opossums obtained in other parts of eastern United States. Although our failure to demonstrate a mixed lymphocyte interaction *in vitro* could be attributed to faulty culture conditions, it seems more likely that North American opossums lack an MLC locus.

Response to infection

The apparent lack of sophistication of the immune system of North American opossums may account for its seeming extraordinary susceptibility to certain infections. Although opossums are typically heavily infested with parasites (Krupp & Quillin 1964, Krupp 1966, Barbero 1960, Barbero 1957, Dickerson 1930, Volk 1938, Sherwood *et al.* 1969) these are usually associated with lesions such as chronic bronchitis or superficial gastric erosions but rarely with fatal illnesses.

However, bacterial infections seem to be a major cause of death in opossums maintained in captivity. In particular, there is a high incidence of bacterial endocarditis in captive opossums, often a result of infection with gram positive cocci (Fox 1924, LaPlante & Burrell 1966, Sherwood *et al.* 1968). Bacterial endocarditis is seen infrequently in the wild and can be essentially eliminated in captive opossums if unusual care is taken in the maintenance of these animals (Sherwood *et al.* 1968). It is likely that multiple factors (e.g. diet, crowding) are operative in causing such infections, but it will also be important to seek a relationship between the opossums's immune system and its susceptibility to infectious diseases.

Summary

Marsupials would appear to be significantly more advanced than monotremes as regards the structure of their lymphoid tissues. The studies identifying differences between various marsupials with respect to their ability to respond to various antigens are of special interest since available data, although admittedly sparse, suggests that the more ancient marsupials (e.g. North American opossums) respond less vigorously than do more phylogenetically advanced marsupials. Should these observations be confirmed, it would seem to represent an instance of evolution of marsupials parallel to that of eutherian mammals with the two lines having common ancestry.

Acknowledgments

The author is indebted to Dr E. Diener for his generosity in providing Figs 1 and 2 and to Dr R. Burrell for his critical review of the text in its early stage of preparation. This work was supported in part by USPHS Grants AM-14372 and HE 13931.

References

ADAMS M.H. (1959) *Bacteriophages*, Interscience, New York.

ADLER F.L. (1956) Studies on mouse antibodies. II. Mercaptoethanol-sensitive 7S antibodies in mouse antisera to protein antigens. *J. Immunol.* **95**, 39.

ATWELL J.L., MARCHALONIS J.J. & EALEY E.H.M. (1973) Major immunoglobulin classes of echidna (*Tachyglossus aculeatus*). *Immunology* **25**, 835.

BARBERO B.B. (1957) Some Helminths from Illinois opossums. *J. Parasit.* **43**, 232.

BARBERO B.B. (1960) Further studies on Helminths of the oppossum, *Didelphis virginiana*, with a description of a new species from this host. *J. Parasit.* **46**, 455.

DICKERSON L.M. (1930) A new variety of *Harmostonum opisthotrias* from the North American opossum, *Didelphis virginiana*, with a discussion of its possible bearing on the origin of its host. *J. Parasit.* **22**, 37.

DIENER E. & EALEY E.H.M. (1965) Immune system in a monotreme: Studies on the Australian echidna (*Tachyglossus aculeatus*). *Nature* **208**, 950.

DIENER E. & NOSSAL G.J.V. (1966) Phylogenetic studies on the immune response. I. Localization of antigens and immune response in the toad, *Bufo marinus*. *Immunology*, **10**, 35.

DIENER E., WISTAR R. & EALEY E.H.M. (1967a) Phylogenetic studies on the immune response. II. The immune response of the Australian Echidna *Tachyglossus aculeatus*. *Immunology* **13**, 329.

DIENER E., EALEY E.H.M. & LEGGE J.S. (1967b). Phylogenetic studies on the immune response. III. Autoradiographic studies on the lymphoid system of the Australian Echidna *Tachyglossus aculeatus*. *Immunology* **13**, 339.

DIENER E. (1970) Evolutionary aspects of immunity and lymphoid organs in vertebrates. *Transplant. Proc.* **2**, 309.

FOX D., WILSON D.W., ROWLANDS D.T. JR. Proliferate reaction of opossum peripheral blood leukocytes to allogeneic cells, mitogens, and to specific antigens. *Transplantation*, in press.

FOX H. (1924) *Disease in Captive Wild Mammals and Birds; Incidence, Description, Comparison*. Lippincott, Philadelphia.

GENCO R.J. & LIEBERT B. (1970) Immunoglobulins of the opossum. *Fed. Proc.* **29**, 704.

KRONVALL G., SEAL U.S., FINSTAD J. *et al.* (1970) Phylogenetic insight into evolution of Mammalian Fc fragments of Gamma-G globulin using Staphyloccal protein A. *J. Immunol.* **104**, 140.

KROUGH H.K. (1970) Low molecular weight antibodies in human sera to stratum corneum. *Int. Arch. Allergy* **37**, 104.

KRUPP J.H. & QUILLIN R. (1964) A review of the use of the opossum for research-husbandry, experimental techniques, and routine health measures. *Lab. Animal Care* **14**, 189.

KRUPP J.H. (1966). Parasitic diseases of the opossum. *Lab. Animal Digest* **4**, 12.

KUWAHARA O., SHINKA S., IMANISHI M. *et al.* (1966) Low molecular weight 3·5S antibodies in rabbit antisera. *Biken J.* **9**, 1.

LaPlante E.S. & Burrell R.G. (1966) Bacterial endocarditis in opossums. *Bull. Wildlife Dis. Ass.* **2,** 10.

LaPlante E.S., Burrell R., Watne A.L. *et al.* (1969) Skin allograft studies in the pouch young of the opossum. *Transplantation* **7,** 67.

Marx J.J. Jr (1970) *A comparative study of the afferent and efferent limbs of the immune response in opossums.* Thesis. West Virginia University, Morgantown, West Virginia.

Marx J.J. Jr, Burrell R. & Fisher S.Q. (1971) A study of the afferent and efferent limbs of the immune response in opossums. *J. Immunol.* **106,** 1043.

Munoz J. (1967) Comparison between Hartley and strain 13 guinea pigs—antibody function and delayed hypersensitivity. *J. Immunol.* **99,** 31.

Nossal G.J.V., Ada G.L., & Austin C.M. (1964) Antigens in immunity. IV. Cellular localization of ^{125}I- and ^{131}I-Labelled flagella in lymph nodes. *Aust. J. Exp. Biol. Med. Sci.* **42,** 311.

Rosen R., Wolff S.M., Butler W.T. *et al.* (1967) The identification of low molecular weight bentonite flocculating antibodies in the serum of the rabbit, monkey and man. *J. Immunol.* **98,** 764.

Rosenquist G.L. & Campbell G.R. (1966) Characteristics of the 19S and 7S response to bacteriophage ØX-174 in the fowl. *Immunology* **10,** 169.

Rowlands D.T. Jr (1967) Precipitation and neutralization of bacteriophage f2 by rabbit antibodies. *J. Immunol.* **98,** 958.

Rowlands D.T. Jr & Dudley M.A. (1968) The isolation of immunoglobulins of the adult opossum (*Didelphis virginiana*). *J. Immunol.* **100,** 736.

Rowlands D.T. Jr (1970) The immune response of adult opossums (*Didelphis virginiana*) to the bacteriophage f2. *Immunology* **18,** 149.

Sherwood B.R., Rowlands D.T. Jr, Hackel D.B. *et al.* (1968) Bacterial endocarditis, glomerulonephritis, and amyloidosis in the opossum (*Didelphis virginiana*). *Am. J Path.* **53,** 115.

Sherwood B.R., Rowlands D.T. Jr, Hackel D.B. *et al.* (1969) The opossum, *Didelphis virginiana*, as a laboratory animal. *Lab. Animal Care* **19,** 494.

Taylor D.L. (1968) *An immunologic study of the North American opossum.* Thesis, West Virginia University, Morgantown, West Virginia.

Taylor D.L. & Burrell R. (1968) The immunologic responses of the North American opossum (*Didelphis virginiana*). *J. Immun.* **101,** 1207.

Thomas W.R., Turner K.J., Eadie M.E. *et al.* (1972) The immune response of the Quokka (*Setonix brachyurus*). The production of low molecular weight antibody. *Immunology,* **22,** 401.

Volk J.J. (1938) *Isospora broughtoni.* New species from the American opossum, *Didelphis virginiana. J. Parasit.* **24,** 547.

Wagner G.G. & Freemen M.J. (1970) Heterogeneity of the antibody response of rabbits to bacteriophage ØX-174. *Int. Arch. Allergy* **37,** 449.

Walker E.D. (1964) *Mammals of the World.* Johns Hopkins Press, Baltimore.

Wirtz G.H. & Westfall S.A. (1967) Immune complement of the opossum. *Immunochemistry* **4,** 61.

Yadav M. & Papadimitriou J.M. (1969) The ultrastructure of the neonatal thymus of a marsupial, *Setonix Brachyurus. Aust. J. Exp. Biol. Med. Sci.* **47,** 653.

Yadav M. (1973) The sensitivity of antibody to 2-mercaptoethanol treatment in three Australian marsupials. *European J. Immunol.* **3,** 359.

Young J.Z. (1962) *The Life of Vertebrates.* Oxford University Press, New York.

Chapter 15. Amphibian Models for Study of the Ontogeny of Immunity

Louis Du Pasquier

Introduction

Genesis of tolerance to histocompatibility antigens
The tolerance induced at embryonic stages
The tolerance during the metamorphic period
Interpretation

The maturation of the thymic function
The thymus and transplantation immunity
The thymus and immunoglobulin synthesis
Origin of lymphocytes in amphibians
Immunoglobulin synthesis by thymus cells

The maturation of the thymic function *continued*
Regulation of immunoglobulin synthesis by the thymus

Origin of antibody diversity
Antibody production during the ontogeny: cellular aspects
Antibody production during the ontogeny: humoral aspects
Discussion

Conclusion

Introduction

During the past 15 years amphibians have become an excellent tool for the study of the ontogeny of the immune system. This trend is due to the following reasons:

(1) Many studies have shown that although a great phylogenetic distance between higher vertebrates and amphibians exists, the latter possess an immune system similar in its basic features to that of mammals.
(2) Their embryonic and larval development have unique characteristics: most of the development takes place in direct contact with the environment which means the lack of materno-fetal interactions and early stimulation by various antigens. The differentiation of the larval immune system is fast. A fully differentiated thymus appears 8 days after fertilization in *Xenopus laevis* for instance. The metamorphosis, during which the new adult specific structures differentiate in contact with the already functional larval immune system, offers a good model for the study of the tolerance to self antigens.

(3) Like all poikilotherms, their immune response may be influenced by the temperature.
(4) Finally, thanks to miniaturization of sensitive antibody assays, or of the mixed lymphocyte reaction assay, the immune responses of very small and young tadpoles possessing as few as 0·5 to 1×10^6 lymphocytes can be analysed.

The purpose of this chapter will be to emphasize the functional rather than the morphological aspects of the ontogeny of immunity in amphibians. The results obtained in this group complement quite well those acquired in mammals, especially in the following areas: the genesis of tolerance to histocompatibility antigens, the maturation of thymus function, and the origin of antibody diversity.

Genesis of tolerance to histocompatibility antigens

Whether tolerance to self and non-self histocompatibility antigens is due to the absence of the reactive cells (forbidden clone hypothesis) or to the blockage of the reactive cells is still unknown. For the elucidation of this problem the amphibians provide the experimenter with two interesting ontogenetic stages. Indeed, tolerance induction is possible:

(1) during their embryonic life when the lymphoid system is not yet developed;
(2) during the metamorphosis period when the animal becomes naturally tolerant to the new adult specific structures which differentiate at this time.

In mammals the study of the embryonic tolerance is rendered difficult by the materno-fetal interactions and by technical problems linked to the necessity of working *in utero*. In amphibians, on the contrary, embryonic grafts and parabiosis have been used for decades by embryologists. These techniques have been considerably improved since the introduction by Volpe & Gebhardt (1966) of the use of a cell marker by using grafts from artificially produced triploid animals (Dasgupta 1962) on normal diploid embryos. This allows, for instance, the detection of blood cell chimeras following embryonic transplantation. The existence of defined pigment pattern mutants especially in *Rana pipiens* also allows the tracing of embryonic grafts such as neural folds, some derivatives of which are pigment cells of the skin.

The tolerance induced at embryonic stages

When the embryonic tissues are exchanged within the same species, most authors agree that there is no rejection at this early stage of the ontogeny. The grafted tissues differentiate in a normal manner and one can trace their derivatives provided the grafts come from a recognizable mutant. When the host has reached larval stages, the fate of the grafted tissue may be either tolerance or rejection. Triplett (1958) always observed that an embryonic graft from a neural fold of *Hyla regilla* on *Rana aurora* was first accepted and then rejected in the larval life. In allogeneic combination, the experiments by Davison (1963, 1966) and Volpe and his co-workers (since 1964) in *Rana pipiens*, and by Clark and Newth in *Xenopus* (1972) yield more information.

Davison made chimeric recombinations in *Rana pipiens* embryos. His major finding was that chimeric recombinations made anterior to the heart presumptive field were incompatible and did not survive to maturity. The more posterior recombinations were found to be compatible. The two chimeras obtained for each experiment accepted subsequent skin allografts from the homologous recombinant. Another experiment made by Davison was the prevention of rejection of neural crest derivatives by putting the host and donor in parabiosis after the exchange of grafts. The same result was obtained if instead of parabiosis an exchange of ventral belly region was achieved. Ex-parabionts accepted subsequent skin exchanges from the homologous ex-parabiont. The interpretation of Davison was that there exists a link between tolerance and blood cell chimerism. He formulated the hypothesis 'no blood cell chimerism—no tolerance' on the basis that chimeric recombination made anterior to the heart presumptive tissue contained blood cells of one of the individuals. On the contrary, all the other combinations involved the exchange of blood stem cells which are known in amphibians not to belong to a single discrete island (Slonimsky 1931). It should be proved, however, that the incompatibility was really due to the lack of blood cell chimerism, for instance, by experiments involving injection of lymphocytes together with a usually non-tolerogenic graft.

Volpe and his colleagues have contributed very much to this field since 1964. His first experiments (Volpe 1964) were quite similar to those of Triplett (1958). The graft of one neural fold is accepted by the host embryo, self differentiates and is rejected in the larval life. This leads to a sensitization of the host as can be seen from the second set reaction which occurs when the host is challenged later by a skin graft from the same donor. More puzzling were the results obtained after the transplantation of two neural folds (Volpe & Gebhardt 1965). When transplantation of two complete neural folds is performed, the host becomes tolerant to subsequent skin allografts from the donor. The author interpreted this as a dose effect. This would seem a rather peculiar dose effect where only a two-fold increase of the dose leads to tolerance instead of immunity. On the other hand, the fact that the two transplanted neural folds must be complete (Volpe 1971) to induce tolerance suggests that their tissues contain primordia of fundamental immunological elements. If one witnesses, for instance, an exchange of the cells bound to populate the thymus, or of the thymus primordia themselves, tolerance is indeed expected.

However, Gebhardt and Volpe (1973) have repeated these experiments with tail tissue in *Rana pipiens* 10 days after fertilization (neural fold exchanges were performed at the neural stage, much earlier). They could again observe that small allografts of tail tissue evoke an immune response since 29/32 were rejected in sibling larvae and 55/55 in non-siblings. On the contrary, large tail fragments induced a state of tolerance. These tolerant animals, like the other ones obtained by the same authors following parabiosis and neural fold transplants, were found to be blood-cell chimeras (Volpe & Gebhardt 1966). Since the chimerism can be estimated by counting triploid cells in Phytohaemagglutinin stimulated blood cultures, one might even propose that the chimerism exists at the level of lymphocytes sharing properties with mammalian T cells. This finding was in agreement with Davison's (1966) hypothesis. The tolerance which has been induced is specific; the animals which had been sensitized after the rejection of a small tail graft showed second-set rejection of a subsequent skin transplant from the same donor (median survival time 10·2 days instead of 14·7 for the unrelated donor) in all cases (18/18) (Gebhardt & Volpe 1973).

In *Xenopus*, embryonic ectoderm allografts can also induce tolerance to subsequent skin allografts (Clark and Newth 1972) but no data are available about an eventual chimerism in this species.

The tolerance during the metamorphic period

This period offers a unique opportunity to study the genesis of tolerance to autologous antigens in an immunologically competent organism. The experiments of Triplett (1962) had shown that this tolerance was the result of an interaction between the antigens and the immune system. In *Hyla regilla* the pituitary from a tail bud embryo can be transplanted in young larvae (2 weeks old) without any rejection. The organ will grow in the recipient. If at a more advanced stage (beginning of metamorphosis) the pituitary is grafted back to its original owner, this autograft is rejected in 10 cases out of 13, as testified by the modification of the skin pigmentation controlled by the pituitary pars intermedia. The following control has been performed to show that the rejection was not due to alloantigens acquired by the pituitary during its transient stay in the host: the graft of half a pituitary should be rejected when grafted back to its owner if it had acquired some of the temporary host antigens. In fact, such grafts were tolerated.

Similar observations showing that tolerance to adult specific structures is the result of the interaction between these antigens and the larval immune system were done by Maniatis *et al.* (1969). Larval *Rana catesbiana* when injected with haemoglobin of adults of the same species can make specific antibodies against it, whereas during their normal development the tadpole becomes tolerant to the adult haemoglobin. Injection to the animals of antibodies specific to the adult haemoglobin will prevent them from making this molecule.

The biology of grafts also has bcen surveyed at the time of metamorphosis. In the Urodele *Pleurodeles waltlii* the skin of recently metamorphosed animals (juveniles) is tolerated in a significant percentage of the cases. The highest percentage of tolerance recorded 8 months after grafting, is observed when juvenile skin is grafted on old larvae (10 cases of tolerance for 39 grafts = 26 per cent). Control grafts of larval skin or fully grown adult skin were rejected respectively in 93 per cent (53/57) and 100 per cent (24/24) of the cases (Orfila & Deparis 1970).

In the bullfrog tadpoles Bovbjerg (1966) noticed that when the grafts were performed at the time of metamorphosis, the graft was invaded 1 or 2 weeks later than in the immunologically competent larvae. Ruben (1970) in *Xenopus* noticed that tumour grafts were more readily accepted if achieved in animals in the process of metamorphosing. A related phenomenon is the observation in *Rana catesbiana* of a depressed antibody synthesis at the moment of metamorphosis (Moticka *et al.* 1973).

Recently, a more specific study of the phenomenon has been published (Chardonnens & Du Pasquier 1973) on the basis of the previous work of Bernardini *et al.* in *Xenopus* (1969, 1970). *Xenopus* individuals having just completed their metamorphosis (juvenile) have been used either as donor or recipient of allograft within a sibship. Such animals tolerate the skin allograft in 30 per cent of the cases. The use of anachronic grafts (i.e. old adult skin on juvenile and vice versa) showed that the unresponsiveness of the animals was not due to a lack of antigenicity as it seemed to be the case in *Pleurodeles*. In *Xenopus*, the host immune system seems to be affected since juvenile skin was perfectly well rejected by grown up adults whereas adult skin was tolerated by juvenile hosts.

In their first series of experiments, Bernardini *et al.* (1969a,b, 1970) thought that they were witnessing an ontogenic appearance of the graft immunity in *Xenopus*. However, Horton (1969) has shown that this species as all other anurans until now tested (for review see Cohen 1971, Du Pasquier 1973) is capable of rejecting grafts at early larval stages. This suggested that the impairment of the *Xenopus* immune system was transient. Indeed, the study of allograft rejection in a sibship of *Xenopus* showed that tadpoles and adults rejected grafts in nearly 100 per cent of the cases while at the time of metamorphosis about 25–50 per cent of the grafts were tolerated (Chardonnens & Du Pasquier 1973). This tolerance to skin allograft induced by skin allograft has the characteristics of an immunological tolerance. It is specific, and a third party graft is normally rejected except in some cases where it can lead to the break-down of tolerance to the first tolerogenic transplant. In other cases the third party graft can be tolerated. Both experiments suggest a sharing of histocompatibility antigens rather than a non-specific tolerance. The tolerance lasts much longer than the period during which it can be induced. It seems permanent. In no case is one able to predict the ultimate fate of these grafts. Some have been tolerated for 2 years and are still viable, some have been rejected after 1 year. An important characteristic of this tolerance is the presence of lymphocytes near the transplanted skin, as evidenced by histological examination (Bernardini *et al.* 1970).

The interpretation that one can give to this phenomenon depends on other experiments concerning: (1) the size effect in graft rejection at metamorphosis, (2) the genetic relationship of individuals, (3) the state of the lymphoid system during the period when tolerance induction is possible.

Bernardini *et al.* (1970) have shown that the percentage of graft rejection at metamorphosis was size-dependent. A medium sized (4 mm^2) graft led to about 46 per cent of tolerance whereas the reduction of the graft surface to 2 mm^2 was followed by about 25 per cent of tolerance cases. A further decrease in the size (up to 1 mm^2) did not modify significantly this 25 per cent figure. On the other hand, increasing the surface of the graft up to 9 mm^2 provoked about 70 per cent of tolerance and further increase was impossible for technical reasons. It seems that a certain percentage of tolerance cases are size-independent: the first 25 per cent. The others from 25 per cent to 70 per cent appear to be highly size-dependent. The hypothesis has been proposed that the size-independent 25 per cent of tolerance cases were due to genetic reasons (Chardonnens & Du Pasquier 1973). Indeed, 25 per cent tolerance would be the expected percentage of compatible siblings in the progeny of parents, both of whom are likely to be heterozygotes and to differ at the four haplotypes of a main histocompatibility genetic region. It is also the percentage of non-stimulating MLR combinations which can be recorded in similar *Xenopus* siblings (Du Pasquier & Miggiano 1973). It was therefore tempting to consider that at the time of metamorphosis the main histocompatibility antigens are still immunogenic but that their effect is linked to the size of the grafts, as in cases where weak histocompatibility differences are involved in Mammals (Billingham & Silvers 1974).

The major histocompatibility locus of the *Xenopus* would then have some properties of weak histocompatibility loci of higher vertebrates. It has been suggested that the 25 per cent tolerance, which seems to be the one essentially depending on the metamorphosis, would concern other histocompatibility antigens, essentially allogeneic variants of adult specific structures to which the animal becomes tolerant during this period.

To understand the mechanism of the induction and the maintenance of this tolerance, the modifications of the lymphoid system and the reactivity of the lymphocytes in the MLR assay have been followed during the ontogeny (Du Pasquier & Weiss 1973).

As shown in Fig. 15.1, the growth of the thymus and to a lesser extent of the spleen, are very much affected by the metamorphosis. The thymus loses about 80–90 per cent of its lymphocytes before starting a new growth period. It appeared that the impaired allograft responsiveness is detected precisely during this depletion and new growth of the thymus (Fig. 15.1b). This phenomenon has to be related to the finding by Riviere and Cooper (1973) of a thyroxin induced regression of lymph glands in *Rana catesbiana*. Lymphocyte depletion and histogenesis of the thymus are two conditions which are known to be favourable to tolerance induction in higher vertebrates (MacGregor & Gowans 1964).

The reactivity of lymphocytes in unidirectional MLR has been followed during the ontogeny either between siblings or between unrelated individuals (Du Pasquier and Weiss 1973). As summarized in Fig. 15.1c one can observe that the reactivity of thymic lymphocytes is practically not affected by the metamorphosis when the stimulating cells come from unrelated individuals. On the contrary, when stimulating cells come from sibs, the reactivity of thymic lymphocytes is very much depressed. From 75 per cent the number of stimulating combinations goes down to about 20 per cent. The difference of reactivity according to the genetic characteristics of the stimulating cells suggested the hypothesis: at the time of metamorphosis not only tolerance to weak histocompatibility antigens can be observed but also tolerance to some main histocompatibility antigens and in parallel, to MLR determinants. It seems likely that at this time a one-haplotype difference at the level of the main histocompatibility locus would be insufficient in prompting graft rejection in the cases of large grafts. They would need a two-haplotype difference to provoke the rejection. This would be the same in the MLR where the number of cells are 1×10^5 for both the stimulator and the responder, which would correspond to a very large graft. It is not surprising therefore that between siblings the percentage of tolerated large grafts and the percentage of non-stimulating MLRs are relatively close (30 per cent–20 per cent) and at any rate statistically compatible with each other.

A further indication is obtained when looking at the graft rejection at metamorphosis between unrelated individuals. Although there is a discernible effect, it is much more discrete than within a sibship (Chardonnens & Du Pasquier 1973). Some combinations may yield to 5 per cent tolerance. Similarly, MLR reactivity was subnormal. Such a result was expected since it is likely that most of the combinations between unrelated individuals involve two-haplotype differences. Nevertheless, some rare unrelated families showed high percentages of tolerance at metamorphosis similar to those observed within a sibship. This may be due to the fact that the animal comes

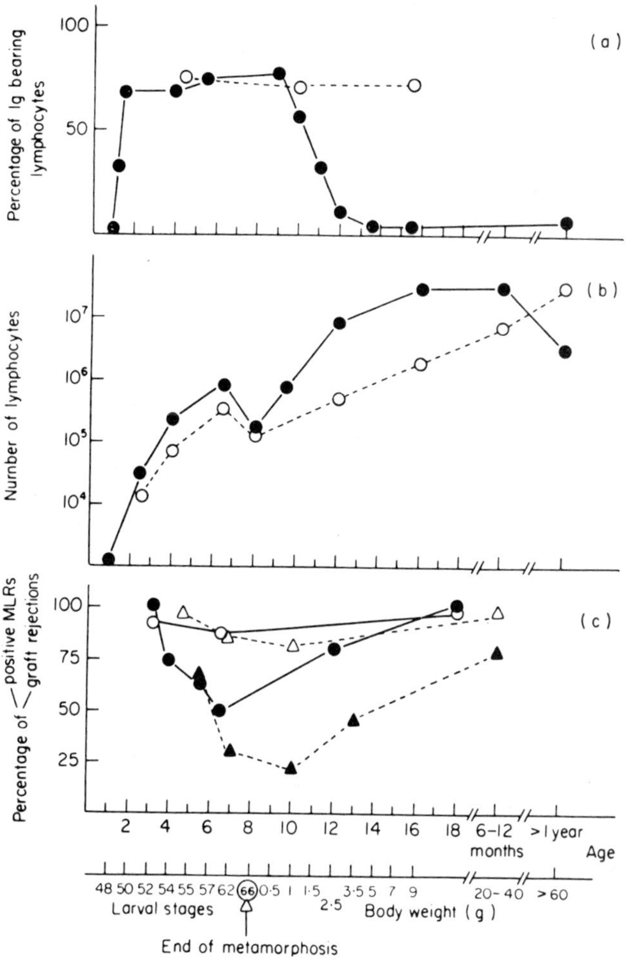

Fig. 15.1. Ontogenic changes in the lymphoid complex of *Xenopus laevis*. (1A) Evolution of the percentage of thymic lymphocytes with membrane bound immunoglobulins, detected by spot test (●——●) or by cap test (○- - - -○). (See text for explanations.) (1B) Evolution of the number of lymphocytes in the thymus (●——●) and in the spleen (○- - - -○) during the ontogeny of *Xenopus laevis*. (1C) Evolution of the reactivity of thymus lymphocytes in the mixed lymphocyte reaction (MLR) compared to the evolution of the reactivity to skin allograft during the ontogeny.

△- - - -△ MLR between genetically unrelated animals.
○——○ Graft rejection between genetically unrelated animals.
▲- - - -▲ MLR between F_1 siblings.
●——● Graft rejection between F_1 siblings.

from one geographic region and it is likely that they represent a restricted pool of the histocompatibility haplotypes of the species.

Interpretation

The interpretation of Volpe on the tolerance state following large grafts performed at embryonic stage is that no tolerant cells exist in the tolerant animals (Volpe 1971). The blood cell chimerism which is about 50 per cent in ex-parabiotic larvae would be possible only if reactive cells have been eliminated. The finding that after metamorphosis the proportion of donor blood cells falls down to 5 per cent was interpreted as the occurrence of the growth of a new population of blood cells of host origin which could incidentally lead to the breakdown of tolerance.

More recently, Gebhardt and Volpe (1973) have also suggested that blocking serum factor could play a role in the tolerance induction and maintenance. In fact, the tolerance state which exists in chimeric frogs must be compared to the state of tolerance existing in allophenic mice rather than to the neonatal tolerance which can be induced in an animal the lymphoid system of which is already partially developed. Indeed, in these peculiar chimeras the situation is far from being clear, since the finding of serum blocking factor is not constant and seems to depend on the genetic characteristic of the strains used to make chimera (for review see Meo *et al.* 1973). The study of the reactivity in MLR of lymphocytes from animals in which tolerance was induced at metamorphosis may provide some further indication (Du Pasquier & Chardonnens, unpublished). The lymphocytes from tolerant animals irradiated at 2000 r were used to stimulate siblings responding cells and their stimulating capacity was compared to that of non-tolerant siblings. In another experiment, the cells from tolerant animals were used as responding cells towards stimulating cells coming from the tolerogenic partner or from other siblings. Lymphocytes from tolerant animals did not respond to the lymphocytes coming from the tolerogenic donor but could respond in 13 of 45 (29 per cent) combinations between siblings. Cells from non-tolerant animals were able to respond in 64 per cent of the cases (29 of 45 combinations). The puzzling finding is that, when the stimulating capacity is studied, the lymphocytes from the tolerant animals also behave as poor stimulators since the percentage of cases where these cells did stimulate lymphocytes from siblings was also 33 per cent whereas the stimulating capacity of normal sibling cells was again 65 per cent. This finding can be interpreted as the evidence for a blocking factor released from tolerant cells and showing some degree of specificity since all MLR combinations are not inhibited. It may also be compared to the finding in humans of the poor stimulating capacity of lymphocytes coming from pregnant women (Ceppellini *et al.* 1971). Finally it may suggest, as experiments by Jones and Lafferty (1969) and Killby *et al.*

(1972) also suggest, that in the MLR involving tolerant stimulating cells, these lymphocytes do not produce a hypothetical factor responsible for the cell divisions of the responding cells. On the other hand, it may indicate that the tolerance at metamorphosis cannot be simply explained by a blood cell chimerism, but the existence of chimerism has not yet been looked for in *Xenopus*. However, removal of a tolerated graft followed 60 days later by regrafting a skin graft from the same donor is followed by rejection in about 50 per cent of the cases (Chardonnens, personal communication). This argues against the general existence of a blood cell chimerism when tolerance is induced by skin graft at metamorphosis. There seems, therefore, to be some suggestive data about the existence of a blocking factor. Whether it is similar to blocking agents from pregnant women, to the blocking factors of Hellström and Hellström (1972) or to enhancing antibodies (Voisin *et al.* 1972) is not known. Nevertheless, one can derive some hypothesis from the work of Marchalonis (1971) who found in *Rana pipiens* a serum component likely to be an immunoglobulin (neither IgM nor IgG) which appeared in the serum at the time of metamorphosis. It was less abundant in fully grown adults; it could be a candidate for the blocking factor. The existence of a blocking factor would allow to interpret the apparently conflicting results obtained in *Pleurodeles* and in *Xenopus*. In *Pleurodeles* the blocking factor could stick to the antigen, while in *Xenopus* it would act on effector cells, perhaps via antigen–antibody complexes.

The results of Clark and Newth (1972) in *Xenopus* provide more indications that tolerance is an active phenomenon. Specific tolerance was obtained by grafting *Xenopus* embryos at stage 22 of Nieuwkoop and Faber (1967). These grafts include presumptive skin, gut, and blood-forming cells. In one experiment two animals called B and C were made mutually tolerant and one of them, B, unilaterally tolerant to a third animal A. In post-metamorphic life, A gave a tolerated skin graft to B and two immunizing ones to C. Then the spleen of C was transferred to B which tolerated it. Of 12 sets of such triplets only one could elicit an anti-A reaction in the host B which was tolerant to A. This strongly suggests that the tolerant state of B has been transferred to the anti-A spleen of the animal C. It resembles very much the experiments of Martinez *et al.* (1960) in the mouse, where tolerance could be transferred from one animal to another by the means of parabiosis.

In summary, only suggestive data has been provided until now concerning the mechanism of tolerance induction in amphibians. Most of the data of Davison and Volpe on tolerance induced at embryonic stages were compatible with the existence of blocking factor. Moreover, they suggest that the chimerism at the blood cell level is responsible for the tolerance. Data on tolerance at metamorphosis in *Xenopus* seem not to be well explained by the blood cell chimerism. It is very likely that the two types of tolerance are not identical.

Some properties of the lymphocytes of tolerant animals suggest the existence of a blocking factor. Finally, data presented by Clark and Newth (1972) strongly suggest that tolerance is an active phenomenon and is not due to the absence of responding cells, unless this absence is due to a specific suppression mechanism. Whatever the theoretical output, amphibians remain excellent technical models for obtaining chimera and parabionts, while these techniques are quite delicate in mammals.

The maturation of the thymic function

The study of thymus function is relatively easy in amphibians for the following reasons:

(1) The thymus is usually easily accessible (mainly in the *Xenopus*). Thymectomy can therefore be practised with a good yield. The fact that embryonic development takes place outside the mother also allows easy removal of thymus primordia (Turpen *et al.* 1973). Later the ablation of the epithelial anlage is quite possible before the organ gets populated with lymphocytes (Horton & Manning 1972). In some species such as *Rana pipiens* (Curtis & Volpe 1971) *R. catesbiana* (Baculi & Cooper 1973), *Alytes obstetricans* (Du Pasquier 1968) the thymus may regenerate after extirpation, whereas in *Xenopus* no sign of regeneration can be detected, except in 5 per cent of the cases, when the thymus is removed with the techniques of Horton and Manning (1972).

(2) In some species such as *Xenopus* (Manning 1971) or *Triturus alpestris* the thymectomy is not followed by any runting disease (Tournefier 1973). This allows long-term studies of the effect of thymectomy.

(3) Thymus lymphocytes react in the mixed lymphocyte culture assay (MLR) (Weiss & Du Pasquier 1973, Du Pasquier & Miggiano 1973).

(4) Thymus lymphocytes exhibit immunoglobulin molecules, the expression of which varies with ontogenic stages (Du Pasquier *et al.* 1972).

The thymus and transplantation immunity

If one is going to use amphibians as a model for the study of ontogeny of immune response one has to be sure that the thymus of amphibians is really the equivalent of the thymus in mammals. It is now well known that the thymectomy in Urodeles and in Anurans is effective in preventing graft rejection (for review see Cooper 1973, Du Pasquier 1973). A few experiments bearing on graft studies in thymectomized animals or in animals having a particular development of the thymus show how new insights can be made thanks to amphibians.

(1) The case of *Triturus alpestris* (Tournefier 1973a,b, see also Charlemagne

1973, Houillon 1973). This is a particularly interesting Urodele since its thymus becomes lymphoid very late, 9–10 weeks after fertilization. This allows the study of the effect of graft before the thymus becomes competent in controlling allograft rejection which may be useful for the study of tolerance. The removal of the thymus in the tenth week of life led to the observation of 72 per cent tolerance. For the 28 per cent of the animals which rejected grafts the mean survival time was 36 days instead of 23 for control animals.

(2) The case of *Ambystoma tigrinum* (Cohen 1969). The maturation of the allograft immunity in this species seems to be gradual and interesting variation of parameters such as age of the animal at thymectomy, age of the donor can be used. The most striking phenomenon observed by Cohen which can eventually be further investigated is the fact that in many cases after thymectomy the grafts were first apparently rejected but then recovered. There was a direct relationship between the percentage of recovery of fully viable stage and the age of the animal at thymectomy: 'the earlier the thymectomy the higher the percentage of recovery'. It is tempting to relate this recovery to the phenomenon of tolerance observed at metamorphosis in *Pleurodeles* and *Xenopus*. In the absence of the thymus the graft rejection is incomplete and slow, therefore the antigens of the grafts may persist until the animal will start its pre-metamorphic period and then induce tolerance.

(3) The case of *Xenopus* (Horton & Manning 1972). The lack of any runt disease has permitted Horton and Manning to study long term effect of thymectomy in this species. The removal of the thymus at stage 48 of Nieuwkoop and Faber, i.e. about 9 days after fertilization, does not modify the development of the animal. The thymectomy however, affects the graft rejection capacity of the larvae in 100 per cent of the cases when thymectomy was practised between 8 and 11 days after fertilization. Oddly enough, when grafting is performed in the adult life of those thymectomized animals, the grafts are rejected in a somewhat chronic fashion (28 days instead of 9–13 days). It can be concluded from these experiments involving thymectomy 8 days after fertilization that thymus-derived lymphocytes have already settled in the spleen for instance. This result may also suggest that part of graft rejection is thymus-independent in *Xenopus* and could eventually be mediated by antibodies. Or there could exist other organs generating cells with properties similar to those of thymus-derived lymphocytes. However, recent experiments (Du Pasquier & Horton, 1976) have shown that in about 1-year-old *Xenopus* thymectomized in larval life, the MLR of blood lymphocytes was apparently abolished.

Another approach in *Xenopus* consisted in studying the ontogeny of the

MLR reactivity in thymus lymphocytes (Du Pasquier & Weiss 1974) according to the degree of immunoglobulin expression at the surface of these cells. What can be the influence of such modifications on the MLR? In order not to deal with the modification of MLR reactivity at the metamorphosis, due to genetic reasons (see Sections on tolerance during the metamorphic period and interpretation) one has to look to MLR combinations between unrelated individuals which give practically a constant and high percentage of positive response. Thymuses were removed from animals at various stages of the ontogeny. The youngest tadpoles tested were at stage 54 of Nieuwkoop and Faber (about 4 weeks old) the oldest were fully grown adults taken after the involution of the thymus. The level of thymidine incorporation was measured in non-stimulated cultures and in stimulated cultures and the numbers were compared from one stage to another. No significant differences could be found when the same numbers of cells were used at each stage. Stimulation indices and numbers of counts were spread within the same range in larvae and adults, which seems to indicate that once acquired, the reactivity of lymphocytes in MLR is not any more modified. In particular, it is not much modified by the ontogenic changes of thymocytes' immunoglobulin expression. Further studies on the effect of anti-immunoglobulin sera on MLR showed that this sera were not inhibitory of the reaction. The results in *Xenopus* would suggest that immunoglobulin molecules are not the receptors involved in MLR stimulation. However, more studies are needed to prove this point. The absence of inhibitory role of anti-immunoglobulin sera can be well explained if one admits that the interactions between one cell and another MLR involve many receptor-antigen reactions leading to an extremely high apparent affinity of the receptors' molecules. The affinity of the anti-immunoglobulin antisera could not be high enough to compete with the cell to cell-binding affinity (M. Cohn, personal communication). From the experiments made until now one can just say that immunoglobulins need not be present in large amounts or need not be expressed in a way easily detectable by immunofluorescence to achieve their function in MLR.

The constancy of the thymus cells' reactivity in the MLR assay suggests that the proportion of cells reacting is not much modified from the early stages of ontogeny onwards. In a thymus containing 2×10^5 or 6×10^7 cells the proportion of blasts which can be counted is the same, i.e. about 12–15 per cent on days 3–4 for a reaction between unrelated individuals. The stability of this figure shows that there is no dilution of MLR reactive cells by other types of cells during the ontogeny.

In summary, it is clear that thymus mediates graft immunity in amphibians. *Xenopus* thymus show ontogenic changes in the expression of immunoglobulins at the surface of thymocytes which can be used as a tool to study the role of these molecules in the MLR stimulation. Thymocytes from a very small thymus (2×10^5 cells) of a young larva can react in the mixed lymphocyte cultures, and further improvement of the technique should allow to assay for this reactivity in younger thymus to determine at which stage of the lymphoid development of the thymus occurs the commitment of the lymphocytes to react with products of the histocompatibility genetic region.

Thymus and immunoglobulin synthesis

Recent experiments in the Urodele *Triturus viridescens* tend to demonstrate that cellular cooperation between equivalent of thymus-derived (T) and bursa type or bone marrow type (B) cells is required for obtaining a response to a hapten carrier complement (Ruben *et al.* 1973). The particularly advantageous characteristics of larval and embryonic models of amphibians offer a good opportunity to look at the early differentiation of the two lines of cells.

ORIGIN OF LYMPHOCYTES IN AMPHIBIANS

The experiments by Volpe and Gebhardt (1966) showed the chimerism of parabionts or tolerant *Rana pipiens* at the level of PHA-stimulable cells. In recent experiments done in *Xenopus* (Du Pasquier & Horton 1976) it was found that lymphocytes from thymectomized animals do not respond at all to PHA. This suggests that chimeric animals are chimeric at the level of T cells which could mean that peripheral lymphoid precursors can enter the thymus and become T cells. Recent experiments however seem to indicate that in the normal situation most of the lymphocytes are of thymus origin and that they differentiate in the thymus from stem cells present in this area. This was already suggested by observations by Sterba (1950) (in *Xenopus*), Slonimsky (1931) and Deparis (1968) in *Pleurodeles*, who found that the thymus was populated by mesenchymatous precursor cells (essentially present in the head) entering the thymus and differentiating into lymphocytes.The elegant experiments by Turpen *et al.* (1973) bring more information about this point. Thymus anlage from *Rana pipiens* embryo are exchanged between triploid and diploid individuals of the same stage. The resulting animals are then screened for the degree of ploidy of their lymphocytes in the thymus, spleen, kidney and bone marrow of the adult: about 95 per cent of the adult transplanted thymus cells are of donor type, which clearly indicates that thymocytes of the adult frog are derived from the thymus presumptive tissue of the donor. The fact that in unilateral exchanges the host thymus is populated with host type lymphocytes suggests on the other hand that each thymus is occupied by a self-perpetuating population of lymphocytes. Another finding in bilaterally transplanted animals was that about 78 per cent of the cells in an adult frog are of thymic origin, suggesting that the thymus is likely to be the source of various types of lymphocytes (of B- or T-cell type).

IMMUNOGLOBULIN SYNTHESIS BY THYMUS CELLS

Amphibians have in fact the peculiarity to express immunoglobulin on the membrane of the thymic lymphocytes in a way which makes them easily detectable by immunofluorescent techniques (Du Pasquier *et al.* 1972). Moreover, during the ontogeny the expression of these molecules changes. Figure 15.1a shows the evolution of the percentage of thymus lymphocytes bearing immunoglobulin molecules during the ontogeny of *Xenopus*. When the 'spot' technique is used which detects clusters of immunoglobulin molecules at the surface of lymphocytes, one finds a sharp decrease in the percentage of fluorescent lymphocytes in the thymus of post-metamorphic animals. If the 'cap' technique is now used, where all fluorescence is accumulated at one pole of the cells thanks to the absence of NaN_3 (which in the spot assay inhibits the modulation), then the same percentage of immunoglobulin positive lymphocytes is detected in the larvae and in the adult thymus. It is simply less easy to detect them in adult thymus. The spleen shows a constant level of highly fluorescent cells (60 per cent) during the whole life. Fluorescence of thymocytes is always less bright than that of spleen cells, therefore revealing a heterogeneity of the lymphocytes population with respect to surface immunoglobulins.

REGULATION OF IMMUNOGLOBULIN SYNTHESIS BY THE THYMUS

(1) The effect of thymectomy on natural rosette-forming cells and on the level of 'normal' immunoglobulins. It has been shown in *Alytes obstetricans* thymectomized during the first month of larval life that the proportion of natural splenic rosette-forming cells from sheep or human red cells was about 25–50 per cent of that of intact animals (Du Pasquier 1970b). In the same species the level of protein having the electrophoretic mobility of immunoglobulins was increased by a factor of 2 (Du Pasquier 1965). More recent and more precise experiments in *Xenopus* (Weiss *et. al.* 1973) have shown that early thymectomy led: (i) to a similar increase of the absolute level of immunoglobulins which were later in the life characterized as IgM; (ii) an increase of the proportion of Ig positive lymphocytes. A qualitative analysis showed that this increase was not only due to the disappearance of a population of Ig negative cells but also if not essentially to increased amounts of immunoglobulin detected per cell. On the whole, these results would suggest that T-derived cells are an important fraction of natural splenic rosette-forming cells and that the thymus could normally exert an inhibitory activity on Ig synthesis, a fact which would be in accord with some results obtained in mammals such as those of Kerbel and Eidinger (1972).

(2) The effect of thymectomy on antibody synthesis. It has been studied in *Alytes obstetricans* (Du Pasquier 1970c) and in *Rana catesbiana* (Baculi & Cooper 1973) and *Xenopus* (Manning 1972 personal communication). *Alytes obstetricans* individuals, thymectomized as young larvae, gave a rosette response to human red blood cells which was not different from the background. Response to sheep red cells was also diminished as evidenced by the absence of plaque-forming cells or by their low numbers in thymectomized animals. In *Rana catesbiana* (Baculi & Cooper 1973) the results were in agreement with what was found in *Xenopus* at the level of normal immunoglobulins, namely a somewhat increased titre of the anti-bovine serum albumin antibody. But *Alytes* and *Rana* are not the best models for thymectomy experiments, their thymus can regenerate. Results obtained in *Xenopus* are therefore more reliable since no regeneration occurs. Thymectomized *Xenopus* failed to respond to injections of human γ-globulin (Turner & Manning 1974).

(3) Thymus and IgG synthesis. It is well established in mammals that IgG synthesis and IgG memory are two thymus-dependent functions (Taylor and Wortis 1968). In young amphibian larvae, although two classes of immmunoglobulins are produced (Geczy *et al.* 1973, for review see Du Pasquier 1973, see also Fig. 15.2 and Fig. 15.3), it is clear that larvae produce less IgG than adults under normal resting conditions. Larval spleen from young tadpoles produce under culture conditions two classes of immunoglobulins whereas under the same conditions thymus cells will produce only IgM molecules (Feinstein & Du Pasquier unpublished, Fig. 15.2). In adults IgG is much more abundant. However, although they are able to make IgG, the tadpoles will practically not make IgG antibodies upon stimulation by the antigen (Fig. 15.3). This has been found in *Rana catesbiana* for sheep red cells (Moticka *et al.* 1972) for phages (Geczy *et al.* 1973) for 2,4-dinitrophenyl (DNP) and 2,4,6-trinitrophenyl (TNP) groups (Haimovich & Du Pasquier 1973). In the latter case, however, sucrose gradient analyses have revealed that the 7S fraction from immune sera containing IgG molecules contained some anti-DNP antibodies, but they were 100 times less abundant than in the 19S fraction and were of very poor affinity (Du Pasquier & Haimovich 1974). The production of IgM antibodies to DNP and TNP was observed whether keyhole limpet haemocyanin (KLH) or Pneumococcus carriers were used. On the contrary, in *Rana catesbiana* the nature of anti-DNP antibodies depends very much on the carrier. DNP on keyhole limpet haemocyanin will elicit an IgG response while DNP Salmonella will elicit only an IgM response (Rosenquist & Hoffmann 1972). KLH is considered in mammals to be a thymus-dependent antigen while Salmonella is not. It seems therefore that part of the thymus function has not matured in the larval form. It is tempting to relate this precise maturation step to the ontogenic

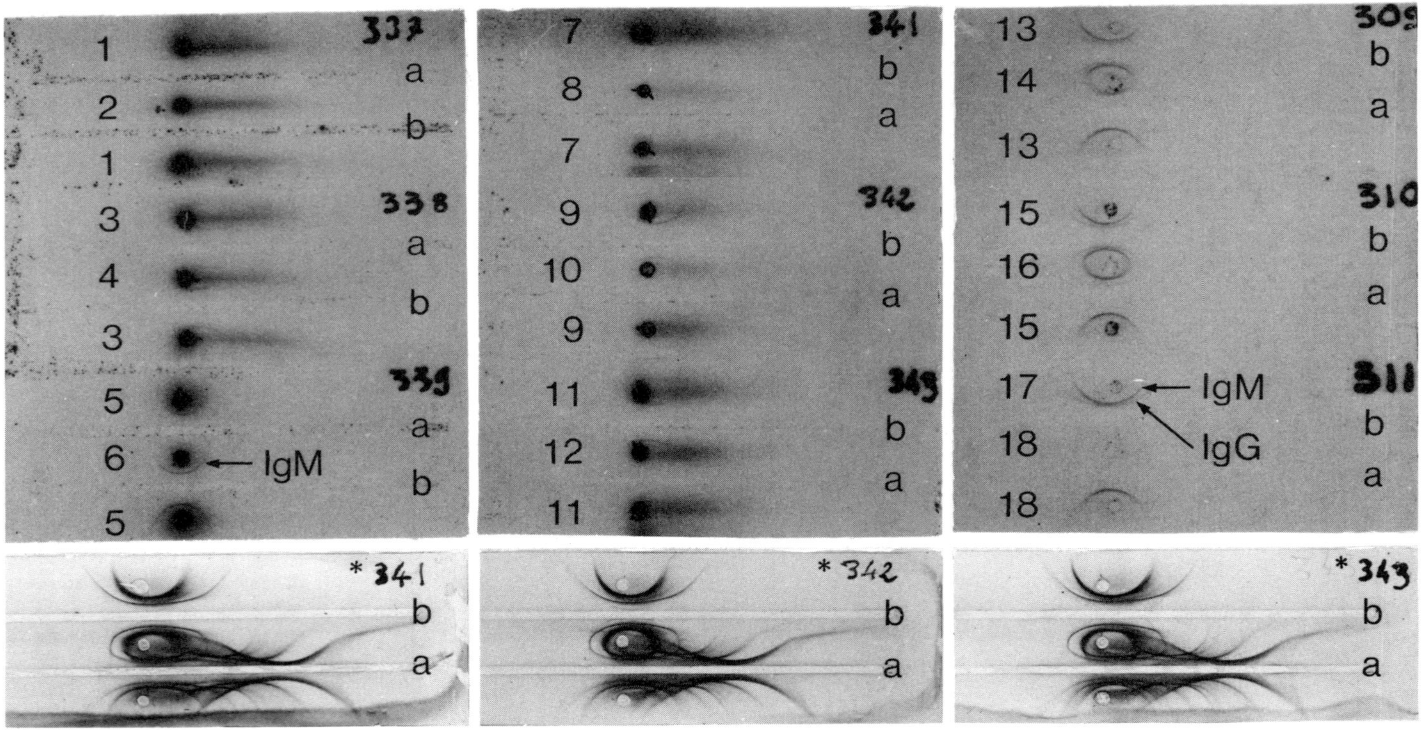

Fig. 15.2. Immunoglobulin production by thymus and spleen cells from young (5 months old) adult *Xenopus laevis*. ***In vitro*** biosynthesis (Du Pasquier & Feinstein, unpublished).

Culture conditions: 5×10^5 lymphocytes in 0·1 ml of L_{15} Medium. 28°C. ^{14}C Leucine pulse: Day 2 to 3, 4 μCi per culture. Supernatant analysed by immunoelectrophoresis after addition of 20 per cent carrier *Xenopus* serum. Autoradiography: Kodirex film, 3 weeks' exposure.

Numbers 1–18 correspond to different individuals.

(2A) *337–343*: Thymus cell cultures. Production of small amounts of IgM only.

(2B) *309–311*: Spleen cell cultures. Production of IgM and IgG (IgG is distinct only when samples were revealed with anti-Ig antiserum (b)). All samples were revealed by rabbit anti-total *Xenopus* serum proteins antiserum (a) and by rabbit anti-total *Xenopus* Ig antiserum (b). Compare slides 309 and 339 where similar amounts of Ig were produced. However, only IgM can be detected in the thymus.

(2C) *341–343*: Immunoelectrophoresis stained with Amido-Schwarz stain.

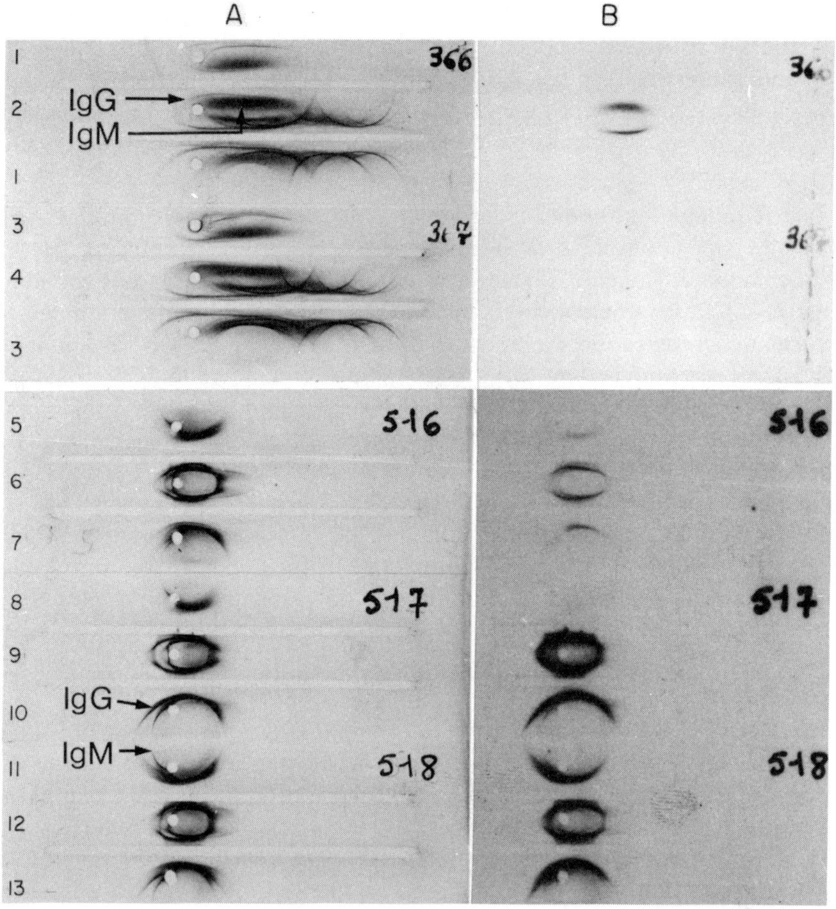

Fig. 15.3. Production of anti-DNP antibodies by *Rana catesbiana* detected by autoradiography (according to Rosenquist & Hoffman 1972): iodinated (^{131}I) α-N-(3,5 diiodo-4-hydroxyphenacetyl)-ε-N-DNP-lysine (kindly provided by Dr G. Roelants) is reacted with the anti-DNP antibodies precipitated by anti-immunoglobulin serum in immuno-electrophoresis. (A) Precipitation pattern. (B) Autoradiographs. *1–3*: Primary response of bullfrog tadpoles, 4 weeks after injection of 40 μg of DNP-KLH. Each serum has been precipitated with anti-total Ig antiserum and with anti-total serum antiserum to detect eventual non-specific binding. Note: (1) the presence of IgM and IgG in tadpole serum, (2) the occurrence of IgM antibodies only in the corresponding autoradiographs, (3) the apparent restricted heterogeneity of the anti-DNP antibodies. *4*: Unimmunized control. *5–8*: Primary response of adults 3 months after metamorphosis. Peritoneal fluid 3 weeks after injection of 2 μg of DNP-KLH. Notice animal 6 producing IgG and IgM antibodies. Animals 5, 7 and 8 produce only IgM. *9–13*: Adults' secondary response. These animals were primed during larval life with 40 μg of DNP-KLH and boosted 3 months after metamorphosis with 2 μg of DNP-KLH. Peritoneal fluids 3 weeks after the second injection. All animals produce large amounts of IgG antibodies.

changes of the expression of Ig on thymocytes. This may suggest either the differentiation of a new population of thymus cells able to cooperate and expressing less Ig on their surface or the modification of surface characteristics due to an external influence. There seems to be the correlation 'the more mature the less immunoglobulins detectable on thymus derived cells'.

In Urodeles, antibodics from larval and adult individuals are always of the IgM type (Fougereau & Houdayer 1968, Houdayer & Fougereau 1972, Marchalonis & Cohen 1973) and no natural IgG can be detected. It would be interesting to see whether this is due to the lack of a thymus function and to repeat in Urodeles the experiments done in *Xenopus* on surface immunoglobulins, the prediction being that thymus immunoglobulins would be detected equally well during the whole life.

In summary, the amphibian development thus offers a model where two thymus-dependent functions mature at different times. Reactivity in MLR is the earliest to appear in larval life and is independent of Ig expression on thymocytes. Thymic function mediating IgG antibody synthesis seems to develop in adults after metamorphosis and in relation with the post-metamorphic lower expression of Ig at the surface of thymus lymphocytes.

Origin of antibody diversity

Whether the acquisition of antibody diversity is due to a germinal or to a somatic process can be suggested by experiments done during the ontogenetic development of the individuals (e.g. Silverstein 1973, Spear *et al.* 1973). The fact that many species of amphibians have larvae displaying immune capacity together with a simple lymphoid system (i.e. with a small number of lymphocytes) makes these animals a very suitable model for this type of approach. For a few years, thanks to miniaturization and adaptation of amphibians of antibody assays at the cellular level (plaque and rosette technique) or humoral level (phage inactivation) such studies are possible in very young animals, possessing less than 1×10^6 lymphocytes.

Antibody production during the ontogeny: cellular aspects

That tadpoles were able to synthesize antibodies to various antigens has been well demonstrated by Cooper *et al.* (1964) and Cooper and Hildemann (1965) but real ontogenic studies have been achieved only more recently in *Xenopus* (Kidder *et al.* 1973) and in *Alytes obstetricans* (Du Pasquier 1970a,b,c). In these two species the ontogeny of the immune response to various red cell antigens has been followed by the means of cellular techniques. Spleen cells removed from animals at various stages of their ontogeny were assayed for antigen binding either without previous immunization, or after injections of red cells. In both species the spleen of non-immune tadpoles contained cells which bound the red cells and in both species the proportion of these natural rosette-forming cells were higher in the younger and smaller spleens (containing as few as 10^3 cells). A decrease from about 1 per cent to 1 per thousand was observed in the proportion of natural rosette-forming cells to human red cells in *Alytes obstetricans* spleens. Whereas no natural rosette-forming cells were found in *Alytes* thymus, such cells were observed in *Xenopus* but their frequency was about 10 per cent of that measured in the spleen.

In both species injections of red cells have been performed at various stages of the development of the lymphoid system and the results were quite similar in the two species. There exists a period before the number of splenic lymphocytes reaches 10^4 during which no response to the antigen can be detected. Whether the injections of red cells at that time induce tolerance is not yet known. From the moment the spleen reaches 10^4 cells, increased numbers of rosettes can be detected a few days after injection (4 to 8 days according to the route of injection). In *Alytes obstetricans* the occurrence of plaque-forming cells coincided with that of increased numbers of rosettes after injection. No background plaque-forming cells could be observed in young tadpoles. In both species the rosette-forming cells bound the antigen specifically (for review see Du Pasquier 1973). The proportion of rosette, forming cells or plaque-forming cells, and the kinetics of the response seems to be the same in young larvae (about 3 weeks old) and in adults. According to the species and the technique, the responses during larval life may vary. Moticka *et al.* (1973) for instance reported a number of the order of 3×10^3 plaques per million in *Rana catesbiana*, whereas only 10^2 plaques per million were found in *Alytes*; high antigen dose, and source of amphibian complement may be sufficient to explain the improved results of Moticka *et al.* (1973) as well as the detection of plaque-forming cells in the thymus.

Secondary response has been studied at the cellular level in *Alytes obstetricans* (Du Pasquier 1970). Seventeen days after an intraperitoneal injection which had led to a primary response of 5×10^5 rosettes of sheep red cells per million on day 10, the animals were reinjected with the same antigen. The peak of the response was reached on day 4 after the second injection but the number of rosettes was not very much higher than in the primary response (9×10^2 per million instead of 5×10^2).

Antibody production during the ontogeny: humoral aspects

The rather gross specificity of the immune responses determined by the cellular assays could not allow a precise estimation of the quality of antibodies produced by animals possessing small numbers of lymphocytes. Therefore, the specificities of tadpoles antibodies to single nitrophenyl haptenic determinants were examined (Haimovich & Du Pasquier 1973). This could be achieved with the technique of inactivation of dinitrophenylated (DNP)-bacteriophage T_4 (DNP-T_4) and trinitrophenylated T_4 (TNP-T_4) and its inhibition with various concentrations of hapten coupled to lysine. This assay does provide a reliable relative estimate of the relative affinities and cross-reactivity of antibodies. Inhibition tests were performed with the peritoneal fluid of tadpoles of *Rana catesbiana* tadpoles weighing between 0·6 and 1·8 g and having about $1\text{–}2 \times 10^6$ lymphocytes. The data (Table 15.1) showed that anti-DNP antibodies (almost exclusively IgM as stated in the section on thymus and immunoglobulin synthesis) obtained after a single injection of DNP-keyhole limpet haemocyanin (DNP-KLH) in complete Freund's adjuvant were more effectively inhibited by DNP-lysine than by TNP-lysine. In contrast, TNP-lysine and DNP-lysine were almost exclusively equally efficient in inhibiting anti-TNP antibodies. In practically all cases mononitrophenyl-lysine (MNP) was the poorest inhibitor of both anti-TNP and anti-DNP antibodies. In summary, antibodies elicited by immunization with DNP-pneumococci and DNP-KLH were highly specific for the DNP group. Antibodies from tadpoles immunized with TNP-KLH showed a different pattern of specificity. Relative affinities of anti-DNP on anti-TNP antibodies were 12·0 and 1·3 respectively. The difference is highly significant ($p < 0{\cdot}001$) and is similar to that observed in guinea-pigs or rabbits (Little & Eisen 1967, Yoshida *et al.* 1970). Moreover, inhibition of inactivation of DNP-T_4 by anti-DNP IgM antibodies from goat required the same concentration of hapten as in the tadpole system (Haimovich & Fuchs, unpublished).

More recently maturation of the antibody response has been investigated in this species (Du Pasquier & Haimovich, 1974). In *Rana catesbiana* natural anti-DNP antibodies are of low affinity: 3×10^4 M of inhibitor are needed to obtain about 50 per cent inhibition of the inactivation of the modified phage. During the 3 weeks following one injection of 20 μg of DNP-KLH the affinity of IgM antibodies will increase about 10 times. Cross-reaction with TNP will decrease concomitantly. Adult bullfrogs upon the same stimulation behave in a similar fashion although after 4 weeks IgG antibodies are detected. In tadpoles the small amount of IgG antibodies which can be detected (see the thymus and immunoglobulin synthesis) do not increase in affinity.

Multiple injections of antigen to tadpoles did not promote a significant secondary response. Red cell antigens provoke an accelerated response but not higher than the primary response in *Rana catesbiana* (Moticka *et al.* 1973).

During metamorphosis the response is weaker than in larvae, as measured by the variations of haemagglutination titres (Moticka *et al.* 1973). The response was at least three titres less than that of control tadpoles. There is little doubt that the decrease in the number of lymphocytes detected in *Xeno-*

Table 15.1. Inhibition with nitrophenyl derivatives of lysine of the inactivation of DNP-T_4 and TNP-T_4 by peritoneal fluids from *Rana catesbiana* individuals immunized with DNP-Pneumococci, DNP-KLH and TNP-KLH. All samples taken 3 weeks after injections.

	Inhibition concentration ($\times 10^6$ M) required for 50 per cent inhibition $\pm$ S.E.								
	Larvae $< 2 \times 10^6$ lymphocytes			Larvae $> 2 \times 10^6$ lymphocytes			Adults 3 months after metamorphosis		
	DNP-lys	TNP-lys	MNP-lys	DNP-lys	TNP-lys	MNP-lys	DNP-lys	TNP-lys	MNP-lys
Anti-DNP antibodies	2·4 ± 0·6	14·4 ± 4·3 (16)*	65 ± 12·1	1·1 ± 0·6	7·0 ± 1·8 (12)	> 100	2·1 ± 3·5	13·0 ± 4.2 (4)	> 100
Anti-TNP antibodies	33·5 ± 8·3	24·3 ± 4.7 (23)	204 ± 56	120 ± 60·2	49·3 ± 19·5 (5)	> 200		Not done	

* Number of animals

pus also occurs in *Rana catesbiana* and has an influence on the antibody response. Further studies should elucidate whether the response is weakened because of an overall loss in lymphocytes or because selective type of cells involved in cooperation disappear at this time. From the curve of Fig. 15.16 it seems that thymus cells are more affected than splenic cells by the metamorphosis. The important changes of metamorphosis do not seem to affect the pool of memory cells in *Rana catesbiana*. Excellent secondary responses were obtained in adults which had been previously injected with 20 μg of DNP-KLH during larval life. A second injection of 2 μg three months after metamorphosis led to an accelerated response (peak at 20°C: 2 instead of 3 weeks) and 10 times higher (constant of phage neutralization K (minutes) = 100 instead of 10).

This response is characterized by early appearance of IgG (Fig. 15.3) and high specificity and affinity of the antibodies as soon as they are detected.

Discussion

The development of the immune system in tadpoles is characterized: (1) by its fast development (about 21 days from fertilization) and (2) by the small number of lymphocytes present when apparently full immunological competence is reached. These are the two points which deserve attention from the point of view of general immunology since they indirectly suggest mechanisms involved in acquisition of antibody diversity.

The immunologically competent tadpoles, able to reject cell grafts, to give mixed lymphocyte reaction, to synthesize specific antibodies have about 1 to 2 million lymphocytes, at least in *Rana catesbiana*, *Alytes obstetricans* and *Xenopus laevis*. In trying to estimate the number of clones available to respond to any particular antigenic determinant one must consider that only a fraction of these cells have immunoglobulin molecules on their surface (Du Pasquier *et al.* 1972) and that some of them are already engaged in the secretion of immunoglobulins and therefore not likely to function as precursor antigen sensitive cells. Furthermore, each clone is likely to be composed of a few cells (perhaps ten in resting clones, and a few hundreds in expanding ones). All the remaining lymphocytes have probably not reached the proper stage of maturity allowing them to function as antigen sensitive cells. Altogether the number of potentially responding clones in a single tadpole may amount to fewer than 10^4. Other studies have shown that a primary antibody response can be obtained in an *in vitro* system where the number of lymphocytes was of the order of 10^4 (Auerbach 1970). However, the fine specificity of the antibodies was not determined and it remained possible that the potential number of antibodies produced was quite small but that the antibodies cross-reacted extensively with other antigenic determinants. The study on DNP-

TNP cross-reactivity in *Rana catesbiana* excludes this possibility at least for anti-DNP and anti-TNP antibodies. How can a system with about 10^4 clones of antigen-sensitive cells produce antibodies discriminating antigens as well as higher vertebrates where the minimum number of different kinds of antibody molecules required to cover the vast spectrum of antigen specificities has always been estimated to be at least 1 million (Jerne 1955, Haurowitz 1967). The difficulty is emphasized by the apparent unipotentiality of each cell which produces only a single kind of antibody molecule at least at one time. It seems necessary to consider seriously the possibility that a given cell or its progeny expresses different specificities at different times, thereby increasing the number of specificities over a period of time. According to Cunningham (1973) the antigen would be responsible for the increase in antibody diversity. The hypothesis is based on the changes which take place during the maturation of an antibody response after the injection of antigen. If this hypothesis is correct an adult animal which has encountered more natural antigens than the young larvae should probably have a larger repertoire than the larva. For the DNP-TNP system it does not seem to be the case since natural anti-DNP and anti-TNP antibodies are apparently as bad in larvae and adult. Moreover, the maturation of the response follows the same pattern in larvae and adults.

The very fast development of the immune system in tadpoles (about 15 days or less from the day of appearance of the first lymphocytes) together with the small number of cells, lets one expect that the number of cell divisions necessary to produce the pool of immunologically competent lymphocytes is of the order of 15–18 if one starts with one lymphocyte precursor. If the primary repertoire is acquired by somatic mutation mechanisms the characteristic of amphibian development would demand an extremely high and unrealistic rate of successful mutations since the 5×10^5 cells of the animal should represent 10^3 or 10^4 different clones to account for the specific responses which have been recorded. Therefore, results obtained in amphibians would be easier to reconcile with a germ-line mechanism for acquisition of the antibody diversity at least as far as primary IgM repertoire is concerned. Because of the small number of lymphocytes present in the larval animals, it is also suggested that the primary antibody repertoire does not represent the whole set of antibody specificities which the animal can make. Therefore the maturation process that has been observed in tadpoles could mean that the antibody diversity is increased after the triggering of cell divisions by antigens.

Conclusion

Ontogenic studies in amphibians seem to have produced data on immunological tolerance, thymus function, origin of antibody diversity which are of good standard from the theoretical point of view. However, it is clear that most immunologists put a barrier between mammalian and lower vertebrate immunology. Obviously amphibians are not yet as good models as some mammalian or bird species, mainly because of the paucity of inbred strains*. The other reason why many immunologists do not take an interest in amphibians is what can be called the 'phylogenetic prejudice' which leads everyone to doubt about the general value of results obtained in lower vertebrates. It is clear from the present chapter that this prejudice does not apply to ontogenic studies in amphibians and moreover many experiments such as long-term observations of thymectomized animals without runt, embryonic development without materno-fetal interaction, preparation of chimeras are *easier* to perform in amphibians. This could stimulate further studies in this field.

References

AUERBACH R. (1970) Cellular differentiation and antibody variability. *Amer. Zool.* **10,** 319.

BACULI B.S. & COOPER E.L. (1973) Lymphoid changes during antibody synthesis in larval *Rana catesbiana. J. Exp. Zool.* **183,** 185.

BERNARDINI N., CHARDONNENS X. & SIMON D. (1969a) Développement après la métamorphose de compétences immunologiques envers les homogreffes cutanées chez *Xenopus laevis. C. R. Acad. Sci. Paris (D).* **269,** 1011.

BERNARDINI N., CHARDONNENS X. & SIMON D. (1969b) Etude du comportement immunologique chez *Xenopus laevis* en prèsence de deux greffes cutanées différentes. *C. R. Acad. Sci. Paris (D).* **269,** 1107.

BERNARDINI N., CHARDONNENS X. & SIMON D. (1970) Tolérance des allogreffes cutanées chez *Xenopus laevis* Influence de la taille et de l'âge du greffon. *C. R. Acad. Sci. Paris (D).* **270,** 2351.

BILLINGHAM R. & SILVERS W. (1971) *The immunobiology of transplantation*, p. 41. Prentice-Hall, Englewood Cliffs, N.J.

BOVBJERG A.M. (1966) Rejection of skin homografts in larvae of *Rana pipiens. J. Exp. Zool.* **161,** 69.

CEPPELLINI R., BONNARD G.D., COPPO P., MIGGIANO V.C., POSPISIL M., CURTONI E.S. & PELLEGRINO, M. (1971) Mixed leukocyte cultures and HLA antigens. I. Reactivity of young fetuses, newborns and mothers at delivery. *Transplant. Proc.* **III,** 58.

CHARDONNENS X. & DU PASQUIER L. (1973) Induction of skin allograft tolerance during metamorphosis of the toad *Xenopus laevis*: a possible model for studying generation of self-tolerance to histocompatibility antigens. *Eur. J. Immunol.* **3,** 569.

* **Note added in proofs:** Work has recently been published on

(1) Production of large clones of histocompatible fully identical clawed toads (*Xenopus*), H.R. KOBEL & L. DU PASQUIER (1975) *Immunogenetics*, **2,** 87.

(2) Obtention of histocompatible strains in the urodele amphibian *Pleurodeles waltii* Michali (Salamandridae). J. CHARLEMAGNE & A. TOURNETIER (1974) *J. Immunogenetics*, **1,** 125.

(3) Transplantation immunogenetics and MLC reactivity of partially inbred strains of Salamanders (A. Mericanum): preliminary studies. L.E. DE LANNEY, N.H. COLLINS, N. COHEN & R. REID (1975) *in Immunologic Phylogeny* W.H. HILDEMANN and A.A. BENEDICT (eds.) Plenum Press N.Y. 315.

CHARLEMAGNE J. (1973) Les réactions immunitaires chez les Amphibiens Urodèles. I. Résultats acquis et possibilités expérimentales, p. 86. In *L'Etude phylogénique et ontogénique de la réponse immunitaire et son apport à la théorié immunologique.* INSERM, Paris.

CLARK J.C. & NEWTH D.R. (1972) Immunological activity of transplanted spleens in *Xenopus laevis. Experientia* **28,** 951.

COHEN N. (1969) Immunogenetic and developmental aspects of tissue transplantation immunity in Urodele amphibians, p. 153. In *Biology of amphibian tumors*, ed. Mizell M. Springer-Verlag, New York.

COHEN N. (1971) Amphibian transplantation reaction: a review. *Amer. Zool.* **11,** 193.

COOPER E.L., PINKERTON W. & HILDEMANN W.H. (1964) Serum antibody synthesis in larvae of the bullfrog *Rana catesbiana. Biol. Bull.* **127,** 232.

COOPER E.L. & HILDEMANN W.H. (1965) Allograft reaction in bullfrog larvae in relation to thymectomy. *Transplantation* **3,** 446.

COOPER E.L. & HILDEMANN W.H. (1965) The immune response of larval bullfrog *Rana catesbiana* to diverse antigens. *Ann. N.Y. Acad. Sci.* **126,** 647.

COOPER E.L. (1973) The thymus and lymphomyeloid system in poikilothermic vertebrates, p. 13. In *Contemp. Top. in Immunol.* **2,** eds Davies A.J.S. & Carter R.L. Plenum Press, New York.

CUNNINGHAM A.J. & PILARSKI, L.M. (1974) Antibody diversity: a case for its generation after antigenic stimulation. *Scand. J. Immunol.* **3,** 5.

CURTIS S.K. & VOLPE E.P. (1971) Modification of responsiveness to allografts in larvae of the leopard frog by thymectomy. *Devl. Biol.* **25,** 177.

DASGUPTA S. (1962) Induction of triploidy by hydrostatic pressure. *J. exp. Zool.* **151,** 105.

DAVISON J. (1963) Gene action mechanisms in the determination of color and pattern in the frog (*Rana pipiens*) *Science* **141,** 648.

DAVISON J. (1966) Chimeric and ex-parabiotic frogs (*Rana pipiens*): Specificity of tolerance. *Science* **152,** 1250.

DEPARIS P. (1968) Hématopoièse embryonnaire et larvaire chez l'Amphibien Urodèle *Pleurodeles waltlii Michah. Ann. Embryol. Morph.* **1,** 107.

DU PASQUIER L. (1965) Recherches sur les aspects cellulaires et humoraux de l'intolérance aux homogreffes chez le têtard d'*Alytes obstetricans* Thèse 3ᵉ cycle Enseignement Supérieur no. 336, Bordeaux.

DU PASQUIER L. (1968) Les protéines sériques et le complexe lymphomyéloide chez le têtard d'*Alytes obstetricans* normal et thymectomisé. *Ann. Inst. Pasteur* **114,** 490.

DU PASQUIER L. (1970a) Ontogeny of the immune response in animals having less than one million lymphocytes: the larvae of the toad *Alytes obstetricans. Immunology* **19,** 353.

DU PASQUIER L. (1970b) Immunologic competence of lymphoid cells in young amphibian larvae. *Transplant. Proc.* **2,** 293.

DU PASQUIER L. (1970c) L'acquisition de la compétence immunologique chez les Vertébrés. Etude chez la larve du crapaud accoucheur *Alytes obstetricans.* Thèse Doctorat ès Sciences no. 290, Bordeaux.

DU PASQUIER L., WEISS N. & LOOR F. (1973) Direct evidence for immunoglobulins on the surface of thymus lymphocytes of amphibian larvae. *Eur. J. Immunol.* **2,** 366.

DU PASQUIER L. (1973) Ontogeny of the immune response in cold blooded vertebrates. *Cur. Top. Microbiol. Immunol.* **61,** 37.

DU PASQUIER L. & MIGGIANO V.C. (1973) The mixed leucocyte reaction in the toad *Xenopus laevis*: a family study. *Transplant. Proc.* **4,** 1457.

DU PASQUIER L. & WEISS N. (1973) The thymus during the ontogeny of the toad *Xenopus laevis*: growth, membrane bound immunoglobulins and mixed lymphocyte reaction. *Eur. J. Immunol.* **3,** 773.

Du Pasquier L. & Haimovich J. (1974) Changes in affinity of IgM antibodies in amphibian larvae. *Eur. J. Immunol.* **4,** 580.

Du Pasquier L. & Horton J.D. (1976) The effect of thymectomy on the mixed leukocyte reaction and phytohemmagglutinin responsiveness in the clawed toad *Xenopus laevis. Immunogenetics* **3,** 105.

Fougereau M. & Houdayer M. (1968) Immunoglobulines et réponse immunitaire chez l'Axolotl, *Ambystoma mexicanum. Ann. Inst. Pasteur* **115,** 968.

Gebhardt B.M. & Volpe E.P. (1973) Immunity and tolerance to embryonic tail allografts in the leopard frog. *Transplantation* **15,** 189.

Geczy C.L., Green P.C. & Steiner L.A. (1973) Immunoglobulins in the developing amphibian *Rana catesbiana. J. Immunol.* **111,** 1261.

Haimovich J. & Du Pasquier L. (1973) Specificity of antibodies in amphibian larvae possessing a small number of lymphocytes. *Proc. Nat. Acad. Sci. USA* **70,** 1898.

Haurowitz F. (1967) The evolution of selective and instructive theories of antibody formation. *Cold Spring Harbor Symp. Quant. Biol.* **32,** 559.

Hellström K.E. & Hellström I. (1972) The role of serum factors (blocking antibodies) as mediator of immunological non-reactivity to cellular antigens, p. 133. In *Ontogeny of acquired immunity*, eds Porter R. & Knight J. Ciba Found. Symp. Elsevier. Excerpta Medica, North-Holland Publishing Co., Amsterdam.

Horton J.D. (1969) Ontogeny of the immune response to skin allografts in relation to lymphoid organ development in the Amphibian *Xenopus laevis* Daudin. *J. Exp. Zool.* **170,** 449.

Horton J.D. & Manning M.J. (1972) Response to skin allografts in *Xenopus laevis* following thymectomy at early stages of lymphoid organ maturation. *Transplantation* **14,** 141.

Houdayer M. & Fougereau M. (1972) Phylogénie des Immunoglobulines: La réaction immunitaire de l'axolotl *Ambystoma mexicanum.* Cinétique de la réponse immunitaire et caractérisation des anticorps. *Ann. Inst. Pasteur* **123,** 3.

Houillon C. (1973) Les réactions immunitaires chez les Amphibiens Urodèles. II. Interventions microchirurgicales sur les embryons, p. 97. In *L'Etude phylogénique et ontogénique de la réponse immunitaire et son apport à la théorie immunologique.* INSERM, Paris.

Kerbel R.S. & Eidinger D. (1972) Enhanced immune responsiveness to a thymus independent antigen early after thymectomy: evidence for a short-lived inhibitory thymus-derived cell. *Eur. J. Immunol.* **2,** 114.

Jerne N.K. (1955) The natural selection theory of antibody formation. *Proc. Nat. Acad. Sci. USA* **41,** 849.

Jones M.A.S. & Lafferty K.J. (1969) Characteristics of lymphocyte transfer reactions produced in sheep. *Aust. J. exp. Biol. Med. Sci.* **47,** 159.

Kidder G.M., Ruben L.N. & Stevens J.M. (1973) Cytodynamics and ontogeny of the immune response of *Xenopus laevis* against sheep erythrocytes. *J. Embryol. exp. Morph.* **29,** 73.

Killby V.A.A., Lafferty K.J. & Ryan M. (1972) Interaction of embryonic chicken spleen cells and adult allogeneic leucocytes. *Aust. J. exp. Biol. Med. Sci.* **50,** 309.

Little J.R. & Eisen H.N. (1967) Specificity of the immune response to the 2,4-dinitrophenyl and 2,4,6-trinitrophenyl groups. *J. Exp. Med.* **129,** 247.

MacGregor D.D. & Gowans J.L. (1964) Survival of homografts of skin in rats depleted of lymphocytes by chronic drainage from the thoracic duct. *Lancet* **i,** 629.

Manning M.J. (1971) The effect of early thymectomy on histogenesis of the lymphoid organs in *Xenopus laevis. J. Embryol. exp. Morph.* **26,** 219.

MANIATIS G.M., STEINER L.A. & INGRAM V.M. (1969) Tadpoles antibodies against frog hemoglobin and their effect on development. *Science* **165,** 67.

MARCHALONIS J.J. (1971) Ontogenetic emergence of immunoglobulins in *Rana pipiens. Develop. Biol.* **25,** 479.

MARCHALONIS J.J. & COHEN N. (1973) Isolation and partial characterization of immunoglobulin from a Urodele amphibian (*Necturus maculosus*). *Immunology* **24,** 395.

MARTINEZ C., SMITH J.M., SHAPIRO F. & GOOD R.A. (1959) Transfer of acquired immunological tolerance of skin homografts in mice joined in parabiosis. *Proc. Soc. Exp. Biol. Med.* **102,** 413.

MEO T., MATSUNAGA T. & RIJNBEEK A.M. (1973) On the mechanism of self-tolerance in embryo-fusion chimeras. *Transplant. Proc.* **4,** 1607.

MOTICKA E.J., BROWN B.A. & COOPER E.L. (1973) Immunoglobulin synthesis in bullfrog larvae. *J. Immunol.* **110,** 855.

NIEUWKOOP P.D. & FABER J. (1967) *Normal table of* Xenopus laevis *Daudin,* 2nd ed. Amsterdam North Holland Publishing Company.

ORFILA C. & DEPARIS P. (1970) Influence de l'âge du donneur et du receveur sur l'évolution des homogreffes cutanées chez les larves du triton *Pleurodeles waltlii* Michah. *Path. Biol.* **18,** 1033.

RIVIERE H.B. & COOPER E.L. (1973) Thyroxine-induced regression of tadpole lymph glands. *Proc. Soc. Exp. Biol. Med.* **143,** 320.

ROSENQUIST G.L. & HOFFMANN R.Z. (1972) The production of anti-DNP antibody in the bullfrog *Rana catesbiana. J. Immunol.* **108,** 1499.

RUBEN L.N. (1970) Immunological maturation and lymphoreticular cancer transformation in larval *Xenopus laevis* the South African clawed toad. *Develop. Biol.* **43,** 58.

RUBEN L.N., VAN DER HOVEN A. & DUTTON R.W. (1973) Cellular cooperation in hapten carrier responses in the Newt *Triturus viridescens. Cell. Immunology.* **6,** 300.

SILVERSTEIN A.M. An ontogenetic view of the generation of immunological diversity, p. 221. In *Phylogenic and ontogenic study of the immune response and its contribution to the immunological theory.* INSERM, Paris.

SLONIMSKY P. (1931) Recherches expérimentales sur la genèse du sang chez les Amphibiens. *Arch. Biol.* (*Liège*) **32,** 415.

SPEAR P.G., WANG A.L., RUTISHAUSER U. & EDELMAN G.M. (1973) Characterization of splenic lymphoid cells in fetal and newborn mice. *J. exp. Med.* **138,** 557.

STERBA G. (1950) Uber die morphologischen und histogenetischen Thymus probleme bei *Xenopus laevis* (Daudin) nebst einigen Bemerkungen über die Morphologie der Kaulquappe. *Abh. sächs. Akad. Wiss.* **44,** 1.

TAYLOR R.B. & WORTIS H.H. (1968) Thymus dependence of antibody response: variation with dose of antigen and class of antibody. *Nature,* **220,** 927.

TOURNEFIER A. (1973) Développement des organes lymphoides chez l'Amphibien Urodèle *Triturus alpestris* Laur; tolérance des allogreffes après la thymectomie larvaire. *J. Embryol. exp. Morph.* **29,** 383.

TOURNEFIER A. (1973b) Les réactions immunitaires chez les Amphibiens Urodèles III. Rôle du thymus dans l'immunité de transplantation. Capacité d'immunisation aux antigènes particulaires chez le Pleurodèle et le Triton alpestre adultes, p. 105. In *L'Etude phylogéniqe et ontogénique de la réponse immunitaire et son apport à la théorie, immunologique.* INSERM, Paris.

TRIPLETT E.L. (1958) The development of the sympathic ganglia, sheath cells and the meninges in amphibians. *J. Exp. Zool.* **138,** 283.

TRIPLETT E.L. (1962) On the mechanism of immunologic self recognition. *J. Immunol.* **89,** 505.

TURNER R.J. & MANNING M.J. (1974) Thymic dependence of amphibian antibody response. *Eur. J. Immunol.* **4,** 343.

TURPEN J.B., VOLPE E.P. & COHEN N. (1973) Ontogeny and peripheralization of thymic lymphocytes. *Science* **182,** 931.

VOISIN G.A., KINSKY R.G. & DUC H.T. (1972) Immune status of mice tolerant of living cells. II. Continuous presence and nature of facilitation enhancing antibodies in tolerant animals. *J. exp. Med.* **135,** 1185.

VOLPE E.P. (1964) Fate of neural crest homotransplants in pattern mutants of the leopard frog. *J. Exp. Zool.* **157,** 179.

VOLPE E.P. & GEBHARDT B.M. (1965) Effect of dosage on the survival of embryonic homotransplants in the leopard frog *Rana pipiens. J. Exp. Zool.* **160,** 11.

VOLPE E.P. & GEBHARDT B.M. (1966) Evidence from cultured leucocytes of blood cell chimerism in ex-parabiotic frogs. *Science* **154,** 1197.

VOLPE E.P. (1971) Immunological tolerance in Amphibians. *Am. Zool.* **11,** 207.

WEISS N. & DU PASQUIER, L. (1973) Factors affecting the reactivity of amphibian lymphocytes in a miniaturized technique of the mixed lymphocyte culture. *J. Immunol. Methods* **3,** 273.

WEISS N., HORTON J.D. & DU PASQUIER, L. (1973) The effect of thymectomy on cell surface associated and serum immunoglobulins in the toad *Xenopus laevis* (Daudin): A possible inhibitory role of the thymus on the expression of immunoglobulins, p. 135. In *L'Etude phylogénique et ontogénique de la réponse immunitaire et son apport à la théorie immunologique*. INSERM, Paris.

YOSHIDA T., PAUL W.E. & BENACERRAF B. (1970) Genetic control of the specificity of anti-DNP antibodies. I. Differences in the specificity of anti-DNP antibody produced by mammalian species. *J. Immunol.* **105,** 306.

Chapter 16. Ontogenesis of the Immune System in Birds

A. Szenberg

Introduction

Role of thymus derived cells in antibody production in the chicken
Lymphoid organs in the fowl

Development of lymphoid organs in ontogenesis
Bursa of Fabricius
Modification of bursa development by testosterone

Development of lymphoid organs in ontogenesis *continued*
Thymus
Bone marrow
Spleen

Development of immune competence

Antibody production

Introduction

The ability to produce specific immune responses, which appears first in the cyclostomes, is based anatomically on the presence of lymphoid organs and tissues—the immune system. In birds this system stands in its development between the one in reptiles and the one in mammals (Good & Finstad 1967). As in mammals, we can distinguish between primary (central) and secondary (peripheral) lymphoid organs.

The definition of a primary lymphoid organ which we use in this paper is as follows: (1) the first organ in which lymphopoiesis takes place in ontogenesis; (2) the lymphopoiesis is independent from antigenic stimulation; (3) elimination of the primary lymphoid organ early in ontogenesis inhibits the normal development of secondary lymphoid organs and development of immune responses; (4) under normal circumstances the immune response does not develop in a primary lymphoid organ.

In birds there exist two primary lymphoid organs: thymus and bursa of Fabricius. Their characterization as primary lymphoid organs and their function in ontogenesis of the immune system has been well established (Szenberg & Warner 1962, Warner *et al.* 1962, Isakovic *et al.* 1963, Cooper *et al.* 1965, 1966). As in mammals, the thymus produces precursors of cells involved in specific cell-mediated immune responses. Early removal of the thymus causes defects in ability of the bird to reject allogenic skin-grafts and produce delayed type skin reactions. Anatomically the defect is expressed in depletion of lymphocytes from the peri-arteriolar sheath in the white pulp of the spleen.

Role of thymus derived cells in antibody production in the chicken

Early experiments on the antibody production in thymectomized chicken produced contradictory results. Production of antibodies to human gamma-globulin (Szenberg & Warner 1962) and to human red cells (Isakovic *et al.* 1963) was found to be normal. Graetzer *et al.* (1963) studying large numbers of thymectomized chickens found that 6 per cent failed to respond to BSA. Similarly, Cooper *et al.* (1965) found no response to *Brucella abortus* in 5 out of 12 thymectomized chickens.

In more recent experiments using adoptive cell transfer into irradiated recipients synergistic effects have been found between thymus and bursa cells from 1-week-old donors. In older recipients this effect was less evident (McArthur *et al.* 1974).

Clear evidence for collaborative effect of carrier-sensitized T cells and hapten-immunized B cells was obtained in experiments of Weinbaum *et al.* (1973) and Sarvas *et al.* (1974).

In our experiments (Szenberg, unpublished results) incompletely thymectomized chickens (12 out of 14 lobes removed) produced 2–4 times more plaque-forming cells to sheep erythrocytes than age-and-sex matched normal controls.

Rouse and Warner (1974) did show that peripheral blood cells obtained from chicken, made tolerant to histocompatibility antigen, will reduce significantly the graft versus host reaction of normal blood lymphocytes when inoculated together with the active cells. They considered this finding as evidence for existence of repressor cells in tolerant birds.

The bursa of Fabricius exist only in birds and produces the precursors of antibody-forming cells. The equivalent of bursa of Fabricius in mammals has not been identified. Early and complete inhibition of bursal development causes complete inability to produce antibody responses and immunoglobulins. Absence of germinal centres in the spleen is the morphological mark of this deficiency.

Most of the work on the immune system in birds has been done on domestic fowl and our description will be based on this species.

Lymphoid organs in the fowl

Lymphoid organs in the domestic fowl have been described in detail by Payne (1971). In an adult chicken the thymus is comprised of 14 lobes, 7 located on each side of the neck, closely following the jugularis. The most proximal lobes are located just distal to the thyroid and parathyroid glands. Thymus reaches its maximal size at approximately 4 months of age and starts to atrophy shortly afterwards (Wolfe *et al.* 1962). Recrudescence of the thymus has been described in some birds (Hohn 1956) and in the fowl after treatment with thyroid hormone (Hohn 1959, Warner 1964). Bursa of Fabricius is a round or oval organ located behind the cloaca and connected with it by a short duct. It is usually larger in hens than in cockerels and reaches its maximal size at approximately 10 weeks of age and becomes completely atrophic (Wolfe *et al.* 1962) at between 5–6 months.

The secondary lymphoid organs in the chicken are: the spleen; various agglomerations of lymphoid cells along the intestinal tract, the largest being the coecal tonsil located at the caudal end of the coecum, with germinal centres. According to Bäck (1970, 1971) they contain both thymus-dependent and bursa-dependent lymphocytes. Mammalian type lymph nodes have been described in some bird species (Jolly, quoted by Payne 1971), but are absent in others, including chickens.

Other lymphoid structures common to all bird species are small agglomerations of lymphoid cells in the lumen of lymphoid vessels. They are known under the name of mural nodules (Biggs 1957). After local antigenic stimulus these nodules can develop germinal centres (Good *et al.* 1967).

Development of lymphoid organs in ontogenesis

Bursa of Fabricius

Bursa rudiment starts to form on the 4th day of incubation as epithelial proliferation along the ventral–caudal area of contact between cloacal rudiment and ectodermal surface epithelium (Ruth *et al.* 1964). Between 6 and 8 days of incubation the epithelial cord develops a central lumen which connects with the lumen of cloacal rudiment. The bursa rotates to a vertical position and grows on a cylindrical stalk (Payne 1971). The first epithelial plicae develop between days 9–10 of incubation and increase in number till days 17–18.

The following results have been obtained in our laboratory (Szenberg unpublished observations). The first haemopoietic stem cells can be seen in the mesenchyme of the bursal rudiment at 11th day of incubation and start moving into the epithelium between 11th and 12th days (Fig. 16.1). Their arrival via circulation and origin from the yolk has been documented, in parabiosis and culture experiments (Moore & Owen 1966).

Entry of the stem cell into the epithelium starts multiplication of both epithelial and lymphoid cells in this area, which produces a follicular structure (Fig. 16.2). The follicle grows fast and pushes into the sub-epithelial

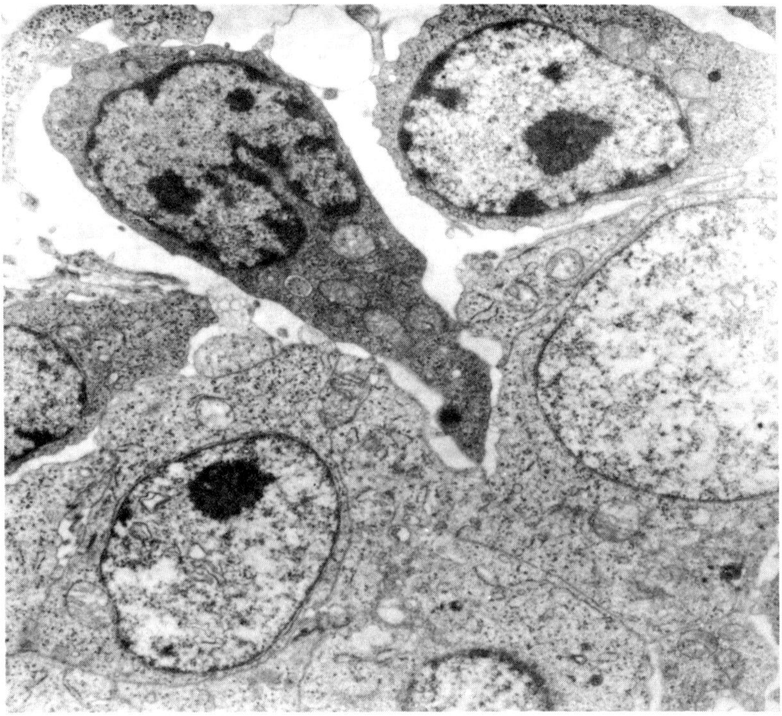

Fig. 16.1. 12-day-old chick embryo bursa. Two stem cells entering the epithelium.

mesenchyme and finally separates from the epithelium (Fig. 16.3). The increase in the number of lymphoid cells in the developing bursa has been assessed by preparing cell suspensions from 50–100 organs of different age embryos and counting the cells with blast and lymphocyte morphology.

The 12-day-old bursa contains approximately 13×10^3 cells. The largest increase, approximately 10-fold, takes place between the 13th and 14th days of incubation. Most probably this corresponds to the largest influx of stem cells from the circulation. At the 20th day already approximately 6×10^6 lymphocytes are present in the bursa.

Similar cell suspensions have been used to establish the appearance and number of cells carrying surface immunoglobulins. The total of Ig positive cells and cells positive for IgM and IgG have been enumerated in autoradiographs using sandwich technique: rabbit anti-chicken IgG and I^{125}, sheep anti-rabbit immunoglobulins. Anti-chicken IgA was not available at that time. The results are presented in Table 16.1. Two points of interest emerge. First, the surface Ig-positive cells appear only a few hours after the first stem cells arrive in the epithelium of the bursal rudiment. The stem cell population from 10- and 12-day embryonic yolk does not contain any Ig-positive cells.

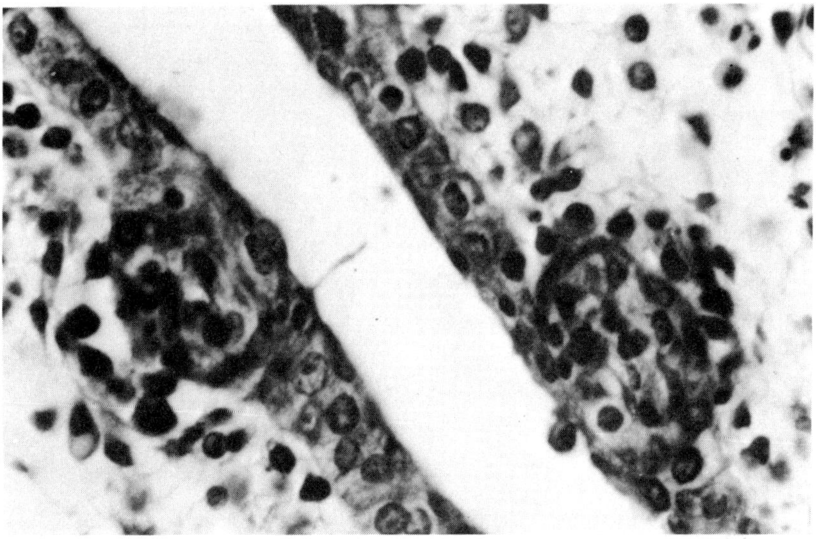

Fig. 16.2. 12-day-old chick embryo bursa. Two early stages of follicle development.

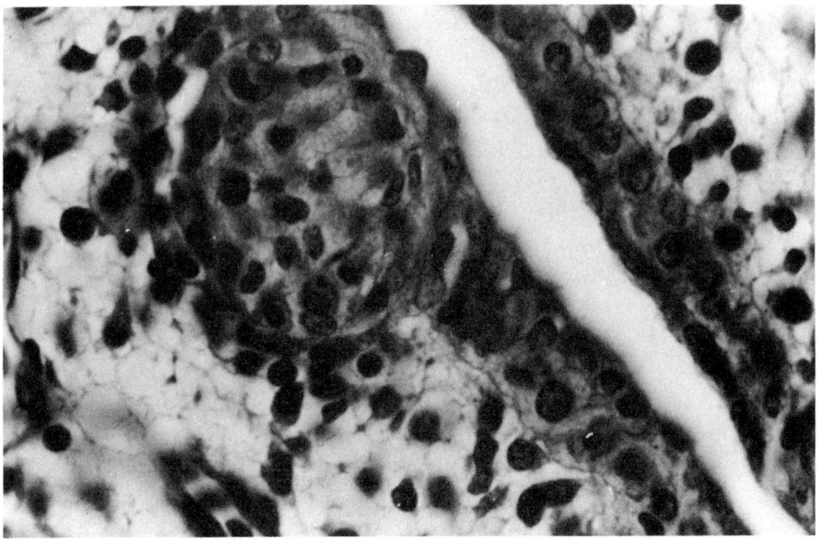

Fig. 16.3. 12-day-old chick embryo bursa. Follicle now located mostly in the mesenchyme. Notice the cuboidal type of the epithelial layer.

Table 16.1. The appearance and number of cells in suspension carrying surface immunoglobulins.

Day of incubation	Lymphoid cells/bursa × 10^{-4}	Ig positive (%)	Percentage of Ig-positive cells binding antibodies to IgM	IgG	Both*
12	1·33	7·5	100	0	0
13	1·64	10	65	40	0
14	18·2	20	73	30	0
15	53·0	46	71·5	7	0
16	114·7	65	76·5	5	0
17	238·5	53	91	75	66
18	510	59	80	96	76
20	575	88	90	70	60

* (Percentage cells positive for IgM + percentage cells positive for IgG) − Percentage cells positive for Ig.

This means that one, or at a maximum, two divisions are enough to differentiate the stem cells into committed precursor cells. The second point of interest is that at days 17–20 of incubation the total of IgM plus IgG-positive cells is approximately 160 per cent of the number of Ig-positive cells. This indicates that at this stage of development a massive switch from IgM to IgG cells takes place. Kincade & Cooper (1971a), using immunofluorescent techniques on bursal section, did observe, directly, cells staining for both IgG and IgM. Their results, if corrected for difference of sensitivity between autoradiographic and fluorescent techniques are essentially the same as ours. The IgM-positive cells in ontogenesis of the antibody-forming system seem to be the precursors of both IgG and IgA producing cells. This has been shown in experiments of Kincade *et al.* (1970), Martin and Leslie (1972) and Leslie and Martin (1973), in which treatment of the embryos at appropriate times with heterologous anti-IgM serum prevented development of IgG- and IgA-producing cells in chickens grown from such treated embryos.

Modification of bursal development by testosterone

Mayer *et al.* (1959) observed that injection of chicken embryos with 19-nor-testosterone will inhibit partially or completely the development of the bursa. Warner and Burnet (1961) obtained the same results using testosterone propionate. We have observed (Szenberg & Warner 1962) that in approximately 30 per cent of the treated embryos variable degrees of inhibition of thymus development did take place. In approximately 3 per cent of the hormone-treated embryos a complete atrophy of the thymus was produced.

In experiments described below (Szenberg 1970 and unpublished results) embryos were injected at 8th day of incubation with 2 mg of testosterone propionate (Schering, A.G.) into the allantoic cavity. The first visible effect, apparent already in 10-day bursal rudiments, was a change in the morphology of the epithelium lining the bursal lumen. In normal embryos this lining consists of two layers of undifferentiated cuboidal cells (Fig. 16.3). In the treated embryos the rudiment consists of columnar type cells (Fig. 16.4). PAS stain reveals that these cells secrete a mucous material.

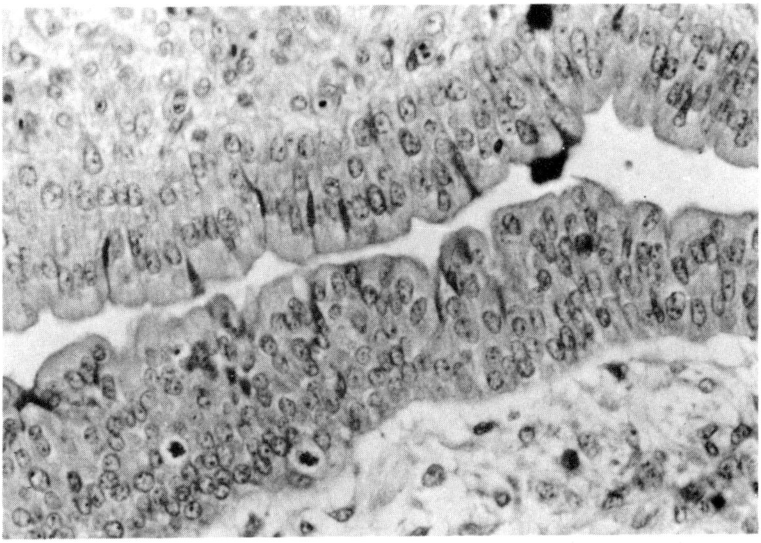

Fig. 16.4. 12-day-old chick embryo bursa. Embryo injected into the allantoic cavity with 2 mg of testosterone propionate at 8th day of incubation. Notice the columnar type of epithelium.

In electronmicrographs taken at 12th day of incubation haemopoietic stem cells can be seen in the mesenchyme of the bursa rudiment but no cells can be observed entering the epithelial layer. The obvious explanation of this finding is that testosterone forcibly matured the epithelium of the bursal rudiment to an adult type intestinal epithelium and in this way removed the proper microenvironment for multiplication and differentiation of stem cells into lymphocytes.

The possibility that the stem cell population itself has been modified by the action of testosterone has been excluded by the following experiments. Ten-day-old bursal rudiments from normal and hormone-treated embryos were placed on the chorioallantoic membranes of 10-day-old normal recipients and incubated for 7–8 days. As has been described by Moore and Owen (1966) normal rudiments become colonized by host stem cells and developed lymphoid follicles. The rudiments from testosterone treated embryos remained purely epithelial and the change of epithelial cells from cuboidal to columnar was obvious. The action of testosterone seems to be very fast and irreversible because bursa rudiments removed and placed in normal recipients only 3 hours after hormone injection did show significant suppression of lymphoid development.

These observations indicate that development and function of the lymphoid system may be influenced by action of hormones on the epithelial part of primary lymphoid organs. Examples of such a situation have been quoted on page 421 (Hohn 1956, 1959, Warner 1964), and others have been described in mammals (Pierpaoli *et al.* 1969, Castro 1974).

Thymus

The thymus rudiment develops from the third and fourth pharyngeal pouches (Hamilton 1952). According to Hammond (1958) both ectoderm and entoderm participate in formation of epithelial cord extending along the jugularis on the fifth day of incubation. The cords separate from the pharynx in the next 12 hours and at 6 days have a basement membrane dividing them from the mesenchyme.

The first haemopoietic stem cells are visible in the mesenchyme surrounding the rudiment at 7 days and at 8 days migrate into the epithelium. The origin of these cells from the yolk have been experimentally documented by Moore and Owen (1967c). After 9 days of incubation the thymus rudiment becomes vascularized and is predominantly lymphoidal from the 12th day.

The differentiation of the stem cells into lymphocytes in the chicken thymus has not been timed because of lack of appropriate markers.

In the mouse, 13-day-old embryonic thymus rudiment contains already θ-positive cells (Mandel, personal communication). This would correspond to approximately 9-day-old chick embryo thymus.

The time of the beginning of migration of lymphocytes out of the thymus has not been established but as discussed later, cells competent to produce graft versus host reaction seem to be present in 17–18-day-old embryonic spleen after antigenic stimulation.

Bone marrow

The bone marrow cavity develops in the calcified cartilage of long bones through penetration of perichondrial mesenchyme and blood vessels (Bloom 1938). This takes place between the 8th and 9th days of incubation. At the 12th day of incubation large basophilic cells can be observed in the marrow capillaries. Parabiosis experiments of Moore and Owen (1965, 1967a,b) using chromosome markers indicate that these cells arrive from the circulation and most probably originate in the yolk. The presence of lymphoid stem cells in the bone marrow has been investigated by Moore and Owen (1967b). They found that bone marrow cells from 17-day-old embryos can repopulate lymphoid tissues of irradiated embryos. As in mammals, the bone marrow is the source of haemopoietic stem cells during the lifespan of the fowl (Bäck 1972). Antibody-forming cell precursors can be found in the bone marrow of normal chickens, but not in bursectomized ones (Ivanyi *et al.* 1972) which indicates that they do not originate in the marrow itself.

Spleen

A detailed description of the development of splenic rudiment in the chick embryo has been provided by DeLanney (DeLanney & Ebert 1962). It appears as mesenchymal condensation at day 4 of incubation and capillaries begin to penetrate this area at the same time. Already at this early stage cells with morphologic characteristics of haemopoietic stem cells are frequent in both vascular and perivascular areas. From the 11th day of incubation granulopoiesis and erythropoiesis are extensive. The areas of future white pulp, reticulum cell sheaths around the central arterioles, become visible from the 17th day, when the granulopoietic activity subsides. The first lymphocytes appear in the white pulp at the 19th day of incubation. A full population of the white pulp by lymphoid cells takes place during the first week after hatching. Injected labelled thymic lymphocytes located in small numbers in 12–16-day-old splenic rudiments but their number increased rapidly from day 17 onwards (Moore, in Metcalf & Moore 1971).

Development of immune competence

In mammals, immune competence can develop under influence of early contact with antigen long before birth (Silverstein, 1964). Cellular immune competence of 19-day-old embryos and 1- and 5-day-old chickens has been assessed by measuring the ability of their spleen cell suspensions to produce splenomegaly in recipient 14-day-old embryos. Those cell suspensions failed to produce any significant splenomegaly in the recipients. Owen (Owen & Maudsley 1969) found that thymuses from 20–21-day-old embryos transplanted on the chorioallantoic membrane of a 10-day-old recipient produced severe graft versus host reaction.

Adult levels of graft versus host activity were found at approximately 3 weeks of age (Seto 1968). In our experience (Szenberg, unpublished results) 1-week-old chickens were able to reject allogeneic skin grafts in 7–8 days, which is the time of graft rejection in adults of the same flock.

Experiments of Simonsen (1965) did indicate that early contact with antigen can accelerate the maturation immunocompetence. In these experiments Simonsen injected i.v. 17-day-old embryos with allogeneic adult lymphocytes. Seven days later the recipient's spleen had been used to inoculate a second set of recipients and produced significant splenomegaly. Such serial passage could have continued an apparently unlimited number of times. The important point in these observations was that the active cells in the second and further passages were of the host origin. If the recipient embryos were 14 days old, the activity disappeared after 1–2 passages. Obviously, 17-day-old embryo spleens contain some thymus-derived cells, or the presence of allogeneic inoculum accelerates the influx of such cells from the thymus.

Another result pointing in the same direction is the fact that the older the recipient embryo the less splenomegaly is produced. This would indicate that older embryos may be able to mount a host versus graft reaction.

Antibody production

According to Solomon and Tucker (1963) injection of sheep erythrocytes into 16-day and older embryos and 1-day-old chickens resulted in induction of tolerance. Two-day-old chickens responded with low level of antibody. The dose of antigen injected was rather high, and such experiments should be repeated with lower doses.

In experiments of Wolfe and Dilks (1948) a proportion of 1-day-old chickens was able to produce antibodies to a protein antigen. Full adult responsiveness was achieved at 6 weeks of age.

The fact the immune responses in chicken mature only some time after hatching is interesting, considering that precursors of immunocompetent cells are present in the bursa and thymus at least 6–7 days before hatching.

An explanation for this discrepancy may possibly be in the fact that the major secondary lymphoid organ, spleen, becomes lymphoidal only late in ontogenesis and the microenvironment of the spleen may be necessary to complete the maturation of precursor cells into immunocompetent lymphocytes. The environment of embryonic spleen seems also to be not suited to support development of antibody response by immunocompetent cells transferred from adult birds (Isacson 1960, Papermaster *et al.* 1962).

Experiments performed in our laboratory were supported by grants from NHMRS (Canberra) and Volkswagen Stiftung, West Germany.

References

Bäck O. (1970) Studies on the Lymphocytes in the Intestinal Epithelium of the Chicken. III. Effect of Thymectomy. *Int. Arch. Allergy* **39**, 192.

Bäck O. (1970) Studies on the Lymphocytes in the Intestinal Epithelium of the Chicken. IV. Effect of Bursectomy. *Int. Arch. Allergy* **39**, 342.

Bäck R. (1972) Influence of antigenic stimulation on lymphoid cell traffic in the chicken. II. Increased homing of bone-marrow-derived cells to the Bursa of Fabricius after human serum albumin administration. *Int. Arch. Allergy* **43,** 921.

Biggs P.M. (1957) The association of lymphoid tissue with the lymph vessels in the domestic chicken (Gallus domesticus). *Acta Anat.* **29,** 36.

Bloom W. (1938) Embryogenesis of Mammalian Blood, vol II, p. 863. In *Handbook of Haematology*, eds Downey H. Hoeber, New York.

Castro J.E. (1974) Orchidectomy and the immune response. I. The effect of orchidectomy on the lymphoid tissues of mice. *Proc. R. Soc. Lond.* **B185,** 425.

Cooper M.D., Peterson R.D.A. & Good R.A. (1965) Delineation of thymic and bursal lymphoid systems in the chicken. *Nature* **205,** 143.

Cooper M.D., Peterson R.D.A., Soutch M.A. & Good R.A. (1966) The function of the thymus system and the bursa system in the chicken. *J. Exp. Med.* **123,** 75.

DeLanney L.E. & Ebert J.D. (1962) Carnegie Institution of Washington Publication 621. *Contribution to Embryology*, **37,** 57.

Good R.A. & Finstad J. (1967) *Germinal Centers in Immune Response*, pp. 4–27, eds Cottier H., Odartchenko N., Schindler R. & Congdon C.C. Springer-Verlag, Berlin.

Graetzer M.A., Wolfe H.R., Aspinall R.L. & Mayer R.K. (1963) Effect of thymectomy and bursectomy on precipitin and natural hemagglutinin production in the chicken. *J. Immunol.* **90,** 878.

Hamilton H.L. (1952) *Lillie's development of the chick*. Henry Holt, New York.

Hammond W.S. (1954) Origin of the thymus in the chick embryo. *J. Morph.* **95,** 501.

Hohn E.O. (1956) Seasonal recrudescence of the thymus in adult birds. *Can. J. Physiol.* **34,** 90.

Hohn E.O. (1959) Action of certain hormones on the thymus of the domestic fowl. *J. Endoc.* **19,** 282.

Isacson P. (1959) Cellular transfer of antibody production from adult to embryo in domestic fowl. *Yale J. Biol. Med.* **32,** 209.

Isakovic K., Jankovic B.D., Pospekovic L. & Milosevic D. (1963) Effect of neonatal thymectomy, bursectomy and thymo-bursectomy on haemagglutinin production in chickens. *Nature*, **200,** 273.

Ivanyi J., Murgatroyd L.B. & Lydyard P.M. (1972) Bursal origin of bone marrow cells with competence for antibody formation. *Immunology* **23,** 107.

Kincade P.W., Lawton A.R., Bockman D.E. & Cooper M.D. (1970) Suppression of immunoglobulin G synthesis as a result of antibody-mediated suppression of immunoglobulin M synthesis in chickens. *Proc. Nat. Acad. Sci.* **67,** 1918.

Kincade P.W. & Cooper M.D. (1971a) Development and distribution of immunoglobulin-containing cells in the chicken: an immunofluorescent analysis using purified antibodies to μ, γ and light chains. *J. Immunol.* **106,** 371.

Leslie G.A. & Martin L.N. (1973) Modulation of immunoglobulin ontogeny in the chicken: effect of purified antibody specific for μ chain on IgM, IgY and IgA production. *J. Immunol.* **110,** 959.

Martin L.N. & Leslie G.A. (1974) IgM-forming cells as the precursors of IgA producing cells during the ontogeny of the immunoglobulin-producing system of the chicken. *J. Immunol.* **113,** 120.

Mayer R.K., Rao M.A. & Aspinall R.L. (1959) Inhibition of the development of Bursa of Fabricius in the embryo of the common fowl, by 19-nor-testosterone. *Endocrinology* **64,** 820.

McArthur W.P., Gilmour D.G. & Thorbecke G.J. (1973) Immunocompetent cell in the chicken. II. Synergism between thymus cells and either bursa or bone marrow cells in the humoral response to sheep erythrocytes. *Cell. Immunol.* **8,** 103.

METCALF D. & MOORE M.A.S. (1971) *Haemopoietic Cells*, eds Tatum E.L. & Neuberger A. North-Holland, Amsterdam and London.

MOORE M.A.S. & OWEN J.J.T. (1965) Chromosome marker studies on the development of the hemopoietic system in the chick embryo. *Nature* **208,** 956.

MOORE M.A.S. & OWEN J.J.T. (1966) Origin of bursal lymphocytes. *Dev. Biol.* **14,** 40.

MOORE M.A.S. & OWEN J.J.T. (1967a) Chromosome marker studies in the irradiated chick embryo. *Nature*, **215,** 1081.

MOORE M.A.S. & OWEN J.J.T. (1967b) Stem cell migration in the developing myeloid and lymphoid system. *Lancet*, **ii,** 658.

MOORE M.A.S. & OWEN J.J.T. (1957c) Experimental studies on the development of the thymus. *J. Exp. Med.* **126,** 715.

OWEN J.J.T. & RITTER M.A. (1969) Tissue interaction in the development of thymus lymphocytes. *J. Exp. Med.* **129,** 431.

PAPERMASTER B.W., BRADLEY S.G., WATSON D.W. & GOOD R.A. (1962) Antibody producing capacity of adult chicken spleen cells in newly hatched chicks. *J. Exp. Med.* **115,** 1191.

PAYNE L.N. (1971) The lymphoid system, pp. 985–1037. In *Physiology and Biochemistry of Domestic Fowl*, eds Bell D.J. and Freeman B.M. Academic Press, New York.

PIERPAOLI W., BARONI C., FABRIS N. & SORKIN E. (1969) Hormones and immunological capacity. II. Reconstitution of antibody production in hormonally deficient mice by somatotropic hormone, thyrotropic hormone, and thyroxin. *Immunology* **16,** 217.

ROUSE B.T. & WARNER N.L. (1974) The role of suppressor cells in avian allogenic tolerance: implications for pathogenesis of Marck's Disease. *J. Immunol.* **113,** 904.

RUTH R.F., ALLEN C.P. & WOLFE H.R. (1964) In *The Thymus in Immunobiology*, pp. 183–205, eds Good R.A. & Gabrielson A.E. Harper & Row, New York.

SARVAS H., MÄKELÄ O., TOIVANEN P. & TOIVANEN A. (1974) Effect of carrier preimmunisation on the anti-hapten response in the chicken. *Scand. J. Immunol.* **3,** 455.

SETO F. (1968) Variations in the Graft-versus-Host reaction capacity of growing chickens. *Transplantation* **6,** 771.

SILVERSTEIN A.M. (1964) Ontogeny of the immune response. *Science* **144,** 1423.

SIMONSEN M. (1965) Recent experiments on the graft-versus-host reaction in the chick embryo. *Brit. Med. Bull.* **21,** 129.

SOLOMON J.B. & TUCKER D.F. (1963) Ontogenesis of immunity to erythrocyte antigens in the chick. *Immunology* **6,** 592.

SZENBERG A. (1970) Influence of testosterone on the primary lymphoid organs in the chicken. In *Hormones and the immune response*, eds Wolstenholme G.E. & Julie Knight. Ciba Foundation Study Group No. 36. J. & A. Churchill, London.

SZENBERG A. & WARNER N.L. (1962) Dissociation of immunological responsiveness in fowls with hormonally arrested development of lymphoid tissues. *Nature* **194,** 146.

THORBECKE G.J., WARNER N.L., HOCHWALD G.M. & OHANIAN S.H. (1968) Immune globulin production by the bursa of Fabricius of young chickens. *Immunology* **15,** 123.

WARNER N.L. (1964) The immunological competence of different lymphoid organs in the chicken. II. The immunological competence of thymic cell suspensions. *Aust. J. Exp. Biol. Med. Sci.* **42,** 401.

WARNER N.L. & BURNET F.M. (1961) The influence of testosterone treatment on the development of the Bursa of Fabricius in the chick embryo. *Aust. J. Biol. Sci.* **14,** 580.

WARNER N.L. & SZENBERG A. (1962) Effect of neonatal thymectomy on the immune response in the chicken. *Nature* **196,** 784.

WARNER N.L., SZENBERG A. & BURNET F.M. (1962) The immunological role of different lymphoid organs in the chicken. I. Dissociation of immunological responsiveness. *Aust. J. Exp. Biol.* **40,** 373.

Weinbaum F.I., Gilmour D.G. & Thorbecke G.J. (1973) Immunocompetent cells of the chicken. III. Cooperation of carrier sensitized cells from agammaglobulinemic donors with hapten immune B cells. *J. Immunol.* **110,** 1434.

Wolfe H.R. & Dilks E. (1948) Precipitin production in chickens. *J. Immunol.* **58,** 245.

Wolfe H.R., Sheridan S.A., Bilstad N.M. & Johnson M.A. (1962) The growth of lymphoid organs and testes of chickens. *Anat. Records* **142,** 485.

Chapter 17. Ontogeny of Immunity in Mammals

David T. Rowlands, Jr

Introduction

Development of lymphoid tissues
Thymus
Peripheral lymphoid tissues
Plasma cells

Lymphocyte subpopulations

Immune responses

Development of serum proteins

Summary

Introduction

Similar conclusions regarding development of immune responsiveness may be reached using either phylogenetic or ontogenetic models, but one or the other may offer special advantages in particular cases. For example, only the ontogenetic approach, using inbred animals, permits an unequivocal identification of the relative importance of B and T classes of lymphocytes in the development of acquired immunity. The present chapter is concerned with the ontogeny of immunity in mammals with a view towards illuminating various critical experimental studies and observations which have been made and towards identifying areas in which progress is likely to be made toward our understanding of developmental immunology in the near future.

Development of lymphoid tissues

Thymus

The thymus, splenic white pulp, and lymph nodes along with lymphoid masses associated with the gastrointestinal tract make up the organized lymphoid tissues of mammals. Among these lymphoid tissues the thymus is the first to appear in each species of mammal which has been studied in detail; an observation which suggested the primacy of the thymus in lymphoid tissue development to early embryologists. The earliest identifiable anlage of the thymus is a sheet of epithelioid cells which soon becomes associated with lymphocytes. This can be seen in man at 9 weeks of gestation and in mice at 9 days of gestation. Proliferation of the lymphocytes and organization of the thymic tissue results in the formation of distinct cortical and medullary components of the thymus. The thymic cortex is composed of abundant, closely-packed lymphocytes (Fig. 17.1) while the medulla is more loosely

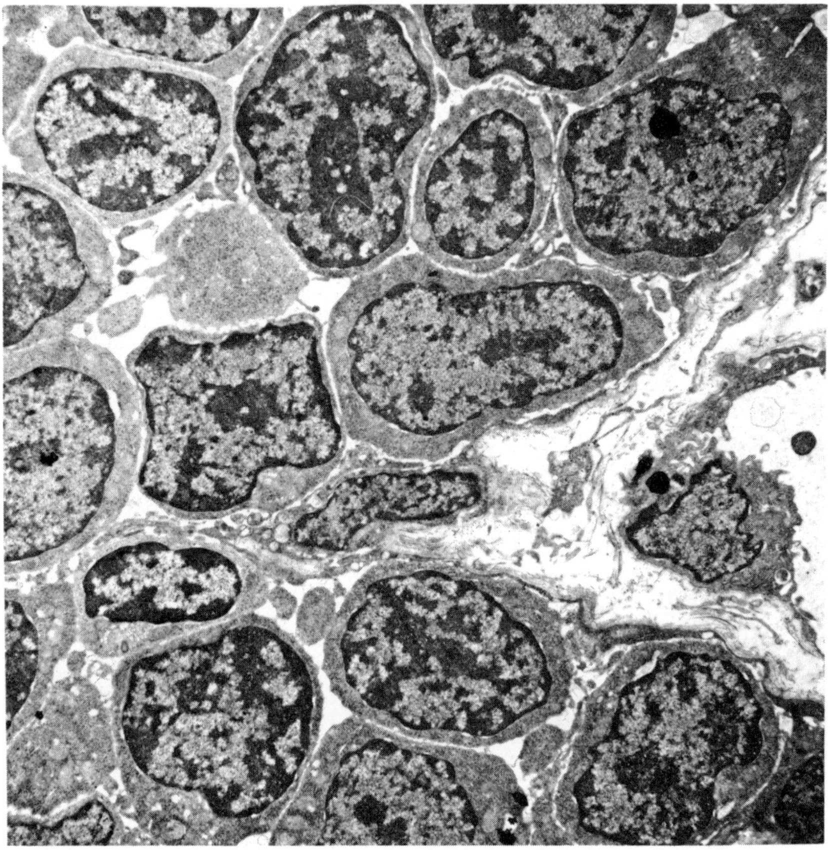

Fig. 17.1. This electron micrograph shows the closely packed lymphocytes in the most superficial portions of the cortex. One of the vessels beneath the capsule is seen on the right.

organized containing relatively few lymphocytes but many epithelioid cells and macrophages. Hassall's corpuscles, variously believed to be aggregates of epithelioid cells or effete blood vessels, appear early in the course of development of the thymus and persist into adult life. The growth rate of the thymus is most rapid in young mammals with the gland reaching its maximal size in adolescence or young adulthood. Thereafter, there is a gradual involution of the thymus the rate of which may be amplified by systemic illnesses.

Peripheral lymphoid tissues

As was suggested earlier, development of the thymus is essential to the differentiation of other, peripheral, lymphoid tissues (Miller 1962, Martinez *et al.* 1962). In the earliest phases of development of the splenic component of the peripheral lymphoid tissues, lymphocytes appear adjacent to splenic blood vessels and then rapidly increase in number. Similarly, lymphocytes appear early among mesenchymal cell anlage of lymph nodes. After rapid proliferation of the lymphocytes in these primitive lymph nodes, distinct cortical and medullary segments of lymph nodes appear. Lymphocytes of the gastrointestinal tract are first found in the lamina propria. Germinal centers appear late in development of each of these peripheral lymphoid tissues (e.g. spleen, lymph nodes, gastrointestinal tract).

Plasma cells

As in the case of germinal centres, plasma cells appear to be largely localized to peripheral lymphoid tissues and to appear in these tissues only late in the course of development. For example, plasma cells are not ordinarily seen in human infants which are younger than full term. However, studies of the time of appearance of plasma cells may be used as an argument favouring the role of antigen in driving maturation of the lymphoid system. Benirschke and Bourne (1958) observed plasma cells in a 22-week placenta of an infant with syphilis and Silverstein and Lukes (1962) noted that plasma cells appeared in the earliest fetus examined by them (29 weeks) in a study of human fetuses infected with syphilis or with toxoplasmosis. The plasmocytosis in the lymphoid tissues of the infants studied by Silverstein and Lukes (1962) appeared to correlate with the severity of the infection of the fetus and the remaining lymphoid tissue (e.g. lymph nodes) also appeared to have been accelerated in their development but the extent of proliferation of plasma cells and the development of other lymphoid tissues did not necessarily correspond to each other. A similar phenomenon of antigen-dependent maturation of plasma cells has been suggested by experimental work in cattle with the early appearance of plasma cells in fetal calves infected with *Leptospira saxkoebing* (Fennestad & Borg-Petersen 1962).

Both of these observations suggest that the ontogeny of certain elements of the lymphoid system is antigen driven. In apparent contrast to these situations is the failure to identify an accelerated maturation of plasma cells in the tissues of young marsupials exposed to antigens (Rowlands *et al.* 1964). Because of important anatomical and physiological differences between the *in utero* position of eutherian mammals and the pouch of marsupials, it may be possible to reconcile these observations. First, the failure to recognize accelerated maturation of plasma cells in opossums could be because changes due to the superimposed exposure to antigens are obscured by the rapid differentiation going on normally in the reticuloendothelial system of these animals. Secondly, the accelerated differentiation of plasma cells may be better seen when the antigens are living, proliferating agents. In these connections it is most important to recognize that because of the unique position of newborn opossums, in the maternal pouch, they may be exposed to many more antigens than may fetal sheep protected in the uterus.

Lymphocyte Subpopulations

Recently, there has been increasing interest in defining the maturation of subpopulations of lymphoid cells in terms of their particular functions. Press and Klinman (1973a,b, 1974) have provided data bearing on this aspect of the ontogeny of B cells (antibody-producing cells) in the immune response. They utilize a method which permits enumeration of precursor cells, quantification of antibodies produced by splenic foci established *in vitro*, and evaluation of the degree of heterogeneity of antibodies harvested from these foci. In essence, the method employed by these investigators is a transfer of cells to carrier primed, irradiated recipients. Chunks of tissue from the reconstituted animals are stimulated *in vitro* and antibody is recovered from those containing antibody-producing cells. With this technique it was possible to show that precursors of DNP-producing cells are available in the mouse spleen as early as the 17th day of gestation, that the quantity of antibody produced by these cells is appreciably less than that obtained in a similar way from adult mice, and that the antibodies appearing in young animals are less diverse than are those of adult animals. The observation that the numbers of precursor cells for the haptens DNP and TNP in the spleens of 17-day-old mouse embryos were identical to the frequency of such precursors in adult mice was of particular interest. In contrast, the incidence of precursor cells for the hapten fluorescein, was materially less than that for other haptens. That these three hapten precursor cells represent separate populations of cells was suggested by the observation that the numbers of precursor cells detected when the haptens were used together were the same as the sum of the numbers arrived at by independent stimulations. Other investigators (Spear *et al.* 1973) have evaluated developing populations of B lymphocytes with respect to their antigen-binding abilities. These investigators have shown that well-differentiated B cells appear early in intrauterine life.

An overview of the studies of the ontogeny of B cells suggest that precursor cells for specific antibodies appear relatively early in development but that not all cells which can bind specific antigens are able to be stimulated by these same antigens to produce antibodies. On account of this, several alternative views may be taken of the process of cellular development and the generation of immunologic diversity. For example, it could be either that antigen is required to drive and direct maturation of lymphoid cells or that the processes of cellular maturation are entirely at the genetic level. The fact that similar numbers of precursor cells can be detected in germ free mice and in normal animals speaks against an antigen-driven process (Press & Klinman 1974). There is at present no clear indication of the essential differences between those antibody-binding cells which go on to produce antibodies and those which do not produce antibodies in the face of an adequate antigenic stimulus.

These studies outlined above have spoken especially of topics of B-cell maturation. Attention has now also been directed toward T cell, thymus-derived cell, maturation as regards the participation of these cells in the immune response (Spear *et al.* 1973, Spear & Edelman 1974). Chiscon and Golub (1972) showed convincingly that, although there are ample specific B-cells present in neonatal mice for response to sheep red blood cells, these animals are deficient in functioning T cells and it is only several days after birth that mature T cells become sufficiently abundant to operate in the immune response. Spear *et al.* (1973), in contrast, found both B and T cells in the spleens of Swiss-L mice as early as the 15th day of gestation. In spite of this, these investigators were not able to demonstrate an immune response either *in vivo* or *in vitro* until 1 week later. Spear and Edelman (1974) then produced evidence suggesting that a subset of T cells essential to the generation of some forms of humoral immunity appears later than the 15th day of gestation.

Immune Responses

It was thought for many years that embryonic life was a null period during which there was essentially no immunologic activity. This has, of course, proved not to be the case so that differentiation of the lymphoid cells and tissues described above is accompanied by development of the embryos' capacities to recognize antigens and to react immunologically to a wide variety of antigens (Riha 1962, Sterzl & Silverstein 1967, Uhr 1960, Eichwald & Shinefield 1963).

Among the key questions that have concerned immunologists during the last decade, is the manner in which the immune response is 'turned on'. In particular, emphasis has been placed on discovering whether immune responsiveness is activated simultaneously to all antigens or whether there is a hierarchy of responsiveness to the various antigens.

Studies were cited earlier in this chapter suggesting that fetal cattle may respond to an infection while still *in utero* (Fennestad & Borg-Petersen 1962). In this case, fetal calves infected with *L. saxkoebing* showed antibodies when infected as early as day 132 of the cow's 200-day gestation. More recently, the question of the relationship between development of lymphoid tissues and the responses of embryos to antigens has been approached more systematically. Silverstein and his associates have carried out extensive studies of sheep *in utero* (1963a,b, 1964). Sheep have a gestation period of 149 days and show no evidence of transfer of maternal antibodies across the placenta to the fetus. Because these embryos can be successfully approached through a uterotomy relatively early in development, they represent a useful model for the study of the ontogeny of immunity. They have the added characteristic of a high incidence of twinning so that satisfactory control and experimental animals can be had in the same uterus. The results of studies using this model suggested that the immune responses of fetal animals to various antigens is in the form of a hierarchy. Fetal lambs responded to the bacteriophage ØX 174 when immunization was carried out as early as the 39th day *in utero* (Sterzl & Silverstein 1967), with ferritin by 80 days and ovalbumin at 120 days (Silverstein *et al.* 1963a). At no time did these fetuses respond to injections of diphtheria toxoid, *Salmonella typhosa*, or BCG. Skin allografts applied at any time after the 77th day of gestation were readily rejected while grafts applied at earlier times remained in place without stimulating a detectable immune response (Schinkel & Ferguson 1953, Silverstein *et al.* 1964). The rate of graft rejection in these fetuses was similar to that in adults. In addition, the morphological changes in the graft and in related lymph nodes were like those of other mammals except that a superficial layer of epithelial cells was often retained after graft rejection. Silverstein *et al.* (1964) postulated that maintenance of these cells might result from the peculiarity of the graft lying within the amniotic sac.

The immune response of sheep embryos to the various antigens used by Silverstein is of special interest in several respects. First, the immune response to bacteriophage can be seen in sheep when the thymus is free of lymphocytes. Secondly, the relative amounts of antibodies formed in response to the antigens followed the same order as the qualitative responses to the various antigens. That is, fetal sheep produced larger amounts of antibodies against bacteriophage than they did against ovalbumin. In addition, limited numbers of studies suggested that an anamnestic response appeared in sheep primed *in utero* and given a booster injection of antigen after birth (Silverstein *et al.* 1963b).

The opossum (*Didelphis virginiana*) has provided another model for the study of immune responses in developing mammals. This marsupial has a 12·5-day gestation period after which the young enter the maternal pouch where they are readily available for study (Block 1963). Opossum young are essentially embryos with respect to the development of their lymphoid tissues when they enter the maternal pouch and the thymus is an epithelioid anlage devoid of lymphocytes. Lymphocytes appear first in the thymus at 2 days, in a cervical lymph node at 3 days, and in thoracic lymph nodes at 6 days (Block 1963, Rowlands *et al.* 1964). Splenic lymphocytes are found centred about splenic anterioles after 17 days (Block 1963, Rowlands *et al.* 1964) and as organized tissue in the lamina propria of the gastrointestinal tract after 35 days (Rowlands *et al.* 1974).

Our experiments (LaVia *et al.* 1963, Rowlands *et al.* 1964, Rowlands & Dudley 1969, Rowlands *et al.* 1974) using the fetal opossum were designed to test the hypothesis that there is a well ordered hierarchy of responsiveness to a wide variety of antigens in the intact animal. In order to standardize the sensitivity of the antibody assays the antibodies to all but one antigen were measured by bacteriophage neutralization (Adams 1959, Rowlands 1967) or by an appropriate modification of the bacteriophage neutralization assay (Blakeslee *et al.* 1973, Rowlands *et al.* 1974). Antibodies to *S. typhosa* were measured by agglutination, a method which is less sensitive than bacteriophage neutralization.

The responses of opossum embryos to antigens used by us and others (La Plante *et al.* 1969) are included in Figure 17.2. The age of the animals when

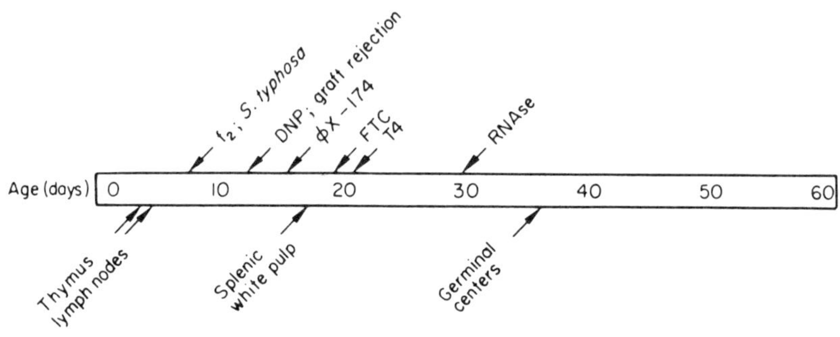

Fig. 17.2. This diagram illustrates the development of immune responses in opossums. The age of the animals in days in the maternal pouch is indicated in the centre, the time of onset of responsiveness to individual antigens is shown above the box, and the time of onset of lymphocyte development in various tissues is indicated below the box.

introduction of antigens results in immune responses is compared to development of various components of the lymphoid system of the opossum. These embryos responded to both *S. typhosa* and to bacteriophage f2 by the end of their first week in the maternal pouch. They responded to bacteriophage ØX 174, to the hapten DNP and to skin grafts at a later time. This was followed by responsiveness to the hapten fluorescein (FTC) and still later to responses to both the bacteriophage T4 and a small protein (RNAase).

Taken together these studies in several animal species indicate that a hierarchy of responsiveness to antigens can be demonstrated in intact animals and that this hierarchy seems to be independent of the chemical or physical characteristics of the antigens.

The models outlined above which have been used to reach this conclusion have the disadvantage that the animals are not inbred so that the roles of their lymphocyte sub-populations in establishing this hierarchy cannot be readily defined. For this reason, a model utilizing reconstitution of the lymphoid system of mice with syngeneic fetal liver or neonatal cells has been developed (Sherwin & Rowlands 1974). In our preliminary efforts we have utilized the bacteriophages f2, ØX 174, and T4; the hapten-carrier complexes DNP-BSA and FTC-BSA; and three small proteins, hen egg lysozyme (LYS), sperm whale myoglobin (Myo) and bovine pancreatic ribonuclease (RNAse). As in the experiments utilizing the opossum, the antibodies to these antigens were assayed by direct bacteriophage neutralization or its appropriate modification (Blakeslee *et al.* 1973).

Individual mice responded to these antigens in a sequential fashion. The mice responded to both bacteriophage f2 and ØX 174 when immunized 3 days after reconstitution and to bacteriophage T4 when immunized 7 days after reconstitution. Similarly, it was necessary to delay immunization until day 10 to see a response to the hapten DNP and to day 14 for the response to FTC. The mice began to respond to Lys at 3 weeks, to RNase at 4 weeks, and to Myo at 5 weeks. The hierarchy in these animals would then be bacteriophage f2 and ØX 174 > bacteriophage T4 > DNP > FTC > Lys > RNase > Myo. Further study utilizing this system should permit us to establish the roles of lymphocyte sub-populations in establishing this hierarchy.

Development of serum proteins

Analyses of the properties of the serum of the fetus is often complicated because of its attachment to the mother leading to the possibility that serum proteins and, more importantly, immunoglobulins of the mother have contributed to those of the fetus by either transplacental or colostral-mediated transfer of immunoglobulins from mother to fetus. The extent of these contributions are, therefore, essential to know before reaching conclusions regarding the immunoglobulin synthesizing capabilities of the intact fetus.

Sheep, as was implied previously, offer an advantage in this regard since these fetuses are not contaminated with maternal immunoglobulins *in utero*. Silverstein and his colleagues (1963b) utilized this property of sheep, in the course of their previously described studies, to analyse the ability of fetal sheep to produce immunoglobulins. Since antibody activity could be found in animals immunized during their second month *in utero*, it seems obvious that immunoglobulins must be produced at this early stage of development. It was shown that B_2M immunoglobulins could be detected in fetal lambs which were as young as 70 days of age (immunized at 60 days of age). Quantitation of the 7S γ-globulin in animals stimulated by injection of antigen showed a progression in serum levels from 66-day fetuses to older animals. Fetuses less than 66 days of age seem not to have been studied.

In most other animals which have been studied in detail, synthesis of immunoglobulins appears at about the time of parturition. In the case of rabbits, the synthesis seems not to begin until after birth (Diechmiller & Dixon 1957). Guinea-pigs, however, first synthesize IgM immunoglobulins by day 58 of their gestation with production of other immunoglobulins beginning 2 weeks after birth. The order of appearance of immunoglobulins in the serum of guinea-pigs is the same as the order of appearance of immunoglobulins during the immune response of adult guinea-pigs (Dancis & Shafran 1958, Thorbecke 1964). As pointed out by Solomon (1971), although rabbits and guinea-pigs differ in the time of onset of antibody synthesis with respect to parturition, the onset of antibody synthesis at 58 days from conception is equivalent in these two species.

Evaluation of immunoglobulins in opossums have been carried out from birth through adult life. Table 17.1 shows representative data selected from a

Table 17.1. Development of serum proteins in opossums

Age (days)	Total*	γ*	β*	α_2*		α_1*	Albumin*
7	2·9	0·16	2·21		0·23		0·3
15	2·0	0·14	1·08		0·14		0·62
25	2·2	0·18	1·85	0		0	0·18
32	3·2	0·22	0·35	0·70		0·61	1·31
44	3·0	0·24	1·02		0·24		1·50
65	4·8	0·82	0·76	1·06		0·14	2·11
80	5·8	0·53	1·57		0·51		2·20
Adult	6·4	0·77	1·81	1·21		0·33	2·32

* Values expressed as g/100 ml.

larger volume of material which has been previously published (Rowlands & Dudley 1969). This data illustrates that the total serum proteins and most of its constituents increase progressively from birth to adult life. The early appearance of β-globulins is currently unexplained but the available evidence suggests that the β-globulin is not derived from maternal colostrum (Rowlands & Dudley 1969). There is no data available indicating as to whether or not similar proteins are available in the opossum *in utero*. When the serum of opossum embryos was evaluated by sucrose gradient centrifugation, it was evident that the earliest immunoglobulin detected which was similar to that in adults was IgM-like. As will be discussed below, there is a possibility that the formation of IgM in opossum embryos is actually preceded by the appearance of another class of immunoglobulins.

The influence of fetal or neonatal serum immunoglobulin levels of proteins which have been passed transplacentally (Brambell 1966) or through the colostrum is well illustrated in mice and in humans. The effect of passively transferred immunoglobulins in mice may be best seen through quantitation of serum γG in newborn mice during their neonatal period. An elevation in this level is reached at 1 week of age but it returns to a low level after an additional 2–3 weeks. The most likely explanation for the series of events in the level of serum γG of mice is selective gastrointestinal absorption of maternal colostral γG by newborn mice in their first month of life (Hemmings & Morris 1959). The gastrointestinal absorption by young rats is more general than in mice with albumin, transferrin, and γ-globulin being readily absorbed in the first week of life, albumin less readily in the next two weeks, and cessation of absorption of these proteins being evident at 21 days (Jordan & Morgan 1968).

The most thoroughly studied instance of modification of levels of fetal immunoglobulins appears to be that of the human. In this case maternal IgG is passed transplacentally to the fetus, accounting for the depressed level of this immunoglobulin throughout fetal and early neonatal life. Because of this, it was generally believed that the human fetus and the human newborn were incapable of synthesizing immunoglobulins. Subsequent evidence has shown this concept to be in error. The major alterations in our views about the immunological capabilities of the human fetus came about because of the careful *in vitro* work of van Furth and his colleagues (1965). These investigators evaluated the ability of tissues obtained from human abortions to synthesize immunoglobulins. In the case of the spleen, synthesis of both IgM and IgG could be identified after 19 weeks of gestation but synthesis of neither IgA nor IgD could be found. In these early stages of development, the splenic lymphocytes were few and remained confined to perivascular locations but these foci of lymphopoieses in the spleen enlarged thereafter. In addition, IgM was found in the serum of 20-week or older fetuses. Other investigators have also identified the production of IgM and IgG by the human fetus (Matsen *et al.* 1967, Martensson & Fudenberg 1965, Rothberg 1969).

More recently, studies of the synthesis of human immunoglobulins have been extended to include IgE synthesis (Miller *et al.* 1973). These investigators showed that IgE and IgG began to be synthesized by the lung and liver of the human fetus as early as the 11th week of gestation. It was felt most likely that synthesis by the lung depends on hilar lymph nodes included in the preparations. Synthesis by the liver is, in contrast to the negative findings of van Furth *et al.* (1965), but is not surprising since, as the authors point out, this organ is the seat of active haematopoiesis at this stage of development of the fetus (Arey 1954).

Synthesis of IgA or IgD have not, as yet, been demonstrated in the human fetus although IgA has been detected in human cord serum.

The role of antigens in driving early antibody formation is not clearly understood but several studies have suggested the importance of bacteria and viruses which enter the respiratory and gastrointestinal tract (McCracken & Shinefield 1965, Rothberg 1969, Janeway 1968, Allensmith *et al.* 1968). In addition, it is conceivable that maternal antigens which cross the placental barrier and cause stimulation of the immune system of the fetus are significant factors in initiating immunoglobulin synthesis *in utero.* Although these antigens may be in the form of infectious agents (Silverstein & Lukes 1962, McCracken & Shinefield 1965, Stiehm *et al.* 1966) they may also be part of conventional physiological experiences. For example, it has been shown that the human fetus can react to antigenic determinants of maternal IgG (Fudenberg & Fudenberg 1964).

Cooper *et al.* (1971) have produced evidence in experimental animals suggesting that there is an ordered sequence of development of cells producing specific immunoglobulins. Miller *et al.* (1973) have inferred from their studies that this is not the case in the human. They believe, instead, that IgM-, IgG-, and IgE-producing cells arise as separate cell lines and differentiate independently. It would seem to this author that, although the data produced by Miller *et al.* (1973) is undoubtedly correct, it cannot be seriously considered to exclude the hypothesis of sequential development of immunoglobulin synthesizing potential suggested by Cooper *et al.* (1971) since it could be that an ordered sequence of development was already completed when Miller *et al.* (1973) made their observations.

Most studies suggest that IgM is the earliest immunoglobulin to appear in the circulation of developing vertebrates. However, there is now some evidence to suggest that production of IgM may be preceded or accompanied by synthesis of other forms of immunoglobulin. In the case of the opossum (Rowlands and Dudley 1969) the earliest immunoglobulins to appear in the circulation of the embryo are intermediate in size between IgM and IgG. These antibodies appear in exceptionally small quantities and disappear from the circulation of the fetus early in development. It remains to be determined whether this 'embryonic antibody' represents a distinct class of antibodies or whether it is related to the conventional IgM and IgG immunoglobulin classes. In a similar vein, Marchalonis (1971) has found a protein which resembles IgG in the serum of developing amphibia. This protein, however, has not been shown to have antibody activity.

The most extensive observations on the presence of 'non-classical' immunoglobulins have been done with the pig (Sterzl *et al.* 1960). It is generally agreed that these animals are free of conventional immunoglobulins at birth. However, when fetal pigs, near term, are removed from the uterus and their serum greatly concentrated, it can be shown that the serum contains a protein of small molecular size which is precipitable with anti-γ-globulin. Kim *et al.* (1966) have demonstrated that, under appropriate conditions, antibody formation can be seen in newborn miniature pigs. In this case the first immunoglobulin is 19S in size but is antigenically identical to 7S immunoglobulins.

Summary

The ontogeny of the immune system in every animal species which has been studied in detail displays a well ordered maturation of lymphoid tissues and immunoglobulins. In every case the development of these components begins early in ontogeny (e.g. before the end of the first half of gestation in man) and it appears that either IgM or a fetal immunoglobulin make up the first antibodies produced. Recent evidence suggests that there is a hierarchy of responsiveness to a variety of antigens. Although it seems likely that B cells reach maturity more rapidly than do T cells, the maturation events among the sub-populations of lymphocytes has not been fully explored.

Acknowledgments

This work has been supported in part by USPHS Grants AM 14372 and HE 13931.

References

ADAMS M.H. (1959) *Bacteriophages*. Interscience, New York.

ALLANSMITH M., MCCLELLAN B.H., BUTTERWORTH M. & MALONEY J.R. (1968) The development of immunoglobulin levels in man. *J. Pediat.* **72**, 276–90.

AREY L.B. (1954) *Developmental anatomy*. W. B. Saunders Co., Philadelphia, PA.

BENIRSCHKE K. & BOURNE G.L. (1958) Plasma cells in an immature human placenta. *Obstet. Gynec.* **12**, 495.

BLAKESLEE D., ANTCZAK D.F. & ROWLANDS D.T. JR (1973) Detection of antibodies specific for FTC, DNS and myoglobin by neutralization of conjugated bacteriophage T4. *Immunochem.* **10**, 61–3.

BLOCK M. (1963) The blood forming tissues and blood of the newborn opossum (Didelphys virginiana). I. Normal development through about the one hundredth day of life. *Ergebn. Anat. Entwicklungsgesch* **37**, 237–366.

BRAMBELL F.W.R. (1966) The transmission of immunity from mother to young and the catabolism of immunoglobulins. *Lancet* **ii**, 1087–93.

CHISCON M.O. & GOLUB E.S. (1972) Functional development of the interacting cells in the immune response. I. Development of T cell and B cell function. *J. Immun.* **108**, 1379–86.

COOPER M.D., KINCADE P.W. & LAWTON A.R. (1971) Thymus and bursal function in immunological development. In *Immunologic Incompetence*, eds Kagan B. & Stiehm E.R. Year Book Medical Pub. Inc., Chicago.

DANCIS J. & SHAFRAN M. (1958) The origin of plasma proteins in the guinea pig foetus. *J. Clin. Invest.* **37**, 1093–9.

DEICHMILLER M.P. & DIXON F.J. (1960) The metabolism of serum proteins in neonatal rabbits. *J. Gen. Physiol.* **43,** 1047–59.

EICHWALD H.F. & SHINEFIELD H.R. (1963) Antibody production by the human fetus. *J. Pediat.* **63,** 870.

FENNESTAD K.L. & BORG-PETERSEN C. (1962) Antibody and plasma cells in bovine fetuses infected with Leptospira saxkoebing. *J. Infect. Dis.* **110,** 63–9.

FUDENBERG H.H. & FUDENBERG B.R. (1964) Antibody to hereditary human gammaglobulin (Gm) factor resulting from maternal fetal incompatibility. *Science* **145,** 170–1.

HEMMINGS W.A. & MORRIS I.G. (1959) An attempt to affect the selective absorption of antibodies from the gut in young mice. *Proc. Roy. Soc. London* (*B*) **150,** 403–9.

JANEWAY C.A. (1968) Progress in Immunology. Syndromes of diminished resistance to infection. *J. Pediat.* **72,** 885–903.

JORDAN S.M. & MORGAN E.H. (1968) The development of selectivity of protein absorption from the intestine during suckling in the rat. *Aust. J. Exp. Biol. Med. Sci.* **46,** 465–72.

KIM Y.B., BRADLEY S.G. & WATSON D.W. (1966) Ontogeny of the immune response. II. Characterization of 19S γG- and 7S γG-immunoglobulins in the true primary and secondary responses of piglets. *J. Immunol.* **97,** 189–96.

LAPLANTE E.S., BURRELL R., WATNE A.L., TAYLOR D.L. & ZIMMERMAN B. (1969) Skin allograft studies in the pouch young of the opossum. *Transplantation* **7,** 67–72.

LAVIA M.F., ROWLANDS D.T. JR & BLOCK M. (1963) Antibody formation in embryos. *Science* **140,** 1219–20.

MARCHALONIS J.J. (1971) Ontogenetic emergence of immunoglobulins in *Rana pipiens* larvae. *Develop. Biology* **25,** 479–91.

MARTENSSON L. & FUDENBERG H.H. (1965) Gm genes and γG-globulin synthesis in the human fetus. *J. Immun.* **94,** 514–20.

MARTINEZ C., KERSEY J., PAPERMASTER B. & GOOD R.A. (1962) Skin homograft survival in thymectomized mice. *Proc. Soc. Exp. Biol. Med.* **109,** 193–6.

MATSEN J.M., HEIMLICH E.M. & BUSSER R.J. (1967) Fetal Immunoglobulins; Immunofluorescent identification and localization in bone marrow. *Ann. Allergy* **25,** 607–10.

MCCRACKEN G.H. & SHINEFIELD H.R. (1965) Immunoglobulin concentrations in newborn infants with congenital cytomegalic inclusion disease. *Pediatrics* **36,** 933–7.

MILLER D.L., HIRVONEN T. & GITLIN D. (1973) Synthesis of IgE by the human conceptus. *J. Allergy Clin. Immunol.* **52,** 182–8.

MILLER J.F.A.P. (1962) Effect of neonatal thymectomy on the immunological responsiveness of the mouse. *Proc. Roy. Soc. B,* **156,** 415–28.

PRESS J.L. & KLINMAN N.R. (1973a) Enumeration and analysis of antibody-forming cell precursors in the neonatal mouse. *J. Immun.* **111,** 829–35.

PRESS J.L. & KLINMAN N.R. (1973b) Isoelectric analysis of neonatal monofocal antibody. *Immunochem.* **10,** 621–7.

PRESS J.L. & KLINMAN N.R. (1974) Frequency of hapten specific B cells in neonatal and adult murine spleens. *Eur. J. Immunol.* **4,** 155.

RIHA I. (1962) *Mechanisms of Immunological Tolerance*, ed. Hasek M. Publishing House of the Czechoslovak Academy of Science, Prague.

ROTHBERG R.M. (1969) Immunoglobulin and specific antibody synthesis during the first weeks of life of premature infants. *J. Ped.* **75,** 391–9.

ROWLANDS D.T. JR, LAVIA M.F. & BLOCK M.H. (1964) The blood forming tissues and blood of the newborn opossum (Didelphys virginiana). II. Ontogenesis of antibody formation to flagella of *S. typhi*. *J. Immun.* **93,** 157–64.

ROWLANDS D.T. JR (1967) Precipitation and neutralization of bacteriophage f2 by rabbit antibodies. *J. Immun.* **98,** 958–64.

ROWLANDS D.T. JR & DUDLEY M.A. (1969) The development of serum proteins and humoral immunity in opossum 'embryos'. *Immunol.* **17,** 969–75.

ROWLANDS D.T. JR, BLAKESLEE D. & ANGALA E. (1974) Acquired immunity in opossum (*Didelphis virginiana*) embryos. *J. Immun.* **112,** 2148–2153.

SCHINKEL P.G. & FERGUSON K.A. (1953) Skin transplantation in the fetal lamb. *Aust. J. Biol. Sc.* **6,** 533–46.

SHERWIN W.K. & ROWLANDS D.T. JR (1974) Development of humoral immunity in lethally-irradiated mice reconstituted with fetal liver. *Fed. Proc.* **33,** 735.

SILVERSTEIN A.M. & LUKES R.L. (1962) Fetal response to antigenic stimulus. I. Plasma-cellular and lymphoid reactions in the human fetus to intra-uterine infection. *Lab. Invest.* **11,** 918–32.

SILVERSTEIN A.M., UHR J.W., KRANER K.L. & LUKES R.J. (1963a) Fetal response to antigenic stimulus. II. Antibody production by the fetal lamb. *J. Exp. Med.* **117,** 799–812.

SILVERSTEIN A.M., THORBECKE G.J., KRANER K.L. & LUKES R.J. (1963b) Fetal response to antigenic stimulus. III. γ-globulin production in normal and stimulated fetal lambs. *J. Immun.* **91,** 384–95.

SILVERSTEIN A.M., PRENDERGAST R.A. & KRANER K.L. (1964) Fetal response to antigenic stimulus. IV. Rejection of skin homografts by the fetal lamb. *J. Exp. Med.* **119,** 955–64.

SOLOMON J.B. (1971) *Foetal and Neonatal Immunology.* Am. Elsvier Pub. Co. Inc., New York.

SPEAR P.G., WANG A.L., RUTISHAUSER U. & EDELMAN G.M. (1973) Characterization of splenic lymphoid cells in fetal and newborn mice. *J. Exp. Med.* **138,** 557–73.

SPEAR P.G. & EDELMAN G.M. (1974) Maturation of the humoral immune response in mice. *J. Exp. Med.* **139,** 249–63.

STERZL J., KOSTKA J., RIHA I. & MANDEL L. (1960) Attempts to determine the formation and character of gamma globulin and of natural and immune antibodies in young pigs reared without colostrum. *Folia Microbiol.* **5,** 29–40.

STERZL J. & SILVERSTEIN A.M. (1967) Developmental aspects of immunity. *Adv. Immunol.* **6,** 337–459.

STIEHM E.R., AMMANN A.J. & CHERRY J.D. (1966) Elevated cord macroglobulins in the diagnosis of intrauterine infections. *N. Eng. J. Med.* **275,** 971–7.

THORBECKE G.J. (1964) Development of immune globulin formation in fetal, newborn and immature guinea pigs. *Fed. Proc.* **23,** 346.

UHR J.W. (1960) Development of delayed hypersensitivity in guinea pig embryos. *Nature* **187,** 957–9.

VAN FURTH R., SCHUIT H.R.E. & HIJMANS W. (1965) The immunological development of the human fetus. *J. Exp. Med.* **122,** 1173–87.

Index

Acanthocephala, tumours 174
Acoelomates, organelle transplantation 37
Acropora, graft survival 42, 43
Actinopterygii 9
Adenocarcinomas, renal, *Rana pipiens* 179, 183, 196
Adenomas 170
Adjuvants, effects
  on chicken antibody production 363
  on reptilian antibody production 328
Agammaglobulinaemia
  B lymphocyte lack and 26
  delayed hypersensitivity, RFC absence in chickens and 130
Agglutination, in anura 214
Agglutinins
  coelomocytes and 71
  opsonin function in *Aplysia californica* 26
Aggregation, cellular
  in porifera 39
  mixed, anthozoa and porifera 43
  non-specific 40
  see also Reaggregation
Agnatha 7
  transplantation immunity 106
  tumours 178, 179
    immunity 106
Agrionemys horsfieldi
  antibodies 300
    effect of antigen type 327
  anti-DNP antibodies, affinity 325, 326
  haemolytic plaque-forming cells 314
    electron microscopy 315
  HMW anti-DNP antibodies, binding capacity 315
  IgM antibodies, valence 319
  5·7S antibodies, valence and binding site 319, 321
Albumin, serum
  bovine, dinitrophenylated 123
  increase in neoplastic *Xenopus* 195
Alligator mississipiensis
  antibodies 299
  antitoxins 298
  diphtheria antibody production, temperature effects 228
Alligators, immunoglobulins, molecular weights 301
Alloantibodies, absence after allografts in *Heterodontis* 107
Alloantigens
  histocompatibility, effects of thymectomy 220
  lack of differences in annelids 54
  transplant, urodele skin graft rejection and 215
Allogenic cells, response to 100
Allografts
  between *Stentor* sp. 38
  first-set, rejection in earthworms 53
  hydrozoa, edge cell pseudopodial activity and 41
  kidney, humoral antibody effects 111
  quasi-immunorecognition 36
  rejection
    anamnesis and 146
    bursectomized and X-irradiated chickens and 110
    delayed hypersensitivity reaction and 104
    in opossums 386
    reptiles and 109
  skin
    latent tumour activation and 191
    successive, in *Heterodontis* 107
  survival times, in different organs 112
Alloimmunity, role of T lymphocytes 108
Alytes obstetricans
  larval thymectomy

Alytes obstetricans (*cont.*)
antibody synthesis and 405
anti-SRBC responses and 124
splenic RFC and 404
spleen, PFC and RFC 409
thymus regeneration 400
Amaroecium constellatum, regeneration in 48
Ambystoma mexicanum
immunoglobulin characterization 281
lymphosarcomas 108, 183, 196
Ambystoma tigrinum, allograft immunity 401
Ameirus melas, T_2-phage antibody production, temperature effects 230
Amia calva
delayed hypersensitivity and 104
LMW immunoglobulins, mass deficiencies 248
response to KLH 146
Amino acids
immunoglobulin 240, 243, 248, 249, 260
sequence 261
genetic implications 262
N-terminal 256, 262
5·7S immunoglobulin H-chain 357
Amoeba
as 'prototype macrophage' 105
immunological specificity and 38
Amoeba discoides, nuclei transfer to *A. proteus*, clone non-development and 38
Amoeba proteus
enucleated cytoplasm, nuclei transfer effects 38
flagellare and ciliate ingestion 81
hydra elicited chemotactic response 81
Amphibia
annelid, convergent evolution and 16
antibodies
nature of antigen and 278
origin of diversity 408
response 278
evolution and taxonomy 10, 210, 211, 212
histocompatibility antigen tolerance 391
embryonic 392
metamorphosis and 393
percentage tolerance 395
Volpe theory 398
histoincompatible graft rejection, causes 210, 215
immunocompetence maturation 220
immunological differences 209
immunoglobulins
diversity 211
physicochemical characterization 280
types 291
larval ix, xi
lymphocyte origins 403
lymphoid organ diversity 217
ontogeny of immunity 390
phylogeny 211
reticuloendothelial system 220
spleens, PFC and RFC 409
7S non-IgM antibodies 277
thymus
antibody and immunoglobulin synthesis 404
function maturation 400
transplantation immunity and 400
transplantation immunity 108, 400
tumours 178, 179, 180, 181
advantages of study 198
immunity and 108, 193
limb regeneration and 185
Amphioxus 7
Ampullaris australis
methylcholanthrene induced tumours 176
Anamnesis, immunological 31, 37, 98, 144
absence
opossums 385
various species 146
Alytes obstetricans 409
antigen type and 313
Bufo marinus 146
coelomocyte-mediated, xenografts and 65
earthworm histoincompatibility and 58
long-term, annelid 51
negative 51, 59
positive 51, 59
short-term, second-set xenografts and 60
reptilian 313
second-set xenograft rejection and 58
short-term 60
annelid 51
echinodermata 51
Eptatretus 107
typical 67
xenograft, temperature effects 65
Xenopus laevis 146
Anaphylaxis, avian
cutaneous, passive 349, 353
temperature effects 351

Anaphylaxis, avian (*cont.*)
  systemic 349
Anaploma fimbria, immune response, temperature effects 230
Anapsida 12
Anas platyrhynchos, immunoglobulins 336
Anemonia sulcata (Pennant), porifera and, mixed-cell aggregation 43
Anguilla anguilla, vibrio antibodies, temperature effects 229
Annelida ix, 4
  amphibian convergent evolution and 16
  cell-mediated immunity 52
    primordial 37
  coelomocytes 72
    function 70
  first-set allograft rejection 53, 57
  first-set xenograft rejection 57
  humoral immunity 4
  immunological anamnesis and 51
  immunological specificity
    diverse, intrafamilial 57
    self-recognition and 56
  regeneration 172
Anseriformes
  antibodies 362
  immunoglobulins, properties 360
  methylcholanthrene induced tumours, incidence 110
  5·7S immunoglobulins 357, 366
    biological properties 358
    phylogenetic formula 357
    structure 357
  7S immunoglobulins
    biological properties 353
    structure 352
  17S immunoglobulins, carbohydrate content 355
Anthozoa
  histoincompatibility in 42
  porifera and, mixed cell aggregation 43
Antibodies
  active sites 263, 266
  affinity maturation 364
  amphibian
    production during ontogeny
      cellular aspects 408
      humoral aspects 410
    thymectomy effects on synthesis 405
  assay 87
  avian 335
  blocking, tumour cell protection 191
  combining sites 263
  cytophilic, false rosette generation and 138, 140
  cytotoxic, tumour cell destruction 111
  discovery of 84
  DNP derivatives and 265
  DNP specific 127
  heterogeneity, electrophoretic 259
  homocytotropic 291
  humoral
    kidney allograft survival and 111
    thymectomy and ATS effects 123, 124
    tumours and 190
  'natural' 21
    antibody-combining sites and 266
  paired-iodinated peptide isolation 339
  plaque forming cells and 128
  producing cells
    activity measurement 143
    antigen recognizing cells and 135, 136
    temperature effects 138
  production
    B lymphocyte pathway 98
    cellular basis 314
    Gallus domesticus 428
    reptilia 298, 325
    selection and 21
      clonal theory 21
    temperature effects 138, 228
  reptilian
    adjuvant effects 328
    antigen binding sites 320
    factors influencing production 298, 325
    ontogeny 312
    seasonal influences 329
    temperature effects 328
    valence and affinity 315
  specific macrophage bound 105
  Testudo, ME-sensitive 307
  thymic synthesis, regulation 404
  transfer into eggs 312
Anti-BSA antibodies
  avian 359
  Chelonia mydas 362
  haemagglutinin titres in high salt 348
Anti-DNP antibodies
  affinity, *Rana catesbiana* 410
  Chelonia mydas 362
  fluorescence quenching 322, 324, 339
  HMW 315
  inhibition by DNP- and TNP-lysine 410, 411
  Rana catesbiana 405, 407, 408
Anti-DNP $F(ab')_2$, precipitation in high salt 348
Anti-erythrocyte response
  immunogen dosage

Anti-erythrocyte response (*cont.*)
in *Rana* 148
in *Triturus* 131
experimental study method (Ruben) 132
spleen lymphocyte differentiation and 124
Antigen-antibody complexes
phagocyte recognition 85
reptilian 312
Antigens
binding
after SRBC dosage in *Rana* 152, 153
in anura 214
techniques 347
binding cells
embryonic bursa and thymus and 123
Greaves and Möller theory 129
carcino-embryonic, retrogenesis and 188
determinants 21
'carrier' 30
glycocalxes and 39
elimination, in reptilia 311
fetal, tumour autoantigens and 188
histocompatibility
amphibian tolerance 391
embryonic induction 391
metamorphosis and 393
avian transplantation immunity and 110
Darwinian natural selection and 16
IgM-like receptors, macrophage antigen-IgT adsorption and 30
IgT, adsorption by macrophages 30
localization sites in echidna 377, 380
lymphocyte-defined, MLC reactions and 100
macrophages and 105
polymerization, B lymphocyte stimulation and 126
receptor affinity, lymphocyte 27, 28
recognizing cells, antibody producing cells and 135, 136
RNA complexes, lymphocyte triggering and 27
serologically defined, MLC reactions and 100
soluble, avian antibody production and 358
tumour-specific, transplantation 188
types
anamnesis and 313
reptilian antibodies and 325
Anti-hapten antibodies, synthesis 125, 143
Anti-HSA antibodies, adjuvant effects on production 363
Anti-immunoglobulin serum, thymus RFC sensitivity and 130
Anti-thymocyte serum, thymectomy and, humoral antibody
depression and 123, 124
Anti-TNP antibodies, inhibition by DNP- and TNP-lysine 410, 411
Anti-ϕ treatment, MLC reactions and 100
Anti-X antibodies 21
Anura 11, 210, 212
antibody production, time course 279
coelom, lymph node-like structures 106
histoincompatible graft rejection 214
immunity
cell-mediated 108
humoral 278
immunoglobulin M, inter-species antigenicity and 281
immunoglobulins 282
molecular weight and electrophoretic behaviour 283
lymphoid system 217
lymphomyeloid complex 277
major histocompatibility complex evolution 215
positive MLC reactivity 216, 217
7S immunoglobulins, relatedness to avian and reptilian 7SIg 289
transplantation immunity 108
thymectomy and 401
tumours 179
immunity 109
Aplysia californica, opsonin function of agglutinins 86
Apoda 11, 210, 211, 212
transplantation immunity 108
Arachnida
as vertebrate ancestors 4
regeneration 172
Arbacia, injection into *Asterias*, circulating amoebocyte effects 50
Archaeopteryx 12
Archosauria 12
Arowana, transplantation immunity 107
Arthropoda 4
as vectors for viral tumours 182
regeneration 172
transplantation immunity, pests and 46
Arthus reactions, *Gallus* 350, 351
Artiodactyls 14
Ascidia
non-fusion reaction 48
transplantation specificity, genetic control 48

Asterias forbesi
haemagglutinins
HRBC and 93
molecular weight and size 93
transplant discrimination 49
Asterias rubians, coelomocyte foreign matter ingestion 82
Asteroidea, transplants
cell and tissue 49
cell responses, self-recognition and 50
'ATXBM' mice, B lymphocytes 26
Australorbis glabratus, cephalopedal sinus allografts 45
Autectomy, invertebrate 172
Autoantigens, tumour 188
Autografts 36
coelomocyte response 70
invertebrate recognition 37
Lumbricus, *histocompatibility* 55
Azathioprine, RFC sensitivity to 130

Bacteriophage
antibodies in sheep 437
clearance by non-human vertebrates 105
Bacteriophage f2, immunization
Petromyzon response 241
temperature effects on antibodies 235
Bacterium salmonicada, temperature effects on antibody production 229
Birds
antibody production 335
soluble antigens and 358
immunoglobulins 335
types 291
immunology, phylogenetic studies 122
seashore, guinea pig complement fixation 353
transplantation and tumour immunity 110
Blaberus cranifer, haemocytes, bacteria phagocytosis 88
B lymphocytes 22
antibody production and 98
antigen binding and 435
anti-tumour activity 191
'ATXBM' mice and 26
central and peripheral 26
differentiation from T lymphocytes 24
hapten immunized, carrier sensitized T lymphocytes and 420
lack, in agammaglobulinaemia 26
mammalian, surface immunoglobulin 155
multiple types, evolution 106
phytohaemagglutinin stimulation of 126
rosettes, thymectomy effects 131
thoracic duct lymph 27
Bone marrow, *Gallus domesticus*, development 426
Botryllus primigenus, transplantation specificity, genetic control 48
Bovine serum albumin
as carp antigen 231
penicillin conjugate, carrier enhancement 233
temperature effects on antibody production 232
Brucella abortus
immunization, *Eptatretus* response 241
temperature effects on antibody production 230
B–T lymphocyte cooperation 156
antibody production and 235, 236
ICA assays and carrier-hapten immunization and 128
phylogeny 120
Bufo, lymphoid systems 217, 218, 219
Bufo marinus
anamnesis and 146
bacteriophage f_2 immunization
HMW antibody response 279
temperature effects on antibodies 235
IgM response to *Salmonella* 213
immune response to *Salmonella* 278
immunoglobulin fractions, molecular weights 283
lymphocytes, response to mitogens 216
MLC reactivity 216
Bufonidae 211
organ transplant rejection 215
Burkitt's lymphoma
arthropods as vectors 182
Epstein-Barr virus isolation 197
Bursa of Fabricius 419
development inhibition, antibody production and 420
embryonic, antigen binding cells 123
Gallus domesticus, development 421
testosterone effects 424
lymphocyte formation 22
Bursectomy
allograft rejection and 110
SRBC immunization and, splenic effects 123
surgical, RFC and PFC effects 130

Caecilia *see* Apoda
Caiman sclerops, antibody production 299
Calcichordata 6

Calcispongiae, demonspongiae and, bispecific aggregation 40
Calf antigen, carp antibody production, temperature effects 230
Calliphora, tissue rejection by *Periplanata* 47
Calotes versicolor
  antibody production 299
    ontogeny 312
  splenectomy, effects 12
Carassius auratus, T_1 bacteriophage clearance 105
Carbohydrates, immunoglobulin 242, 244, 245, 246, 248, 249, 254, 256
Carboxymethyl cysteines
  immunoglobulin 252
  5·7S immunoglobulin 358
Carcinogens, chemical 176, 182, 185, 186, 189
Carcinoma 170
Cardiochiles nigriceps, haemocyte recognition of eggs 86
Carp
  agglutinins to *Pseudomonas*, temperature effects 228
  Brucella antibody production, temperature effects 230
  non-microbial antigen immunized, antibody production and temperature 231
  thymus lymphocytes xi
'Carrier determinants' 30
Carrier-hapten conjugate
  immunization 232
    temperature effects 233, 234
Caudata *see* Urodela
CD *see* Dichroism, circular
Cells, malignant
  invertebrate 171
  proliferation 169
Cephalochordata 6, 7
Cephalopoda, auto and allograft success 46
Chelonia
  antibodies 300, 301
    transfer into eggs 312
  immunoglobulin production 303
  transplantation immunity 109
  tumours 179
Chelonia mydas
  antibody types 309
  anti-BSA and anti-DNP antibodies 362
Chelydra
  antibody production 300
  immunoglobulins, structure 309
Chelydra serpentina
  antibodies
    ontogeny 312
    types 309
  grant versus host reaction and 109
  5·7S antibody, affinity labelling 323
  5·7S anti-DNP antibody, valence 320
Chicken
  bursectomy, RFC and PFC effects 130
  embryonic, thymus and bursa AB cells 123
  see also Galliformes; *Gallus domesticus*
Chimerism, blood cell, immune tolerance and (Davison) 392, 393
C^h histocompatibility, lymphosarcoma spread in *Ambystoma* and 196
Chlamydia, soluble antibody, complement fixation and 349
Cholera, antitoxins, production in *Alligator mississipiensis* 298
Chonacocytes, porifera nutrition and 81
Chondostrei 9
Chondrichthyes 9
  immunoglobulin M responses 106
  immunoglobulin size classes 243
  lymphoid system 217
  transplantation immunity 106
  tumours 178, 179
    immunity 106
Chondromas 170
Chondrosarcomas 170
Chondrostea, immunoglobulin size classes 243
Chordata 4
  regeneration 172
  tumours 174
Chromatography, affinity, haemagglutinin purification and 93, 94
Chrysemys elegans, antibodies, production 300
Chrysemys picta
  antibodies
    adjuvant effects 328
    production 300
  immunoglobulin structure 303, 307
Ciliata, organelle transplantation 38
Ciona intestinalis, blood cells, phytohaemagglutinin effects 102
Cistudio lutaria
  antibody production 300
  antigen elimination 311
  antitoxin and agglutinin production 298
Clathrina coriacea (Montagu), anthozoa and, mixed cell aggregation 43
Clemmys capsica, antibody production 300
Cliona celata, antisera, cell aggregation and 39

Clones
abortion, immunological tolerance and 33
reproduction, relatedness of cell transferred parts and 38
selection theory, antibody formation and 21
CMI *see* Immunity, cell-mediated
Cnidaria *see* Coelenterata
Coelenterata 2
histoincompatibility in 40
quasi-immunorecognition in 102
regeneration 172
Coelocanthini 10
Coelom, invertebrate formation 3
Coelomocytes
anamnesis and, xenografts and adoptive transfer 65
earthworm 72
autograft and xenograft distinguishability 56
functions 70
graft rejection and 61, 63
humoral factor release and 71
interrelationships 70
invertebrate, functions 81
origin, radiolabelling and 72
receptors and recognition units 37
self- versus not-self recognition 73
xenografts and, non-specific injury effects 66
Colostrum, materno-fetal immunoglobulin transfer 439, 441
Columba livia
anti-BSA antibody structure 353
7S immunoglobulins, structure and biological properties 353
Complement
binding
antibody transfer into chelonia eggs and 312
Gallus antibodies and 348
marsupial 386
Concanavalin A, mitogens, T lymphocyte reactivity and 100
Condylarthia 14
Conformations, immunoglobulin 255
Coturnix coturnix, 7S immunoglobulin, molecular weight 337
Cotylosauria 12
Crassostrea commercialis, epithelial tumours 176
Crassostrea gigas
allografts 44
epithelial tumours 176
ganglioneuromas 176
Crassostrea virginica
allografts 45
amoebocytes, rabbit erythrocyte ingestion 87
coelomocyte foreign matter ingestion 82
herpes-type virus tumours 182
mesenchymal tumours 176
sheep erythrocyte agglutinin and 90, 92
CRBC, adherence to *Periplanata* haemocytes 88
Crocodilia
antibody production 299
immunoglobulin production 301
transplantation immunity 109
Crossopterygii 10, 210, 211
water-land transition characteristics 10
Crustacea 4
regeneration 172
Cucumaria tricolor, histoincompatibility in 50
Cyclophosphamide immunosuppression, tumours and 189
Cyclostomes 8
limited humoral response to antigens 241
ostracoderm-derived xii
Cysteines
carboxymethyl, 5·7S immunoglobulin 357
immunoglobulin 252
Cytotoxicity, antibody mediated, in *Bufo marinus* 213

Dansyl chloride, immune response lack in oppossums 383
Darwin's theory 14, 15
Dasyatis say, response to KLH 146
Davison's tolerance hypothesis 392, 393
Demonspongiae, calcispongiae and, bispecific aggregation 40
Dendritic cells 27
Dendrocoelum lacteum, regeneration and tumours 186
Dendrostomum zostericolum, egg transplantation 44
Dichroism, circular 253, 255, 267
Didelphis virginiana
cell-mediated immunity 386
immune responses 383
comparison with rabbit 384
fetal 437
immunoglobulin subclasses 442
infection response 387
lymphoid tissue 382
serum proteins, development 440

Diemictylus viridescens, mycobacterial granulomas 183
Di George syndrome, T lymphocyte lack and 26
Dimethylnitrosamine, hepatoma induction in fish 182
Dimetrodon 12
Dinitrophenol haptens
- response to 264
  - in *Rana catesbiana* 279

Dinitrophenol-L-lysine, absorption spectra 265, 266
Diphtheria toxin, temperature effects on antibody production 228
Dipnoi 10
Dipsosaurus dorsalis
- anamnesis, antigen type and 313
- antibody production 299
- *Salmonella* antibody production, temperature effects 229

Diptera, ovarian xenotransplantations 46
Direct complement fixation test (Brumfield and Pomeroy) 349
Discoglossidiae 211
- sub-acute graft rejection 215

Disulphides, interchain, immunoglobulin 241, 249, 251
- location 251

DNA synthesis, phytohaemagglutinin effects 102
DNP_{20} BSA, HRBC and, humoral antibody depression 123
DNP-lysine, anti-DNP antibody inhibition 410
DNS chloride conjugates, immunoglobulin 258
Drosophila, ovarian xenotranplantation 46
Drosophila melanogaster, neuroblastomas 174

Echidna
- antibodies, 2-mercaptoethanol reduction 380
- immune responses 380
- immunoglobulins 381
- lymph nodes
  - anatomy and physiology 377
  - cell radio-labelling 377, 379
  - cellular arrangement 377
- lymphocytes 376

Echinodermata x, 4
- anamnesis, short-term 49
- primordial cell-mediated immunity 37
- protochordate evolution and 5
- regeneration 172
- tornaria larvae 6

Echinoidea transplantation cell responses and 50
Ectothermata, immunosuppression, temperature effects 112
EDTA, haemagglutinin inactivation 93
Effectors, lymphocyte, transplantation and tumour immunity 111
Egrets, anti-ornithosis antibodies 353
Eisenia
- cell-mediated immunity 52
- xenografts 62
  - rejection, *Lumbricus* and 54
  - second-set, *Lumbricus*, anamnesis and 58

Eisenia foetida, allografts, first-set 53
Elasmobranchii 9
- IgM responses 106
- immunoglobulin size classes 243
- lymphoid system 106
- transplantation immunity 106
- tumours 178, 179
  - immunity 106

Electrophoresis, SDS-acrylamide, immunoglobulin 287, 303, 310
Eledone cirrosa
- phagocytes, human erythrocyte ingestion 87
- phagoytic-type cells in 106

Emys meleagris, antibodies 300
Emys orbicularis
- antibodies 300
  - diphtheria, temperature effects 228
  - types 309
- antigens, elimination 311

Encapsulation, macrophageal 105
Encephalitis, allergic, *Didelphis virginiana* cell-mediated immunity and 386
Endocarditis, bacterial, *Didelphis virginiana* 387
Enteropneusts 5, 6
Enzymes
- digestion, galliforme 7S immunoglobulins and 342
- immunoglobulin 250
- proteolytic, macrophage secretion of 105

Epinephelus itaira
- 5·7S immunoglobulin 366
- LMW immunoglobulins, mass deficiencies 248

Epitheliomas 170
- *Ampullaris australis* 176
- *Crassostrea* 176

Epstein-Barr virus 197

Eptatretus stoutii 8
anamnesis, short-term 107
antibodies, human 'O' erythrocyte, physicochemical properties 241
blood cells, phytohaemagglutinin effects 102
immune response 106
immunoglobulins, physicochemical characterization 241
KLH and SRBC immunization responses 241
9S immunoglobulins, invertebrate agglutinating glycoproteins and 242
tumour immunity 107
Equilibrium dialysis, antigen-binding 347
Erythrocytes
agglutination, *Panulirus* haemolymph and 90
binding
lymphocyte microvilli and 131
Parachaereps haemocytes and 89
heterologous
B-T lymphocyte cooperation and 123
humoral specific antibodies and 120
human, ingestion by *Eledone* phagocytes 87
human A, *Helix* haemagglutinin and 92
human 'O', *Petromyzon* response 241
see also Anti-erythrocyte response; CRBC; HRBC; RRBC; SRBC
Escherichia coli ix
antibody production in *Ginglymostoma* 231
Ethylenediaminotetra-acetate, haemagglutinin inactivation 93
Eucumaria laevigata, sexual differentiation and 83
Euglobulins, enzymatic digestion 342
Euryapsida 12
Eurypterids 4
Eutheria, reproduction 14
Evolution
environment and 16
principles 14

Fabricius' bursa *see* Bursa
$F(ab')_2$
anti-DNP, pepsin-produced 348
precipitation in high salt 348
f_2 bacteriophage *see* Bacteriophage f_2
Farr antigen-binding technique 347
Fc immunoglobulin, human fetal transfer 312
Fetus, membranes, immunoglobulin transfer 312
Fibromas 170
viruses, transmission 182
Fibrosarcomas 170
Fishes
lymphocytes x
transplantation immunity 106
tumours 180, 181
chemical carcinogen-induced 182
haematopoietic 180, 184
immunity 106
water pollution and 182
Forbidden clone hypothesis 391
Freund's adjuvants
effects, in galliformes 365
antibody production 363
hypersensitivity reaction testing and 103
Fluorescence polarization, immunoglobulin subunit flexibility and 258
Fluorescence quenching 347
anti-DNP antibodies 322, 324, 339
Furunculosis, trout
natural immunity development 229
Aeromonas antibodies and 231

Galliformes
antibodies, adjuvant effects 363
anti-BSA antibodies 359
FCA effects 365
IgA-like immunoglobulins 356
structure 357
immunoglobulins, properties 360
7S immunoglobulins 336
aggregation 344
allotypes 346
antigenic relationships 344
binding site 339
biological properties 346
carbohydrate composition 340
complement fixation 348
egg yolk 351
electrokinetic properties 336
enzymatic digestion 342
H-chains 338
homogeneity 339
immediate-type hypersensitivity 349
L-chains 337
molecular weights 337
precipitin reaction 346
effect of high salt 346
reductive dissociation 342
structure 336
17S immunoglobulins 353
binding site 355
biological properties 355
carbohydrate composition 354

Galliformes (*cont.*)
molecular weights 354
reductive dissociation 355
structure 353
thymectomy, antibody production and 420
Gallus domesticus
antibody production 428
histamine sensitivity 349, 350
immune competence development 427
lymphoid organs 420
ontogenesis 421
mammalian IgG-like antibodies 336
7S IgG 336
sedimentation coefficient 344
Gamma globulins
human, mammalian IgG heavy chains and 285
serum, increase in neoplastic *Xenopus* 195
Ganglioneuromas 170
Crassostrea 176
Gastropoda, histoincompatibility in 45
Genes
immune response 29, 30
immunoglobulin structural 30
Ginglymostoma cirratum, antibody production 231
Gliomas 170
Glycocalyxes, sponge cell aggregation and 39
Glycoproteins
agglutinating, lamprey 9S immunoglobulins and 242
lymphocyte, carbohydrate moieties, plant lectin binding 100, 101
Gorgonacea
histoincompatibility in 42
'pre-immunology' theory (Theodor) 42
Grafts *see* Allografts; Heterografts; Transplants; Xenografts
Granulomas
FACA induced 363
effect of thymectomy and irradiation 363
mycobacterial, tumour induction in amphibia 183
Graptolites, fossil, pterobranchii and 6
Growth, determinate and indeterminate, invertebrate tumours and 172
Guanidine-HCl, disulphide reduction 251
Gymnophiona *see* Apoda

Haeckel's law 16
Haemagglutinins
amino acid composition 91, 93
from invertebrates
molecular weight and size 93
physicochemical properties 89
IgM as, bullfrog 213
Parachaereps, purification 93
titres, after HRBC dosage in newts 146, 147, 148, 149
Haemocyanin
antibodies, in rhynchocephalia 299
Dipsosaurus anamnestic response and 314
keyhole limpet
as thymus-dependent antigen 408
Eptatretus response to 241
Rana response to 279
Haemocytes
Blaberus cranifer, bacteria phagocytosis 88
Cardiochiles nigriceps egg recognition 86
effects of trypsin 88
insect tumours and 184
mollusc, role 184
Parachaereps bicarinatus, bacteria elimination 86, 88
erythrocyte binding and 89
Periplanata, adherence of chicken erythrocytes to 88
receptors and recognition units 37
see also Coelomocytes
Haemolymph, recognition factors, bacteria removal and 86
cytophilic 99
Haemopoietic tissues, tumours 170
distribution and incidence 183
lower vertebrate 180, 181
mollusc 176
research rationale 184
Haliclona elegans (Bow), anthozoa and, mixed cell aggregation 43
Haplotype differences, graft rejection and 396
Haptens
antibody production in chickens 362
B-T lymphocyte cooperation and 125
dinitrophenol 264
immune response in opossums 383
Harmontella, bacteria agglutination 81
Hassall's corpuscles
Didelphis virginiana 382
mammalian 433
Helisoma, xenograft and allograft reactions 45, 46

Helix pomatia, haemagglutinin
human A erythrocytes and 92
molecular weight 92
Hellstöm blocking factors 399
Hemichordata 4, 6
Heptaginia, haemocyte disease 184
Hepatoblastomas 171
Hepatomas, chemical carcinogen induced 182
Herons anti-ornithosis antibodies 353
Herpes-type virus tumours 179, 182, 196
Rana renal adenocarcinoma and 179, 196, 197
Heterodontis francisci
delayed hypersensitivity and 103
transplantation immunity 107
Heterografts
Stentor, chimerae and incompatibilities 39
survival in *Acropora* 43
Hexosamine: hexose ratio, 72
7S immunoglobulin 340
Hexose, *Gallus* 7S immunoglobulin content 340
H-2 genes, murine, amphibian MLC reaction and 216
Histidine, immunoglobulin, modification by nitrobenzenefluoroborate 266
Histoincompatibility 61
coelenterata and 40
complex
amphibian 214
major, oncogenesis and 217
immunoglobulin heavy chains and 22
MLC reactions and 99, 100
mollusca and 44
orthoptera and 47
HLA complex 22
Hodgkin's disease 195
Holocephali 9
Holostei 9
immunoglobulin size classes 243
Holothuria 6
HRBC
antibody production, temperature effects 235
anti-erythrocyte response by *Triturus* and 131
Asterias haemagglutinin and 93
DNP_{20} BSA and, humoral antibody depression 123
dosage
primary immune response 134, 144
secondary immune response 144
Limulus haemagglutinin and 90, 93
3H-thymidine, lymph node cell labelling 377, 379
Hydra, amoeba chemotectic response and 81
Hydractinia echinata, histoincompatibility in 41
hyperplastic stolon overgrowth and 41
Hydrozoa
allografts and xenografts, edge cell pseudopodial activity 41
histoincompatibility in 41
Bibb and Campbell theory 42
Hyla regilla
metamorphosis, immune tolerance and 394
neural fold graft on *Rana aurora* 392
Hyla viridis, typhoid antibody production, temperature effects 228
Hyperplasia versus neoplasia, invertebrate 174
Hypersensitivity, delayed, vertebrate 103

Ictalurus nebulosus, salmonella antibody production, temperature effects 228
Iguana iguana, antibody production 299
Immune competence, *Gallus domesticus*, development 427
Immune recognition
primitive animal 106
transfer from non-susceptible to susceptible host 86
Immune response
amphibian lymphoreticular tumours and 184
anamnesis and 144
cell-mediated
suppression, humoral responses and 128
thymectomy and 124
echidna 338
genetic factors 30
humoral
B-T lymphocyte cooperation and 124, 125
unnatural immunogen theory 121
macrophages and 105
mammalian
comparison with amphibian 154
development 436
marsupial 383
maturation 323
phylogeny 112
primary, SRBC dosage
in mice 154
in *Rana* 152, 153
temperature effects 51, 52

Immune response (*cont.*)
thymus dependent 279
tumours and 187, 191
vertebrate evolution and 153
visualization 126
'Immune surveillance' 198
tumours and 190
Immune system, development in tadpoles 413
Immunity
cell-mediated 20, 98
amphibian and mammalian compared 155
avian 110
deficiency in neoplastic *Xenopus* 195
definition 22
in free-living *Xenopus* 197
mammalian 106
amphibian and 155
marsupial 386
primordial 49, 68, 72, 102
echiderm and annelid 37
reptilian cancer and 110
thymus and 22
definition 20
depression, Marek's disease and 110
humoral
bursa of Fabricius and 22
cell-mediated immunity suppression and 128
definition 22
immunogens and 120
in opossums 384
mammalian, cell-mediated immunity and 98
theory (von Behring) 84
temperature effects 227
Bisset's hypothesis 228, 232, 234, 235
transplantation 106
tumours 107
Immunocyto-adherence
after HRBC dosage in newts 147
antigen and antibody cells and 129
assays 128
spleen lymphocyte differentiation and 124
Immunodeficiency, tumours and 189
Immunofluorescence xi
Immunogenicity, definition 28
Immunogens
anti-erythrocyte response, *Triturus viridescens* and 131
dosage, immune response and 125
humoral specific antibodies and 120
unnatural, humoral immune response and 121
Immunoglobulin A
human fetal 442
J chain 254, 255
Immunoglobulin A-like immunoglobulins
galliformes 356
structure 357
Immunoglobulin D 442
Immunoglobulin E, human, synthesis 441
Immunoglobulin G 29
amphibian, synthesis, thymus and 405
antibodies, non-production in urodeles 408
anuran 213
Didelphis, 2-mercaptoethanol reduction 386
mammalian 242, 247
chelonia 7S immunoglobulin and 310
heavy chain, human gamma globulin and 285
reactions, humoral antibodies and 111
spleen levels, SRBC immunization and 123
Immunoglobulin M 29
amphibian 281
antibodies, urodele 408
anuran 213
elasmobranchii response to 106
fetal 442
human, disulphides 251
mammalian 242, 247
chelonia HMW immunoglobulin and 310
marsupial 383, 384
placoderm-derived vertebrate 240
reactions, humoral antibodies and 111
reduction into heavy and light chains 252
solvent perturbation difference 259
spleen levels, SRBC immunization and 123
sub-classes 293
thymus-independent antigens and 279
Immunoglobulin M-like immunoglobulins, mammalian 243
evolution 243, 248
Immunoglobulin RAA 291
chicken, duck IMW antigenic relationship 249
Immunoglobulin T, antigens, adsorption by macrophages 30
Immunoglobulin Y 291
chicken, duck IMW antigenic relationship 249

Immunoglobulins 29, 74
adsorption, immune recognition and 85
amino acids 240, 243, 248
amphibian
diversity 211
thymus cell synthesis and 404
anseriformes, properties 360
avian 335
B and T lymphocyte, mammalian 155
carbohydrates 242, 244, 245, 246, 248
chains
evolution 263
molecular representation 190
chelonia HMW, mammalian IgM and 310
conformation 255
development in *Didelphis virginiana* 440
disulphide bonds 241, 249
echidna 381
egg transfer 351
Eptatretus
molecular weight estimation 241
preliminary characterization 241
sub-unit composition 242
evolution 277
tandem duplication of genes and 292
galliformes, properties 360
Gallus domesticus
homocytotropic 350
IgA-like 249
heavy chains, histocompatibility and 22
homologies 366
human, fetal 441
IMW, mammalian, physicochemical properties 249
relationship to HMW and LMW 249
interchain noncovalent binding 252
LMW, mammalian, molecular structure 244, 247, 249
lower vertebrate, classification 240
lymphocyte surface location 128
macrophage receptors and 105
mammalian
physicochemical properties 244, 249
polymer state 243, 244
marsupial 385
materno-fetal transfer 439
ostrachoderm-derived vertebrates 240
physical properties, phylogenetic comparison 239
placoderm-derived vertebrates 242
enzymatically-derived subunit structure 250
reduction-derived subunit structure 242
primary structure 259
paucigene and multigene theories 263
reduced, SDS-acrylamide electrophoresis 303, 310
reptilian 301
serum, increase
in multiple myeloma 195
in plasmacytoma 196
synthesis, thymus and 403
T lymphocyte antigens and 130
see also S immunoglobulins
Immunosuppression
ectotherms and, temperature effects 112
side-effects 189
tumours and 189
Immunotherapy, tumours 192
Indirect complement fixation test (Rice) 349
Inflammation, chronic, cell-mediated immunity and 22
Insecta
regeneration 172
tumours 174
Invertebrates
autograft recognition 37
circulation, foreign particle removal 86
evolution 3
haemagglutinins
molecular weight and size 93
physicochemical properties 89
malignant cells 171
phagocytosis and, *in vitro* studies 87
phylum, taxonomy 2
size, tumours and 173
tumour development, features affecting 172
Ir genes, lymphocyte receptors and 29
isoantigen, T lymphocyte studies and 129

Keyhole limpet haemocyanin
anti-DNP antibodies in *Rana* 279
as thymus-dependent antigen 408
immunization
Amia response 146
Dasyastis response 146
Eptatretus response 241
Rhinobatus response 146
Kidneys, allografts, humoral antibody effects 111
Kimura, non-Darwinian evolution theory 15

Labyrinthodontia 11

Lacerta muralis
antibody production 299
antigen elimination 312
Lacerta viridis, antibody production 299
Lacertilia
antibody production 299
immunoglobulins, structure 302, 303, 304
Lamprey 8
Latimeria 10
LD antigens, MLC reactions 100
Lectins, plant, mitogens, T lymphocyte reactivity and 100
Lepidosauria 12
Lepidosiren 10
Lepospondyli 11, 210
Leucocytes, mixed culture reactions 113, 216
biphasic 100
lack in *Didelphis virginiana* 387
non-specific mitogen responsiveness and 99
phylogeny 101
thymic dysplasia and 101
T lymphocytes and 100
Xenopus metamorphosis and 396, 397
Leukaemia
activation by immune reactions 191
cattle 183
cytotoxic antibody effects 111
fish 184
Limulus sp., T_2 bacteriophage clearance 105
Limulus polyphemus ix, 4
haemagglutinins, molecular weight and size 93
HRBC agglutination and 90, 93
Lipopolysaccharides, peripheral lymphocytes and 220
Lissamphibia 11, 210
Longevity, invertebrate tumours and 173
Lumbricus
autografts 62
histocompatibility 55
cell-mediated immunity 52
xenografts
first-set, rejection 56, 57
rejection, *Eisenia* and 54
second-set, *Eisenia* and, anamnesis 58
Lumbricus terrestris
coelomocyte foreign matter ingestion and 82
first-set allografts 53
Lungfish, immunoglobulins xii
Lymph, thoracic duct, B lymphocytes and 27
Lymph nodes
coelomocyte function and 63
echidna, anatomy and physiology 377
T lymphocyte colonization 23
Lymphocytes
aggregation in porifera 39
β_2-microglobulin and 293
Didelphis virginiana 382
evolution from epithelium 106
fetal liver
MLC reactions and 101
phytohaemagglutinin response and 101
glycoprotein carbohydrate moieties, plant lectin binding 100, 101
'helper' 125
immunoglobulin surface locations 128
mammalian, sub-populations, development 435
origins in amphibia 403
PHA response, thymectomy and 403
protochordate, radiosensitivity 102
Rana and *Bufo*, response to mitogens 216
role in immunity 22
Thamnophis allograft rejection and 109
see also B and T lymphocytes
Lymphoid system
amphibian
diversity 217
urogenital associated tissues 220, 221
central (primary), definition 419
components 23
Gallus domesticus 420
gut associated tissues 217
peripheral (secondary), mammalian 434
tissue evolution 105
Lymphokines 29
macrophage secretion of 105
production effects of thymectomy 220
Lymphomas
Burkitt's
arthropods as vectors 182
Epstein-Barr virus 197
cytotoxic antibody effects 111
spontaneous, *Xenopus laevis* transplantation 109
Lymphoreticular tumours 179
amphibian, immunity 184
cell-mediated immunity deficiency and 195
growth-necrosis-growth recycling 194, 195
Xenopus laevis 194

Lymphosarcomas
  allograft-induced in *Xenopus* 185
  Ambystoma mexicanum 183, 196
  development, temperature effects 109
  fish 184
  spontaneous, immunity in *Ambystoma mexicanum* 108
  water lizard 110
Lysins, coelomocytes and 71
Lysis, complement-mediated, in anura 214

Macrophages
  B-T lymphocyte cooperation and 121
  echidna lymph glands 377
  evolution 105
  role in immunity 26
  Thamnophis allograft rejection and 109
  tumour cell destruction 111
  vertebrate, immunoglobulin receptors 105
Macropus eugenii, immune responses 385
Malaria parasites, effects on mammalian IgM-like immunoglobulins 243
Malformations, developmental 170
Mammalia
  as successful vertebrates 13
  immune phenomena 20
  immune responses, development 436
  immunoglobulin placental transfer 352
  lymphocytes, sub-populations 435
  lymphoid tissues
    development 432
    peripheral (secondary) 434
  ontogeny 432
  plasma cells, development 434
  quasi-immunorecognition 37
  serum proteins, development 439
  therapsid ancestry 13
  T lymphocyte surface immunoglobulin 155
  transplantation and tumour immunity
Mannose: galactose ratio
  7S immunoglobulin 340
  17S immunoglobulin 354
Marek's disease, bursa degeneration and necrosis 110
Marsupials
  cell-mediated immunity 386
  complement 386
  immune responses 383
  immunoglobulins 385
  infection response 387
  lymphoid tissues 382
  plasma cells, antigens and 434
  'pouch young' x
  reproduction 14
Mast cell release, antigen–antibody reactions in *Gallus* 350
Melanomas 171
  humoral antibodies and 190
Melanosarcomas 171
Meleagris gallapavo, 7S immunoglobulin L-chains 337
Memory *see* Anamnesis, immunological
Meningopneumonitis antigen, complement fixation and 349
2-mercaptoethanol
  antibody reduction
    Didelphis 386
    echidna 380
  Gallus 7S Ig reduction 342, 243
  Ophisaurus immunoglobulin sensitivity to 302
Mercenaria mercenaria, reproductive system tumours 176
Mesoderm, invertebrate formation 3
Mesothuria intestinalis, sexual differentiation and 83
Metanitrobenzene diazonium fluoroborate, antibody affinity labelling studies 323
Metastasis, tumour 169
Metazoa, organelle transplantation 37
Methylcholanthrene, tumour induction
  in *Ampullaris* 176
  in anseriformes 110
  lymphoid 186
Microconia prolifera
  antisera, cell aggregation and 39
  cell sorting 39
β_2-microglobulin, lymphocyte surface 293
Microvilli, lymphocyte, erythrocyte binding and 131
Migration inhibitory factor 71
Mitchison's 'local concentration' hypothesis 126
Mitogens
  non-specific responsiveness, MLC reactions and 99
  plant lectin, T lymphocyte reactivity and 100
  response to, phylogeny 101
MLC *see* Leucocytes
Mollusca
  haemopoietic tumours 175, 184
  haemocytes, role 184
  histoincompatibility in 44
  trocophore larvae 4
  tumours 173, 174, 175, 176, 198
Montremata
  immune responses 380
  immunoglobulins 286, 287, 381

Montremata (*cont.*)
lymphoid system, anatomy 376
reproduction and 14
Morphogenesis, malignant tumour development and 169
Morphostasis, malignant tumour development and 169
Multiparity, human, MLC reactivity and 101
Mustelus canis, immunoglobulin classification (Marchalonis and Edelman) 240
Mycobacteria, tumour reduced immunity and 195
Mycobacterium avium, 7S Ig production and 364
Myeloma
IgG_{2a}, murine, complement binding and 312
multiple, serum immunoglobulin increase and 195
Myriapoda, regeneration 172
Mytilus edulis, sarcoma 176, 182
Myxine glutinosa, delayed hypersensitivity and 103
Myxofibroma, *Vipera russelli* 181

Natural selection, Darwin's theory 14
Nauphoeta cineria, tissue rejection by *Periplanata* 47
Necturus, response to phytohaemagglutinin 217
Necturus maculosus
immunoglobulin characterization 281
LMW immunoglobulin lack 243, 245
Nemertea 4
Neoceradotus 10
Neoceradotus forsteri, 5·7S immunoglobulin 363
Neoplasia *see* Tumours
Nephroblastomas 171
Nervous system, tissue tumours 170
Neurilemmoma-like tumours, *Petromyzon marinus* 178
Neuroblastomas, *Drosophila melanogaster* 174
Newcastle disease virus, antibodies, in galliformes 356
Newts, response to HRBC dosage 146
Nitrobenzenefluoroborate, immunoglobulin tyrosine and histidine modification 266
Nitrobenzyl compounds, binding by *Gallus* anti-DNP antibody 339
Non-fusion reaction, ascidia and 48
Non-haematopoietic mesenchymal tissues, tumours 170

Ontogeny
phylogeny and (Haeckel's law) 16
phylogeny recapitulation and (Haeckel) 74
Ophiocomina nigra, tumours 174
Ophisaurus apodus
antibodies 299
monovalency 319, 320
anti-DNP antibodies
affinity 325
HMW binding properties 315
immunoglobulin structure 302, 304
LMW antibodies, effects of antigen types 327
6·8S LMW antibody 318, 320
Opossums
plasma cell maturation 434
'pouch young' x
Opsonins 85
coelomocytes and 71
Opsonization, in anura 214
Organelles, transplantation in protozoa 37
Ornithorhynchus paradoxus, lymphocytes 376
Ornithosis
antibodies, heron and egret 353
complement fixation tests and 349
Orthoptera
enzyme treated allograft rejection 47
histoincompatibility in 47
Osteichythes 9
tumours 178, 179
Osteomas 170
Osteosarcomas 170
Ostracodermata 7
Ostria lurida, sarcomas 176
Ovalumin, antibodies in sheep 437
Ovaries, xenotransplantation, in diphthera 46

Paddlefish, transplantation immunity development 107
Panulirus interruptus, haemolymph, erythrocyte and spermatozoa agglutination 90
Papillomas 170
Parachaereps bicarinatus
haemagglutinins, purification 93
haemocytes
bacteria elimination and 86, 88
erythrocyte binding and 89
host defence 83
Patiria miniata, transplant discrimination 49
Pecten irridens, transplants in 44

Pecten maximus, histoincompatibility in 44
Pelecypoda, histoincompatibility in 44
Pelycosauria, 12, 13
Peptides
immunoglobulin proteolysis and 250
mapping, immunoblobulin 261
Periplanata americana
haemocytes, CRBC adherence to 88
hormones 47
xenograft encapsulation 47
Perissodactyls 14
Petromyzon marinus
antibody production 241
delayed hypersensitivity and 103
neurilemmoma-like lesions 178
T_1 bacteriophage clearance 105
Peyer's patches, T lymphocyte colonization 23
Phagocytes
disease defence, Metchnikoff theory 84
invertebrate
exogenous material recognition 80, 84
functions 81
non-living particle ingestion 85
'wandering', host nutrition and 82
Phagocytosis 105
Agrionemys antibody producing cells and 315
invertebrate, *in vitro* studies 87
sexual differentiation and 83
Phagolysosomes 27
Phasianus colchicus, 7S immunoglobulins
L-chains 338
molecular weights 337
Phenylalanine, H-chain C-terminal residue, anseriformes, 5·7S immunoglobulin 357
Phrynosoma solave, antibody production 299
Phyla, invertebrate, nutrition and 81
taxonomy 2
Phylogeny
B-T lymphocyte cooperation and 120
mammalian, immunity and 98, 99
mitogen responses and 101
MLC reactions and 101
ontogeny and (Haeckel's law) 16
Phytohaemagglutinins
effect on blood cells 102
invertebrate evolution and 102
impaired response to, thymic dysplasia and 101
mammalian T lymphocyte reactivity and 100
T lymphocyte blastosis and 126
Piglets, 'non-classical' immunoglobulins 442
Pigment cells, tumours 171
Pinctada margaritifera, mantle tissue transplantation 45
Pinocytosis 105
Agrionemys antibody producing cells and 315
Pipidae 211
Placenta, immunoglobulin transfer 352
Placentals, reproduction 14
Placoderms 8
Planaria, transplantation reactions between species 43
Planorbius corneus, histoincompatibility in 45
Plant lectins, mitogens, T lymphocyte reactivity and 100
Plaque forming cells 125
antibodies, antigen dosage and 128
assay (Jerne and Nordin) 128
bursectomy effects 130
haemolytic, sites 315, 316, 317, 318
rosette forming cells and 130
spleen levels, SRBC immunization and 123
Plasma cells
antibody secretion 22
mammalian, development 434
Plasmacytoma, serum immunoglobulin increase and 196
Platyhelminthes 3
regeneration 172
transplantation reactions 43
Pleomorphism, cellular, malignant tumours and 169
Pleurodeles waltlii, metamorphosis, immune tolerance and 394
Pogonophora 6
Poikilotherms
bacterial resistance 178
B-T lymphocyte cooperation and 124
tumours 178, 179
Polymorphism, intraspecies, histocompatibility genes and 22
Polymorphonuclear cells
non-living particle ingestion 85
phagocytosis and 85
Polyodon spathula, delayed hypersensitivity and 103
Polyoma virus induced tumours, immune spleen cells and 112
Polypeptides
immunoglobulin
chain differences 259

Polypeptides (*cont.*)
solvent perturbation difference spectroscopy 259
molecular weight 281
synthetic, antibody production in birds 358
three-dimensional folding 252
Polypterus 9
Polysaccharides, pneumococcal, chicken antibody production 362
Porifera
anthozoa and, mixed cell aggregation 43
lymphocyte aggregation in 39
reaggregation specificity 39
Precipitins
C-reactive protein-like 267
high salt, RPA reactions and 351
Pregnancy, lymphocyte stimulation and 398
Proteins
acute phase, mammalian 268
inhibitors, rosette formation and 129
serum
antibody production in birds 358
development in mammals 439
structure, phylogenesis and 239
Proteolysis, enzymatic, immunoglobulin structure comparisons 250
Protochordata x, 4, 6
evolution 5
lymphocytes, radiosensitivity 102
Protopterus 10
Protoreaster nodosus, histoincompatibility in 50
Prototheria *see* Monotremata
Protozoa
organelle transplantation 37
phyla 2
regeneration 172
Pseudemys, immunoglobulins, structure, 309, 310
Pseudemys scripta
antibody production 300
types 309
Pseudoglobulins, enzymatic digestion 342
Pseudomonas fluorescens, antibodies in fishes 231
Psittacosis, complement fixation tests and 349
Pterobranchs 5, 6
Pygoscelis adeliae, anti-BSA antibody production 359

Quasi-immunorecognition 36, 72, 101, 102

Rabbits, immune responses, comparison with opossums 384
Radioelectrocomplexing 347
Rana, lymphoid systems, 217, 218, 219
Rana aurora, *Hyla regilla* neural fold graft 392
Rana catesbiana
anti-DNP and TNP antibodies 410, 411
affinity 410
anti-$f_2$phage antibodies 282
clones 412
IgG antibody non-production to antigens 405
IgM antibody production to DNP and TNP 405, 407, 408
immunoglobulins, gel electrophoresis 213
larval, antibody production, thymectomy and 405
LMW antibody response to bacteriophage f_2 279
lymph gland regression, thyroxin induced 396
metamorphosis, immune tolerance and 394
thymus regeneration 400
Rana esculenta, antibody production, temperature effects
diphtheria 228
typhoid 228
Rana pipiens
anti-erythrocyte response, immunogen dosage and 148
embryonic, blood cell chimeric recombinations 392
lymphocytes, response to mitogens 216
MLC reactivity 216
renal adenocarcinoma 179, 183, 196, 197
tail tissue allografts, immune response induction 393
thymus regeneration 400
Rana temporaria
antibody production, temperature effects 228, 299
IgM structure 285
Ranidae 211
Reaggregation, cellular
calcium effects 40
porifera antisera and 39
Receptors
lymphocyte 22
antigen affinity 28
antigen interaction 27
collaboration 28

Receptors (*cont.*)
cross-linkage, excessive 32
IgM-like 29
immune response genes and 29
'Red leg' disease, temperature effects on resistance to 228
Regeneration
invertebrate tumour formation and 172
limb, amphibian tumours and 185
Registry of Tumours in Lower Animals 168, 197
Reproduction, asexual, invertebrate tumours and 172
Reproductive system, *Mercenaria*, tumours 176
Reptilia
antibodies 298
adjuvant effects 328
affinity, effect of antigen types 327
antigen binding sites 320
biological properties 311
ontogeny 312
production factors 325
seasonal influences 329
temperature effects 328
valence and affinity 315
antigen elimination 311
evolution 11
immunoglobulins 301
types 291
immunological anamnesis 313
therapsid xii
transplantation immunity 109
tumours 179, 180, 181
lymphoreticular 180, 183
Reticuloendothelial system, amphibian 220
Reticulum, endoplasmic, *Agrionemys* plasma cells and 315
Retrogenesis, carcino-embryonic antigens and 188
RFC *see* Rosettes, forming cells
Rhinobatos productus
delayed hypersensitivity and 103
response to KLH 146
Rhipidistia 10
Rhithrogena, haemocyte disease 184
Rhyncocephalia 12
antibody production 299
immunoglobulin production 301
RNA, macrophage derived, antibody formation and 27
Rous sarcoma viruses, antibody production in *Ginglymostoma* 231
Rosettes
assay
antigen binding and producing cells and 129
spleen lymphocyte differentiation and 124
forming cells 129
activity measurement 140, 141
HRBC dosage in newts and 148
aggamaglobulinaemia effects 130
anti-immunoglobulin serum inhibition of 130
azathioprine sensitivity 130
bursectomy effects 130
mammalian cells and 129
morphological distinctions between ARC and APC 135
non-secretory and secretory, in newts, HRBC and 147, 148
PFC and 130
temperature effects 129, 138, 139
temperature insensitive 238
thymectomy effects 131
thymus dependent in *Rana* 153
type identification importance 138
hydrocortisone resistant 129
protein inhibition and 129
secretory and non-secretory
HRBC in newts and 147, 148
morphological studies 157
T lymphocyte, visualization 129
RRBC, ingestion by *Crassostrea* ameobocytes 87
Russell's viper, myxofibroma 181

Salamanders
allograft rejection and anamnesis 146
lymphoid system 217
negative MLC reactivity 216
causes 217
Salmo, *Bacterium salmonicada* antibodies, temperature effects 229
Salmo gardineri, delayed hypersensitivity and 104
Salmonella adelaide, antigen localization site in echidna 377
Salmonella typhimurium
dinitrophenylated, antibody response to 279
mouse macrophage interaction, Ig antibodies and 86
Salvelinus fontinalis, lymphoid tumours 194
Sarcodina, organelle transplantation 38
Sarcomas
humoral antibodies and 190
mollusca 176

Sarcomas (*cont.*)
Mytilus edulis 183
reticulum cell, mosquito as vector 182
Sarcopterygii 9, 10
Sauromalus obesus, antibody production 299
SD antigens, MLC reactions and 100
SDS-acrylamide electrophoresis, immunoglobulin 287, 303, 310
Sepharose, phytohaemagglutinin polymerization 126
Serpentes
antibody production 300
immunoglobulins 303
Setonix brachyurus
IgA- and IgE-like immunoglobulins 288
immune responses 385
Seymouria 11
S−FRC 135
S+FRC 135
Sharks, negative MLC reactivity 216, 217
Sheep, materno-fetal antibody transfer lack 437
see also SRBC
Shope fibroma virus 182
'Signal 1 only' theory, immunological tolerance and 32
5·7S immunoglobulin
anseriformes 357, 366
biological properties 358, 360
phylogenetic formula 357
structure 357
transfer into chelonia egg 312
7S immunoglobulin
amphibian, as evolutionary pattern of human IgG 291
anseriformes
biological properties 353
structure 352
anuran 213
chelonia, mammalian IgG and 310
comparisons in vertebrates 285
contamination of 17S immunoglobulin 354
evolution and 288
galliformes 336
aggregation 344
allotypes 346
anti-BSA 359
antigen relationships 344
binding sites 339
biological properties 346
carbohydrate composition 340, 341
complement fixation 348
electrokinetic properties 336
enzymatic digestion 342
H-chains 338
homogeneity 339
immediate-type hypersensitivity 349
L-chains 337
molecular weights 337
precipitin reaction 346
reductive dissociation 342
structure 33
heavy chains, SDS gel mobility 286
hexosamine: hexose ratio 340
mammalian, molecular weights 288
mannose: galactose ratio 340
pig 443
production, effect of adjuvants 363
17S immunoglobulin
anseriformes, carbohydrate content 355
galliformes 353
anti-BSA 359
binding site 355
biological properties 355
carbohydrate composition 354
molecular weights 354
reductive dissociation 355
structure 353
7S immunoglobulin contamination 154
19S immunoglobulin
anuran 213
pig 443
Sipunculida, eggs as xenografts 44
Siredon mexicanum, primary and secondary immune response 281
Skin
graft rejection, in opossums 386
passive anaphylaxis 349, 350, 353
Snapper, lymphocyte-lymphocyte effects 216
Sodium chloride, antigen binding and 346, 347
Specificity, immunological 98
Lumbricus histoincompatibility and 58
vertebrate response and 36
Spectroscopy, solvent perturbation difference 258
Spermatozoa, agglutination, *Panulirus* haemolymph and 90
Sphenodon 12
Sphenodon punctatum
immunoglobulin production 301
Salmonella antibodies 299
Spleen
Gallus domesticus, development 427
immune cells, T lymphocyte depleted, cytotoxicity and 112

Spleen (*cont.*)
plasma cells, *Agrionemys* 315, 316
SRBC immunization effects 123
T lymphocyte colonization 22
Xenopus laevis, immunoglobulin production 406
Splenectomy, *Agrionemys*, SRBC antibodies and 315
Sponges *see* Porifera
Squalus acanthus, T_1 bacteriophage clearance 105
Squamata
transplantation immunity 109
tumours 179
Squirrel fibroma virus 182
SRBC immunization
Crassostrea haemagglutinin and 90, 92
Eptatretus response 241
murine response 154
Rana response 149, 151
spleen and
after bursectomy and radiation 123
after thymectomy and radiation 123
Staphylococcus aureus, phagocytosis (Wright and Douglas) 85
Stentor, allografts between 38
Sulphhydryl reducing agents, *Gallus* antibodies and 343
Synapsida 12
Syphilis, placental plasma cells and 434

Tachyglossus aculeatus
gamma globulin electrophoresis 286
lymphocytes 376
T_1 bacteriophages, clearance by non-human vertebrates 105
T-B lymphocyte cooperation *see* B-T lymphocyte cooperation
Teleostei 9
antigen-antibody reactions 106
immunoglobulin size classes 243
positive MLC reactivity 216
Temnocephala, tumours 174
Teratomas 171
Terrapene carolina, antibody production 300
Testosterone, lymphoid organ developmental effects 424
Testudo
antibodies 300, 305, 206
types 308, 309
antigen elimination 311
immunoglobulins, structure 309, 310
Testudo hermanni
antibodies
adjuvant effects 328
seasonal influence 329
immunization schedule (Ambrosius) 304
immunoglobulin structure 305
immunological anamnesis 313
Testudo ibera
Brucella antibody production, temperature effects 229
immunoglobulin structure 303
Tetanus, antitoxins, production in *Alligator mississipiensis* 298
Tethya aurantium (Pallas), anthozoa and, mixed cell aggregation 43
Therapsida 12, 13
Thamnophis sirtalis, allograft rejection, lymphocyte and macrophage infiltration and 109
Thy 1 (ϕ) alloantigen, murine thymus cells xi
Thymectomy
Alytes, effect on splenic RFC 404
amphibian
regeneration after 400
transplantation immunity and 400
anti-thymocyte serum, humoral antibody depression and 123, 124
avian, spleen lymphocyte depletion and 420
cell-mediated immune response and 124
galliformes, antibody production and 420
immunocompetence and 220
incomplete, PFC formation and 420
neonatal
Ambystoma lymphosarcoma and 196
delayed hypersensitivity and 103
FCA induced granulomata and 363
MLC reactions and 100
RFC effects 131
SRBC immunization and, effect on spleen 123
urodele larvae and, immune response loss 108
Thymidine, tritiated, lymph node cell labelling 377, 379
Thymus
amphibian
function maturation 400
IgG synthesis and 405
immunocompetence maturation and 220
avian 419
congenital dysplasia, MLC reactions and 101

Thymus (*cont.*)
development
amphibian metamorphosis and 396
arrest, gene mutation and 26
Xenopus laevis 390
Didelphis virginiana 382
embryonic, antigen binding cells 123
Gallus domesticus 421
development 426
testosterone effects 424
immunoglobulin synthesis and 403
lymphocytes *see* T lymphocytes
mammalian, development 432
marsupial 382
primordium, lymphocyte production in frogs 108
transplantation immunity 400
Xenopus laevis
development 390
immunoglobulin production 406
Tidacna maxima, foreign matter ingestion and 82
Tiliqua, immunoglobulin structure 304
Tiliqua rugosa
antibodies 299
CFA effects 329
Tiliqua scincoides, antibodies 299
T lymphocytes 22
alloimmunity and 108
amphibian metamorphosis and 396
antibody affinity and 364
as effectors in mammals 111
blocking antibody tumour cell protection from 191
B lymphocyte triggering and 30
carrier-sensitized, hapten-immunized B lymphocytes and 420
cell-mediated immunity and 98, 99
central and peripheral 26
chicken antibody production and 420
deficiencies
congenital, MLC reactions and 100
gene mutations and 26
in di George syndrome 26
tumour growth and 112
delayed hypersensitivity and 103, 104
differentiation from B lymphocytes 24
frog, origins 108
'helper' 106
activity measurement 140, 141
IgG production and 29
IgM-like receptors 29
immunocompetent 23
immunoglobulin synthesis 404
Ir gene receptors and 29
mammalian, surface immunoglobulin 155
response
primordial 73
evolution 102
to allogeneic cells and 100
rosettes
thymectomy effects 131
visualization 129
SRBC dosage and 151, 152
suppressor, effect on B lymphocytes 32
target tumour cell destruction 111, 112
Xenopus, ontogeny of MLC reactivity 402
see also B-T lymphocyte cooperation
Tolerance, immunological 28, 31
amphibian 391
blood cell chimerism and (Davison) 382, 383
clonal abortion and 33
receptor cross-linkage, excessive and 32
'signal 1 only' theory 32
tumours and 190
Tornaria larvae 6
Toxoplasmosis, fetal plasma cells and 434
T_2-phage, temperature effects on antibody production 230
Trachystomata 210, 211, 212
Transplantation immunity 106
amphibia 108
avian 110
fishes 106
histocompatibility gene evolution versus inherent immune response 108
mammalian 111
reptilian 109
thymus and 400
Transplants
rejection
histocompatibility antigens and 215
histopathology 61
re-vascularization 63
Trichosurus vulpecula
immune responses 385
immunoglobulin characterization 287
Triturus alpestris, thymectomy
runting disease absence 400
transplantation immunity and 401
Triturus cristatus, regeneration and tumours in 186
Triturus pyrrhogaster, mycobacterial granulomas 183

Triturus viridescens
B-T lymphocyte cooperation and 124, 403
immunogen dosage
anti-erythrocyte response and 131
ARC(S−)RFC and APC(S+) RfC response and 136
methylcholanthrene-induced lymphoid tumours 185, 186
Trout, MLC reactivity 216
Trypanosomes, temperature effects on antibody production 229
Trypsin, effect on haemocytes 88
Tryptophan
interaction at antibody binding site 322
polypeptide 259, 267
Tyrosine, immunoblobulin, modification by nitrobenzenefluorborate 266
Tuberculin sensitivity
delayed 103
marsupial 386
Tumours
amphibian, limb regeneration and 185
antigens, genetic factors and 30
autoantigens 188
benign 169
case distribution 181
development
immune response and 191
normal development and 186
T lymphocyte depletion and 112
epidemiology 182
haematopoietic 170, 180, 181
distribution and incidence 183
research rationale 184
host relationships and 169
humoral antibodies and 190
'immune surveillance' and 190
immunity 107, 167, 187
amphibian 108
avian 110
effect of tumour size 192
fishes 107
low vertebrates 193
mammalian 111
reptilian 109
immunodeficiency and 189
immunological tolerance and 190
immunosuppression and 189
immunotherapy 192
invertebrate
features affecting 172
occurrence 174
research value 173
lymphoreticular 179, 180, 183
immune response and 184
a major histocompatibility complex and 217
malignant
aberrant cell activity 169
characteristic features 169
classification 170
definition 168, 169
host death and 170
metastases 169
occurrence 181
phylogeny 167
Registry, in lower animals (RTLA) 168, 197
vertebrate 176
occurrence 178
research rationale 176, 177
viruses 179, 181, 182, 196
Willis' definition 169
Tunicates x, 6, 7
quasi-immunorecognition 37
regeneration in 48
transplantation specificity, genetic control 47
Typhoid bacterium, antibodies, temperature effects 228

Urn cells 82
trees 83
Urochordata x, 6, 7
quasi-immunorecognition 37
regeneration in 48
transplantation specificity, genetic control 47
Urodela 11, 210, 211, 212
antibodies 214, 278, 408
B-T lymphocyte cooperation and 125
histoincompatible graft rejection 214
IgG and IgM antibodies 408
immunoglobulins 280
lymphoid system 217
major histocompatibility complex 217
lack 215
thymectomy
larval, immune response loss and 108
transplantation immunity and 401
transplantation immunity 108
tumours 179
immunity 108

Velesunio ambiguus, haemagglutinins 92
Vertebrates
delayed hypersensitivity 103
ectothermic x
immunity, temperature effects 227
evolution 7

Vertebrates (*cont.*)
  lower
    malignant cells 176
    tumour immunity and 193
  ostrachoderm-derived, immunoglobulins 240
  placoderm-derived
    IgM-like molecules 240
    immunoglobulins 242
Vibrio, temperature effect on antibody production 229
Vipera ammodytes, antigen elimination 312
Vipera russelli, myxofibroma 181
Viruses, tumours and 179, 181, 182, 196
  immunosuppression effects 189
Viscera, embryonic tumours 171

Waddington-Needham hypotheses 172, 185, 186, 198
Wattle reactions, FCA-induced 366

Xenografts
  coelomocyte response 71
    anamnesis and 65
  first-set rejection 59
    in interfamilial annelids 57
    in *Lumbricus* 56
  hydroxoa, edge cell pseudopodial activity 41, 42
  quasi-immunorecognition 36
  second-set
    positive short-term anamnesis and 59, 60
    rejections 59, 60
  Stentor, chimeras and incompatibilities 39
Xenopus, lymphoid system 217, 218
Xenopus laevis
  allogeneic and syngeneic, immune response to grafts 196
  allografts, rejection 146
  antibody response to bovine gamma globulin 280
  clones 412
  free-living, thymus-dependent immunity and 197
  HMW immunoglobulins, hexameric 243
  IgM structure 285
  immunized, 7S and 19S immunoglobulins 213
  immunoglobulins
    gel electrophoresis 213
    molecular weight of fraction 283
  lymphoid complex, ontogenic changes 396, 397
  lymphoma transplantation from 109
  lymphoreticular tumours 194
    cell-mediated immunity deficiency and 195
  lymphosarcomas, allograft-induced 185
  metamorphosis
    immune tolerance and 394
      graft size and 395
  methylcholanthrene-induced tumours 185, 186
  MLC reactivity 216
  mycobacterial granulomas 183
  non-stimulating MLR combinations 395
  spleen, PFC and RFC 409
  thymectomy
    human gamma globulin response 405
    larval 124
    long-term effect (Horton and Manning) 401
    runting disease absence 400
  thymus, development 390

Zonurus giganteus, antibody production 299